Blood Cell Biochemistry

Volume 8

Hematopoiesis and Gene Therapy

Blood Cell Biochemistry

Series Editor

J. Robin Harris, *Institute of Zoology, University of Mainz, Mainz, Germany*

Volume 1 **Erythroid Cells**
Edited by J. R. Harris

Volume 2 **Megakaryocytes, Platelets, Macrophages, and Eosinophils**
Edited by J. R. Harris

Volume 3 **Lymphocytes and Granulocytes**
Edited by J. R. Harris

Volume 4 **Basophil and Mast Cell Degranulation and Recovery**
Ann M. Dvorak

Volume 5 **Macrophages and Related Cells**
Edited by Michael A. Horton

Volume 6 **Molecular Basis of Human Blood Group Antigens**
Edited by Jean-Pierre Cartron and Philippe Rouger

Volume 7 **Hematopoietic Cell Growth Factors and Their Receptors**
Edited by Anthony D. Whetton and John Gordon

Volume 8 **Hematopoiesis and Gene Therapy**
Edited by Leslie J. Fairbairn and Nydia G. Testa

A Continuation Order Plan is available for this series. A continuation order will bring delivery of each new volume immediately upon publication. Volumes are billed only upon actual shipment. For further information please contact the publisher.

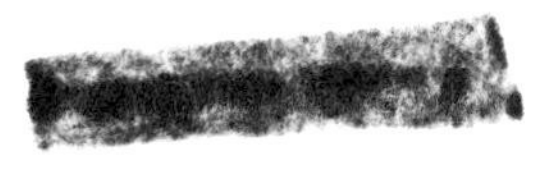

Blood Cell Biochemistry

Volume 8
Hematopoiesis and Gene Therapy

Edited by

Leslie J. Fairbairn and
Nydia G. Testa

Christie CRC Research Centre
Paterson Institute for Cancer Research
Christie Hospital NHS Trust
Manchester, United Kingdom

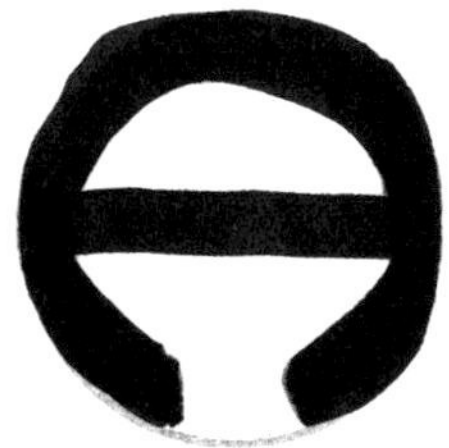

Kluwer Academic / Plenum Publishers
New York, Boston, Dordrecht, London, Moscow

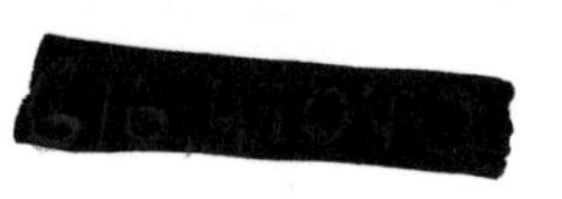
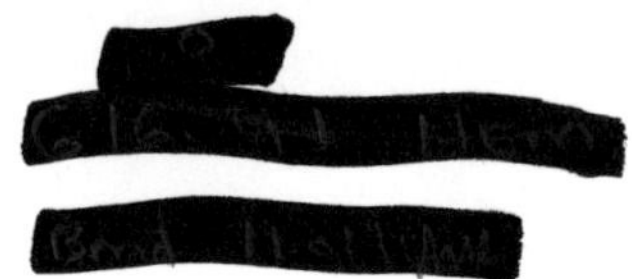

ISSN 1078-0491

ISBN 0-306-45962-0

233 Spring Street, New York, N.Y. 10013

10 9 8 7 6 5 4 3 2 1

A C.I.P. record for this book is available from the Library of Congress.

Printed in the United States of America

Contributors

Michael Antoniou Department of Experimental Pathology, GKT Medical and Dental School, King's College, London, Guy's Hospital, London SE1 9TR, United Kingdom

Cynthia L. Brazolot Millan Loeb Health Research Institute, Ottawa Civic Hospital, Ottawa, Ontario K1Y 4E9, Canada

Colin Casimir Department of Haematology, Imperial College School of Medicine at St. Mary's, Norfolk Place, London W2 1PG, United Kingdom

Mary Collins CRC Centre for Cell and Molecular Biology, Chester Beatty Laboratories, London SW3 6JB, United Kingdom

Heather L. Davis Loeb Health Research Institute, Ottawa Civic Hospital, Ottawa, Ontario K1Y 4E9, Canada, and Faculties of Health Sciences and Medicine, University of Ottawa, Ottawa, Canada

Rosa Maria Diaz Richard Dimbleby/ICRF Department of Cancer Research, Rayne Institute, St. Thomas' Hospital, London SE1 7EH, United Kingdom

A. Djeha CRC Department of Experimental Haematology, Paterson Institute for Cancer Research, Manchester M20 4BX, United Kingdom

I.D. Dubé Departments of Medicine, Medical Biophysics, Pediatrics, and Pathology, The University of Toronto, and the Toronto Hospital Oncology Gene Therapy Program, Toronto, Ontario M5G 2C4, Canada

L. J. Fairbairn Paterson Institute for Cancer Research, Christie Hospital (NHS) Trust, Manchester M20 4BX, United Kingdom

Frank Grosveld Department of Cell Biology, Erasmus University-Rotterdam, 3000DR Rotterdam, The Netherlands

R. G. Hawley Departments of Medicine, Medical Biophysics, Pediatrics, and Pathology, The University of Toronto, and the Toronto Hospital Oncology Gene Therapy Program, Toronto, Ontario M5G 2C4, Canada

Anthony D. Ho Blood and Marrow Transplant Program, Department of Biology and Medicine, University of California, San Diego, La Jolla, California 92093

J. Hows University of Bristol, Division of Transplantation Sciences, Bristol, United Kingdom

L. S. Lashford Paterson Institute for Cancer Research, Christie Hospital (NHS) Trust, Manchester M20 4BX, United Kingdom

Ping Law Blood and Marrow Transplant Program, Department of Biology and Medicine, University of California, San Diego, La Jolla, California 92093

Xinqiang Li Blood and Marrow Transplant Program, Department of Biology and Medicine, University of California, San Diego, La Jolla, California 92093

Stephen G. O'Brien Department of Haematology, University of Wales College of Medicine, Cardiff CF4 4XN, Wales, United Kingdom

Colin Porter CRC Centre for Cell and Molecular Biology, Chester Beatty Laboratories, London SW3 6JB, United Kingdom

J. A. Rafferty Paterson Institute for Cancer Research, Christie Hospital (NHS) Trust, Manchester M20 4BX, United Kingdom

Arun Srivastava Departments of Microbiology and Immunology, Walther Oncology Center, Indiana University School of Medicine, and Walther Cancer Institute, Indianapolis, Indiana 46202-5120

Colin G. Steward Department of Pathology and Microbiology, Bristol University Medical School, and Bristol Royal Hospital for Sick Children, Bristol BS2 8BJ, United Kingdom

A. K. Stewart Departments of Medicine, Medical Biophysics, Pediatrics, and Pathology, The University of Toronto, and the Toronto Hospital Oncology Gene Therapy Program, Toronto, Ontario M5G 2C4, Canada

N. G. Testa CRC Section of Haemopoietic Cell and Gene Therapeutics, Paterson Institute for Cancer Research, Manchester M20 4BX, United Kingdom

Richard G. Vile Molecular Medicine Program, Guggenheim 18, Mayo Clinic, Rochester, Minnesota 55905

Flossie Wong-Staal Blood and Marrow Transplant Program, Department of Biology and Medicine, Universtity of California, San Diego, La Jolla, California 92093

E. A. de Wynter CRC Section of Haemopoietic Cell and Gene Therapeutics, Paterson Institute for Cancer Research, Manchester M20 4BX, United Kingdom

Preface

Since the first concepts of gene therapy were formulated, the hemopoietic system has been considered the most natural first target tissue for genetic manipulation. The reasons for this include the fact that a very large number of inherited disorders (including some of the most common disorders, such as the hemoglobinopathies) are disorders of the hemopoietic system, and the large amount of experience in hematopoietic transplantation biology. The consequence of this resulted in the first clinical trial of gene therapy in 1989, where two children suffering from severe combined immune deficiency (ADA-SCID) were transplanted with T-cells expressing adenosine deaminase (the defective enzyme in patients with this disorder). The partial success of this treatment was perhaps responsible for undue optimism among those proposing other gene therapy treatments within the hematopoietic system, and it has since become clear that there are a number of technical and biological difficulties to overcome before hematopoietic gene therapy becomes a mainstream therapeutic strategy. The chapters in this book evaluate the need for gene therapy in the hematopoietic system, discuss how efficient gene transfer and expression can be achieved in the target cells, highlight areas of difficulty to be addressed, and examine a number of potential applications of the gene therapy approach.

The book begins with a chapter by Testa and colleagues, discussing the various sources of hematopoietic cells for both transplantation and gene therapy. This is followed by a chapter by Steward, which sets out to challenge the need for gene therapy in the hematopoietic system in the light of current and potential advances in bone marrow transplantation. This chapter also sets some tough goals for gene therapy. Next comes a series of chapters examining the technology surrounding gene transfer into the hematopoietic system. They discuss the potential of current gene transfer methods and highlight the technololgical advances required to transform hematopoietic gene therapy from an experimental to a mainstream treatment. The remainder of the book is given over to examples of the use of gene therapy in the hematopoietic system. These include therapy of inherited disorders of the hematopoietic system and inherited disorders of multiple systems (exemplified by the lysosomal storage disorders). The applications of hematopoietic cell gene therapy to treating and monitoring neoplastic disease are discussed in chapters examining the efficacy of antisense treatment of leukemia, induction of autologous immune responses against tumors, the protection of otherwise sensitive normal tissues against the side effects of chemotherapy, and the use of gene transfer to mark hematopoietic grafts, enabling assessment of graft function and the extent of contamination by metastatic tumor cells. Finally, the use of gene transfer technology to treat AIDS and induce novel immune responses against potential human pathogens (DNA-based immunization) are discussed.

The combination of the experienced views of the various authors amalgamated in this book should introduce the reader to the basic concepts of gene therapy in the hematopoietic system, provide a critical analysis of progress to date with a view of the necessary ways forward to more effective therapy, and demonstrate the wide range of opportunity that exists for using the hematopoietic system in formulating therapeutic approaches to many different clinical problems.

Leslie J. Fairbairn

Contents

Chapter 9

Gene Marking and the Biology of Hematopoietic Cell Transfer in Human Clinical Trials

A. K. Stewart, I. D. Dubé, and R. G. Hawley

Chapter 10

Antisense Strategies to Leukemia

Stephen G. O'Brien

Chapter 13
Molecular Immunotherapy by Gene Transfer
Rosa Maria Diaz and Richard G. Vile

Chapter 14
DNA-Based Immunization
Heather L. Davis and Cynthia L. Brazolot Millan

Chapter 1

Hemopoietic Stem Cells as Targets for Genetic Manipulation

Concepts and Practical Approaches

N. G. Testa, E. A. de Wynter, and J. Hows

1. HOW MANY STEM CELLS DO WE NEED?

1.1. The Experimental Approach

The extensive potential for cell proliferation and differentiation of hematopoietic stem cells is clearly demonstrated in experimental systems. The bone marrow of one mouse repopulates about 2000 potentially lethally irradiated mice. In turn, each of these mice provides cells for a similar number of second generation recipients. In turn under certain conditions these may repopulate a third generation of mice (Harrison and Astle, 1982). In recent experiments, as few as 30 highly purified putative stem cells injected into irradiated mice permanently repopulated the lymphohematopoietic tissue (Spangrude *et al.*, 1995). With only about 20% of the injected cells expected to lodge in the bone marrow (Testa *et al.*, 1972), it is likely that five or six of the cells injected originated all the lymphohematopoietic cells in these animals. Recently, another study demonstrated that one injected cell with a "stem cell" phenotype can reconstitute hematopoiesis in an irradiated mouse (Osawa *et al.*, 1996). Again, the proportion of mice reconstituted after

N. G. Testa and E. A. de Wynter CRC Section of Haemopoietic Cell and Gene Therapeutics, Paterson Institute for Cancer Research, Manchester M20 4BX, United Kingdom. **J. Hows** University of Bristol, Division of Transplantation Sciences, Bristol, United Kingdom.

Blood Cell Biochemistry, Volume 8: Hematopoiesis and Gene Therapy, edited by Fairbairn and Testa. Kluwer Academic/Plenum Publishers, New York, 1999.

injection with a single cell agrees with the expected proportion of cells that seed in the bone marrow. Transplantation studies with marked murine cells have demonstrated that monoclonal or oligoclonal hematopoiesis occurs for long periods of time (Capel *et al.*, 1989; Keller and Snodgrass, 1990). Only limited data are available in larger mammals. In experiments with cats a small number of syngeneic putative stem cells maintain hematopoiesis (Abkowitz *et al.*, 1995).

1.2. Patient Data

Normal hematopoiesis is polyclonal, and polyclonal hematopoiesis is also usually observed after allogeneic transplantation. Nevertheless, there are anecdotal reports of oligo- or monoclonal hematopoiesis, determined by examining X -chromosome-linked polymorphisms, after allogeneic transplantation. This was observed in 2/12 cases by Turhan *et al.* (1989). One of them was limited to myeloid cells and the other also comprised lymphoid cells. Unfortunately the observations were made shortly after transplant, and the long-term features of hematopoiesis in those patients are not known. Limited data on atomic bomb survivors, however, indicate that oligoclonal hematopoiesis, as determined by cytogenetic markers, occurs for several years (Amenomori *et al.*, 1988; Kusunoki *et al.*, 1995). In one interesting patient, a single identifiable clone provided about 10% of all lymphohaemopoietic cells for a period of 10 years, starting about 40 years after the radiation exposure and in the absence of any detectable signs of abnormal hematopoiesis. A more recent study of normal subjects showed that about 30% of females of 70 or more years of age had oligoclonal hematopoiesis in the myeloid but not the lymphoid lineages. Whether this is caused by altered regulation of cell production or a limited supply of stem cells in the aged is not known. What is known, however, is that progressive telomere shortening of CD34+ cells (among which the stem cells are found) occurs with age (Vaziri *et al.*, 1994), and we have shown that in paired studies of donors and recipients of allogeneic transplantation, the telomere length in the blood cells in the recipient is significantly shorter than that of their donors. Such shortening is equivalent to that observed during 15 years of normal aging (median value) and in the worst case is equivalent to 40 years (Wynn *et al.*, 1998).

The data summarized previously are compatible with the concept that in humans, as in experimental systems, only a fraction of the vast reserve population of stem cells needs to proliferate and differentiate in a normal lifetime. In successful transplantation, however, where the whole tissue is regenerated from a relatively small number of stem cells, the proportion of cells recruited to proliferate and differentiate is likely to be higher. How many of the available stem cells are likely to do so is an important consideration after genetic manipulation if only a minority of the target cells are successfully modified. Thus, because the aim of treating the maximum possible number of target (stem) cells becomes critical, the search for the best source of cells is of great logistical importance.

2. SELECTION AND IDENTIFICATION BY PHENOTYPE AND FUNCTION

It is possible to separate the most primitive hematopoietic cells from their close progeny of progenitor cells. The former have a distinct phenotype of cell membrane markers (Table I) and are also characterized by low metabolic activity. This latter feature allows isolating primitive cells by negative selection using dyes, such as rhodamine-123, which concentrates in active mitochondria, or nucleic acid dyes like Hoechst 33342 (Ratajczak and Gewirtz, 1995; Spangrude *et al.*, 1994). One of the most useful membrane markers for selecting primitive cells has been the CD34 antigen, and this feature has been exploited in a number of different positive cell selection procedures (Table II). However, the CD34+ cells comprise a wide population encompassing stem cells, progenitor cells, and the more differentiated hematopoietic cells. In fact, only 0.1–1% of the CD34+ cells have the most primitive phenotype, whereas about 10–30% are progenitor cells, and the rest are more differentiated cells (Table III). Because of this, it is important to try and assess the proliferative and differentiation capacity of the selected cell subpopulations.

The clonogenic *in vitro* assays detect mainly the progenitor cells which are more mature than stem cells but some of the clonogenic assays may partially overlap

Table I
Phenotypic Markers of Primitive Cells

Stem cells	Progenitor cells
CD34+	CD34+
CD38−	CD38+
CD33−	CD33+
Lineage−	Lineage+
HLA-DR− or weakly+	HLA-DR weakly+
CD71−	CD71+
Thy 1 *low*	Thy 1+
CD45RA *low*	CD45RA+
c-kit+	c-kit *low* or −

Table II
Results of Positive Selection of CD34 Cells Using Different Selection Procedures[a]

Selection procedure	Purity (%)	Yield (%)	CFC-enrichment (× fold)
FACS	73.6	39.2	31.8
DYNAL	26.3	5.0	12.3
CEPRATE	72.0	41.4	68.0
CELLector	32.5	17.0	17.0
MiniMACS	72.2	62.6	102.0

[a] Data taken from de Wynter *et al.*, 1995.

Table III
Percentage of CFC in the Different CD34+ Subpopulations Expressing Stem and Progenitor Cell Phenotype

Phenotype	Percentage of cells	Percentage CFC
CD34+38+DR+	90.2	30.6
CD34+38+DR−	3.8	N.D.[a]
CD34+38−DR+	5.6	1.0
CD34+38−DR−	0.3	0.2

[a] Not determined.

with the stem cell compartment because of the continuous spectrum of proliferation and differentiation in the hematopoietic tissue. The blast colony assay (Bl-CFC; Leary and Ogawa 1987; Suda *et al.*, 1983) or the high proliferative potential colony assay (HPP-CFC; Bradley and Hodgson, 1979) are within this category (Table IV).

Functional assays are crucial to identify the phenotype that characterizes the most primitive cells and their progeny. Thus, only transplantation experiments can define stem cells strictly by their capacity to repopulate the hematopoietic tissue permanently (Table III). Currently, the most primitive human cells which can be assayed *in vitro* are the long-term culture initiating cells (LTC-IC). These cells have certain "stem cell" characteristics, but it is not yet clear how they are related to the repopulating cells. Using an animal model, Ploemacher (1994) showed that murine LTC-IC repopulate irradiated mice and therefore can be regarded as equivalent to the mouse repopulating cell. In efforts to study human stem cells both qualitatively and quantitatively, a number of animal models have been developed for transplantation studies. Sublethally irradiated severe combined immunodeficient, nonobese diabetic (SCID/NOD) mice were used to test the engraftment and repopulating potential of putative human stem cell populations (Vormoor *et al.*, 1994; Pflumio *et al.*, 1996; Turner *et al.*, 1996). The cells that engrafted and repopulated the marrow of these SCID/NOD mice were mainly located in the CD34+ population. However, limiting dilution repopulation assays indicated that the frequency of a SCID mouse repopulating cell was 1 in 10^6 cord blood mononuclear cells, whereas 1 in 3×10^3–10^4 mononuclear cells was an LTC-IC (Denning-Kendall, 1997; Pettengell, 1994). Clearly, the human repopulating cells assessed in the NOD/SCID model are more primitive than the human LTC-IC. Further evidence that these cells are distinct was provided by a gene transfer study (Larochelle *et al.*, 1996) using a retroviral adenosine deaminase (ADA) vector. In this system 30–40% of colony-forming cells (CFC) and LTC-IC are transduced with the ADA vector, but when the vector-transduced mononuclear cells were transplanted into NOD/SCID mice, none of the colony-forming cells generated were positive for ADA. Although high numbers of CFC and mature cells were obtained, the transfected cells contributed little to the graft, and the cells responsible for repopulation were not transfected, a further indication that the repopulating cell may be more primitive than the ADA positive LTC-IC. However, the incidence of 1 in 10^6 cells for the putative repopulating cells in the NOD/SCID model is much lower than the widely accepted incidence of long-term repopulating cells in murine studies of 1 in 10^5 bone marrow cells. Thus, there may

Table IV
Assays for Primitive Stem and Progenitor Cells

Cells	Assay
Long-term repopulating cells (*LTRC*)	Reconstitution of haemopoietic tissue
Long-term culture initiating cells (*LTC-IC*)	Generation of progenitor cells (CFC) after 5–8 weeks of culture
Clonogenic colony forming (CFC)	Colony formation in vitro
HPP-CFC	
Bl-CFC	
CFC-Mix or CFU-GEMM	

be yet unknown features of this model leading to an underestimation of the numbers of repopulating cells.

3. SOURCES OF PRIMITIVE HEMATOPOIETIC CELLS

3.1. Bone Marrow

It is generally accepted that the safe numbers of stem cells required for autologous transplantation after ablation are present in grafts that contain 2×10^8 nucleated cells per kg of body weight. The primitive cell populations in this cell number are about 2×10^6 CD34+ cells and 10^5 GM-CFC (progenitors of granulocytes, G, and macrophages, M), and about 10^4–2×10^4 LTC-IC (Table V). These numbers are usually obtained in conventional bone marrow harvests.

3.2. Peripheral Blood

One of the startling by-products of using hematopoietic cytokines in the clinic was the observation that primitive cells are mobilized into the circulation in large numbers after administeving cytokines. The cytokine most widely used for that purpose is G-CSF which induces the migration of stem and progenitor cells in such numbers that the mononuclear cells in the peripheral blood at the time of maximum mobilization can be considered equivalent to nucleated bone marrow cells on a cell per cell basis (Baumann *et al.*, 1993). Indeed, this source of cells is adequate for allogeneic transplantation with cells collected in two to three aphereses (usually processing 10–15 liters of blood for each apheresis) to reconstitute hematopoiesis in ablated recipients (Dreger *et al.*, 1996; Kobbe *et al.*, 1997). More recently Flt3 (Molineux *et al.*, 1997) and stem cell factor (SCF, also called c-*kit* ligand) in combination with G-CSF were also shown capable of mobilizing large numbers of primitive cells. When administered together with G-CSF and cyclophosphamide, the latter produces cell mobilization of such magnitude that a median volume of 512 ml would be sufficient to provide enough cells for an allogeneic transplantation to an individual of 70 kg of body weight (Table VI). Even more interestingly, when patients were treated with G-CSF and cyclophosphamide, the variation between

Table V
Approximate Median Frequency of LTC-IC in the Mononuclear Cell Fraction of Cord Blood and Normal Bone Marrow[a]

	Cord blood	Bone marrow
Week 5 LTC-IC	1:4,000	1:9,000
Week 8 LTC-IC	1:22,000	1:34,000

[a] Data from Pettengell *et al.*, 1994.

individual patients was much larger than when the protocol included SCF. In the latter case, only 73 ml of blood would be needed for allogeneic transplantation from the patient who showed the highest mobilization (Weaver *et al.*, 1998). Although patients in these series received cyclophosphamide, it is likely that G-CSF + SCF treatment without chemotherapy would result in comparable cell mobilization because previous work has shown that G-CSF plus cyclophosphamide induces a similar mobilization compared with treatment with G-CSF alone (Weaver *et al.*, 1996).

3.3. Cord Blood

Collections of cord blood contain about 10% of the numbers of progenitors present in the average bone marrow harvest. With such low progenitor cell numbers, cord blood transplants run the risk of either slow engraftment or even failure to engraft, and this is already of clinical concern in pediatric transplantation (Hows *et al.*, 1986; Rabian Hertzog *et al.*, 1992). Any processing of these cord blood collections, such as preparation of mononuclear cells or isolation of CD34+ cells will result in further substantial cell losses, including the mature T cells and NK cells (Denning-Kendall *et al.*, 1997). In transplantation this is of concern because removal of donor T-cells increase the risk of graft failure after marrow transplantation, probably caused by reduction of T-cell derived cytokines. Another potential problem could be delayed immune reconstitution of T and B cells with the possibility of a permanently reduced T and B cell repertoire if a full ablation regime is used before autologous transplantation. The combined effects of CD34+ cell losses during processing, T-cell removal, immune reconstitution and *in vitro* culture with hematopoietic growth factors to enhance transfection for gene therapy are currently unknown. A partial solution to these problems might be to retain both the CD34+ and the lymphoid-containing CD34 negative populations, transfect the CD34+ cells, and reinfuse both populations into the recipient.

4. HOW CAN WE MAXIMIZE THE NUMBER OF TARGET CELLS?

In the last few years, there has been great enthusiasm for the *ex vivo* expansion of hematopoietic cells in response to cytokine treatment. Indeed, a vast expansion of progenitor cells can be achieved (Table VII). However, expansion of more

Table VI
Median Volume of Unseparated Whole Blood (in Milliliters) that Contain Specified Numbers of Cells at the Time of Peak Mobilisation[a]

Target number of cells/kg	Cyclophosphamide 3 g/m^2 followed by G-CSF	Cyclophosphamide 3 g/m^2 followed by G-CSF SCF
GM-CFC (1×10^5)	490	138
CD34+ (2×10^6)	2602	512

[a] Data calculated from Weaver and Testa (1998) and Weaver *et al.*, 1996, for a patient of 70 kg body weight.

Table VII
***Ex vivo* Expansion of Progenitor Cells**

Initial cell population	SCF	G	GM	IL1	IL3	IL6	IL11	EPO	Fold expansion of CFC
CD34+ (human)[a]	•	•	•	•	•	•			50–60×
CD34+ (human)[b]	•	•	•	•	•	•			33×
CD34+ (human)[c]	•			•	•	•		•	190×
CD34+ (human)[d]	•			•	•	•			30–50×
CD34+ (human)[e]	•			•	•	•			79×
NBM (mouse)[f]	•			•		•			100×
NBM (mouse)[g]	•				•	•	•		3×

[a] Bohbot *et al.*, 1994.
[b] Haylock *et al.*, 1992.
[c] Brugger *et al.*, 1993.
[d] Heimfeld *et al.*, 1994.
[e] Moore and Hoskins, 1994.
[f] Muench *et al.*, 1992.
[g] Peters *et al.*, 1996.

primitive cells like LTC-IC has been more problematic. Early experiments showed at best, maintenance of the input numbers and not infrequently, a decline with time in culture (Henschler *et al.*, 1994). Recently, however good expansion of LTC-IC has been achieved (Table VIII), and calculations from our own data on cultured single cells from human cord blood indicated that LTC-IC may have expanded as much as 280-fold (de Wynter *et al.*, 1996). To date, the most exciting data shows amplification of 2×10^5-fold over initial input numbers (albeit after several weeks of culture), using a combination of Flt3 ligand and thrombopoietin (Piacibello *et al.*, 1997). These results were achieved using human cord blood. It will be of interest to investigate whether similar expansion of LTC-IC can be obtained from bone marrow cells. The combination of cytokines and the concentrations used may be important because the protocols that achieve the best expansion of LTC-IC differ from those that allow the best progenitor cell expansion (Zandstra *et al.*, 1997). Thus the *ex vivo* manipulation necessary for improved early regeneration (probably effected by CFC and more mature populations) is likely to be different from that required to

Table VIII
***Ex vivo* Expansion of LTC-IC in Response to Different Cytokines**

Initial cell population	FL[g]	G	IL3	IL6	SCF	NGF[h]	TPO[i]	Fold expansion	(days)
CD34+38−33−DR+[a]	•		•	•	•			4×	(14–21)
CD34+38−[b]	•		•		•			ND	
CD34+[c]	•		•		•			7–26×	(10–14)
CD34+38−[d]	•	•	•	•	•			5×	(5–8)
CD34+38−[e]	•	•	•	•	•	•		30–50×	(10–31)
CD34+[f]	•						•	160×	(35)

[a] Conneally *et al.*, 1996.
[b] Dooley *et al.*, 1996.
[c] Mobest *et al.*, 1996.
[d] Petzer *et al.*, 1996.
[e] Piacibello *et al.*, 1996.
[f] Zandstra *et al.*, 1996.
[g] FL, Flt ligand.
[h] NGF, Nerve growth factor.
[i] TPO, Thrombopoietin.

expand more immature cells including stem cells. Thus, results obtained will depend on the particular protocol and the choice of cytokines to be used for *ex vivo* cell expansion.

Although early experimental studies showed that transplantation of expanded cells may result in accelerated recovery (Muench, 1992), definitive data on the functional capacity of the expanded cells to repopulate the hematopoietic tissue permanently are not yet available (Table VIII). Although a primitive phenotype may be conserved, the repopulation capacity may be decreased (Spangrude *et al.*, 1995). Because of this, it is not known whether the same threshold numbers of cells needed for transplantation using freshly harvested cells will apply for cells expanded *in vitro*. In ablated mice, cell grafts with equivalent numbers of expanded or freshly harvested GM-CFC were not equivalent in their ability to regenerate hematopoiesis. Indeed, experiments in these mice indicated that 6- to 50-fold higher numbers of *in vitro* generated GM-CFC are required to achieve equivalent numbers of leucocytes in the circulation (Albella *et al.*, 1997). In addition, we can expect that shortening of telomere length with increased proliferative history of a cell population is likely to be accompanied by some loss of stem cell characteristics and increased risk of genetic instability in a cell population which will also undergo very marked proliferative stress if transplanted (Wynn *et al.*, 1997, in preparation). Indeed, data from experimental systems and from patients indicate that cytotoxic treatment (with the accompanying proliferative stress exerted by the need for endogenous regeneration of the haemopoietic tissue) results in a serious and permanent defect in the numbers of hematopoietic stem cells (Testa *et al.*, 1996). A sensible alternative approach is to increase the offer of available cells for manipulation. This is indeed achieved by using the best mobilization regimes. For example, the data in Table VI suggest that, in adults, it should be possible to obtain well in excess of 100-fold more than the number of stem cells required for a successful

Table IX
***In Vivo* Repopulation with Expanded Cells**

Initial cell[a] population	Cytokines for expansion[i]								Engraftment (months)	
	SCF	IL-1	IL-3	IL-6	IL-11	EPO	MIP	FL	Short-term <6 months	Long-term >6 months
WGA+,15.1−, Rho−[b]	•		•				•		5	No
5FU−,Sca+,c-kit+,Lin−[c]	•				•			•	4	nd[i]
NBM[d]	•		•	•	•				2.5	No
NBM[e]	•				•				1	?
CD34+(monkey)[f]	•		•	•					1.5	No
CD34+(human)[g]	•	•	•	•		•			1	?
CD34+(human)[h]	•		•	•					6	?

[a] Where not otherwise specified, murine cells were used. Human cells were assessed in immunosuppressed mice. Murine cells were used in[b–e].
[b] Data taken from references Tanosaki *et al.*, 1996.
[c] Yonemura *et al.*, 1996.
[d] Peters *et al.*, 1996.
[e] Holyoake *et al.*, 1996.
[f] Tisdale *et al.*, 1996.
[g] Brugger *et al.*, 1995.
[h] Brown & Zanjani, 1996.
[i] MIP, macrophage inflammatory protein 1α; FL, Flt ligand, NBM, normal bone marrow; nd, not determined.

transplantation from cells harvested in two to three aphereses (the number at present performed for allogeneic and for many autologous transplants). The situation with cord blood may differ and *ex vivo* expansion may be more effective than when using bone marrow cells, as suggested by the large expansion of LTC-IC already achievable (Piacibello *et al.*, 1997), and also safer because of the shorter proliferative history of the cord blood cells.

5. CONCLUDING COMMENTS

The present knowledge of stem cell biology and the state-of-the-art methodologies for genetically manipulating them make a judicious choice necessary of both the target cell population and the manipulation protocols to achieve specific aims. This chapter has presented the available choices for selecting target cells, ways to deal with the constraints that limited cell numbers may pose, and the potential problems which may arise from *in vitro* manipulation of stem cells.

6. REFERENCES

Abkowitz, J. L., Persik, M. T., Shelton, G. H., Ott, R. L., Kiklevich, J. V., Catlin, S. M., and Guttorp, P., 1995, Behaviour of hematopoietic stem cells in a large animal, *Proc. Natl. Acad. Sci. USA* **92:**2031–2035.

Albella, B., Segovia, J. C., and Bueren, J. A., 1997, Does the granulocyte-macrophage colony forming unit content in ex-vivo expanded grafts predict the recovery of the recipient leucocytes? *Blood* **90:**464–470.

Amenomori, T., Honda, T., Otaka, M., Tomonoga, M., and Ichimaru, M., 1988, Growth and differentiation of circulating hemopoietic stem cells with atomic bomb irradiation—induced chromosome abnormalities, *Exp. Hematol.* **16:**849–853.

Baumann, I., Testa, N. G., Lange, C., de Wynter, E. A., Luft, T., Dexter, T. M., van Hoef, M. E., and Howell, A., 1993, Haemopoietic cells mobilised into the circulation by lenograstim as alternative to bone marrow for allogeneic transplants, *Lancet* **341:**369.

Bohbot, A., Lioure, B., Faradji, A., Schmitt, M., Cuillerot, J. M., Laplace, A., and Oberling, F., 1996, Positive selection of CD34+ cells from cryopreserved peripheral blood stem cells after thawing: Technical aspects and clinical use, *Bone Marrow Transplant.* **17:**259–264.

Bradley, T. R., and Hodgson, G. S., 1979, Detection of primitive macrophage progenitor cells in mouse bone marrow, *Blood* **54:**1446–1450.

Brown, R. L., and Zanjani, E., 1996, CD34+ cultured in the presence of serum lose their long-term marrow repopulating ability, *Blood* **88**(Suppl. 1)**:**607a, abstract 2415.

Brugger, W., Heimheld, S., Berenson, R. J., Mertelsman, R., and Kanz, L., 1995, Reconstitution of hematopoieis after high-dose chemotherapy by autologous progenitor cells generated ex-vivo, *N. Engl. J. Med.* **333:**283–287.

Brugger, W., Mocklin, W., Heimfeld, S., Berenson, R. J., Mertelsman, R., and Kanz, L., 1993, Ex vivo expansion of enriched peripheral blood CD34+ progenitor cells by stem cell factor, interleukin-1 beta (IL-1 beta), IL-6, IL-3, interferon-gamma, and erythropoietin, *Blood* **81:**2579–2584.

Capel, B., Hawley, R., Covarrubias, L., Hawley, T., and Mintz, B., 1989, Clonal contributions of small numbers of retrovirally marked hematopoietic stem cells engrafted in unirradiated neonatal W/W^v mice, *Proc. Natl. Acad. Sci. USA* **86:**4564–4568.

Champion, K., Glibert, J. G. R., Asimakopoulos, F. A., Hinshlewood, S., and Green, A. R., 1997, Clonal haematopoiesis in normal elderly women: Implications for the myeloproliferative disorders and myelodysplastic syndromes, *Br. J. Haematol.* **97:**920–926.

Conneally, E., Cashman, J., Petzer, A. L., and Eaves, C. J., 1996, In vitro expansion of human lymphomyeloid stem cells from cord blood demonstrated using a quantitative in vivo repopulating assay, *Blood* **88**(Suppl. 1)**:**628a, abstract 2501.

Denning-Kendall, P. A., Horsley, H., Donaldson, C., Nicol, A., Bradley, B., and Hows, J. M., 1997, Is in vitro expansion of human cord blood cells clinically relevant? *Bone Marrow Transplantat.*, in press.

de Wynter, E. A., Nadali, G., Coutinho, L. H., and Testa, N. G., 1996, Extensive amplification of single cells from CD34+ subpopulations in umbilical cord blood and identification of long-term culture initiating cells present in two subsets, *Stem Cells* **14:**566–576.

de Wynter, E. A., Coutinho, L. H., Pei, X., Marsh, J. C. W., Hows, J., Luft, T., and Testa, N. G., 1995, Comparison of purity and enrichment of CD34+ cells from bone marrow, umbilical cord and peripheral blood (primed for apheresis) using five different separation systems, *Stem Cells* **13:**524–532.

Dooley, D. C., Oppenlander, B. K., Plunkett, J. M., and Xiao, M., 1996, FLT3 ligand (FL) stimulates long-term culture initiating cells (LTC-IC) and preferentially enhances the growth of $CD34^+CD38^{dim}CD33^{dim}HLA\text{-}DR^+$ cells compared to $CD34^+CD38^{dim}CD33^{dim}HLA\text{-}DR^{dim}$ cells, *Blood* **88**(Suppl. 1)**:**540a, abstract 2149.

Dreger, P., Glass, B., Uharek, L., and Schmitz, N., 1996, Allogeneic peripheral blood progenitor cells: Current status and future directions, *J. Hematother.* **5:**331–337.

Harrison, D. E., and Astle, C. M., 1982, Loss of stem cell repopulating ability upon transplantation. Effects of donor age, cell number and transplantation, *J. Exp. Med.* **156:**1767–1779.

Haylock, D. N., To, L. B., Dowse, T. L., Juttner, C. A., and Simmons, P. J., 1992, Ex-vivo expansion and maturation of peripheral blood CD34+ cells into myeloid lineage, *Blood* **80:**1405–1412.

Heimfeld, S., Kalamasz, D. F., Fogarty, B. L., Fei, R., Tsui, Z. N., Jones, H. M., and Berenson, R. J., 1994, Isolation and ex-vivo expansion of CD34+ cells from cord blood using dextran sedimentation and avidin column selection, *Blood Cells* **20:**397–403.

Holyoake, T. L., Freshney, M. G., McNair, L., Parker, A. N., McKay, P. J., Steward, W. P., Fitzsimons, E., Graham, G. J., and Pragnell, I. B., Ex-vivo expansion with stem cell factor and interleukin 11 augments both short-term recovery post transplant and the ability to serially transplant marrow, *Blood* **87:**4589–4595.

Keller, G., and Snodgrass, R., 1990, Life span of multipotential hematopoietic stem cells in vivo, *J. Exp. Med.* **171:**1407–1418.

Kobbe, G., Soehngen, D., Heyll, A., Fischer, J., Thiele, K. P., Aul, C., and Wernet, P., 1997, Large volume leukapheresis maximises the progenitor cell yield for allogeneic peripheral blood progenitor donation, *J. Hematother.* **6:**125–131.

Kusunoki, Y., Kodama, Y., Hirai, Y., Kyoizumi, S., Nakamura, N., and Akiyama, M., 1995, Cytogenetic and immunologic identification of clonal expansion of stem cells into T and B lymphocytes in one atomic- bomb survivor, *Blood* **86:**2106–2112.

Larochelle, A., Vormoor, J., Hanenberg, H., Wang, J. C., Bhatia, M., Lapidot, T., Moritz, T., Murdoch, B., Xiao, X. L., Kato, I., Williams, D. A., and Dick, J. E., 1996, Identification of primitive human hematopoietic cells capable of repopulating NOD/SCID mouse bone marrow: Implications for gene therapy, *Nature Med.* **2:**1329–1337.

Leary, A. G., and Ogawa, M., 1987, Blast colony assay for umbilical cord blood and adult bone marrow progenitors, *Blood* **69:**953–956.

Mobest, D., Winkler, J., Garbe, A., Schulz, G., Lange, W., Mertelsman, R., and Henschler, R., 1996, Kinetics of long term bone marrow culture—initiating cell (LTC-IC) amplification during culture of CD34+ blood progenitor cells (BPC) at a clinical scale, *Blood* **88**(Suppl. 1)**:**111a, abstract 431.

Molineux, G., McCrea, C., Yan, X. Q., Kerzic, P., and McNiece, I., 1997, Flt-3 ligand synergises with granulocyte colony-stimulating factor to increase neutrophil numbers and to mobilise peripheral blood stem cells with long-term repopulating potential, *Blood* **89:**3998–4004.

Moore, M. A., and Hoskins, I., 1994, Ex-vivo expansion of cord blood-derived stem cells and progenitors, *Blood Cells* **20:**468–479.

Muench, M. O., Schneider, J. G., and Moore, M. A., 1992, Interactions among colony-stimulating factors, IL-1 beta, IL-6 and kit-ligand in the regulation of primitive murine hematopoietic cells, *Exp. Hematol.* **20:**339–349.

Osawa, M., Hanada, K., Hamada, H., and Nakauchi, H., 1996, Long-term lymphohematopoietic reconstitution by a single CD34-low/negative hematopoietic stem cell, *Science* **273:**242–245.

Peters, S. O., Kittler, E. L., Ramshaw, H. S., and Quesenberry, P. J., 1996, Ex vivo expansion of murine marrow cells with interleukin-3 (IL-3), IL-6, IL-11 and stem cell factor leads to impaired engraftment in irradiated hosts, *Blood* **87:**30–37.

Pettengell, R., Luft, T., Henschler, R., and Testa, N. G., 1994, Direct comparison by limiting dilution analysis of long-term culture initiating cells in human bone marrow, umbilical cord blood and blood stem cells, *Blood* **84:**3653–3659.

Petzer, A. L., Zandstra, P. W., Piret, J. M., and Eaves, C. J., 1996, Differential cytokine effects on primitive (CD34+38-) human hematopoietic cells: Novel responses to FLT3-ligand and thrombopoietin, *J. Exp. Med.* **183:**2551–2558.

Pflumio, F., Izac, B., Katz, A., Shultz, L. D., Vainchenker, W., and Coulombel, L., 1996, Phenotype and function of human hematopoietic cells engrafting immune-deficient CD17-severe combined immunodeficiency mice and non-obese diabetic-severe combined immunodefiency mice after transplant of human cord blood mononuclear cells, *Blood* **88:**3731–3740.

Piacibello, W., Sanavio, F., Garetto, L., Severino, A., Bergandi, D., Ferrario, J., Fagioli, F., Berger, M., and Aglietta, M., 1997, Extensive amplification and self-renewal of human primitive hematopoietic stem cells from cord blood, *Blood* **89:**2644–2653.

Ploemacher, R., 1994, Cobblestone area forming cell (CAFC) assay, in *Culture of Haematopoietic Cells* (R. I. Freshney, I. B. Pragnell, and M. G. Freshney, eds.), Wiley-Liss, New York, pp. 1–21.

Rabian Hertzog, C., Lesage, S., and Gluckman, E., 1992, Characterisation of lymphocyte populations in cord blood, *Bone Marrow Transplant.* **9:**64–••.

Ratajczak, M. Z., and Gewirtz, A. M., 1995, The biology of hematopoietic stem cells in *Semin. Oncol.* **22:**210–217.

Spangrude, G. J., 1994, Biological and clinical aspects of hematopoietic stem cells, *Ann. Rev. Med.* **45:**93–104.

Spangrude, G. J., Brooks, D. M., and Tumas, D. B., 1995, Long term repopulation of irradiated mice with limiting numbers of purified hematopoietic stem cells: In vivo expansion of stem cell phenotype but not function, *Blood* **85:**1006–1016.

Suda, T., Suda, J., and Ogawa, M., 1983, Single-cell origin of mouse hemopoietic colonies expressing multiple lineages in variable combinations, *Proc. Natl. Acad. Sci. USA* **80:**6689–6693.

Tanosaki, R., Asihara, E., Migliaccio, G., and Migliaccio, A. R., 1996, Macrophage inflammatory protein-1α (MIP-1α) and leukemia inhibitory factor (LIF) protect the engraftment potential of enriched murine hematopoietic stem cells (HSC) during *ex-vivo* expansion with interleukin-3 (IL-3) and stem cell factor (SCF), *Blood* **88**(Suppl. 1)**:**345a, abstract 1369.

Testa, N. G., Lord, B. I., and Shore, N. A., 1972, The in vivo seeding of haemopoietic colony forming cells in irradiated mice, *Blood* **40:**654–661.

Testa, N. G., de Wynter, E. A., and Weaver, A., 1996, The study of haemopoietic stem cells in patients: Concepts, approaches and cautionary tales, *Ann. Oncol.* **7**(Suppl. 2)**:**5–8.

Tisdale, J. F., Sellers, S. E., Agricola, B. A., Donahue, R. E., and Dunbar, C. E., 1996, Gene marking studies indicate that ex-vivo expansion of mobilised rhesus peripheral blood cells results in rapid initial engraftment but diminished long-term repopulating ability, *Blood* **88**(Suppl. 1)**:**300a, abstract 1188.

Turhan, A. G., Humphries, R. K., Phillips, G. L., Eaves, A. C., and Eaves, C. J., 1989, Clonal hematopoiesis demonstrated by X-linked DNA polymorphisms after allogeneic bone marrow transplantation, *N. Engl. J. Med.* **320:**1655–1661.

Turner, C. W., Yeager, A. M., Waller, E. K., Wingard, J. R., and Fleming, W. H., 1996, Engraftment potential of different sources of human haematopoietic progenitor cells in BNX mice. *Blood* **87:**3237–3244.

Vaziri, H., Dragowska, W., Allsopp, R. C., Thomas, T. E., Harley, C. B., and Lansdorp, P. M., 1994, Evidence for a mitotic clock in human hematopoietic stem cells: Loss of telomeric DNA with age, *Proc. Natl. Acad. Sci. USA* **91:**9857–9860.

Vormoor, J., Lapidot, T., Pflumio, F., Risdon, G., Patterson, B., Broxmeyer, H. E., and Dick, J. E., 1994, Immature human cord blood progenitors engraft and proliferate to high levels in severe combined immunodeficient mice, *Blood* **83:**2489–2497.

Weaver, A., Wrigley, E., Watson, A., Chang, J., Collins, C. D., Jenkins, B., Gill, C., Pettengell, R., Dexter, T. M., Testa, N. G., and Crowther, D., 1996, A study of ovarian cancer patients treated with dose-intensive chemotherapy supported with peripheral blood progenitor cells mobilised by filgrastim and cyclophosphamide, *Br. J. Cancer* **74:**1821–1827.

Weaver, A., Ryder, D., Crowther, D., Dexter, T. M., and Testa, N. G., 1996, Increased numbers of long-term culture initiating cells in the apheresis product of patients randomised to receive increasing doses of stem cell factor administered in combination with chemotherapy and a standard dose of granulocyte colony-stimulating factor, *Blood* **88:**3323–3328.

Weaver, A., Testa, N. G., 1998, Stem cell factor leads to reduced blood processing during apherisis or the use of whole blood aligusts to support dose intensive chemotherapy, *Bone Marrow Transp.* **22:**33–38.

Wynn, R. F., Cross, M. A., Hatton, C., Will, A. M., Lashford, L. S., Dexter, T. M., and Testa, N. G., 1998, Accelerated telomere shortening in young recipients of allogeneic bone marrow transplants, *Lancet*, in press.

Yonemura, Y., Ku-H., Lyman, S. D., and Ogawa, M., 1997, In vitro expansion of hematopoietic progenitors and maintenance of stem cells: Comparison between FLT3/FLK2 ligand and KIT ligand, *Blood* **89:**1915–1921.

Zandstra, P. W., Conneally, E., Petzer, A. L., Piret, J. M., and Eaves, C. J., 1997, Cytokine manipulation of primitive human hematopoietic cell self-renewal, *Proc. Natl. Acad. Sci. USA* **94:**4698–4703.

Chapter 2

Bone Marrow Transplantation for Genetic Diseases

Colin G. Steward

1. INTRODUCTION

Successful bone marrow transplantation (BMT) for treating genetic diseases in animals and man was first performed in the late 1960s. Steinmuller and Motulsky (1967) corrected hereditary spherocytosis in an animal, closely followed by successful treatment of boys with severe combined immunodeficiency (SCID) (Gatti *et al.*, 1968). The relative absence of T-cell function in the SCID patients allowed engraftment without chemotherapy to prevent immune rejection. However, it soon became apparent that only a limited number of diseases (all of them immunodeficiency states) could be treated so simply, and work began to develop effective chemotherapy conditioning regimes.

Although high dose radiotherapy was effective, its long term consequences, especially in young children, were considered unacceptable. Therefore, no real progress was made, until Santos demonstrated that chemotherapy with busulphan and cyclophosphamide produces effective marrow ablation (Santos *et al.*, 1983). Then Hobbs used this combination to perform BMT successfully in a patient with Hurler's disease (Hobbs *et al.*, 1981), leading to his proposal for the wider use of these drugs for conditioning before BMT for treating genetic diseases (Hobbs, 1981). Since then busulphan/cyclophosphamide conditioning has enabled more than 1500 transplants to be performed for more than 50 different genetic diseases.

Colin G. Steward Department of Pathology and Microbiology, Bristol University Medical School, and Bristol Royal Hospital for Sick Children, Bristol BS2 8BJ, United Kingdom.

Blood Cell Biochemistry, Volume 8: Hematopoiesis and Gene Therapy, edited by Fairbairn and Testa. Kluwer Academic/Plenum Publishers, New York, 1999.

The particular relevance of these transplant procedures is that they effectively establish the limits of hematopoietic gene therapy by acting as *in vivo* therapy with long-term, fully regulated gene expression at normal levels. They define which specific diseases can be treated and which tissues will respond best in multiorgan diseases. They also provide occasional examples of how normal enzymes present after BMT may be seen as immunologically novel to a patient who has previously produced only abnormal enzyme, thereby eliciting an immune response capable of neutralizing the therapy.

This chapter gives a brief overview of the theory underlying BMT for genetic diseases, aspects of patient and donor selection, and the mechanics of the transplant process, including short- and long-term complications. However, its main function is to review the results in the disease groups considered primary candidates for transplantation. Particular attention will also be paid to those diseases where a differential tissue response occurs, for example, in Hurler's disease where BMT ameliorates neurological deterioration, hepatosplenomegaly, and corneal clouding but has little impact on the progression of bony disease.

The reader should remember that, where transplants have failed to effect improvement either in whole diseases or in particular organ systems, these failures have usually occurred despite complete normalization of enzyme levels post-BMT. Hematopoietic gene therapy may only be able to match, and certainly will only improve on these results, if high levels of engraftment of gene-modified cells are obtained and if the relevant genes are expressed at supranormal levels.

2. GENERAL PRINCIPLES OF BMT

2.1. Classes of Diseases Treated

In general terms BMT is therapeutic either in hematological diseases involving intrinsic defects in hemopoietic cells or in metabolic diseases where donor hemopoietic cells can donate normal enzyme to nonhematopoietic tissues. These can be conveniently grouped as follows:

1. Those diseases in which hematopoiesis is disordered and leads to defective production or function of red cells, platelets, lymphocytes or granulocytes, for example, *thalassemia*, *Wiskott–Aldrich syndrome*, *SCID*, *chronic granulomatous disease*
2. Those diseases in which fixed tissue cells of monocyte/macrophage lineage are defective, for example, *osteopetrosis*, *Gaucher's disease*
3. Metabolic diseases in which blood-derived cells provide exogenous enzyme to nonhematopoietic tissues, for example, *X-linked adrenoleukodystrophy (ALD)*, *Hurler's disease*

2.2. Enzyme Transfer

In 1968 Fratantoni *et al.* first observed the potential for fibroblasts from patients with Hurler's and Hunter's diseases to cross-correct their respective storage defects when grown together in culture. This observation was later extended to fibroblasts from metachromatic leukodystrophy (Porter *et al.*, 1972; Wiesmann *et al.*, 1971). Subsequently it was shown that both normal human serum and lymphocyte extracts correct disease in fibroblasts, implying that the relevant factors transferred from fibroblasts were also produced by lymphocytes (Olsen *et al.*, 1981). More recently these observations have been extended to show specific enzyme transfer from cells of donor bone marrow origin into CNS microglia (Walkley *et al.*, 1994). Now it is appreciated that mannose-6-phosphate receptors on cell membranes mediate enzyme uptake in these disorders, and bound enzyme is internalized by way of endosomes and stored in lysosomes.

These experiments led to diverse attempts to administer enzyme therapy via methods, such as regular blood/plasma transfusions or fibroblast/placental tissue implants (Barranger, 1984). All resulted either in no response or only transient improvements, mainly because of the short half-lives of the relevant enzymes or the rejection of tissue grafts. Only with the development of therapy for Gaucher's disease using mannose-terminated placental glucocerebrosidase (GC), an enzyme modified specifically to allow uptake by mannose-6-phosphate receptors, has enzyme therapy become a routine clinical treatment (Barton *et al.*, 1991). This has been followed by successful modification of adenosine deaminase (ADA) to treat SCID due to ADA deficiency (Hershfield *et al.*, 1987). Now similar therapies are under development for other diseases, notably mucopolysaccharide (MPS) disorders. However, enzyme therapies are required life long, involve regular intravenous injections, and have proven extremely expensive (a consequence of high development costs but use in relatively rare diseases). A further concern is that they could potentially be compromised by antibody formation, analogously to that in which factor VIII antibodies impair the treatment of hemophilia A, although this is not supported by experience to date in either Gaucher's disease or ADA-SCID.

2.3. Animal Models

Good animal models exist for globoid cell leukodystrophy (Krabbe disease), Niemann–Pick disease, fucosidosis, and MPS types I, VI and VII. Usually experiments in the relevant animal model precede experimental treatment, such as BMT, in man. However, the human diseases in question carry very poor prognoses and mostly have no alternative treatment. For this reason human BMT has largely been performed in parallel with or before the equivalent animal experiments.

Despite this some basic information on the potential utility, limitations, and mechanism of enzyme transfer after BMT has come from animal experiments. The details of these experiments, which are given in Table I, are summarized as follows:

1. BMT increases enzyme levels in blood, visceral organs, and the CNS resulting in mobilization of storage material, clinical improvement, and prolongation of survival compared to control animals. *This effect is highly dependent on the specific condition treated and the stage of the animal's disease. Better results are obtained when treatment is performed at a presymptomatic stage.*

Table I
Animal Models of BMT for Metabolic Disease

Human disease	Animal model	Findings	References
Fucosidosis	Springer spaniel	• No effect on advanced disease despite good CNS enzyme levels • Amelioration of disease when presymptomatic at BMT	Taylor *et al.*, 1986, 1989
Globoid cell leukodystophy (Krabbe disease)	Twitcher mouse	• Increased galactosylceramide and decreased psychosine levels in CNS • CNS macrophages of donor origin	Yeager *et al.*, 1984 Hoogerbrugge *et al.*, 1988
Mannosidosis	Cat	• Normal enzyme detected in glial cells and neurons after BMT	Walkley *et al.*, 1994
Hurler's disease (MPS I)	Platt hounds	• Glycosaminoglycans cleared from CSF and brain	Breider *et al.*, 1989
Maroteaux–Lamy disease (MPS VI)	Siamese cat	• Improved CNS signs despite no change in CNS enzyme levels	Wenger *et al.*, 1986
Sly disease (MPS VII)	Mouse	• Decreased visceral storage material • Bone disease and CNS not improved	Hoogerbrugge *et al.*, 1987
Niemann–Pick disease	Spm/Spm mouse	• Decreased visceral storage material • CNS deterioration not arrested	Sakiyama *et al.*, 1986

2. CNS macrophages and microglia of donor origin can be demonstrated post-BMT. *At least a proportion of CNS microglia are derived from monocytes and therefore are gradually replaced by donor cells after BMT. It is postulated that cell-to-cell transfer of enzyme occurs from donor microglia to affected neurons.*
3. In neurovisceral diseases, better resolution of storage material is seen from visceral organs than from the CNS. *This may result in progression of CNS disease despite improvement in other organs.*
4. Progression of neurological disease is slowed without measurable changes in overall CNS enzyme levels. *Amelioration of neurological symptoms occur in cats with arylsulphatase-B deficiency without any change in CNS enzyme levels.*

2.4. Mechanism and Speed of Response

A successful bone marrow transplant results in engraftment of donor lymphoid and hematopoietic stem cells. All of the elements of the immune and hematopoietic system become donor-derived, including fixed-tissue macrophages, such as osteoclasts, Kupffer cells, and CNS microglia.

When the target for disease correction is a blood cell itself, it is reasonable to expect a rapid response. In theory, because the typical life span of red blood cells is approximately 120 days, full donor engraftment after BMT for sickle cell anemia or thalassemia should result in clearing residual abnormal cells from the blood after 3–4 months. Considerably slower responses occur when replacement of fixed tissue macrophages is required. Although blood monocytes are principally of donor origin at the time of successful engraftment, it can take up to eight weeks for macrophages in liver, lungs, and skin to begin to be replaced. Furthermore, complete replacement may be protracted. For example, Gaucher cells are still detected in liver biopsies for up to three years after BMT (Ringden *et al.*, 1995).

Response is slowest where enzyme transfer into neurons is required because this relies on the replacement of microglia by cells of donor origin (Hickey and Kimura, 1988). Experiments in mice suggest that this process is relatively slow, and approximately 20% of microglia are replaced within three to four months of transplant (Krall *et al.*, 1994). Presumably this explains the typical delay of 6–12 months before CNS disease begins to stabilize in Hurler's disease or ALD.

The likely speed of response after BMT governs both the decision as to whether transplantation is appropriate and the urgency of the procedure. This is well exemplified by two diseases, both of which may present with visual signs—osteopetrosis and ALD. In osteopetrosis, osteoclast dysfunction causes overgrowth of skull foramina and this may present with absent visual fixation because of optic nerve compression in the early months of life. However, BMT rapidly reverses excess bone deposition due to engraftment of donor osteoclasts and can prevent further loss of vision if performed at this stage (Gerritsen *et al.*, 1994). By contrast, if a child presents with a squint as a first sign of cerebral adrenoleukodystrophy, BMT is generally considered contraindicated. In this disease rapid neurological deterioration often follows development of the first neurological sign(s). The slow replacement of CNS microglia which BMT effects is too slow to prevent this disease progression.

2.5. Displacement BMT

It has been estimated that just 10% of normal enzyme levels prevent symptoms of metabolic disease (Sandhoff, 1984). By a logical extension it may seem that 10% replacement of a patient's diseased bone marrow with that of a normal donor should "cure" the relevant disease. However, this fails to take note of three considerations:

1. Stable low level chimeras are rare entities, and transplants are usually rejected if less than 30% of bone marrow is of donor origin in the early months post-BMT. Early graft rejection is usually immune-mediated. However, rejection may occur silently as late as seven years post-BMT. In such cases "crowding out" of the donor stem cells by regenerating recipient stem cells may be responsible rather than a true immune rejection process (Hobbs, 1981).
2. Patients have often sustained tissue damage by the time of referral for BMT. High levels of enzyme may well be needed to reverse these changes. This is particularly pertinent in neurological diseases, for example, ALD with white matter changes, where only relatively small numbers of donor cells will penetrate the brain.
3. There may be major antigenic differences between the new donor enzyme and the defective enzyme of the patient which could result in forming of neutralizing antibodies. However, the complete replacement of a patient's

marrow usually overcomes this risk by replacing the recipient's immunity with that of the donor.

In consequence BMT must always aim for full "displacement" of the recipient's marrow stem cells with those of the donor (the sole exception are forms of SCID with defective T-cell function). This minimizes the likelihood of graft rejection and antibody formation against donated enzyme while maximizing therapeutic enzyme levels in metabolic diseases. Therefore, the assessment of chimerism (the balance of donor and recipient hematopoietic cells) is of major interest in transplants for genetic disease.

2.6. Conditioning Therapy

The very earliest successes in genetic BMT were in immunodeficiency states in which the patient's immune system could not reject the incoming donor cells. However, it was rapidly appreciated that rejection inevitably followed if BMT was performed in the face of a functional immune system. This led to attempts to condition patients transplanted for a variety of genetic diseases using cyclophosphamide, a powerful immune suppressant. However, all of these were unsuccessful (Bach *et al.*, 1968).

The most informative of these attempts concerned two patients who were transplanted for chronic granulomatous disease (CGD). One was conditioned by using 50 mg/kg cyclophosphamide on four consecutive days, and the other with the same chemotherapy following 10 Gy of selective pelvic irradiation (Hobbs, 1981). The average proportion of donor phagocytes in sternal BM aspirates from both patients after BMT was only 12%, but in marrow from the irradiated pelvic area this figure was 100%. This strongly implied a requirement for stem cell displacement, that is, making space for the incoming donor cells in addition to immunosuppression. It was subsequently shown that total body irradiation (TBI) provides highly effective displacement therapy. However, studies performed primarily in children transplanted for malignant disease showed long term side effects, notably growth and pubertal delay, hypothyroidism, and neuropsychological impairment, especially when TBI was used in very young children (Deeg, 1994).

No further progress was made until Santos' demonstration in rats that busulphan is highly cytotoxic to stem cells, so that, when allied to cyclophosphamide, the two agents comprise a highly effective conditioning regime (Santos, 1989). Busulphan/cyclophosphamide conditioning has since been used in large numbers of transplants for genetic diseases and in smaller numbers for malignant disease. The doses used have gradually been refined. Initially, busulphan was administered at 2 mg/kg/day for four days but this resulted in frequent graft rejection (Fischer *et al.*, 1983; Kamani *et al.*, 1984). This was greatly improved by increasing the dose to 4 mg/kg/day on four days. Higher doses cause unacceptable rates of veno-occlusive disease, a serious early complication of BMT (Grochow *et al.*, 1989; Morgan *et al.*, 1991). Also, children under the age of six years metabolize busulphan more rapidly, giving higher rates of graft rejection or incomplete donor engraftment, and therefore need a higher dose (typically 5 mg/kg/day on four days) (Grochow *et al.*, 1990; Vassal *et al.*, 1992). Cyclophosphamide is typically given at a dose of 50 mg/kg on four consecutive days.

When used to condition patients for BMT from sibling donors, these doses are highly effective and result in graft rejection in less than 5% of cases. Unfortunately, higher rates of rejection are seen in transplants for particular genetic diseases, for example, thalassemia (due to previous sensitization by multiple blood transfusions), Gaucher's disease (massive splenomegaly), and Hurler's disease (splenomegaly ± altered busulphan kinetics).

However, the greatest shortcomings of busulphan/cyclophosphamide conditioning therapy are in non-HLA-identical BMT. Use of T-lymphocyte replete bone marrow grafts from such donors causes unacceptable rates of severe graft versus host disease. This problem is largely overcome by heavy T-cell depletion of the BM inoculum, which unfortunately favors development of mixed chimerism, even if *in vivo* T-cell depletion of the patient prior to BMT is used to redress the T-cell balance. This is illustrated by the first five patients transplanted for genetic diseases in Bristol using marrow from unrelated donors (UD). None of them developed moderate/severe graft versus host disease. Following T-cell depletion using CAMPATH antibodies, two showed total graft rejection within the first year post-BMT, and two others are currently stable 50% and 75% donor chimeras two to three years post-BMT. Only one child is a persistent full donor chimera at 3.5 years post-BMT. Similarly, the first three patients transplanted in Minnesota after T-cell depletion by elutriation all rejected their transplants and autoengrafted (personal communication, Prof. W. Krivit).

These results, together with disappointing rates of complete donor engraftment following sibling BMT for Hurler's disease, have encouraged the North American Storage Disease Collaborative Study Group to modify the conventional regime and to reduce the doses of busulphan (to 320 mg/m^2 over two days) and cyclophosphamide (to 120 mg/kg over two days) but to add 750 cGy of TBI in a single fraction. Early results are encouraging. More than 90% of patients evaluable at one year after UD-BMT showed full donor engraftment despite the T-cell depletion, although the long term impact of irradiation in these young children remains to be seen. Other groups are investigating the addition of the myelosuppressive alkylating agent, thiotepa, to busulphan/cyclophosphamide conditioning.

2.7. Studies of Graft Chimerism after BMT

The results discussed previously emphasize the importance of assessing donor chimerism carefully after BMT. Historically this has relied on enzyme assays, studies of red blood cell polymorphisms, or cytogenetic analysis in sex mismatched transplants (Petz, 1994). These techniques all have limitations, including poor sensitivity, interference from red blood cell transfusions, limited degrees of polymorphism, and lack of sex mismatch between donor and recipient. More recently, techniques involving Southern blot analysis of restriction fragment length polymorphisms (RFLP) (Blazar *et al.*, 1985) and variable number of tandem repeat (VNTR)

(Roth *et al.*, 1990) regions have allowed more accurate and widespread assessment of postgraft chimerism. However, these are limited by the requirement of DNA from at least 10^6 cells for reliable analysis.

Therefore, Southern blot techniques have been superseded by PCR amplification of VNTR regions, especially those comprising di- to tetranucleotide repeats [short tandem repeat (STR) regions]. In UD grafts, where such studies are likely to be of most interest, a panel of primers to just six different STR loci amplify polymorphisms distinct between donor and recipient in more than 90% of cases (a larger panel of markers is frequently needed to reveal informative polymorphisms between siblings). Now these markers allow accurate assessment of chimerism down to 1% sensitivity in a test which takes less than one working day (Hancock *et al.*, 1997). By coupling this technique to immunomagnetic cell selection, engraftment kinetics in different cellular subpopulations can be carefully studied even when the white blood cell count is less than 0.1×10^9/liter.

The detailed study of early engraftment kinetics is currently in its infancy, but it is hoped that better understanding of patterns of chimerism will allow effective postgraft immunotherapy. This is most likely to occur via manipulation of either stem cell doses and/or T-cell populations.

2.8. Immunoprophylaxis

A major aim of total displacement BMT is to efface the immunity of the recipient and replace it with that of the donor, so that antibodies cannot be formed against the donor enzyme or protein. However, if the new (normal) protein is presented to the patient while some recipient memory B cells survive, in the early post-transplant period, this will stimulate the persistence of these cells (Riches *et al.*, 1986) and ongoing antibody production which may compromise the therapy. Furthermore, this concern must extend beyond BMT to clinical gene therapy as currently conceived, because gene therapy will take place against the background of an intact immune system. Evidence already exists that CTL responses neutralize the effect of a transfected transgene *in vivo* because of differences in sequence homology between different species (Yang *et al.*, 1996). Although the intention in human gene therapy trials would not be to introduce genes from different species, this situation might be mimicked by large gene deletions or mutations that alter highly antigenic sites within the native protein product of the patient.

Tolerance to self proteins is established *in utero* before 16 weeks gestation (Wengler *et al.*, 1996) and in a patient with genetic disease includes tolerance to their abnormal protein product. If this protein happens to be antigenically distinct from normal protein, then introducing the normal donor product at any time after 16 weeks gestation will elicit an immune response. The resultant antibody might either interfere with the active sight of the enzyme or tag it so as to affect its transport or breakdown. This chain of events is probably unlikely in mixed allotypes that have defects at separate sites because these result in the presence of cross-reactive immunological material, which would usually prevent antibody formation to the normal product.

The following examples provide two convincing instances of antibody formation following BMT. The first is a girl transplanted for Morquio disease who was investigated when enzyme levels failed to normalize after transplant (Hobbs, 1988). It was found that her plasma contained a persistent IgG fraction which inhibited enzyme activity. The second is a patient transplanted for MLD in Bristol whose arylsulphatase A (ASA) reached normal levels one to three months post-BMT with 100% donor chimerism. Now, at three years post-BMT, the patient has stabilized as a 50% donor chimera, but has a very low ASA level identical to that before BMT. This patient's plasma now inhibits ASA assays of cell extracts from normal individuals, an effect not seen with pre-BMT plasma, and one which implies the presence of antibody.

A further problem is that most enzyme assays are not strictly functional assays but rely on inexpensive and readily accessible artificial substrates. Therefore, it would be possible for antibody formation to affect the function of an enzyme *in vivo* without affecting an *in vitro* assay. This would be particularly likely if the antibody affects transport of the enzyme, for example, across the blood–brain barrier, rather than its active site.

Hobbs strongly advocated "immunoprophylaxis" to minimize the risk of antibody formation (Hobbs, 1988). This comprised administering a donor blood buffy coat fraction after busulphan therapy, followed at precisely 24 and 48 hour intervals by doses of cyclophosphamide, a maneuver designed to delete a primary immune response to the exogenous protein. Although this prevented any further obvious instances of antibody formation in the extensive experience of the Westminster team, this technique has not been widely applied.

3. THE BONE MARROW TRANSPLANTATION PROCESS

3.1. Patient Assessment

The decision to perform BMT in a patient who has a genetic disease is arrived at only after a complex process of medical assessment and counseling. Patients are often referred for transplantation soon after diagnosis, so that they and their families often have only rudimentary knowledge of the disease. In addition, because many diseases are diagnosed only at a relatively advanced stage, patients may have already developed complications which transplantation cannot reverse. Although BMT might offer a chance of lifelong cure it also carries risks, either early (e.g., graft versus host disease, infection) or late (e.g., poor growth, infertility), which causes death or long-term morbidity.

Ideally, patients should be transplanted at as early an age as possible to reduce specific complications of their disease or its treatment (e.g., transfusional sensitization, transmitted viral diseases, sepsis, bony deformity, CNS damage). There is also some evidence that BMT in early life increases the chance of progressing normally through puberty, perhaps indicating less risk of impaired fertility (Obaro and Hobbs, 1995).

In diseases not previously treated by BMT, which lack an appropriate animal model or whose pathogenesis is not understood, it is desirable to attempt *in vitro* correction of measured enzyme deficiency or abnormal cellular morphology. This is done by mixing irradiated candidate donor lymphocytes with target recipient lymphocytes or fibroblasts and assaying the response in the recipient cells. Evidence of successful *in vitro* correction suggests the possibility of correction *in vivo* post-BMT but does not guarantee the scope or long-term success of the procedure. For instance, enzyme transfer can be elegantly demonstrated fibroblast-to-fibroblast or lymphocyte-to-fibroblast in lysosomal storage disorders, yet correction of bony disease is generally poor (possibly as a consequence of poor enzyme penetration of chondrocytes).

3.2. Donor Selection

The availability of suitable donors is of paramount importance. Transplants from HLA-identical sibling donors yield the best results due to a low risk of acute graft rejection and high likelihood of long-term graft stability. However, only one in four siblings represent a full tissue match. Also, because most genetic diseases are inherited in an autosomal recessive manner, one out of any four siblings can be expected to have the same disease, two to be carriers (often with subnormal enzyme levels), and only one to be completely unaffected. Therefore, statistically, the chance of any sibling being an ideal donor, a full tissue match and not a carrier, is only 1 in 16.

When a suitable sibling donor is unavailable, parents, aunts, or uncles, who match half of the patient's tissue type (haplotype matches) or best matched other relatives can act as donors. Generally these transplants are associated with high levels of transplant-related morbidity and mortality. However, in countries where large volunteer UD registries have not been established, they frequently represent the only possibility for BMT.

Fortunately, however, the past decade has seen great advances in UD transplantation with the advent of highly effective T-cell depletion techniques which greatly reduce the incidence and severity of graft versus host disease (GVHD). Although some units rely on the mixed lymphocyte culture to predict probabilities of graft rejection and graft versus host disease and therefore for donor selection, this has little value in heavily T-cell depleted UD transplants. With this proviso it is possible to find suitable donors (fully phenotypically matched or mismatched for one major HLA antigen) for more than 80% of European patients who require BMT and are of European ancestry. Greater use of UD donors has reduced the number of haploidentical transplants performed for those lacking sibling donors. However, this trend may soon be reversed if the early promise shown by high cell dose haploidentical transplants (using heavily T-cell depleted, G-CSF-primed peripheral blood stem cells (Aversa *et al.*, 1994)) is sustained. In the future it seems likely that cord blood transplants will further widen the choice of potential donor tissue and may further reduce the risks of transplantation (see "Future Directions").

Before marrow donation the donor undergoes a thorough medical assessment and is screened for an extensive panel of viral infections. One of the most important considerations for the transplant clinician is the status of the patient and donor with regard to cytomegalovirus (CMV) infection. This is a highly prevalent virus—approximately 70% of adults are seropositive—which remains latent after the original infection. Following BMT, the virus may be reactivated from either recipient or donor tissue causing fatal pneumonitis (Winston *et al.*, 1990). Wherever possible donors are selected on the basis of CMV status and HLA matching.

3.3. Transplantation Protocol

The sections which follow describe a typical protocol used in allogeneic transplant for genetic disease in the BMT Unit at the Royal Hospital for Sick Children, Bristol.

3.3.1. Transplant Preparation and General Care

Before BMT a back-up bone marrow harvest is taken and cryopreserved. In the event of failure of engraftment of the donor marrow, this is used to "rescue" the patient from the aplasia induced by conditioning chemotherapy. An indwelling central venous catheter is inserted to facilitate blood tests and administration of drugs, intravenous nutrition, and blood products.

Because of the long period of anticipated neutropenia, the patient is commenced on regular antibacterial mouthwashes and a diet low in potential pathogens ("clean diet"). Ciprofloxacin is administered orally to reduce rates of gram-negative sepsis and prophylactic antiviral and antifungal agents are also given. Blood products are either obtained preferentially from CMV-negative donors or leucodepleted (to reduce the risk of CMV transmission from transfused leucocytes). Blood products are also irradiated to prevent engraftment by residual leucocytes, causing devastating transfusion-associated GVHD (Greenbaum, 1991).

3.3.2. Conditioning Therapy

The patient then commences a nine day period of conditioning chemotherapy with busulphan (orally) and cyclophosphamide (intravenously). Busulphan is given at a dose of 4 mg/kg/day on days -9 to -6 pretransplant (or 5 mg/kg/day in those less than 6 years old) and cyclophosphamide at 50 mg/kg/day on days -5 to -2. Patients due to receive T-cell depleted marrow from an unrelated donor also receive a five day course of CAMPATH anti-T-cell monoclonal antibody (Hale *et al.*, 1988).

Antiemetic drugs are given to minimize nausea and vomiting, together with an anticonvulsant because busulphan therapy can cause fits (Marcus and Goldman, 1984). Cyclophosphamide can damage the kidney and bladder urothelium causing severe hemorrhagic cystitis. To prevent this it is standard in all BMT units to give high rate intravenous fluids throughout (and for 24 hours after) cyclophosphamide administration, together with diuretic agents if urinary output falls significantly behind fluid input. This is accompanied either by bladder catheterization and/or administration of 2-mercapto-ethane-sulphonate (MESNA), a thiol compound which becomes concentrated in the urine and which binds to activated cyclophosphamide.

No chemotherapy is given for the 24 hours before infusion of donor marrow to allow clearance of cyclophosphamide from the circulation, thereby minimizing damage to donor cells.

3.3.3. Bone Marrow Administration

On the day of the transplant the patient is moved into an isolation unit to reduce the risk of infection. A patient must remain in this room continuously until neutrophil recovery with restricted access by visitors, although several close relatives are allowed access at all times.

Bone marrow is harvested from the pelvic bones of the donor under general anesthetic. The final marrow dose required is calculated on the basis of recipient weight: usually a minimum of 3×10^8 mononuclear cells/kg. Marrow may either be given back to the patient without manipulation (where the donor is matched sibling) or following T-cell depletion when an unrelated donor is used. Procedures to reduce red cell contamination are also employed in cases of major patient/donor ABO incompatibility.

3.3.4. Engraftment

Stem cells and early progenitor cells home rapidly from the blood stream into the marrow cavity where they begin to expand. Now the patient enters a period of maximum risk. The white blood cell count rapidly falls to zero and within 4–5 days most patients develop chemotherapy-induced mucositis. This can be severe enough to prevent swallowing food and secretions and frequently requires pain control with an opiate infusion accompanied by intravenous feeding. Mucositis usually heals within the next seven days. The combination of neutropenia and defective mucosal protection from enteric flora renders the patient at high risk of bacteremia. Therefore, broad spectrum antibiotics are commenced rapidly on development of fever. Many BMT units employ granulocyte colony-stimulating factor to stimulate neutrophil recovery and so reduce the period of major risk.

Patients rarely show signs of engraftment until at least day 10 following BMT, although the majority have a neutrophil count exceeding 0.5×10^9/liter within four weeks of transplant. Patients leave their isolation cubicles when a sustained neutrophil count of 1×10^9/liter has been achieved and they are off intravenous feeding and free of infection.

3.3.5. Posttransplant Care

Patients are gradually weaned from cyclosporin, commencing at 6 months to 1 year. Cotrimoxazole is continued until up to one year post-BMT to prevent pneumocystis infection. Patients are regarded as functionally asplenic and continue on prophylactic penicillin for life. Most require only occasional outpatient visits for review by three months posttransplantation. Endocrine function is assessed with special attention to growth, pubertal development, fertility, and thyroid function.

3.3.6. Management of Rejection

In the event of nonengraftment or early graft rejection, the back-up harvest is returned to the patient without delay. A second transplant can be attempted at a later date, preferably from an alternative donor and after a delay of at least three months to allow the patient to recover. This is generally preferable to awaiting slow autologous reconstitution and the attendant infective risks. If chimeric assessment suggests persisting full donor engraftment in the face of poor blood count recovery or a failing count following initial recovery, patients may benefit from a further infusion of bone marrow or peripheral blood stem cells from the original donor.

4. COMPLICATIONS OF BMT

These can be divided into short- and long-term complications. The former consist primarily of infection and GVHD, and the latter consist of effects on endocrine function, growth, and fertility together with a small risk of chemotherapy-induced malignancy.

4.1. Short- and Medium-Term Complications

4.1.1. Infection

The immunosuppression and destruction of mucosal integrity that follow pretransplantation conditioning render infection one of the major concerns of BMT (Winston *et al.*, 1979). Great strides have been made in the last 20 years in the diagnosis, treatment, and prophylaxis of infection. However, shifting patterns of opportunistic pathogens, changing antimicrobial resistance, and increasing severity of conditioning and immunosuppressive regimens make controlling infection a constant challenge. The period of risk after BMT can be split into the three following broadly distinct periods:

4.1.1a. The Early Recovery Phase. This corresponds to the period before full engraftment, that is, the first month post-BMT. The major agents causing infections during this period are gram-negative and gram-positive bacteria, herpes simplex (HSV) and candida.

Bacterial pathogens account for more than 90% of first infections during neutropenia. Historically, infections with gram-negative organisms have predominated in adults and those with gram-positives in children. The use of prophylactic fluoroquinolones, notably ciprofloxacin and norfloxacin, have dramatically reduced the incidence of gram-negative infections in adults whereas gram-positive bacteremias have become more common in both groups because of the prevalent usage of indwelling central venous catheters. Broad spectrum antibiotic therapy controls most infections if instigated at the first sign of neutropenic fever.

Reactivation of HSV type I occurs in approximately 70% of seropositive patients, usually during the first or second week post-BMT, and leads to localized or diffuse ulceration of the mouth and lower esophagus. The use of prophylactic aciclovir therapy during the early weeks of BMT largely prevents this problem, although the emergence of resistant strains is a cause for concern, particularly following T-cell depleted BMT.

Fungal infections often emerge in the later part of this period when the bacterial gut flora has been altered by broad spectrum antibiotics. Most common fungal infections respond well to treatment with either fluconazole or Amphotericin B, but aspergillus infections carry a high mortality.

4.1.1b. The Early Postengraftment Phase. This covers primarily the second and third month post-BMT when cell-mediated and humoral immunity are still severely deficient. The infections during this time are heavily influenced by graft versus host disease which breaches barriers to infection (notably skin and gut mucosa) and causes immune dysregulation. The major infectious agents are CMV, adenovirus, aspergillus and pneumocystis.

CMV disease typically presents with progressive pneumonitis between 28 and 72 days post-BMT, although it may also present as enteritis, encephalitis, or hepatitis. Well-established disease carries a poor prognosis. The virus may derive from either latent endogenous virus in the patient, from the donor marrow, or from contaminating white cells in blood and platelet transfusions. The latter may be avoided by using blood products exclusively from CMV negative donors or by removal of white cells by filtration (DeWitte *et al.*, 1990). The prevalence of CMV disease is further declining because of aciclovir prophylaxis and earlier detection of viral reactivation, which allows earlier and more effective treatment with agents, such as ganciclovir and foscarnet.

Adenovirus infections affect up to one-fifth of BMT patients and cause respiratory symptoms (including pneumonitis), enteritis, hemorrhagic cystitis, and hepatitis, although the severity of infection varies with serotype. Infections may be either primary or represent reactivation of latent virus. There is no effective form of prophylaxis or treatment. Pneumocystis also causes pneumonitis. This infection can be prevented by prophylactic administration of cotrimoxazole or aerosolized pentamidine.

4.1.1c. The Late Postengraftment Phase. Although both humoral and cellular immunity are gradually recovering, beyond three months post-BMT they are frequently still subnormal. This is especially so after nonidentical allogeneic BMT and in the presence of chronic GVHD. Immunoglobulin deficiencies can occur, either of whole isotypes or of individual subclasses. Response to immunizations may be impaired or absent for up to 18 months after unrelated BMT and indefinitely when chronic GVHD is present.

The major threats are infections with encapsulated bacteria and recurrent Varicella zoster infections. Penicillin is widely used for bacterial prophylaxis, especially in patients with GVHD. Some units use aciclovir for Varicella prophylaxis.

4.1.2. Graft versus Host Disease

GVHD is the most frequent and potentially devastating complication of BMT (Kersey *et al.*, 1971; Sullivan, 1994). It occurs because of the presence of alloantigens in the host that are lacking in the donor, so that the patient appears foreign to the donor graft. This causes donor T lymphocytes contained within the graft to proliferate/differentiate and attack host cells either directly or through secondary mechanisms. Other factors associated with an increased risk of GVHD include older patient age, use of female donors for male patients (especially from parous female donors), and the use of CMV-positive donors for CMV-negative patients.

The resulting disease occurs in two clinically distinct forms, "acute" GVHD which occurs within 100 days post-BMT and "chronic" GVHD beyond this point. Acute GVHD presents as dermatitis, hepatitis, or enteritis, either alone or in combination and is diagnosed histologically by biopsy of the affected tissue(s). Without prophylaxis acute GVHD develops in moderate to severe form in approximately 80% of sibling allogeneic BMT and falls to an average of about 35% with typical current immunosuppression protocols. Even with prophylaxis, rates of 75–80% are seen in full haplotype mismatched transplants from parents or siblings and T-cell replete fully matched UD transplants.

Treatment comprises prednisolone at a starting dose of 2–5 mg/kg/day, tapered according to response. With this treatment the disease often eventually resolves although patients may go on to develop chronic GVHD, especially those with more severe disease. Patients who fail to respond to this therapy have been treated with monoclonal antibodies to CD3, IL-2 receptors, and TNF-α, but with poor long-term success rates. Psoralen and ultraviolet A irradiation (PUVA) can be used in patients with persistent skin GVHD.

Chronic GVHD behaves more like an autoimmune disease, and autoantibodies have been found in up to 62% of patients. The more common problems include skin changes, cholestatic jaundice, oral lesions, keratoconjunctivitis, and weight loss. Delayed immune reconstitution results in increased infections, particularly in the form of bacteremia, sinopulmonary infections, and atypical pneumonitis. Prednisolone, azathioprine, cyclosporin A, and thalidomide have all been used to treat chronic GVHD. However, infections result in death in up to one-half of patients with extensive disease.

The incidence of GVHD is reduced by prophylactic administration of various combinations of cyclosporin A, methotrexate, prednisolone, and anti-thymocyte globulin in the peritransplant period and for 6–12 months thereafter. However, the most effective methods of preventing GVHD rely on removing T-cells from the marrow graft—"T-cell depletion"—either using monoclonal antibodies directed against T-cell epitopes, physical methods (e.g., albumin gradient centrifugation, E-rosette depletion) or a combination of the two. Such methods effect up to a 2–3 log depletion of T-cells but are associated with higher rates of primary graft rejection or later graft loss.

A variety of monoclonal antibodies are used for T-cell depletion. The most commonly used is a rat immunoglobulin M (IgM), CAMPATH-1, which recognizes a glycoprotein (CDw52) expressed by all lymphocytes (T, B, NK cells) and monocytes. To minimize the risk of graft rejection this can be allied to *in vivo* depletion using CAMPATH-1G. After conditioning with TBI and cyclophosphamide, this method resulted in graft failure in only 6% of 50 children transplanted for relapsed ALL from a mixture of fully matched and mismatched unrelated donors. The attendant incidence of moderate to severe acute GVHD was 12% and chronic GVHD 8% (Oakhill *et al.*, 1996).

4.2. Late Effects of BMT

4.2.1. Thyroid Function

Chemotherapy conditioning regimes do not cause thyroid disorders although hypothyroidism is a common complication within two decades of radiation-based conditioning regimens (Katsanis *et al.*, 1990).

4.2.2. Growth

Perhaps the most informative data concerning growth after busulphan/cyclophosphamide conditioned transplants for genetic disease come from studies of children with thalassemia. Of 35 boys and 45 girls transplanted following 14 mg/kg BU and 200 mg/kg CY, all those transplanted at nine years of age or less had normal growth velocity. However, those treated at 10 years or above showed decreased growth velocity and an absent pubertal growth spurt (Manenti *et al.*, 1989). This contrasts with children transplanted for leukemia using BU 16 mg/kg and CY 200 mg/kg who showed decreasing growth velocity (Sanders, 1991a; Wingard *et al.*, 1992).

4.2.3. Puberty

Gonadal function was assessed in 30 prepubertal patients (15 girls, 15 boys, ages 9.3–17.2 years) transplanted for thalassemia following BU 14 mg/kg and CY 200 mg/kg (DeSanctis *et al.*, 1991). Thirteen of the girls had primary ovarian failure, and two had hypogonadotrophic hypogonadism. Responses to gonadotrophin-releasing hormone were reduced in 12 of the 15 boys. It is not known how these figures would compare to children transplanted at much younger age, especially because children with thalassemia may have delayed or absent puberty as a consequence of iron overload.

Women treated with CY 200 mg/kg alone as conditioning for BMT for aplastic anemia when aged less than 26 years at transplant recover ovarian function within three years. However, after BMT conditioning with BU and CY, none of 50 women returned to normal ovarian function within 1–2 years, and all had signs of primary ovarian failure (Sanders *et al.*, 1988, 1991b). Results appear similar for men. Leydig and Sertoli cell function were largely normal 1–15 years after CY alone. However, following BU 16 mg/kg and CY 200 mg/kg, 32 of 34 men had elevated FSH levels. Only one of five had return of spermatogenesis, and this man fathered a child two years post-BMT. The effects on fertility where BU/CY is given early in a child's life therefore remain a matter of conjecture, but families are counseled that infertility is the likeliest outcome of busulphan therapy.

4.2.4. Secondary Malignancy

It is generally agreed that irradiation-based conditioning regimes carry a risk of secondary malignancies, and quoted risks are up to 25% within 10 years (Socie *et al.*, 1991). Very much lower risks result from single-agent cyclophosphamide protocols, for example, 6% in a Seattle series (Witherspoon *et al.*, 1992). Although it is likely that there is a risk of secondary malignancy as a direct consequence of conditioning chemotherapy, data are not available from sufficient numbers of childhood transplants and with adequate follow-up to assess this.

5. RESULTS OF BMT

These are given according to the classification of transplant indications shown in Table II. For ease of reference diseases are listed in alphabetic order within each section. Particular attention is given to those conditions where trials of gene therapy have already commenced.

Table II
Genetic Diseases Treated Successfully by BMT

Disorders of haemopoiesis
Congenital erythropoietic porphyria
Diamond–Blackfan anemia
Dyskeratosis congenita
Familial erythrophagocytic lymphohistiocytosis
Fanconi's anemia
Glanzmann's thrombasthenia
Phagocyte disorders
Shwachman–Diamond Syndrome
Severe combined immunodeficiency disease
Sickle cell anemia
Thalassemia
Wiskott–Aldrich syndrome
Disorders of fixed tissue cells of monocyte/ macrophage origin
Gaucher's disease
Osteopetrosis
Metabolic disorders
Adrenoleukodystrophy
Fucosidosis
Globoid cell leukodystrophy
Metachromatic leukodystrophy (MLD)
Mucopolysaccharidosis Type I (MPS I): Hurler's disease
Mucopolysaccharidosis Type VI (MPS VI): Maroteaux–Lamy syndrome

5.1. Disorders of Hematopoiesis

5.1.1. Congenital Erythropoietic Porphyria (CEP)

This rare autosomal recessive disease results from decreased activity of the enzyme uroporphyrinogen III cosynthase, and results in accumulation and hypersecretion of porphyrins which cause severe cutaneous photosensitivity, hemolysis, and decreased life expectancy (Elder, 1990). Prominent clinical signs are red urine, hirsutism and alopecia, and erythrodontia—blackened teeth which fluoresce red in UV light.

At least five children have been treated by BMT. The first was a girl transplanted from an HLA identical brother in 1990 (Kauffman *et al.*, 1991). Within six months of transplant her symptoms had resolved to the point that she could go into the sunshine without further nodule or sçar formation, but she died unexpectedly of CMV infection at 11 months post-BMT. Since this time an additional three patients have been transplanted, two from bone marrow and one from cord blood (Thomas *et al.*, 1996; Zix-Kieffer *et al.*, 1996). Although one child required retransplantation, all are alive and well and have substantially improved symptoms with follow-up of up to two years.

5.1.2. Diamond–Blackfan Anemia

This typically presents with isolated anemia during the first year of life. The mode of inheritance is either autosomal dominant or recessive, but no gene localizations are known. Treatment with packed cell transfusions carries a long term risk of iron overload although transfusions can be performed less frequently than for thalassemia major. Sixty to seventy percent of patients respond initially to oral corticosteroid therapy and may become transfusion independent. However, the response is steroid dependent in two-thirds of such patients, and some patients eventually become steroid resistant (Janov *et al.*, 1996).

The decision to perform BMT is complicated, even when an HLA-matched disease-free sibling is available. Approximately 20% of patients spontaneously remit, particularly during puberty. Although the number of transplants performed is still relatively small (23 procedures are reviewed in Janov *et al.*, 1996), there is an excessive incidence of moderate to severe GVHD. This suggests the possibility of an underlying DNA repair defect, although none has been formally demonstrated. BMT is probably best reserved for patients who show steroid resistance, a high transfusion requirement, or early symptoms of iron overload.

5.1.3. Dyskeratosis Congenita

This is an X-linked disorder caused in most instances by an unspecified defect in a gene localized to chromosome Xq28 (Connor *et al.*, 1986). The most common presentation is a combination of characteristic changes of the skin, nails, and mucous membranes and pancytopenia, which develops in approximately half of patients during the first or second decade (Sirinavin and Trowbridge,

1975). As in Fanconi's disease (section 5.1.5) there is a predisposition to malignancy. Of 11 patients reported after HLA identical BMT, only four remained alive 8 months to 6 years after grafting (Bordigoni, 1995). Deaths resulted from a combination of factors, including acute GVHD (two), thrombotic microangiopathy after radiotherapy (two), and idiopathic pneumonitis eight years posttransplant.

These results are reminiscent of Fanconi's disease and suggest that modification of conditioning therapy may be necessary to reduce toxicity. Furthermore, there is no evidence that BMT alleviates problems of the integument, and it could potentially increase the risk of malignancy.

5.1.4. Familial Erythrophagocytic Lymphohistiocytosis (FEL)

This rare inherited condition is characterized by generalized activation of the mononuclear phagocyte system. Patients typically present under three years of age with fever, hepatosplenomegaly, and a rash, together with biochemical abnormalities, such as hypofibrinogenemia and hypertriglyceridemia (Henter and Elinder, 1991). Twenty percent of children also have neurological manifestations, such as seizures, irritability, or an altered conscious level. Neither the pathogenesis of the disease nor its genetic basis are understood.

Untreated, the condition has a median survival of six weeks. With the use of chemotherapeutic agents, such as vinca alkaloids, steroids, and epipodophyllotoxins, most patients enter remission. There are also promising results from protocols centered on the use of antithymocyte globulin (Jabado *et al.*, 1997). However, remission is rarely maintained without BMT. A recent review gave details of 19 patients treated by BMT. Nine (47%) were in sustained remission at the time of the report (Goulden *et al.*, 1995). Results were extremely poor where transplants had been performed with active disease or from haploidentical donors. Interestingly, predominant return of recipient hematopoiesis appeared compatible with sustained remission in at least four of these cases, which implies that small numbers of residual donor cells exert disease control.

5.1.5. Fanconi's Anemia

This is a recessively inherited disease which manifests as progressive pancytopenia, a wide variety of congenital anomalies, and predisposition to malignant change (dosSantos *et al.*, 1994; Liu *et al.*, 1994). It is thought to result from a variety of DNA repair defects. Patients can be assigned to one of four different complementation groups, although only one of the responsible genes has so far been identified (for complementation group C) (Verlander *et al.*, 1994). Excess spontaneous chromatid breaks may occur in phytohemagglutinin-stimulated peripheral blood lymphocytes, but incubation with DNA cross-linking agents, such as diepoxybutane or mitomycin result in many more chromatid breaks (Auerbach, 1993; Sasaki and Tonomura, 1973).

Patients may be identified at birth by characteristic defects such as thumb or radial abnormalities, but they are often not identified until the progressive cytopenias develop with macrocytosis at 5–10 years of age. In approximately 75% of patients, cytopenias may respond to treatment with the oral androgenic steroid, oxymethalone. However, this response is often only partial, and patients eventually become refractory to treatment. Even for those responsive to androgens, median survival is only 10 years from commencement of therapy.

Early attempts at BMT resulted in severe toxicity due to the alkylating drugs used in conditioning therapy. Transplantation only became tolerable with the demonstration by Gluckman *et al.* that reduced doses of cyclophosphamide (20 mg/kg total dose) and thoracoabdominal irradiation (5 Gy in a single fraction) allow engraftment from matched sibling donors (Gluckman *et al.*, 1984 & 1995). This has been the mainstay of pre-BMT conditioning ever since, although Gluckman's group has very recently changed to a chemotherapy regime based on busulphan, cyclophosphamide, and ATG. The best figures obtained using cyclophosphamide and TBI rely on the addition of pre- and post-transplant ATG. This has produced an 86% disease free survival rate in a cohort of 20 children with a median follow-up of 4 years, though one of the children required two transplants and three had mild chronic GVHD (Kohli-Kumar *et al.*, 1993 and, Dr. R. Harris personal communication). Results remain good in patients followed up for longer periods although tumors of the tongue and pharynx have been recorded after BMT, suggesting that a predisposition to malignant change may remain (Auerbach and Allen, 1991; Socie *et al.*, 1991; Flowers *et al.*, 1992). These tumors typically appear five years or more after transplant and appear strongly associated with antecedent GVHD (Professor E. Gluckman, personal communication). Interestingly, three patients transplanted in Paris showed mixed chimerism early after BMT but subsequently became full donor chimeras, suggesting that engrafted donor cells may have a competitive advantage over residual recipient cells (Socie *et al.*, 1993).

Relatively few transplants have been performed using nonidentical donors, and the overall results have been disappointing (Hows *et al.*, 1989). This is explained by a combination of high rates of graft rejection and severe GVHD. The latter is not surprising because even HLA-identical transplants cause high rates of acute and chronic GVHD. Current experimental protocols using nonidentical donors are concentrating on the use of alternative conditioning drugs and T-cell depletion for GVHD prophylaxis.

5.1.6. Glanzmann's Thrombasthenia

This disease is inherited in a autosomal recessive fashion and consists of a defect in the platelet membrane glycoprotein IIb/IIIa complex, which leads to a severe bleeding disorder. So far, three patients have been transplanted with good results (reviewed in McColl *et al.*, 1997). BMT is confined to patients with the severest form of the disease.

5.1.7. Phagocyte Disorders

Congenital neutropenia (Kostmann's syndrome), neutrophil actin defects, chronic granulomatous disease (CGD), leukocyte adhesion deficiency (LAD), and Chediak–Higashi syndrome comprise the most commonly recognized diseases of myeloid function. All have been treated successfully by BMT, although only small numbers of patients have been treated in each category.

This particular group of diseases exemplifies particularly well several points made earlier. First, to achieve durable cure of myeloid disorders, conditioning therapy must include either busulphan or irradiation. Use of immunosuppressive drugs alone, for example, cyclophosphamide, procarbazine, or anti-thymocyte globulin, has resulted in failure of cure in cases of neutrophil actin dysfunction, CGD, LAD, and Chediak–Higashi syndrome because the myeloid compartment was reconstituted from surviving recipient stem cells (Camitta *et al.*, 1977; Goudemand *et al.*, 1976). Secondly, patients ideally should be transplanted early in their disease course. A large survey of patients treated for a variety of phagocytic defects revealed disease-free survival of 60% and 67% when BMT was performed before two years of age or between two and four years respectively, but only 18% for those aged greater than four years at the time of transplantation (Fischer *et al.*, 1986). This largely results from a higher infective load at an older age which increases the chance of reactivation infections in the peritransplant period with higher attendant risks of GVHD.

Now, other forms of treatment are largely preferred. Congenital agranulocytosis is treated successfully with G-CSF (Bonilla *et al.*, 1989), so that BMT is usually reserved for those who fail to respond to this treatment, have serious side effects, or do not comply with therapy. Interferon-γ is beneficial in CGD (Woodman *et al.*, 1992), and therefore BMT is reserved for those who fail therapy. Only in LAD does BMT generally constitute the treatment of choice. The irony remains that if patients fail apparently safer treatments, they usually have acquired a sufficient infective load or organ damage to render BMT a high-risk procedure.

5.1.8. Shwachman–Diamond Syndrome

This autosomal recessive disease is characterized by pancreatic exocrine insufficiency, short stature, and cyclic neutropenia. Twenty-five percent of patients develop severe aplastic anemia. Only five transplant procedures are known to the author (Barrios *et al.*, 1990; Tsai *et al.*, 1990). Two patients are reported alive and well nine and 54 months post-BMT, but it is of concern that two patients died of cardiac failure (a comparatively rare event after allogeneic BMT in patients who have not received previous cyclophosphamide chemotherapy) and one other patient died of multiorgan toxicity. It is unclear whether this is a specific toxic effect of full dose cyclophosphamide in this condition or whether cellular repair mechanisms are defective, as in Fanconi's anemia.

5.1.9. Severe Combined Immunodeficiency Disease (SCID)

SCID comprises a broad clinical phenotype in which patients present with recurrent bacterial, fungal, or protozoal infections either together or alone (Gelfand and Dosch, 1983). In all subtypes lymphocytes cannot mount an antigen-specific response. This may be caused by complete absence of lymphoid stem cells, resulting in a lack of circulating T or B lymphocytes, or a defect in lymphocyte differentiation, resulting in an absence of mature T lymphocytes. Notable causes of the latter include absence of the enzyme adenosine deaminase (ADA), defective IL-2 production, and lack of receptors for IL-1. Approximately one-half of all cases of SCID are thought to be X-linked, and the rest have an autosomal pattern of inheritance. ADA deficiency comprises 30–50% of the latter.

In all forms of SCID HLA-identical BMT results in engraftment of normal donor lymphoid stem cells, correction of clinical immunodeficiency, and disease-free survival rates of greater than 90% (Fischer *et al.*, 1990). Because conditioning chemotherapy is not generally used, donor hematopoietic stem cells (HSC) engraft only as a minor population, but in most patients disease is greatly improved by 10–20% replacement of the defective cell series. However, the patient cannot reject the incoming donor T-cells, and all circulating T-cells therefore become of donor origin. B-cells may subsequently either be of donor or recipient origin, depending on the exact type of SCID.

It has been very difficult to obtain comparable results in the majority of patients who lack suitable sibling donors. Typical survival figures are only 50–60% (Fischer *et al.*, 1990). Histoincompatible BMT results in fatal GVHD due to engraftment of mature donor T-cells contained in the marrow inoculum. Transplants using fetal liver/thymus or cultured thymus have also been largely unsuccessful, but several *in utero* transplants using fetal liver cells are notable exceptions (Touraine *et al.*, 1997; Wengler *et al.*, 1996).

Haploidentical parental transplants yield much better results if accompanied by T-cell depletion (by combinations of soybean lectin agglutination and sheep erythrocyte rosetting or by lysis with anti-T cell monoclonal antibodies) and preceded by conditioning therapy with combinations of cyclophosphamide, busulphan, and/or cytosine arabinoside and antithymocyte globulin. Using such techniques, it is possible to achieve successful engraftment in approximately three-quarters of patients with classical forms of SCID (Friedrich *et al.*, 1985). However, immune reconstitution can be very prolonged, recovery of specific antibody synthesis is sometimes never achieved, and some variants, for example, Omenn's syndrome (comprising erythroderma, persistent diarrhea, lymphadenopathy, hepatosplenomegaly, high serum IgE, and eosinophilia), respond poorly.

This is leading increasingly to the use of unrelated donor transplantation. Filipovich *et al.* (1992) obtained good results in patients who received fully matched or one antigen (HLA-A or -B)-mismatched BMT using T-replete bone marrow. Various combinations of busulphan, cyclophosphamide, ATG, fractionated TBI, and etoposide were used for conditioning and combinations of methotrexate, prednisolone, cyclosporin, and anti-CD5 (one patient only) for GVHD prophylaxis. All eight patients so treated engrafted, two died early of post-transplant complications, and only one developed GVHD of grade III which responded to therapy. All six survivors were well and at home with a follow-up of 18–47 months at the time of the report. The incidence of GVHD was remarkably low considering the T-replete nature of the grafts, although this could result from the young age of patients with SCID. The high rate of engraftment may be caused by the T-replete nature of the grafts.

A variety of unrelated donor protocols are under investigation now by other groups. It seems likely that unrelated donor transplants will largely supplant haploidentical transplants when suitable donors are available. An important consideration, however, is the speed of donor availability because children with SCID are often very sick. This is an area where cord blood transplantation may be invaluable when banks reach a sufficient size, because cord blood harvests will be available almost immediately.

5.1.9a. ADA-SCID. This condition is of major interest because, in addition to BMT, now it can be treated by enzyme therapy and is the subject of several important trials of gene therapy. Reported so far in several hundred families, it follows an autosomal recessive pattern of inheritance (Hershfield and Mitchell, 1995; Hershfield *et al.*, 1997). Defects in the gene encoding ADA on chromosome 20q result in low or absent enzyme activity. Deoxyadenosine (dAdo), the normal substrate for ADA, derives from dissolution of DNA within macrophages from cells undergoing apoptosis. Defective enzyme activity leads to a build-up of dAdo in plasma, and this contributes to lymphocyte dysfunction and death, especially in T-cells, via a variety of biochemical pathways.

Severe ADA-SCID presents within the first few months of life with thrush, refractory nappy rash, pneumonia, diarrhea, and failure to thrive. Pneumocystis carinii and viral pneumonia occur often. Complications of infection with viruses (e.g., CMV, Varicella) are the commonest cause of death, which usually occurs by two years of age. Less severe forms of the disease are diagnosed rarely up to the age of 40 years, usually caused by development of unexplained T lymphopenia or chronic pulmonary disorders (Ozsahin *et al.*, 1997).

Supportive care includes vigorous antibiotic therapy for specific infections, regular intravenous immunoglobulin infusions, antifungal and pneumocystis prophylaxis, and management in an isolation cubicle. Vaccination with live viruses and BCG must be avoided. Blood products must be irradiated to avoid the development of fatal transfusion-associated GVHD.

Enzyme replacement therapy with ADA was developed after the finding that the *in vitro* response to mitogen of lymphocytes from an ADA-SCID patient was stimulated by adding purified ADA to the culture medium (Polmar *et al.*, 1975). It was later shown that twice monthly transfusions with irradiated red cells increased blood ADA activity to near normal values, lowering plasma levels of dAdo (Polmar *et al.*, 1976). Then it was that shown covalent bonding of monomethoxypolyethyleneglcol (PEG) stabilizes purified bovine ADA, yielding an enzyme therapy which could be administered as a once weekly intramuscular injection (Hershfield *et al.*, 1987). Metabolic correction by PEG-ADA therapy is more effective than either transfusion therapy or haploidentical BMT (Hershfield, 1995). The major disadvantages are extreme expense and the necessity for repeated intramuscular injections in young children. Now enzyme therapy can be used to stabilize a patient's condition when a suitable donor is available, but the recipient is unfit for BMT because of severe intercurrent infection.

Both HLA-identical and haploidentical BMT have been used successfully in ADA-SCID. After sibling BMT, engraftment of T-cells and improvement of cellular immune function occur within a month, although absolute lymphocyte counts may take years to normalize. B-cell recovery, usually of host origin, is more variable, but long term recovery of immune function is the rule. All eight patients with ADA-SCID who received HLA-identical transplants between 1983 and 1989 in Europe were reported to be cured. The risks of haploidentical transplantation, with or without T-cell depletion, are well illustrated in this disease. All seven patients died who received such transplants up to 1992 at the Hôpital Necker-Enfants Malades in Paris, the world's largest immunodeficiency transplant unit (Fischer *et al.*, 1990).

5.1.10. Sickle Cell Anemia

Severe sickle cell anemia results from a homozygous mutation in the gene encoding β-globin which substitutes valine for glutamic acid at codon 6. This genotype is termed SS. In turn, this predisposes red cells to adopt a sickle conformation which leads to obstruction of small vessels throughout the body and hence to organ dysfunction and pain. However, in contrast to the relatively predictable clinical behavior of thalassemia major, that of sickle cell anemia is highly variable both between patients and throughout the life of an individual patient.

Those who cite SS anemia as an indication for BMT point to the morbidity and mortality of untreated disease. These include stroke (which affects 8% of children and is recurrent in two-thirds), splenic sequestration crises, osteonecrosis of the hip (which develops in 40% by the age of 30 years), recurrent painful crises, acute chest syndrome, chronic renal failure, chronic lung disease, and cor pulmonale. A study from Los Angeles as recently as 1993 reported that the average life expectancy of SS African-Americans is 40 years for men and 49 years for females, approximately a 30 year reduction over that for unaffected members of the equivalent populations (Platt *et al.*, 1994).

Although controversy surrounds selection for BMT, so far, patients have been treated either as a secondary aspect of the treatment of another primary disease (e.g., acute leukemia), following severe disease complications (e.g. stroke) or (as with those coming from African republics) where there were concerns about the quality of primary care. Of a cohort of 42 children transplanted in Belgium and France, 90% were alive with donor engraftment (two after second procedures) 1 to 75 months after BMT, and only one child had died (Vermylen and Cornu, 1994).

Most children with sickle cell disease transplanted from siblings become durable donor chimeras, but interestingly several who have rejected their grafts subsequently developed increased concentrations of fetal hemoglobin (22–33%), as a result of which they have remained symptom free (Brichard *et al.*, 1996). This phenomenon has not been seen after transplants for thalassemia and is unexplained. Neurological complications have been reported in one-third of patients, especially in those who have had a previous stroke. These include seizures, transient ischemic attacks, hemiplegia, and intracranial hemorrhage.

Currently agreed indications for BMT for sickle cell anemia in Britain comprise age less than 16 years and the availability of an HLA matched sibling, preexisting sickle-related neurological defect, cerebrovascular accident or subarachnoid hemorrhage, more than two episodes of acute chest syndrome and stage I chronic sickle lung disease, and debilitating pain due to the disease.

5.1.11. Thalassemia

Thalassemia major comprises the world's commonest indication for BMT (more than 850 procedures have been performed worldwide). However, which patients should receive this form of treatment remains highly contentious.

This disease presents with severe anemia in the first few months of life and, untreated, leads to death in early infancy. Life can be prolonged into the fourth and fifth decades (and possibly beyond) for an increasing number of patients by regular blood transfusion at 15–21 day intervals so as to keep the hemoglobin above 10g/dl—"hypertransfusion therapy" (Piomelli *et al.*, 1969). However, in turn this causes progressive iron overload which eventually leads to endocrine deficiency, liver and pancreatic damage, and cardiomyopathy (Gabutti and Piga, 1996). These effects are minimized by subcutaneous desferrioxamine therapy which must be administered frequently—ideally, 8–12 hours per day at least five days per week (Hershko and Weatherall, 1988). This poses major problems in both compliance and cost. Patients also risk viral infections transmitted in blood transfusions.

The first transplant for thalassemia was performed in 1981, and the patient remains well and disease-free (Thomas *et al.*, 1982). The consistent use of a protocol based on busulphan (14mg/kg) and cyclophosphamide (200mg/kg) in a large cohort of patients aged less than 16 years by Lucarelli *et al.* allowed accurate recognition of patient risk factors (Lucarelli *et al.*, 1995). These include the development of hepatomegaly or portal fibrosis and poor compliance with chelation therapy. On this basis patients can be allocated to risk groups: class 1 for those who have none of these characteristics, class 3 for patients who have all, and class 2 for intermediate patients. Disease-free survival two years post-BMT runs at over 90% for class 1 patients compared to slightly less than 50% for those in class 3. The carrier status of the potential donor appears unimportant in transplant outcome.

Lucarelli's team has gone on to perform transplants in smaller numbers of adults primarily using a less intensive regime with a reduced cyclophosphamide dosage (120mg/kg) and the addition of pre- and posttransplant antilymphocyte globulin to their GVHD prophylaxis protocol. These transplants have also yielded encouraging results. Rejection-free survival rates at two years are more than 70%.

Therefore, proponents of BMT for thalassemia major advocate transplantation at a young age for all patients who have matched siblings, thereby avoiding the complications of hypertransfusion therapy and reducing the risk of graft rejection due to sensitization to previous blood transfusions. This frees patients from the daily tedium of desferrioxamine therapy and prevents development of iron overload or transfusion-related viral infection. There is little doubt that this is the favored option in patients who comply poorly with chelation therapy or transfusion. However, those who favor conventional therapy point to the potential future development of well-tolerated oral chelation therapy and the attendant risks of BMT. Therefore, selection for BMT in this disease requires careful pretransplant evaluation and discussion.

5.1.12. Wiskott–Aldrich Syndrome

This disease presents with eczema, T-cell immunodeficiency, and defective production of carbohydrate antibodies (due to a defect in lymphoid stem cells) and thrombocytopenia (due to a hematopoietic stem cell defect) (Perry *et al.*, 1980; Wolff, 1967). Therefore, full eradication of both hematopoietic and lymphoid stem cells is necessary for cure.

The first sibling BMT was performed in 1968 using cyclophosphamide alone, but this resulted only in T-cell engraftment, so that thrombocytopenia persisted (Bach *et al.*, 1968). The first successful sibling transplant was not performed until 1977. Although only transient T-cell engraftment followed conditioning therapy with cyclophosphamide and cytosine arabinoside (primarily lymphoid ablative chemotherapy), full and permanent engraftment was achieved using procarbazine and antithymocyte globulin (for lymphoid stem cell ablation) and TBI (for HSC ablation) (Parkman *et al.*, 1978). Now, complete correction of disease occurs in more than 90% of patients transplanted from HLA-identical siblings using conventional busulphan/cyclophosphamide conditioning (O'Reilly *et al.*, 1994). There has also been a report of successful transplantation using cord blood cells from a sibling after conditioning therapy with thiotepa and cyclophosphamide (Kernan *et al.*, 1994).

Haploidentical BMT has yielded very poor results even with high dose chemotherapy/TBI conditioning. A particular problem is a very high incidence of posttransplant, EBV-associated, lymphoproliferative disease. Failures in early T-cell depleted matched unrelated donors transplants resulted from inadequate HSC engraftment following busulphan/cyclophosphamide conditioning. The replacement of this with typical antileukemic regimes (cytosine arabinoside or cyclophosphamide plus TBI) has greatly improved results. Up to 75% of patients show full hematopoietic and immunologic reconstitution. However, such transplants are presently limited to patients who have life-threatening thrombocytopenia and/or immunodeficiency.

5.2. Disorders of Fixed-Tissue Cells of Monocyte/Macrophage Origin

5.2.1. Gaucher's Disease

This autosomal recessively inherited lipid storage disorder results from defective activity of glucocerebrosidase (GC). This enzyme is maximally active in cells of the monocyte/macrophage line where it degrades substrates derived from the breakdown of hematopoietic cell membranes. Accordingly, the monocyte/macrophage cells become laden with glycolipid giving them the characteristic appearance of Gaucher cells. They accumulate preferentially in spleen, liver, and bone marrow, causing combinations of hepatosplenomegaly (which may lead to hypersplenism), bone destruction, anemia, thrombocytopenia, and leucopenia.

The major phenotype of the disease (type I, nonneuronopathic) is most common in Ashkenazi Jews and typically presents in late childhood or early adulthood.

Hypersplenism and degenerative bone disease dominate the picture. Types II and III are neuronopathic forms, respectively presenting as a rare acute disease soon after birth, which causes death by the age of two years, and as a subacute disease causing hepatosplenomegaly, slower neurologic deterioration, and death in later childhood. The latter form is commonly caused by a specific GC mutation (L44P) prevalent in the Norbotten area of northern Sweden that gives rise to the alternative name of Norbottnian Gaucher's disease.

The treatment of symptomatic type I disease has been revolutionized by the development of mannose-terminated placental-derived, and recently recombinant, GC which acts as a substrate for the mannose-6-phosphate receptor on macrophages (Barton *et al.*, 1991). This treatment can trigger an antibody response, but this does not compromise therapy. Major disadvantages of the therapy are its high cost and the need for regularly repeated, lifelong, intravenous injections. Enzyme therapy has no impact in type II disease because children are already severely neurologically handicapped at birth, but it ameliorates intellectual deterioration and the other features of type III disease (Bembi *et al.*, 1994; Erikson *et al.*, 1995).

Before enzyme therapy developed, 10 children were transplanted for severe degrees of type I Gaucher's disease at the Westminster Hospital, six from siblings, one from a compatible uncle, and three from unrelated donors (Jones *et al.*, 1989). Two of the first three died because of engraftment problems from hypersplenism. Elective splenectomy was performed just before BMT in the remainder. Only one of the other seven patients went on to reject the graft and was then regrafted successfully from a second unrelated donor. All successful transplants utilized busulphan/cyclophosphamide chemotherapy. Patients felt dramatically better within six weeks, largely cleared bony deposits within six months, and showed marked improvement in growth and activity. Deranged liver function normalized, and hepatomegaly reduced slowly but progressively. One patient cleared pulmonary infiltrates.

An additional six patients have been transplanted in Stockholm, four from matched siblings, one from an HLA-B antigen-mismatched father and one from a matched UD (Ringden *et al.*, 1995). Despite total or partial splenectomy before BMT and conditioning with either cyclophosphamide/TBI or busulphan/cyclophosphamide, one patient rejected the graft and two became 30% and 80% donor chimeras, respectively. Three patients developed worsening or new spinal deformity (kyphosis) despite full engraftment. Hepatomegaly was slow to resolve, took two and three years in two patients, and the liver was palpable up to five and seven years in two others. Gaucher cells were present in bone marrow trephines until 2–3 years post-BMT.

Four of the patients in this group were assessed as having type III disease. Of the three with 80–100% donor engraftment, psychological testing was done to classify them as "above normal", "slightly below normal," and "below normal" for age. The first has completed school with an IQ of 116 at the age of 21 years. These results suggest that successful BMT slows the progress of type III disease, as with enzyme therapy.

Therefore the major indications for BMT in Gaucher's disease are suboptimal response to enzyme therapy, unavailability/inability to afford enzyme therapy and, possibly, development of very severe disease type I disease at a young age (especially with pulmonary, bony, or hepatic complications). Because BMT has not yet been attempted in patients stabilized on enzyme therapy, it remains to be seen whether pre-BMT splenectomy would still be necessary. It also could not be guaranteed that antibody formation which may have occurred with enzyme therapy will not interfere with the efficacy of BMT.

5.2.2. Osteopetrosis

Osteopetrosis (OP) occurs in two main forms: (a) a mild disease of autosomal dominant inheritance which causes increased susceptibility to fractures but no other significant problems; and (b) an infantile malignant form inherited as an autosomal recessive trait which usually results in death within the first decade. Trials of BMT have been restricted to the latter.

Although the mechanism and responsible genes are unknown, infantile malignant OP is most commonly thought to represent a defect of osteoclast function (Coccia, 1984). This causes defective bone resorption resulting in progressive obliteration of bone marrow cavities, extramedullary hematopoiesis, hepatosplenomegaly, and hypersplenism with leucoerythroblastic anemia and thrombocytopenia. Encroachment of bone on cranial foramina results in progressive blindness, deafness, oculomotor and facial nerve palsies, and hydrocephalus. Death usually occurs from infection (to which these children seem more susceptible), bleeding, or severe anemia.

A variety of osteopetrotic mutations have been described in rats, mice, and rabbits. In mice it was first shown that the disease is curable by parabiosis or stem cell transplantation from normal littermates (Walker, 1975). This proved that osteoclasts derive from bone marrow precursors, in contrast to osteoblasts which arise from bone. Then bone marrow infusions were used to treat human disease, although durable engraftment was not sustained in either of the first two children transplanted. Despite this one of these patients, transplanted at five months of age, remains alive and well 16 years later without symptoms of OP except short stature and dense sclerosis of bones.

Successful engraftment typically results in correcting anemia, thrombocytopenia, and bone density within 3–6 months in infants and usually prevents later development of blindness (Gerritsen *et al.*, 1994). However, preexisting visual deficits are rarely corrected. Older children can develop delayed refractory hypercalcemia due to the large mass of calcium to be mobilized (O'Reilly *et al.*, 1984). Cure rates depend on the donor. Approximately two-thirds of children with matched siblings are cured by BMT, compared with one-quarter when alternative donors are employed (Gerritsen *et al.*, 1994). Risks of rejection are considerably higher with the latter, presumably from a combination of lack of bone marrow space for donor cells to populate and hypersplenism, possibly compounded by T-cell depletion.

5.3. Metabolic Disorders

5.3.1. Adrenoleukodystrophy (ALD)

This is an X-linked disorder resulting from a defect in the peroxisomal enzyme lignoceryl-CoA ligase (very long chain fatty acyl-CoA synthetase) which causes accumulation of the very long chain fatty acids (VLCFA), lignoceric acid (C24:0) and hexacosanoic acid (C26:0). The accumulation of VLCFA cause destruction of the adrenal gland and induces a secondary inflammatory reaction in the CNS with destruction of myelin (Powers *et al.*, 1992).

Affected males may progress normally and develop adrenal insufficiency, spastic paraparesis, or psychiatric problems only in their 20s to 40s. This form of the disease is termed adrenomyeloneuropathy (AMN) and has not been treated with BMT. However, 25–50% of affected males develop normally until 4–7 years of age when they present with neuropsychological impairment, usually manifesting as failure in school. Typically, within months these boys go on to develop neurological problems, such as squint, visual loss, hearing impairment, motor problems, or dementia. This heralds a devastating neurodegenerative process which typically renders the patient wheelchair bound and unable to communicate within 12 months. This subtype of ALD is termed childhood onset cerebral adrenoleukodystrophy (COCALD). No specific therapy exists for established disease. Trials of dietary therapy with a low fat diet and "Lorenzo's oil" are ongoing in asymptomatic boys with the hope of delaying or preventing the onset of serious disease (Moser, 1993).

As yet only one patient has shown marked CNS improvement after BMT for COCALD, and increased IQ from a –2 standard deviation (SD) score to +2 SD over a period of four years following transplant (Aubourg *et al.*, 1990). However the rate of deterioration detectable by MRI scan is markedly slowed in most patients, although many have not yet reached four years post-BMT. Krivit estimates that 25 children are alive after BMT who would otherwise have died as a consequence of COCALD. This includes five sets of brothers where the transplanted children are all alive and well 2–5 years beyond the age at which their siblings died (Krivit *et al.*, 1995b). A secondary benefit of BMT is that full donor engraftment usually lowers plasma VLCFA levels greatly, freeing patients from dietary strictures. Important requirements in successful BMT are normalization of VLCFA by dietary manipulation before BMT and avoidance of lipid in intravenous feeding during the transplant period. Unfortunately, if GVHD occurs, this may accelerate CNS deterioration, and therefore, optimal GVHD prophylaxis is essential.

The decision to transplant is complicated by the existence of both forms of the disease (COCALD and AMN) in sets of siblings (Moser *et al.*, 1992) and by the aforementioned trials of dietary therapy. It is presently considered acceptable to perform BMT only when boys show early signs of neuropsychological impairment by sophisticated testing or development of MRI changes (Shapiro *et al.*, 1995). Such tests should ideally be performed at no greater than six month intervals because of the small window of opportunity before serious clinical deterioration.

5.3.2. Fucosidosis

Encouraging results of BMT in a dog model of fucosidosis (Taylor *et al.*, 1986) have been followed up by just one transplant procedure to date (Vellodi *et al.*, 1995). The condition was diagnosed early because of disease in a brother, and UD-BMT was performed at eight months of age when MRI changes were the only sign of disease. When last reported, this patient was exhibiting only mild developmental delay at 18 months of age, in marked contrast to disease progression in his brother.

5.3.3. Globoid Cell Leukodystrophy

This autosomal recessive disorder is caused by deficiency of galactocerebrosidase. Accumulation of psychosine results in forming characteristic giant, multinucleate macrophages (globoid cells) in cerebral white matter, destruction of oligodendroglia, and demyelination. Progressive leukodystrophy eventually leads to decerebrate posturing and death (Kolodny *et al.*, 1991).

Subtypes of the disease are defined by their age at presentation. The classical form, infantile or Krabbe's disease, usually presents between three and six months of age, shows rapid CNS deterioration, and death within a year of presentation. Two patients transplanted for infantile disease both died of BMT complications 24 and 36 months post-BMT without evidence of CNS amelioration. Juvenile and adolescent forms, also recognized, have slower rates of deterioration. A patient with juvenile presentation underwent BMT at 12 years of age. When assessed two years later, her white cell galactocerebrosidase levels remained normal, and she had shown improvement in school performance and in many aspects of neuropsychological testing (Krivil *et al.*, 1995b).

5.3.4. Metachromatic Leukodystrophy (MLD)

This disease is inherited in an autosomal recessive manner and results from a deficiency of arylsulphatase A (ASA). Accumulation of galactosyl sulphatide in the nervous system causes progressive demyelination leading to decreased motor nerve conduction velocities and sensory nerve action potentials. Late infantile, early and late juvenile, and adult forms are recognized. Prognosis is worse for the earlier forms of presentation.

Late infantile disease progresses rapidly to decerebration and death. Seven of eight patients who received BMT for this form of disease have shown disease progression despite normalization of ASA levels (Dhuna *et al.*, 1992; Krivit *et al.*, 1995a). However, in each case the disease pattern and life span were improved over that expected for the disease or shown by affected members of their own family. The only patient to show distinct benefit exhibited a decrease in demyelination (judged from T2-weighted signals on brain MRI) and gains in intelligence when assessed eight years after BMT was performed at the age of four years (Dhuna *et al.*, 1992). However, this child is unable to walk without assistance and has continuous tremor, nystagmus, and truncal ataxia.

The only potential role for BMT in treating of late infantile disease is very early in life at a presymptomatic stage, when diagnosis of the affected patient is made because of a previous index case in the family (Pridjian *et al.*, 1994; Stillman *et al.*, 1994). However, even here compelling evidence is lacking that neurodegeneration can be completely arrested. When diagnosing affected but presymptomatic individuals, it is also essential to perform sulfatide loading studies to exclude pseudodeficiency of ASA, a condition which results in low enzyme levels but does not cause disease.

Results appear more promising in the more slowly progressive, later onset forms of the disease. A patient with juvenile disease has been carefully followed after BMT at 13 years of age (Krivit *et al.*, 1995a). She presented with major behavioral problems, spatial disorientation and failure in school. Three years later she showed no evidence of disease progression and had improved learning and social skills. This outcome was promising compared to a sister who presented at a similar age and whose disease progressed steadily to death at 21 years of age and a brother who was bedridden by 12 years. Another patient with late juvenile disease was transplanted at the age of 28 years and showed stable neurological function 4 years later (Navarro *et al.*, 1996). Three patients with adult forms of the disease have been transplanted. One has improved sufficiently to be discharged from domiciliary care, and the others are stable (Krivit *et al.*, 1995a).

5.3.5. Mucopolysaccharidosis Type I (MPS I): Hurler's Disease

Deficiency of α-L-iduronidase is inherited in an autosomal recessive fashion and gives a wide range of clinical presentation from very mild disease (Scheie) through intermediate (Hurler–Scheie) to severe disease (Hurler) (Roubicek *et al.*, 1985). The latter is a devastating disease which usually presents before 18 months of age and causes death at a median age of five years. Major presenting features are coarse facies, hepatosplenomegaly (due to engorgement with glycosaminoglycan-loaded macrophages), developmental delay, corneal clouding, and multiple bony abnormalities (termed dysostosis multiplex). The skull is large, and patients develop progressive hydrocephalus. Upper respiratory tract problems and ear infections lead to noisy breathing, profuse nasal discharge, and deafness. Patients achieve a maximum functional developmental age of 2–4 years and deteriorate progressively thereafter. Death usually results from obstructive airway disease, respiratory infection, or cardiac complications.

After BMT, leucocyte α-L-iduronidase rapidly stabilizes at donor levels, followed by increased urinary clearance of glycosaminoglycans (GAG) (Hobbs *et al.*, 1981; Peters *et al.*, 1996; Vellodi *et al.*, 1997; Whitley *et al.*, 1986, 1993). Hepatosplenomegaly and obstructive upper airway disease improves (Malone *et al.*, 1988), and progression of liver or cardiac disease is arrested (reversal of severe cardiomyopathy has been seen in one patient). Communicating hydrocephalus, if present, stabilizes or improves. There is marked improvement in facial features, one of the most distressing aspects of the disease. Corneal clouding improves within months but never completely clears (Huang *et al.*, 1996). Overall survival is greatly prolonged by successful BMT, and it now seems likely that many patients will reach their third decade.

Because of the heterogeneity of CNS function at the time of transplant, variable degrees of long-term engraftment, and full or carrier donor enzyme levels, it is difficult to make categorical statements about controlling CNS disease. Patients transplanted beyond 2.5 years of age derive minimal benefit in CNS function, whereas those transplanted before 18 months of age often stabilize or even improve, usually after a delay of 1–2 years following BMT. Seven of 12 patients successfully transplanted at the Westminster Hospital have a sustained IQ of above 70, although they require special educational input to overcome specific physical and sensory problems (Downie *et al.*, 1995; Vellodi *et al.*, 1997). Long-term prognostication is limited by follow-up in a disease first successfully transplanted in 1980.

Primary among the disappointment of BMT has been the poor response of bony disease and progression of spinal and joint problems. Although patients often retain normal mobility until 7–9 years of age, then they start to deteriorate and may eventually need a variety of orthopedic operations including spinal or cervical fusions, femoral osteotomy, and bilateral carpal tunnel releases. It has been postulated that beyond nine years of age the cartilage growth plates exceed 10 cells in thickness, a depth too great for donated iduronidase to penetrate. Skeletal disease is best controlled in those children transplanted before one year of age. Middle ear disease also remains a feature, although the progressive nerve deafness reported in untreated disease does not occur.

More than 80 patients have now been transplanted for Hurler's disease, primarily in London, Minnesota, and Seattle. It is clear from these procedures that BMT should be performed as early as possible and probably not beyond 20 months of age. There is contention as to whether carriers make satisfactory donors (Downie *et al.*, 1995; Vellodi *et al.*, 1997). However, if unrelated donor transplantation continues to improve (allowing full and durable engraftment without serious GVHD), then normal unrelated donors may be preferable to matched carrier siblings in this disease, where responses to BMT are partial at best.

5.3.6. Mucopolysaccharidosis Type VI (MPS VI): Maroteaux–Lamy Syndrome

This disease, caused by a deficiency of arylsulphatase B, is inherited as an autosomal recessive trait. Skeletal changes occur, similar to those seen in Hurler's disease, together with hepatosplenomegaly and corneal clouding, but most patients have normal intelligence. Subsequently pulmonary and cardiac insufficiency and hydrocephalus develop and most patients die in the second to third decade.

One patient, followed up for more than 10 years following BMT, has normal arylsulphatase B levels (Krivit *et al.*, 1984; McGovern *et al.*, 1986). Heart failure, pulmonary hypertension, hepatosplenomegaly, and severe sleep apnea all resolved after BMT, and the patient's facial appearance improved. However, although joint stiffness improved and walking became easier, the skeletal disease has not changed significantly. These findings are mirrored by those in five other patients transplanted for this disease who have been followed up for shorter periods (Jurges *et al.*, 1991;

Krivit *et al.*, 1995b). Therefore, cardiac problems constitute the major indication for BMT in this disease.

5.3.7. Other Forms of Mucopolysaccharidosis

Small numbers of transplants have been performed in the other MPS disorders but have generally yielded disappointing results.

5.3.7a. Hunter's Disease (MPS II) is an X-linked disorder resulting in deficiency of iduronate sulphatase. Neurological disease varies widely in severity. It may be so mild as to allow completion of education and earning a living or so severe as to reduce the IQ to 30 by four years of age. The facial appearance is generally less severe than in Hurler's disease, resulting in relatively later diagnosis, and this may have adversely affected the results of BMT (McKinnis *et al.*, 1996). There is only one report showing stabilized neuropsychological status, and this patient had mild disease and had been followed only for three years post-BMT at the time (Bergstrom *et al.*, 1994). Therefore, BMT should be restricted to patients less than three years old with an IQ of >75 who have a matched sibling. There will be very few patients who meet such criteria.

5.3.7b. Sanfilippo Diseases (MPS III) comprise four distinct enzymatic disorders, all of which follow an autosomal recessive mode of inheritance. Of 28 patients reported to have received BMT for this condition (Krivit *et al.*, 1995b), none of those successfully engrafted has shown stabilized intelligence, although the course of the disease may have been slowed (Vellodi *et al.*, 1992). It seems unlikely that BMT will have a role in managing this condition unless neonatal screening techniques become possible so that transplantation is performed very early in life.

5.3.7c. Morquio's Disease (MPS IV) has clinical features largely confined to the skeleton, notably hypoplasia of the odontoid peg which predisposes patients to atlantoaxial dislocation and cervical myelopathy. As in the other forms of MPS disorder, BMT has little impact on this bone disease (Clink and Ozand, 1991; Krivit *et al.*, 1995b).

5.3.8. Other Metabolic Diseases

Small numbers of BMT procedures have been performed on patients who have a variety of other diseases. There has been no evidence of significant sustained benefit in late infantile Batten's disease (one case), juvenile Batten's disease (one case), Farber disease (one engrafted patient), GM-1 gangliosidosis (one case), type II glycogen storage disease (two cases), I-cell disease (one case), Lesch-Nyhan syndrome (one case), mannosidosis (one case), Niemann–Pick disease type 1A (two cases), type B (one case), or Wolman disease (two cases) (Krivit *et al.*, 1995b). However, most of these patients were transplanted when markedly symptomatic. The background and details of each of these cases would require careful review were a patient to be identified as a neonate because of a previous index case in the family and were an HLA-matched unaffected sibling available as a donor.

6. FUTURE DIRECTIONS

Since BMT was first used to treat a genetic disease in 1968, there have been great changes in our understanding of the pathogenesis and genetic basis of inherited disease, in delineating which diseases respond, and in many technical aspects of the transplantation process. Major challenges for the foreseeable future include, first, development of a conditioning drug or regimen which produces stem cell ablation equivalent to that of busulphan but without a effect on fertility, and secondly, achieving full donor engraftment consistently without significant graft versus host disease. Three approaches are envisaged which may assist the second of these aims: better graft manipulation, *in utero* transplantation, and cord blood transplantation.

6.1. Graft Manipulation

Animal experiments suggest that the higher doses of stem cells may shorten the time to engraftment and reduce the incidence and severity of GVHD (Rao *et al.*, 1997), and the results of bone marrow transplants for acute leukemia and Hurler's disease suggest that a similar mechanism operates in humans (Peters *et al.*, 1996; Sierra *et al.*, 1997). When BMT relied on marrow harvest alone, clinicians could not vary stem cell dose greatly except in small recipients. However, now that it is possible to mobilize large number of early progenitor cells and stem cells into the peripheral blood by using agents such as granulocyte colony-stimulating factor (G-CSF), this problem has been overcome. Over the next few years data from sibling transplants using high doses of mobilized peripheral blood stem cells (PBSC) should confirm whether the benefits seen in animals also extend to humans.

Another area of intense study is T-cell manipulation. In rodents it has been shown that T-cell aliquots administered at approximately 21 days after BMT have a graft versus leukemia effect (and therefore immune competence) but lower rates of GVHD than produced by the same dose of cells given with the original T-cell depleted bone marrow (Johnson and Truitt, 1995). If this can be extrapolated to humans, it suggests that titrated use of T-cell addbacks (based on chimeric assessment) after T-cell depleted BMT may allow equivalent or better engraftment results with less risk of severe GVHD. Furthermore, the donor leukocyte infusions now used for controlling early relapse of chronic myeloid leukemia after BMT provide an excellent model for studying the impact of such T-cell "addbacks" on marrow chimerism (Bacigalupo *et al.*, 1997; Collins *et al.*, 1997; Johnson *et al.*, 1996).

6.2. *In Utero* Transplantation

This approach is based on the concept that the fetus is relatively immunologically incompetent and therefore should be unable to reject infused donor hematopoietic cells. The transplant procedure would also be performed before significant tissue damage, which is particularly important in neurodegenerative disorders. However, although several successful transplants have been performed in SCID where the fetus clearly is immunoincompetent, all others have failed to produce significant long-term engraftment (Haskins, 1996; Touraine, 1996; Wengler *et al.*, 1996) almost certainly because fetal immunity begins to mature at 12–14 weeks of gestation, allowing rejection of any graft given at or after that time. The administration of donor cells before this is technically difficult and carries high rates of fetal loss. Furthermore many parents who know that they carry an affected fetus at that time would opt for abortion.

Therefore, this form of transplantation is greatly hampered by the inability to give conditioning therapy or otherwise manipulate fetal tolerance to the donated cells. It seems likely to remain limited to small numbers of transplants for immune deficiency diseases of sufficient severity to threaten early postnatal life.

6.3. Cord Blood Transplantation

Use of this technique has rapidly expanded since it was first shown in 1988 that a single infusion of human umbilical cord blood contains sufficient progenitors to successfully engraft a five-year-old boy who had Fanconi's anemia (Gluckman *et al.*, 1989). In 1995 the first large report emerged on 44 patients who had received allogeneic sibling UCB transplants, and in 1996 a series of 18 UD-UCB transplants was reported (including technically successful procedures in children with globoid cell leukodystrophy, Diamond–Blackfan anemia, and osteopetrosis) (Wagner *et al.*, 1995, 1996).

Potential disadvantages of cord blood transplantation include low cell doses, the inability to reaccess the donor for further stem cells or donor leukocytes, and a variety of ethical concerns such as (1) the ownership of the UCB, (2) whether clamping the cord early to obtain a better yield can ever compromise the health of the donor baby, (3) what quarantine period should be used before the cord can be used (to allow full testing of the cord blood for infectious agents or common genetic diseases and to make sure that the donors do not themselves develop severe genetic disease) and (4) what parents should be told about the results of such tests (Auerbach, 1994; Burgio and Locatelli, 1997; Gluckman *et al.*, 1993; Sugarman *et al.*, 1995).

Disadvantages are greatly outweighed by the numerous advantages. The cells would be available for almost immediate use, there is no risk to the donor from general anesthesia or blood replacement, and no possibility of the donor becoming too unwell or refusing to donate once conditioning therapy has commenced. Stem cell numbers (which could prove limiting for use in large patients) are usually adequate for small children with genetic diseases. A cord blood bank should exactly reflect the ethnic mix of the community whereas UD registries have a heavy bias toward white Caucasian donors. Furthermore, the maintenance charges of a UCB bank seem likely to prove competitive to that of running an adult UD registry.

However, perhaps the major advantages of UCB transplants apparent now are good engraftment results accompanied by relatively low rates of GVHD from mismatched donors. This is exemplified in the series of UD-UCB referred to previously (Wagner *et al.*, 1996) where all donations were T-replete and 11 of the 18 grafts were mismatched by one to three HLA antigens. All patients, including one of 78.8 kg, engrafted, and no patient developed late graft failure with a median follow-up of 6 months. The rate of serious GVHD (grades III–IV) was only 11%.

It is too early to know all the potential disadvantages of UCB transplants. The relatively low doses of early progenitor cells given (judged according to conventional assays) could result in early graft exhaustion, and there is already data to suggest that immune reconstitution is very poor in mismatched transplants. However, it appears that cord blood offers one of the most exciting developments in genetic disease management since the advent of BMT.

7. REFERENCES

Apperley, J. F., 1994, Umbilical cord blood progenitor cell transplantation, The International Conference Workshop on Cord Blood Transplantation, Indianapolis, November 1993, *Bone Marrow Transplant.* **14:**187–196.

Aubourg, P., Blanche, S., Jambaque, I., Rocchiccioli, F., Kalifa, G., Naud-Saudreau, C., Rolland, M. O., Debre, M., Chaussain, J. L., and Griscelli, C., 1990, Reversal of early neurologic and neuroradiologic manifestations of X-linked adrenoleukodystrophy by bone marrow transplantation, *N. Engl. J. Med.* **322:**1860–1866.

Auerbach, A. D., 1993, Fanconi anemia diagnosis and the diepoxybutane (DEB) test, *Exp. Hematol.* **21:**731–733.

Auerbach, A. D., 1994, Umbilical cord blood transplants for genetic disease: Diagnostic and ethical issues in fetal studies, *Blood Cells* **20:**303–309.

Auerbach, A. D., and Allen, R. G., 1991, Leukemia and preleukemia in Fanconi anemia patients. A review of the literature and report of the International Fanconi Anemia Registry, *Cancer Genet. Cytogenet.* **51:**1–12.

Aversa, F., Tabilio, A., Terenzi, A., Velardi, A., Falzetti, F., Giannoni, C., Iacucci, R., Zei, T., Martelli, M. P., and Gambelunghe, C., 1994, Successful engraftment of T-cell-depleted haploidentical "three-loci" incompatible transplants in leukemia patients by addition of recombinant human granulocyte colony-stimulating factor-mobilized peripheral blood progenitor cells to bone marrow inoculum, *Blood* **84:**3948–3955.

Bach, F. H., Albertini, R. J., Joo, P., Anderson, J. L., and Bortin, M. M., 1968, Bone-marrow transplantation in a patient with the Wiskott–Aldrich syndrome, *Lancet* **2:**1364–1366.

Bacigalupo, A., Soracco, M., Vassallo, F., Abate, M., Van, L. M., Gualandi, F., Lamparelli, T., Occhini, D., Mordini, N., Bregante, S., Figari, O., Benvenuto, F., Sessarego, M., Fugazza, G., Carlier, P., and Valbonesi, M., 1997, Donor lymphocyte infusions (DLI) in patients with chronic myeloid leukemia following allogeneic bone marrow transplantation, *Bone Marrow Transplant.* **19:**927–932.

Barranger, J. A., 1984, Marrow transplantation in genetic disease, *N. Engl. J. Med.* **311:**1629–1631.

Barrios, N., Kirkpatrick, D., Regueira, O., Wuttke, B., McNeil, J., and Humbert, J., 1991, Bone marrow transplant in Shwachman–Diamond syndrome, *Br. J. Haematol.* **79:**337–338.

Barton, N. W., Brady, R. O., Dambrosia, J. M., Di, B. A., Doppelt, S. H., Hill, S. C., Mankin, H. J., Murray, G. J., Parker, R. I., and Argoff, C. E., 1991, Replacement therapy for inherited enzyme deficiency—macrophage-targeted glucocerebrosidase for Gaucher's disease, *N. Engl. J. Med.* **324:**1464–1470.

Bembi, B., Zanatta, M., Carrozzi, M., Baralle, F., Gornati, R., Berra, B., and Agosti, E., 1994, Enzyme replacement treatment in type 1 and type 3 Gaucher's disease, *Lancet* **344:**1679–1682.

Bergstrom, S. K., Quinn, J. J., Greenstein, R., and Ascensao, J., 1994, Long-term follow-up of a patient transplanted for Hunter's disease type IIB: A case report and literature review, *Bone Marrow Transplant.* **14:**653–658.

Blazar, B. R., Orr, H. T., Arthur, D. C., Kersey, J. H., and Filipovich, A. H., 1985, Restriction fragment length polymorphisms as markers of engraftment in allogeneic marrow transplantation, *Blood* **66:**1436–1444.

Bonilla, M. A., Gillio, A. P., Ruggeiro, M., Kernan, N. A., Brochstein, J. A., Abboud, M., Fumagalli, L., Vincent, M., Gabrilove, J. L., and Welte, K., 1989, Effects of recombinant human granulocyte colony-stimulating factor on neutropenia in patients with congenital agranulocytosis, *N. Engl. J. Med.* **320:**1574–1580.

Bordigoni, P., 1995, Bone marrow transplantation for inherited bone marrow failure syndromes, *Int. J. Pediatr. Hematol. Oncol.* **2:**441–452.

Breider, M. A., Shull, R. M., and Constantopoulos, G. C., 1989, Long-term effects of bone marrow transplantation in dogs with mucopolysaccharidosis I, *Am. J. Pathol.* **134:**692.

Brichard, B., Vermylen, C., Ninane, J., and Cornu, G., 1996, Persistence of fetal hemoglobin production after successful transplantation of cord blood stem cells in a patient with sickle cell anemia, *J. Pediatr.* **128:**241–243.

Burgio, G. R., and Locatelli, F., 1997, Transplant of bone marrow and cord blood hematopoietic stem cells in pediatric practice, revisited according to the fundamental principles of bioethics, *Bone Marrow Transplant.* **19:**1163–1168.

Camitta, B. M., Quesenberry, P. J., Parkman, R., Boxer, L. A., Stossel, T. P., Cassady, J. R., Rappeport, J. M., and Nathan, D. G., 1977, Bone marrow transplantation for an infant with neutrophil dysfunction, *Exp. Hematol.* **5:**109–116.

Clink, H., and Ozand, P., 1991, Morquio syndrome treated by displacement bone marrow transplantation, in *Correction of Genetic Diseases by Transplantation 1991* (J. R. Hobbs, and P. G. Riches, eds.), Uxbridge Press, Uxbridge, Middlesex, pp. 21–22.

Coccia, P. F., 1984, Cells that resorb bone, *N. Engl. J. Med.* **310:**456–458.

Collins, R. H. J., Shpilberg, O., Drobyski, W. R., Porter, D. L., Giralt, S., Champlin, R., Goodman, S. A., Wolff, S. N., Hu, W., Verfaillie, C., List, A., Dalton, W., Ognoskie, N., Chetrit, A., Antin, J. H., and Nemunaitis, J., 1997, Donor leukocyte infusions in 140 patients with relapsed malignancy after allogeneic bone marrow transplantation, *J. Clin. Oncol.* **15:**433–444.

Connor, J. M., Gatherer, D., Gray, F. C., Pirrit, L. A., and Affara, N. A., 1986, Assignment of the gene for dyskeratosis congenita to Xq28, *Human Genet.* **72:**348–351.

Deeg, H. J., 1994, Delayed complications after bone marrow transplantation, in *Bone Marrow Transplantation* (S. J. Forman, K. G. Blume, and E. D. Thomas, eds.), Blackwell, Boston, pp. 538–544.

DeSanctis, V., Galimberti, M., Lucarelli, G., Polchi, P., Ruggiero, L., and Vullo, C., 1991, Gonadal function after allogenic bone marrow transplantation for thalassaemia, *Arch. Dis. Child* **66:**517–520.

DeWitte, T., Schattenberg, A., Van, D. B., Galama, J., Olthuis, H., Van, D., Meer, J. W., and Kunst, V. A., 1990, Prevention of primary cytomegalovirus infection after allogeneic bone marrow transplantation by using leukocyte-poor random blood products from cytomegalovirus-unscreened blood-bank donors, *Transplantation* **50:**964–968.

Dhuna, A., Toro, C., Torres, F., Kennedy, W. R., and Krivit, W., 1992, Longitudinal neurophysiologic studies in a patient with metachromatic leukodystrophy following bone marrow transplantation, *Arch. Neurol.* **49:**1088–1092.

dosSantos, C. C., Gavish, H., and Buchwald, M., 1994, Fanconi anemia revisited: Old ideas and new advances, *Stem Cells (Dayt)* **12:**142–153.

Downie, C., Hugh-Jones, K., and Hobbs, J. R., 1995, Up to fourteen years after bone marrow trans-plantation for Hurler's syndrome, in *Correction of Genetic Diseases by Transplantation III* (C. G. Steward, and J. R. Hobbs, eds.), The COGENT Press, Ruislip, Middlesex, pp. 16–24.

Elder, G. H., 1990, The cutaneous porphyrias, *Semin. Dermatol.* **9:**63–69.

Erikson, A., Astrom, M., and Mansson, J. E., 1995, Enzyme infusion therapy of the Norrbottnian (type 3) Gaucher disease, *Neuropediatrics* **26:**203–207.

Filipovich, A. H., Shapiro, R. S., Ramsay, N. K., Kim, T., Blazar, B., Kersey, J., and McGlave, P., 1992, Unrelated donor bone marrow transplantation for correction of lethal congenital immunodeficiencies, *Blood* **80:**270–276.

Fischer, A., Trung, P. H., Descamps-Latscha, B., Lisowska-Grospierre, B., Gerota, I., Perez, N., Scheinmetzler, C., Durandy, A., Virelizier, J. L., and Griscelli, C., 1983, Bone-marrow transplantation for inborn error of phagocytic cells associated with defective adherence, chemotaxis, and oxidative response during opsonised particle phagocytosis, *Lancet* **2:**473–476.

Fischer, A., Griscelli, C., Friedrich, W., Kubanek, B., Levinsky, R., Morgan, G., Vossen, J., Wagemaker,

G., and Landais, P., 1986, Bone-marrow transplantation for immunodeficiencies and osteopetrosis: European survey, 1968–1985, *Lancet* **2:**1080–1084.

Fischer, A., Landais, P., Friedrich, W., Morgan, G., Gerritsen, B., Fasth, A., Porta, F., Griscelli, C., Goldman, S. F., and Levinsky, R., 1990, European experience of bone-marrow transplantation for severe combined immunodeficiency, *Lancet* **336:**850–854.

Flowers, M. E., Doney, K. C., Storb, R., Deeg, H. J., Sanders, J. E., Sullivan, K. M., Bryant, E., Witherspoon, R. P., Appelbaum, F. R., and Buckner, C. D., 1992, Marrow transplantation for Fanconi anemia with or without leukemic transformation: An update of the Seattle experience, *Bone Marrow Transplant.* **9:**167–173.

Fratantoni, J. C., Hall, C. W., and Neufeld, E. F., 1968, Hurler and Hunter syndromes: Mutual correction of the defect in cultured fibroblasts, *Science* **162:**570–572.

Friedrich, W., Goldmann, S. F., Ebell, W., Blutters-Sawatzki, R., Gaedicke, G., Raghavachar, A., Peter, H. H., Belohradsky, B., Kreth, W., and Kubanek, B., 1985, Severe combined immunodeficiency: Treatment by bone marrow transplantation in 15 infants using HLA-haploidentical donors, *Eur. J. Pediatr.* **144:**125–130.

Gabutti, V., and Piga, A., 1996, Results of long-term iron-chelating therapy, *Acta Haematol.* **95:**26–36.

Gatti, R. A., Meuwissen, H. J., Allen, H. D., Hong, R., and Good, R. A., 1968, Immunological reconstitution of sex-linked lymphopenic immunological deficiency, *Lancet* **2:**1366–1369.

Gelfand, E. W., and Dosch, H. M., 1983, Diagnosis and classification of severe combined immunodeficiency disease, *Birth Defects* **19:**65–72.

Gerritsen, E. J., Vossen, J. M., Fasth, A., Friedrich, W., Morgan, G., Padmos, A., Vellodi, A., Porras, O., O'Meara, A., and Porta, F., 1994, Bone marrow transplantation for autosomal recessive osteopetrosis. A report from the Working Party on Inborn Errors of the European Bone Marrow Transplantation Group, *J. Pediatr.* **125:**896–902.

Gluckman, E., Berger, R., and Dutreix, J., 1984, Bone marrow transplantation for Fanconi anemia, *Semin. Hematol.* **21:**20–26.

Gluckman, E., Broxmeyer, H. A., Auerbach, A. D., Friedman, H. S., Douglas, G. W., Devergie, A., Esperou, H., Thierry, D., Socie, G., and Lehn, P., 1989, Hematopoietic reconstitution in a patient with Fanconi's anemia by means of umbilical-cord blood from an HLA-identical sibling, *N. Engl. J. Med.* **321:**1174–1178.

Gluckman, E., Thierry, D., and Traineau, R., 1993, Blood banking for hematopoietic stem cell transplantation, *J. Hematother.* **2:**269–270.

Gluckman, E., Auerbach, A. D., Horowitz, M. M., Sobocinski, K. A., Ash, R. C., Bortin, M. M., Butturini, A., Camitta, B. M., Champlin, R. E., and Friedrich, W., 1995, Bone marrow transplantation for Fanconi anemia, *Blood* **86:**2856–2862.

Goudemand, J., Anssens, R., Delmas-Marsalet, Y., Farriaux, J. P., and Fontaine, G., 1976, Attempt to treat a case of chronic familial granulomatous disease by allogenic bone marrow transplantation, *Arch. Franc. Pediatr.* **33:**121–129.

Goulden, N. J., Steward, C. G., Cornish, J. M., Pamphilon, D. H., and Oakhill, A., 1995, Bone marrow transplantation for familial erythrophagocytic lymphohistiocytosis, in *Correction of Genetic Diseases by Transplantation III* (C. G. Steward, and J. R. Hobbs, eds.), The COGENT Press, Ruislip, Middlesex, pp. 117–125.

Greenbaum, B. H., 1991, Transfusion-associated graft-versus-host disease: Historical perspectives, incidence, and current use of irradiated blood products, *J. Clin. Oncol.* **9:**1889–1902.

Grochow, L. B., Jones, R. J., Brundrett, R. B., Braine, H. G., Chen, T. L., Saral, R., Santos, G. W., and Colvin, O. M., 1989, Pharmacokinetics of busulfan: Correlation with veno-occlusive disease in patients undergoing bone marrow transplantation, *Cancer Chemother. Pharmacol.* **25:**55–61.

Grochow, L. B., Krivit, W., Whitley, C. B., and Blazar, B., 1990, Busulfan disposition in children, *Blood* **75:**1723–1727.

Hale, G., Cobbold, S., and Waldmann, H., 1988, T cell depletion with CAMPATH-1 in allogeneic bone marrow transplantation, *Transplantation* **45:**753–759.

Hancock, J. P., Burgess, M. F., Goulden, N. J., Steward, C. G., Knechtli, C. J. C., Pamphilon, D. H., Potter, M. N., and Oakhill, A., 1997, Same day determination of chimeric status in the immediate period following allogeneic bone marrow transplantation, *Br. J. Haematol.* **99:**403–409.

Haskins, M., 1996, Bone marrow transplantation therapy for metabolic disease: Animal models as predictors of success and in utero approaches, *Bone Marrow Transplant.* **18**(Suppl 3)**:**S25–S27.

Henter, J. I., and Elinder, G., 1991, Familial hemophagocytic lymphohistiocytosis. Clinical review based on the findings in seven children, *Acta Paediatr. Scand.* **80:**269–277.

Hershfield, M. S., 1995, PEG-ADA: An alternative to haploidentical bone marrow transplantation and an adjunct to gene therapy for adenosine deaminase deficiency, *Human Mutat.* **5:**107–112.

Hershfield, M. S., Buckley, R. H., Greenberg, M. L., Melton, A. L., Schiff, R., Hatem, C., Kurtzberg, J., Markert, M. L., Kobayashi, R. H., and Kobayashi, A. L., 1987, Treatment of adenosine deaminase deficiency with polyethylene glycol-modified adenosine deaminase, *N. Engl. J. Med.* **316:**589–596.

Hershfield, M. S., and Mitchell, B. S., 1995, Immunodeficiency diseases caused by adenosine deaminase deficiency and purine nucleoside phosphorylase deficiency, in *The Metabolic and Genetic Bases of Inherited Disease*, 7th ed. (C. R. Scriver, A. L. Beaudet, W. S. Sly, and D. Valle, eds.), McGraw-Hill, New York, pp. 1725–1768.

Hershfield, M. S., Arredondo-Vega, F. X., and Santisteban, I., 1997, Clinical expression, genetics and therapy of adenosine deaminase (ADA) deficiency, *J. Inherit. Metab. Dis.* **20:**179–185.

Hershko, C., and Weatherall, D. J., 1988, Iron-chelating therapy, *Crit. Rev. Clin. Lab. Sci.* **26:**303–345.

Hickey, W. F., and Kimura, H., 1988, Perivascular microglial cells of the CNS are bone marrow-derived and present antigen *in vivo*, *Science* **239:**290–292.

Hobbs, J. R., 1981, Bone marrow transplantation for inborn errors, *Lancet* **2:**735–739.

Hobbs, J. R., 1988, Displacement bone marrow transplantation and immunoprophylaxis for genetic diseases, *Adv. Intern. Med.* **33:**81–118.

Hobbs, J. R., Hugh-Jones, K., Barrett, A. J., Byrom, N., Chambers, D., Henry, K., James, D. C., Lucas, C. F., Rogers, T. R., Benson, P. F., Tansley, L. R., Patrick, A. D., Mossman, J., and Young, E. P., 1981, Reversal of clinical features of Hurler's disease and biochemical improvement after treatment by bone-marrow transplantation, *Lancet* **2:**709–712.

Hoogerbrugge, P. M., Poorthuis, B. J., Wagemaker, G., and van Bekkum, D. W., 1987, Bone marrow correction of lysosomal enzyme deficiency in various organs of beta-glucuronidase deficient mice by allogeneic bone marrow transplantation, *Transplantation* **43:**609–614.

Hoogerbrugge, P. M., Suzuki, K., Poorthuis, B. J., Kobayashi, T., Wagemaker, G., and Van, B. D., 1988, Donor-derived cells in the central nervous system of twitcher mice after bone marrow transplantation, *Science* **239:**1035–1038.

Hows, J. M., Chapple, M., Marsh, J. C., Durrant, S., Yin, J. L., Swirsky, D., and Gordon-Smith, E. C., 1989, Bone marrow transplantation for Fanconi's anaemia: The Hammersmith experience 1977–89, *Bone Marrow Transplant.* **4:**629–634.

Huang, Y., Bron, A. J., Meek, K. M., Vellodi, A., and McDonald, B., 1996, Ultrastructural study of the cornea in a bone marrow-transplanted Hurler syndrome patient, *Exp. Eye Res.* **62:**377–387.

Jabado, N., De Graeff-Meeders, E. R., Cavazzana-Calvo, M., Haddad, E., Le Deist, F., Benkerrou, M., Dufourcq, R., Caillat, S., Blanche, S., and Fischer, A., 1997, Treatment of familial hemophagocytic lymphohistiocytosis with bone marrow transplantation from HLA genetically nonidentical donors, *Blood* **90:**4743–4748.

Janov, A. J., Leong, T., Nathan, D. G., and Guinan, E. C., 1996, Diamond–Blackfan anemia. Natural history and sequelae of treatment, *Medicine* **75:**77–78.

Johnson, B. D. and Truitt, R. L., 1995, Delayed infusion of immunocompetent donor cells after bone marrow transplantation breaks graft-host tolerance allows for persistent antileukemic reactivity without severe graft-versus-host disease, *Blood* **85:**3302–3312.

Johnson, B. D., Hanke, C. A., and Truitt, R. L., 1996, The graft-versus-leukemia effect of post-transplant donor leukocyte infusion, *Leuk. Lymphoma* **23:**1–9.

Jones, S., El-Tumi, M., Abdul-Ahad, A., Hancock, M., Lindsay, I., and Hobbs, J. R., 1989, DBMT for Gaucher's disease, in *Correction of Certain Genetic Diseases by Transplantation 1989* (J. R. Hobbs, eds.), The COGENT Fund, London, pp. 23–29.

Jurges, E., El-Tumi, M., Downie, C., Hancock, M., and Hobbs, J. R., 1991, Metachromatic leukodystrophy 3 years after bone marrow transplantation, in *Correction of Genetic Diseases by*

Transplantation 1991 (J. R. Hobbs, and P. G. Riches, eds.), Uxbridge Press, Uxbridge, Middlesex, pp. 16–20.

Kamani, N., August, C. S., Douglas, S. D., Burkey, E., Etzioni, A., and Lischner, H. W., 1984, Bone marrow transplantation in chronic granulomatous disease, *J. Pediatr.* **105:**42–46.

Katsanis, E., Shapiro, R. S., Robison, L. L., Haake, R. J., Kim, T., Pescovitz, O. H., and Ramsay, N. K., 1990, Thyroid dysfunction following bone marrow transplantation: Long-term follow-up of 80 pediatric patients, *Bone Marrow Transplant.* **5:**335–340.

Kauffman, L., Evans, D. I., Stevens, R. F., and Weinkove, C., 1991, Bone-marrow transplantation for congenital erythropoietic porphyria, *Lancet* **337:**1510–1511.

Kernan, N. A., Schroeder, M. L., Ciavarella, D., Preti, R. A., Rubinstein, P., and O'Reilly, R. J., 1994, Umbilical cord blood infusion in a patient for correction of Wiskott–Aldrich syndrome, *Blood Cells* **20:**245–248.

Kersey, J. H., Meuwissen, H. J., and Good, R. A., 1971, Graft versus host reactions following transplantation of allogeneic hematopoietic cells, *Human Pathol.* **2:**389–402.

Kohli-Kumar, M., Shahidi, N. T., Broxmeyer, H. E., Masterson, M., Delaat, C., Sambrano, J., Morris, C., Auerbach, A. D., and Harris, R. E., 1993, Haemopoietic stem/progenitor cell transplant in Fanconi anaemia using HLA-matched sibling umbilical cord blood cells, *Br. J. Haematol.* **85:**419–422.

Kolodny, E. H., Raghavan, S., and Krivit, W., 1991, Late-onset Krabbe disease (globoid cell leukodystrophy): Clinical and biochemical features of 15 cases, *Dev. Neurosci.* **13:**232–239.

Krall, W. J., Challita, P. M., Perlmutter, L. S., Skelton, D. C., and Kohn, D. B., 1994, Cells expressing human glucocerebrosidase from a retroviral vector repopulate macrophages and central nervous system microglia after murine bone marrow transplantation, *Blood* **83:**2737–2748.

Krivit, W., Pierpont, M. E., Ayaz, K., Tsai, M., Ramsay, N. K., Kersey, J. H., Weisdorf, S., Sibley, R., Snover, D., and McGovern, M. M., 1984, Bone-marrow transplantation in the Maroteaux–Lamy syndrome (mucopolysaccharidosis type VI). Biochemical and clinical status 24 months after transplantation, *N. Engl. J. Med.* **311:**1606–1611.

Krivit, W., Lockman, L., and Shapiro, E., 1995a, Metachromatic leukodystrophy, in *Correction of Genetic Diseases by Transplantation III* (C. G. Steward, and J. R. Hobbs, eds.), The COGENT Press, Ruislip, Middlesex, pp. 41–47.

Krivit, W., Sung, J. H., Lockman, L. A., and Shapiro, E. G., 1995b, Bone marrow transplantation for treatment of lysosomal and peroxisomal storage diseases: Focus on central nervous system reconstitution, in *Principles of Clinical Immunology*, Vol. 2 (R. R. Rich, T. A. Fleisher, B. D. Schwartz, W. T. Shearer, and W. Strober, eds.), Mosby, Louis, MO, pp. 1852–1864.

Liu, J. M., Buchwald, M., Walsh, C. E., and Young, N. S., 1994, Fanconi anemia and novel strategies for therapy, *Blood* **84:**3995–4007.

Lucarelli, G., Giardini, C., and Baronciani, D., 1995, Bone marrow transplantation in thalassemia, *Semin. Hematol.* **32:**297–303.

Malone, B. N., Whitley, C. B., Duvall, A. J., Belani, K., Sibley, R. K., Ramsay, N. K., Kersey, J. H., Krivit, W., and Berlinger, N. T., 1988, Resolution of obstructive sleep apnea in Hurler syndrome after bone marrow transplantation, *Int. J. Pediatr. Otorhinolaryngol.* **15:**23–31.

Manenti, F., Galimberti, M., Lucarelli, G., Polchi, P., De, S. V., Tanas, R., Vullo, C., and Ruggiero, L., 1989, Growth and endocrine function after bone marrow transplantation for thalassemia major, *Prog. Clin. Biol. Res.* **309:**273–280.

Marcus, R. E., and Goldman, J. M., 1984, Convulsions due to high-dose busulphan, *Lancet* **2:**1463.

McColl, M. D., and Gibson, B. E. S., 1997, Sibling allogeneic bone marrow transplantation in a patient with type I Glanzmann's thrombasthenia, *Br. J. Haematol.* **99:**58–60.

McGovern, M. M., Ludman, M. D., Short, M. P., Steinfeld, L., Kattan, M., Raab, E. L., Krivit, W., and Desnick, R. J., 1986, Bone marrow transplantation in Maroteaux–Lamy syndrome (MPS type 6): Status 40 months after BMT, *Birth Defects* **22:**41–53.

McKinnis, E. J., Sulzbacher, S., Rutledge, J. C., Sanders, J., and Scott, C. R., 1996, Bone marrow transplantation in Hunter syndrome, *J. Pediatr.* **129:**145–148.

Morgan, M., Dodds, A., Atkinson, K., Szer, J., Downs, K., and Biggs, J., 1991, The toxicity of busulphan and cyclophosphamide as the preparative regimen for bone marrow transplantation, *Br. J. Haematol.* **77:**529–534.

Moser, H. W., 1993, Lorenzo oil therapy for adrenoleukodystrophy: A prematurely amplified hope, *Ann. Neurol.* **34:**121–122.

Moser, H. W., Moser, A. B., Smith, K. D., Bergin, A., Borel, J., Shankroff, J., Stine, O. C., Merette, C., Ott, J., and Krivit, W., 1992, Adrenoleukodystrophy: Phenotypic variability and implications for therapy, *J. Inherit. Metab. Dis.* **15:**645–664.

Navarro, C., Fernandez, J. M., Dominguez, C., Fachal, C., and Alvarez, M., 1996, Late juvenile metachromatic leukodystrophy treated with bone marrow transplantation: A 4-year follow-up study, *Neurology* **46:**254–256.

O'Reilly, R. J., Brochstein, J., Dinsmore, R., and Kirkpatrick, D., 1984, Marrow transplantation for congenital disorders, *Semin. Hematol.* **21:**188–221.

O'Reilly, R. J., Friedrich, W., and Small, T. N., 1994, Transplantation approaches for severe combined immunodeficiency disease, Wiskott–Aldrich Syndrome, and other lethal genetic, combined immunodeficiency disorders, in *Bone Marrow Transplantation* (S. J. Forman, K. G. Blume, and E. D. Thomas, eds.), Blackwell, Boston, pp. 863–865.

Oakhill, A., Pamphilon, D. H., Potter, M. N., Steward, C. G., Goodman, S., Green, A., Goulden, P., Goulden, N. J., Hale, G., Waldmann, H., and Cornish, J. M., 1996, Unrelated donor bone marrow transplantation for children with relapsed acute lymphoblastic leukaemia in second complete remission, *Br. J. Haematol.* **94:**574–578.

Obaro, S. K., and Hobbs, J. R., 1995, Long term effects of induction regimes for allogeneic BMT in children, in *Correction of Genetic Diseases by Transplantation III* (C. G. Steward, and J. R. Hobbs, eds.), The COGENT Press, Ruislip, Middlesex, pp. 97–108.

Olsen, I., Dean, M. F., Harris, G., and Muir, H., 1981, Direct transfer of a lysosomal enzyme from lymphoid cells to deficient fibroblasts, *Nature* **291:**244–247.

Ozsahin, H., Arredondo-Vega, F. X., Santisteban, I., Fuhrer, H., Tuchschmid, P., Jochum, W., Aguzzi, A., Lederman, H. M., Fleischman, A., Winkelstein, J. A., Seger, R. A., and Hershfield, M. S., 1997, Adenosine deaminase deficiency in adults, *Blood* **89:**2849–2855.

Parkman, R., Rappeport, J., Geha, R., Belli, J., Cassady, R., Levey, R., Nathan, D. G., and Rosen, F. S., 1978, Complete correction of the Wiskott–Aldrich syndrome by allogeneic bone-marrow transplantation, *N. Engl. J. Med.* **298:**921–927.

Perry, G. S., Spector, B. D., Schuman, L. M., Mandel, J. S., Anderson, V. E., McHugh, R. B., Hanson, M. R., Fahlstrom, S. M., Krivit, W., and Kersey, J. H., 1980, The Wiskott–Aldrich syndrome in the United States and Canada (1892–1979), *J. Pediatr.* **97:**72–78.

Peters, C., Balthazor, M., Shapiro, E. G., King, R. J., Kollman, C., Hegland, J. D., Henslee-Downey, J., Trigg, M. E., Cowan, M. J., Sanders, J., Bunin, N., Weinstein, H., Lenarsky, C., Falk, P., Harris, R., Bowen, T., Williams, T. E., Grayson, G. H., Warkentin, P., Sender, L., Cool, V. A., Crittenden, M., Packman, S., Kaplan, P., and Lockman, L. A., 1996, Outcome of unrelated donor bone marrow transplantation in 40 children with Hurler syndrome, *Blood* **87:**4894–4902.

Petz, L. D., 1994, Documentation of engraftment and characterization of chimerism following marrow transplantation, in *Bone Marrow Transplantation* (S. J. Forman, K. G. Blume, and E. D. Thomas, eds.), Blackwell, Boston, pp. 136–148.

Piomelli, S., Danoff, S. J., Becker, M. H., Lipera, M. J., and Travis, S. F., 1969, Prevention of bone malformations and cardiomegaly in Cooley's anemia by early hypertransfusion regimen, *Ann. NY Acad. Sci.* **165:**427–436.

Platt, O. S., Brambilla, D. J., Rosse, W. F., Milner, P. F., Castro, O., Steinberg, M. H., and Klug, P. P., 1994, Mortality in sickle cell disease. Life expectancy and risk factors for early death, *N. Engl. J. Med.* **330:**1639–1644.

Polmar, S. H., Wetzler, E. M., Stern, R. C., and Hirschhorn, R., 1975, Restoration of in-vitro lymphocyte responses with exogenous adenosine deaminase in a patient with severe combined immunodeficiency, *Lancet* **2:**743–746.

Polmar, S. H., Stern, R. C., Schwartz, A. L., Wetzler, E. M., Chase, P. A., and Hirschhorn, R., 1976, Enzyme replacement therapy for adenosine deaminase deficiency and severe combined immunodeficiency, *N. Engl. J. Med.* **295:**1337–1343.

Porter, M. T., Fluharty, A. L., De la Flor S. D., and Kihara, H., 1972, Cerebroside sulfatase determination in cultured human fibroblasts, *Biochim. Biophys. Acta* **258:**769–778.

Powers, J. M., Liu, Y., Moser, A. B., and Moser, H. W., 1992, The inflammatory myelinopathy of adrenoleukodystrophy: Cells, effector molecules, and pathogenetic implications, *J. Neuropathol. Exp. Neurol.* **51:**630–643.

Pridjian, G., Humbert, J., Willis, J., and Shapira, E., 1994, Presymptomatic late-infantile metachromatic leukodystrophy treated with bone marrow transplantation, *J. Pediatr.* **125:**755–758.

Rao, S. S., Peters, S. O., Crittenden, R. B., Stewart, F. M., Ramshaw, H. S., and Quesenberry, P. J., 1997, Stem cell transplantation in the normal nonmyeloablated host: Relationship between cell dose, schedule, and engraftment, *Exp. Hematol.* **25:**114–121.

Riches, P. G., Weatherald, L., Walker, S., and Hobbs, J. R., 1986, Transition to donor type immunoglobulin synthesis following BMT, *Bone Marrow Transplant.* **1:**244

Ringden, O., Groth, C. G., Erikson, A., Granqvist, S., Mansson, J. E., and Sparrelid, E., 1995, Ten years' experience of bone marrow transplantation for Gaucher disease, *Transplantation* **59:**864–870.

Roth, M. S., Antin, J. H., Bingham, E. L., and Ginsburg, D., 1990, Use of polymerase chain reaction-detected sequence polymorphisms to document engraftment following allogeneic bone marrow transplantation, *Transplantation* **49:**714–720.

Roubicek, M., Gehler, J., and Spranger, J., 1985, The clinical spectrum of alpha-L-iduronidase deficiency, *Am. J. Med. Genet.* **20:**471–481.

Sakiyama, T., Tsuda, M., Owada, M., Kitagawa, T., Miyawaki, S., Shinagawa, T., and Tadokoro, M., 1986, Bone marrow transplantation in Niemann-Pick mice, *J. Inherit. Metab. Dis.* **9:**308

Sanders, J. E., 1991a, Endocrine problems in children after bone marrow transplant for hematologic malignancies. The Long-term Follow-up Team, *Bone Marrow Transplant.* **8**(Suppl. 1)**:**2–4.

Sanders, J. E., 1991b, The impact of marrow transplant preparative regimens on subsequent growth and development. The Seattle Marrow Transplant Team, *Semin. Hematol.* **28:**244–249.

Sanders, J. E., Buckner, C. D., Amos, D., Levy, W., Appelbaum, F. R., Doney, K., Storb, Sullivan, K. M., Witherspoon, R. P., and Thomas, E. D., 1988, Ovarian function following marrow transplantation for aplastic anemia or leukemia, *J. Clin. Oncol.* **6:**813–818.

Sandhoff, K., 1984, Function and relevance of activator proteins for glycolipid degradation, in *Molecular Basis of Lysosomal Storage Disorders* (J. A. Barranger, and R. O. Brady, eds.), Academic Orlando, pp. 19–51.

Santos, G. W., 1989, Busulfan (Bu) and cyclophosphamide (Cy) for marrow transplantation, *Bone Marrow Transplant.* **4**(Suppl. 1)**:**236–239.

Santos, G. W., Tutschka, P. J., Brookmeyer, R., Saral, R., Beschorner, W. E., Bias, W. B., Braine, H. G., Burns, W. H., Elfenbein, G. J., and Kaizer, H., 1983, Marrow transplantation for acute nonlymphocytic leukemia after treatment with busulfan and cyclophosphamide, *N. Engl. J. Med.* **309:**1347–1353.

Sasaki, M. S., and Tonomura, A., 1973, A high susceptibility of Fanconi's anemia to chromosome breakage by DNA cross-linking agents, *Cancer Res.* **33:**1829–1836.

Shapiro, E. G., Lockman, L. A., Balthazor, M., and Krivit, W., 1995, Neuropsychological outcomes of several storage diseases with and without bone marrow transplantation, *J. Inherit. Metab. Dis.* **18:**413–429.

Sierra, J., Storer, B., Hansen, J. A., Bjerke, J. W., Martin, P. J., Petersdorf, E. W., Appelbaum, F. R., Bryant, E., Chauncey, T. R., Sale, G., Sanders, J. E., Storb, R., Sullivan, K. M., and Anasetti, C., 1997, Transplantation of marrow cells from unrelated donors for treatment of high-risk acute leukemia: The effect of leukemic burden, donor HLA-matching, and marrow cell dose, *Blood* **89:**4226–4235.

Sirinavin, C., and Trowbridge, A. A., 1975, Dyskeratosis congenita: Clinical features and genetic aspects. Report of a family and review of the literature, *J. Med. Genet.* **12:**339–354.

Socie, G., Henry-Amar, M., Cosset, J. M., Devergie, A., Girinsky, T., and Gluckman, E., 1991, Increased incidence of solid malignant tumors after bone marrow transplantation for severe aplastic anemia, *Blood* **78:**277–279.

Socie, G., Gluckman, E., Raynal, B., Petit, T., Landman, J., Devergie, A., and Brison, O., 1993, Bone marrow transplantation for Fanconi anemia using low-dose cyclophosphamide/thoracoabdominal irradiation as conditioning regimen: Chimerism study by the polymerase chain reaction, *Blood* **82:**2249–2256.

Steinmuller, D., and Motulsky, A. G., 1967, Treatment of hereditary spherocytosis in Peromyscus by radiation and allogeneic bone marrow transplantation, *Blood* **29:**320–330.

Stillman, A. E., Krivit, W., Shapiro, E., Lockman, L., and Latchaw, R. E., 1994, Serial MR after bone marrow transplantation in two patients with metachromatic leukodystrophy, *Am. J. Neuroradiol.* **15:**1929–1932.

Sugarman, J., Reisner, E. G., and Kurtzberg, J., 1995, Ethical aspects of banking placental blood for transplantation, *JAMA* **274:**1783–1785.

Sullivan, K. M., 1994, Graft-versus-host disease, in *Bone Marrow Transplantation* (S. J. Forman, K. G. Blume, and E. D. Thomas, eds.), Blackwell, Boston, pp. 339–362.

Taylor, R. M., Farrow, B. R., Stewart, G. J., and Healy, P. J., 1986, Enzyme replacement in nervous tissue after allogeneic bone-marrow transplantation for fucosidosis in dogs, *Lancet* **2:**772–774.

Taylor, R. M., Stewart, G. J., Farrow, B. R., Byrne, J., and Healy, P. J., 1989, Histological improvement and enzyme replacement in the brains of fucosidosis dogs after bone marrow engraftment, *Transplant. Proc* **21:**3074–3075.

Thomas, C., Ged, C., Nordmann, Y., de, V. H., Pellier, I., Fischer, A., and Blanche, S., 1996, Correction of congenital erythropoietic porphyria by bone marrow transplantation, *J. Pediatr.* **129:**453–456.

Thomas, E. D., Buckner, C. D., Sanders, J. E., Papayannopoulou, T., Borgna, P., De, S. P., Sullivan, K. M., Clift, R. A., and Storb, R., 1982, Marrow transplantation for thalassaemia, *Lancet* **2:**227–229.

Touraine, J. L., 1996, In utero transplantation of fetal liver stem cells into human fetuses, *J. Hematother.* **5:**195–199.

Touraine, J. L., Raudrant, D., and Laplace, S., 1997, Transplantation of hemopoietic cells from the fetal liver to treat patients with congenital diseases postnatally or prenatally, *Transplant. Proc.* **29:**712–713.

Tsai, P. H., Sahdev, I., Herry, A., and Lipton, J. M., 1990, Fatal cyclophosphamide-induced congestive heart failure in a 10-year-old boy with Shwachman–Diamond syndrome and severe bone marrow failure treated with allogeneic bone marrow transplantation, *Am. J. Pediatr. Hematol. Oncol.* **12:**472–476.

Vassal, G., Deroussent, A., Challine, D., Hartmann, O., Koscielny, S., Valteau-Couanet, D., Lemerle, J., and Gouyette, A., 1992, Is 600 mg/m^2 the appropriate dosage of busulfan in children undergoing bone marrow transplantation?, *Blood* **79:**2475–2479.

Vellodi, A., Young, E., New, M., Pot-Mees, C., and Hugh-Jones, K., 1992, Bone marrow transplantation for Sanfilippo disease type B, *J. Inherit. Metab. Dis.* **15:**911–918.

Vellodi, A., Cragg, H., Winchester, B., Young, E., Young, J., Downie, C. J., Hoare, R. D., Stocks, R., and Banerjee, G. K., 1995, Allogeneic bone marrow transplantation for fucosidosis, *Bone Marrow Transplant.* **15:**153–158.

Vellodi, A., Young, E. P., Cooper, A., Wraith, J. E., Winchester, B., Meaney, C., Ramaswami, U., and Will, A., 1997, Bone marrow transplantation for mucopolysaccharidosis type I: Experience of two British centres, *Arch. Dis. Child.* **76:**92–99.

Verlander, P. C., Lin, J. D., Udono, M. U., Zhang, Q., Gibson, R. A., Mathew, C. G., and Auerbach, A. D., 1994, Mutation analysis of the Fanconi anemia gene FACC, *Am J Hum. Genet.* **54:**595–601.

Vermylen, C., and Cornu, G., 1994, Bone marrow transplantation for sickle cell disease. The European experience, *Am. J. Pediatr. Hematol. Oncol.* **16:**18–21.

Wagner, J. E., Kernan, N. A., Steinbuch, M., Broxmeyer, H. E., and Gluckman, E., 1995, Allogeneic sibling umbilical-cord-blood transplantation in children with malignant and non-malignant disease, *Lancet* **346:**214–219.

Wagner, J. E., Rosenthal, J., Sweetman, R., Shu, X. O., Davies, S. M., Ramsay, N. K., McGlave, P. B., Sender, L., and Cairo, M. S., 1996, Successful transplantation of HLA-matched and HLA-mismatched umbilical cord blood from unrelated donors: Analysis of engraftment and acute graft-versus-host disease, *Blood* **88:**795–802.

Walker, D. G., 1975, Bone resorption restored in osteopetrotic mice by transplants of normal bone marrow and spleen cells, *Science* **190:**784–785.

Walkley, S. U., Thrall, M. A., Dobrenis, K., Huang, M., March, P. A., Siegel, D. A., and Wurzelmann, S., 1994, Bone marrow transplantation corrects the enzyme defect in neurons of the central nervous system in a lysosomal storage disease, *Proc. Nat. Acad. Sci. USA* **91:**2970–2974.

Wenger, D. A., Gasper, P. W. Thrall M. A., Dial, S. M., Le Couteur, R. A., and Hoover, E. A., 1986, Bone marrow transplantation in the feline model of arylsulfatase B deficiency, *Birth Defects* **22:**177–186.

Wengler, G. S., Lanfranchi, A., Frusca, T., Verardi, R., Neva, A., Brugnoni, D., Giliani, S., Fiorini, M., Mella, P., Guandalini, F., Mazzolari, E., Pecorelli, Notarangelo, L. D., Porta, F., and Ugazio, A. G., 1996, In-utero transplantation of parental CD34 haematopoietic progenitor cells in a patient with X-linked severe combined immunodeficiency (SCIDXI), *Lancet* **348:**1484–1487.

Whitley, C. B., Ramsay, N. K., Kersey, J. H., and Krivit, W., 1986, Bone marrow transplantation for Hurler syndrome: Assessment of metabolic correction, *Birth Defects* **22:**7–24.

Whitley, C. B., Belani, K. G., Chang, P. N., Summers, C. G., Blazar, B. R., Tsai, M. Y., Latchaw, R. E., Ramsay, N. K., and Kersey, J. H., 1993, Long-term outcome of Hurler syndrome following bone marrow transplantation, *Am. J. Med. Genet.* **46:**209–218.

Wiesmann, U. N., Rossi, E. E., and Herschkowitz, N. N., 1971, Treatment of metachromatic leukodystrophy in fibroblasts by enzyme replacement, *N. Engl. J. Med.* **284:**672–673.

Wingard, J. R., Plotnick, L. P., Freemer, C. S., Zahurak, M., Piantadosi, S., Miller, D. F., Vriesendorp, H. M., Yeager, A. M., and Santos, G. W., 1992, Growth in children after bone marrow transplantation: Busulfan plus cyclophosphamide versus cyclophosphamide plus total body irradiation, *Blood* **79:**1068–1073.

Winston, D. J., Gale, R. P., Meyer, D. V., and Young, L. S., 1979, Infectious complications of human bone marrow transplantation, *Medicine* **58:**1–31.

Winston, D. J., Ho, W. G., and Champlin, R. E., 1990, Cytomegalovirus infections after allogeneic bone marrow transplantation, *Rev. Infect. Dis.* **12**(Suppl. 7)**:**S776–S792.

Witherspoon, R. P., Storb, R., Pepe, M., Longton, G., and Sullivan, K. M., 1992, Cumulative incidence of secondary solid malignant tumors in aplastic anemia patients given marrow grafts after conditioning with chemotherapy alone, *Blood* **79:**289–291.

Wolff, J. A., 1967, Wiskott–Aldrich syndrome: Clinical, immunologic, and pathologic observations, *J. Pediatr.* **70:**221–232.

Woodman, R. C., Erickson, R. W., Rae, J., Jaffe, H. S., and Curnutte, J. T., 1992, Prolonged recombinant interferon-gamma therapy in chronic granulomatous disease: Evidence against enhanced neutrophil oxidase activity, *Blood* **79:**1558–1562.

Yang, Y., Jooss, K. U., Su, Q., Ertl, H. C., and Wilson, J. M., 1996, Immune responses to viral antigens versus transgene product in the elimination of recombinant adenovirus-infected hepatocytes *in vivo*, *Gene Ther.* **3:**137–144.

Yeager, A. M., Brennan, S., Toffamu, C., Moser, H. W., and Santos, G. W., 1984, Prolonged survival and remyelination after hemopoietic cell transplantation in the twitcher mouse, *Science* **225:**1052–1054.

Zix-Kieffer, I., Langer, B., Eyer, D., Acar, G., Racadot, E., Schlaeder, G., Oberlin, F., and Lutz, P., 1996, Successful cord blood stem cell transplantation for congenital erythropoietic porphyria (Günther's disease), *Bone Marrow Transplant.* **18:**217–220.

Chapter 3

Retroviral Vectors

Mary Collins and Colin Porter

1. WHY RETROVIRUSES?

Some aspects of retroviral biology make recombinant retroviruses particularly suitable for delivering foreign DNA. Most such vectors in use for gene delivery to mammalian cells are based on murine C-type retroviruses, which have a small, simple, and well-characterized genome. This allows extensive vector manipulation, for example, to achieve tissue-specific expression. Complementary sequences between vector and packaging constructs can essentially be eliminated, ensuring that recombinant viral preparations are free from replication-competent virus or transferred packaging constructs. Thus, the target cells do not express any viral proteins. Furthermore, because replication-competent C-type retroviruses have never been detected in humans, the risk of vector mobilization following human infection is also minimal. Finally, integrating retroviruses into the target cell genome results in progeny carrying the vector sequence, a property which is desirable if a stem cell is to be infected. Recent research has partly solved some of the well-known drawbacks of recombinant retroviruses, for example, the low titers, the sensitivity to human serum, the requirement for target cell division to allow infection, and the instability of vector expression *in vivo*. In this chapter, we consider the minimal requirements for a retroviral vector and packaging cell and illustrate how they can be modified for specialized applications.

Mary Collins and Colin Porter CRC Centre for Cell and Molecular Biology, Chester Beatty Laboratories, London SW3 6JB, United Kingdom.

Blood Cell Biochemistry, Volume 8: Hematopoiesis and Gene Therapy, edited by Fairbairn and Testa. Kluwer Academic/Plenum Publishers, New York, 1999.

2. THE BASIC VECTOR

2.1. Minimal Vector Requirements

2.1.1. The Viral LTR

A map of a minimal vector based on a murine leukaemia virus (MLV) is shown in Figure 1. Reverse transcription and integration of the recombinant genome in target cells requires some, but not all, sequences of the 600 bp viral long terminal repeats (LTRs). These essential regions are indicated in Figure 1. Two regions, "unique 3′" (U3) and "unique 5′" (U5) are present at the 3′ and 5′ ends, respectively, of the viral RNA but are duplicated following viral DNA synthesis (Figure 2).

The main function of U3 is to act as a transcriptional enhancer and promoter in the 5′ LTR for RNA polII-dependent transcription of the integrated provirus. MLV enhancer function maps to a 75 bp direct repeat (DR) sequence, within which binding sites for six different nuclear factors have been identified (Speck and Baltimore, 1987). The promoter contains a CAAT-box and a TATA-box. Most of the transcription factors involved are ubiquitously expressed, accounting for the lack of any marked cell specificity of the LTR, but motifs controlling expression in lymphoid cells and fibroblasts have been identified (Speck *et al.*, 1990). However, the MLV LTR functions poorly in embryonal carcinoma (EC) and stem (ES) cells (see section 2.2.2). Sequence alterations of the enhancer DR can lead to dramatic changes in viral pathogenesis of MLV *in vivo* (Oliff *et al.*, 1984; Stocking *et al.*, 1986; Vogt *et al.*, 1985). Upstream of the enhancer is a region highly conserved between different type C retroviruses that binds a ubiquitous factor that negatively regulates expression from the LTR (Flanagan *et al.*, 1991). If the viral enhancer is not neces-

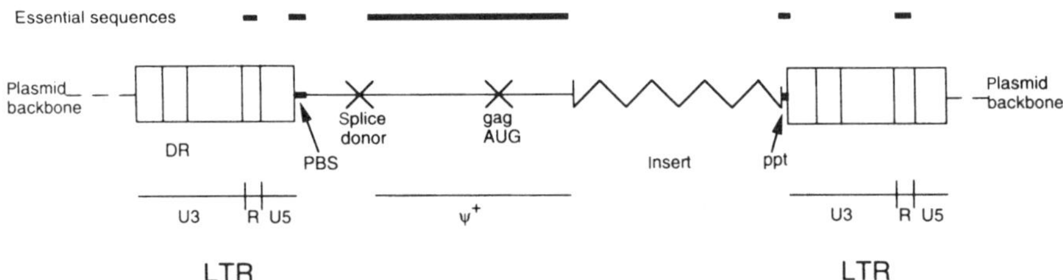

FIGURE 1. Minimal retroviral vector. A schematic representation of retroviral vector DNA. Sequences essential for transmission, completion of reverse transcription, and integration are indicated. The Ψ^+ packaging sequence extends into the *gag* coding region, and so mutations that prevent initiation of translation are inserted. The sequences responsible for initiation of –ve strand and +ve strand synthesis, the primer binding site (PBS), and polypurine tract (ppt), respectively, are shown. The vector contains a copy of the long terminal repeat (LTR) at each end, consisting of the unique 3′ and 5′ (U3 and U5), and repeat (R) regions. The latter is necessary for strand transfer during –ve strand DNA synthesis. A short inverted repeat at the 5′ end of U3 in the 3′ LTR and the 3′ end of U5 in the 5′ LTR is necessary for integration of the provirus. The enhancer direct repeat (DR) is within U3. The splice donor site is commonly mutated, as indicated. Also shown is the position of an insert between the two blocks of *cis*-acting sequences.

sary for vector function, the DR region of U3 can be deleted in the 3′ LTR of the vector. In this way the 5′ LTR still drives vector expression in the packaging cell but, following reverse transcription and integration of the vector in the target cell, the deletion is duplicated in the 5′ LTR (Figure 3). This removal of viral enhancer function may improve the use of exogenous enhancers and promoters (see section 2.2.1). The U3 of MLV also tolerates large sequence insertions, a property that has

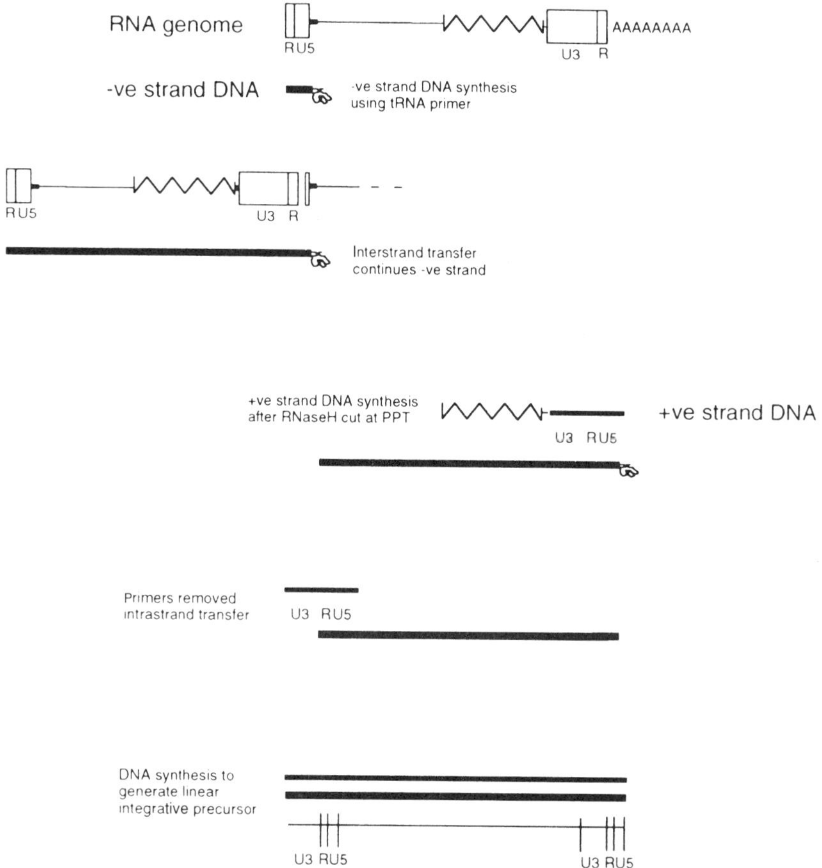

FIGURE 2. Mechanism of proviral DNA synthesis. Synthesis of –ve strand DNA (thick solid line) by reverse transcriptase is primed by a specific tRNA annealed at the primer binding site (PBS) and continues until the 5′ end of the template RNA is reached. RNaseH digests RNA in the RNA/DNA hybrid, leaving unpaired DNA including the R region that can hybridize to R at the 3′ end of the second template RNA to effect an intermolecular jump. –ve strand DNA synthesis continues through the PBS near the 5′ end of the second template. Again RNaseH digests RNA in the duplex, and a specific cleavage at ppt generates a primer for +ve strand DNA synthesis. +ve strand DNA synthesis continues through the PBS, and the tRNA primer is removed. The PBS complementarity at the ends of –ve and +ve DNA strands allows an intramolecular jump, after which synthesis of both strands is completed. The end result is a double-stranded integrative precursor that has a complete LTR at each end.

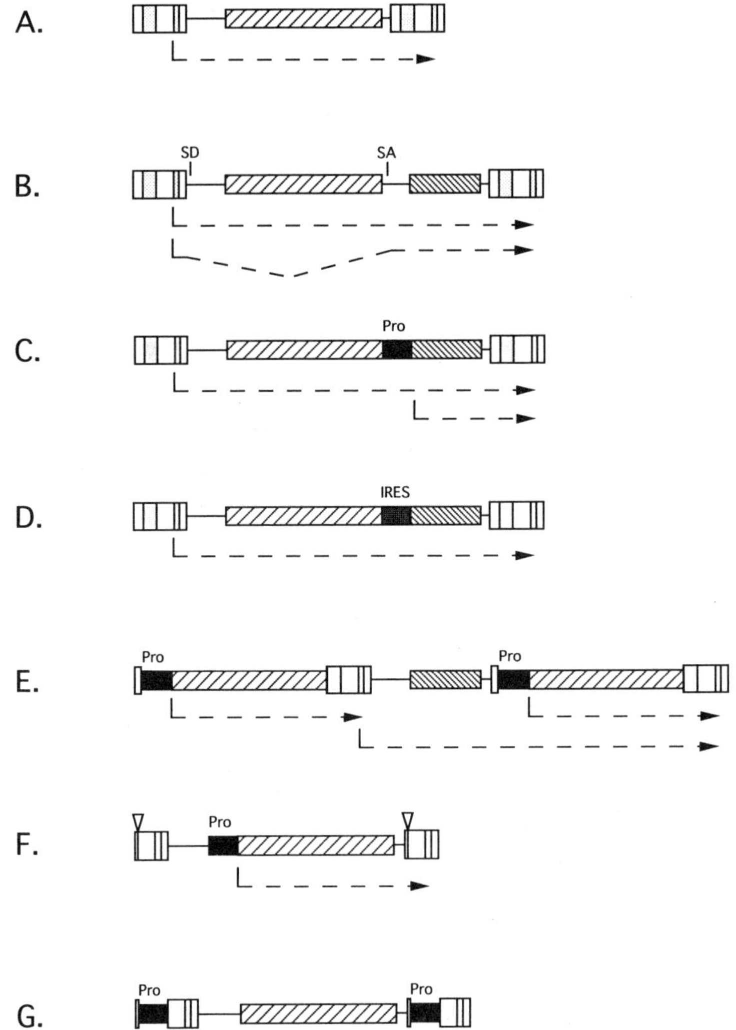

FIGURE 3. Strategies for vector design. A number of retroviral vector designs are illustrated. In each case, the proviral form following infection of the target cell is illustrated. There is a long terminal repeat (LTR) at each end, and the enhancer and R regions are indicated (refer to Figure 1). For vectors involving manipulated LTRs, the modifications are initially made in the 3′ LTR and subsequently copied to the 5′ LTR following proviral synthesis (see Figure 2). The transcripts are indicated beneath each design. In (A) a simple retroviral vector for encoding a single gene (hatched box) is depicted. There is a single LTR-driven transcript. (B) to (E) illustrate strategies for coexpression with a second gene, often a selectable marker, and (F) and (G) illustrate strategies for tissue-specific expression of a single gene. In (B), the second gene is expressed via a spliced mRNA, similarly to the expression of *env* in the wild-type retrovirus. In (C), an internal promoter (Pro) drives expression of the second gene, and an internal ribosomal entry site (IRES) in (D) allows both genes to be expressed via a bicistronic transcript. The double copy strategy is depicted in (E), in which there are two transcriptional units containing the gene inserted into the LTR U3 region. LTR enhancer function is deleted in (F) to prevent intereference with the internal promoter, and in (G) it is replaced with the promoter of interest.

been exploited to generate replication-competent vectors that contain a foreign cDNA (Stuhlmann *et al.*, 1989) or replication-defective vectors that contain an entire expression cassette within U3 (Hantzopoulos *et al.*, 1989).

The R region begins at the transcriptional cap site and is also present at the 3′ end of the viral RNA transcript, preceding the poly(A) tail. Sequences within U3 are required for efficient polyadenylation of the 3′ R region of HIV RNA (Cherrington and Ganem, 1992), and the terminal bases of U3 are necessary for polyadenylation of Moloney murine sarcoma virus RNA (Benz *et al.*, 1980) and spleen necrosis virus RNA (Dougherty and Temin, 1987), possibly because they are involved in RNA secondary structure that activates the polyadenylation signal specifically in the 3′ LTR. R provides a region of sequence homology which allows reverse transcriptase (RT) to transfer between ends of the viral RNA and thus complete viral DNA synthesis (Figure 2). The entire homology of R is not necessary for efficient viral replication (Lobel and Goff, 1985). Deletion of the polyadenylation site in R does not prevent viral replication because "read-through" transcripts are efficiently packaged (Swain and Coffin, 1989). However, it should probably be maintained for optimal gene expression by the integrated provirus. The U5 region forms part of the leader of the viral RNA. Deletions in U5 affect reverse transcription and RNA packaging but some regions of U5 are not essential (Murphy and Goff, 1989).

2.1.2. Other Cis-Acting Sequences

Sequences between the LTRs are also necessary to replicate the minimal retroviral vector (Figure 1). The primer binding site (PBS) binds a cellular tRNA, $tRNA^{Pro}$ in the case of MLV, which acts as a primer for –ve strand DNA synthesis by reverse transcriptase (RT) (Figure 2). This tRNA primer is incorporated into virions bound to the viral RNA(Waters *et al.*, 1980). MLV RT does not require a specific tRNA because mutation of the PBS allows efficient utilization of a variety of tRNA primers (Lund *et al.*, 1993). Other C type retroviral RTs, some of which do not normally use $tRNA^{Pro}$, also replicate MLV vectors efficiently (Takeuchi *et al.*, 1992). This contrasts with HIV, where specific interactions between RT and $tRNA^{Lys}$ have been described (Barat *et al.*, 1989). The PBS was identified as one of the sequences responsible for poor MLV vector expression in EC cells. Mutations which abolish this inhibition can be incorporated into vectors (see section 2.2.2). The retroviral enzyme RNase H, which digests RNA in RNA/DNA hybrids, is essential for viral replication (Tanese *et al.*, 1991). After inititiating –ve strand DNA synthesis, it cuts the template RNA starting within U5 (Schultz *et al.*, 1995), leaving unpaired DNA which can hybridize to R at the 3′ end of the template RNA and allow RT to jump (Figure 2). For -ve strand synthesis this jump is intermolecular between the two RNA genomes packaged in the virion (Panganiban and Fiore, 1988). +ve strand DNA synthesis is initiated at a polypurine tract, first identified as essential in Rous sarcoma virus (Sorge and Hughes, 1982), adjacent to the 3′ LTR (Figure 1). RNase H recognizes features of this sequence and cuts the viral RNA (Rattray and Champoux, 1989) generating a primer for RT (Figure 2). Continuation of +ve strand DNA synthesis requires an intramolecular jump by RT from the 3′ to the 5′ end of the template (Panganiban and Fiore, 1988).

A sequence adjacent to the 5′ LTR, the packaging signal (designated φ) (Figure 1), is required to package MLV vector RNA into viral particles. An extended 824-bp sequence (designated φ^+) gives significantly enhanced packaging efficiency (Bender *et al.*, 1987). Because this optimal packaging signal extends into the gag protein coding region, many vectors include the 5′ end of *gag* but have point mutations in the start codon to prevent synthesizing partial gag products. The packaging signal can be moved within the vector and functions in nonretroviral RNA (Adam, 1988; Mann and Baltimore, 1985). Other C type retroviral particles package MLV vectors efficiently (Takeuchi *et al.*, 1992), and MLV particles package vectors with a considerably shorter packaging signal derived from a cellular virus-like (VL) RNA (Torrent *et al.*, 1994). The packaging signal promotes dimerization of RNA, resulting in a complex secondary structure, which is stabilized by the nucleocapsid (NC) region of the gag polyprotein precursor (Prats *et al.*, 1990). MLV NC encodes a central zinc-finger domain which, with surrounding basic regions, is necessary for efficient and specific RNA packaging (Housset *et al.*, 1993; Meric and Goff, 1989). NC binding to the dimeric genome probably also enhances reverse transcription during infection (Allain *et al.*, 1994). Immediately preceding φ is a splice donor site used to generate a subgenomic mRNA to express the *env* gene. The *gag* and *pol* genes are expressed from the full-length mRNA. This arrangement ensures that only full-length genomic transcripts are packaged. The splice donor is not essential for vector construction. Indeed, it is mutated in many vectors.

2.2. Strategies for Vector Design

The majority of recombinant retroviral vectors that have been used express two genes, one of which is a selectable marker. A number of different strategies have been employed to express this marker in addition to the gene of interest (Figure 3). Depending on the particular application, it may be desirable to maximize expression of the gene of interest or to express this gene in a tissue-specific fashion. These requirements affect optimal design of recombinant retroviral vectors and, in practice, are often at the expense of viral titer. Generation of vectors that work well is still somewhat empirical, necessitating the exploration of alternative strategies.

Because RNAs longer than about 10 kb are not efficiently packaged, this places a limit on vector capacity. Usual practice is to remove any noncoding sequences from the insert to minimize size. Splicing and polyadenylation signals, which would prevent transmission of the full length vector RNA, are also removed from the insert. Specific cDNA inserts may affect viral titer. Thus, it has been reported that neo^R, commonly incorporated in retroviral vectors, possesses transcriptional silencer activity (Artelt *et al.*, 1991). The cDNAs for clotting factor VIII and for cystic fibrosis transmembrane conductance regulator contain inhibitory sequences that block transciptional elongation more than 100-fold, resulting in low expression and poor titers when incorporated into retroviral vectors (Koeberl *et al.*, 1995).

2.2.1. Coexpression and Promoter Interference

MLV proteins are expressed from both the full-length and spliced mRNAs. This strategy was exploited in some of the earliest vectors to enable expression of two genes, one from the full-length mRNA and a second from the spliced mRNA (Cepko *et al.*, 1984) (Figure 3B). However, in many vectors the splice donor site 5′ of the packaging signal (Figure 1) is mutated to prevent instability resulting from splicing to cryptic acceptor sites within the insert (Morgenstern and Land, 1990). An alternative way to express two genes from the same vector is to use an internal promoter in addition to the viral LTR (Figure 3C). Such a vector has two transcriptional units, with LTR-driven expression of one gene and internally driven expression of the second. The internal transcription unit may be placed in the same orientation relative to expression from the LTR, in which case both transcripts terminate by polyadenylation within R of the 3′ LTR or may be in the opposite orientation with its own polyadenylation sequences. However, several studies have shown that the viral LTR and heterologous promoters do not always work efficiently in combination and coexpression may be poor because of promoter interference (Emerman and Temin, 1984, 1986). This is caused by (reversible) epigenetic suppression of one promoter following selection for expression from the other.

The problem of promoter interference has led to the development of vectors using bicistronic transcripts that have picornavirus-derived internal ribosomal entry sites (IRES) to allow expression of two genes from the LTR (Aran *et al.*, 1994; Chen *et al.*, 1993; Ghattas *et al.*, 1991; Morgan *et al.*, 1992) (Figure 3D). This strategy has even been extended to coexpression of three genes from a single LTR-driven transcript (Morgan *et al.*, 1992; Zitvogel *et al.*, 1994). It is also possible to prevent promoter interference by deleting enhancer sequences from the 3′ LTR such that following infection, reverse transcription, and integration, the 5′ LTR is also inactivated, leaving a single transcriptional unit driven by an internal promoter (Cone *et al.*, 1987). An additional advantage of this "self-inactivating" approach is the reduced likelihood that host genes adjacent to the integration site will be expressed from an active LTR. A deletion spanning the enhancer and the CAAT box (Yu *et al.*, 1986), or separate deletions of enhancer, CAAT, and TATA boxes (Yee *et al.*, 1987) have been described. The former still possessed some transcriptional activity, perhaps because of the remaining minimal promoter was activated by internal enhancer sequences, whereas the latter was transcriptionally silent. However, a drawback of these deletion constructs is the low viral titers obtained, avoidable by mutation of the TATA box without enhancer deletion (Nakajima *et al.*, 1993), although the intact enhancer may exert an effect on internal promoters.

A further strategy has been to insert a complete transcriptional unit consisting of heterologous promoter and gene of interest within U3, upstream of the viral enhancer (Figure 3E). Following integration, such a "double-copy" vector results in two complete units, one in each LTR, each outside of the retroviral transcriptional unit to avoid interference (Hantzopoulos *et al.*, 1989). This approach resulted in higher levels of gene expression without significantly reducing titer. However, in a comparison of vectors for coexpressing neo^R and growth hormone, the LTR-driven bicistronic strategy was found optimal. The internal promoter or double-copy strategies compromised expression or viral titers, respectively (Chen *et al.*, 1995). Growth hormone expression was greatest if neo^R was expressed as the second cistron.

2.2.2. Optimized LTR-Based Expression

The MLV LTR functions poorly in ES and EC cells, developmentally the most primitive culturable mammalian stem cells. The block occurs postintegration and is mediated by the cumulative effect of multiple *cis*-acting elements which map to the viral enhancer and PBS in the 5′ untranslated region of the virus (Challita *et al.*, 1995). The viral enhancer is inactive in these cells (Linney *et al.*, 1984), in part because of deficiency in transcription factors necessary for expression (Speck and Baltimore, 1987). Additionally, the enhancer negatively regulates transcription in undifferentiated EC cells (Gorman *et al.*, 1985). Enhancers derived from the mutant myeloproliferative sarcoma virus (MPSV) and a derivative (PCMV) are functional in EC cells (Akgun *et al.*, 1991) owing to the introduction of a new binding site for the transcription factor Sp1 (Grez *et al.*, 1991; Prince and Rigby, 1991). A mutation (termed B2) downstream of the transcriptional cap site also confers activity in EC cells and maps to within the PBS (Barklis *et al.*, 1986). Expression from the PCMV LTR is blocked by the PBS in ES cells but can be relieved by modifying the PBS to use $tRNA^{Glu}$ instead of $tRNA^{Pro}$ (Grez *et al.*, 1990; Peterson *et al.*, 1991). A stem-cell-specific transcriptional silencer is coincident with the wild-type PBS and binds a nuclear factor present in undifferentiated EC cells (Kempler *et al.*, 1993; Yamauchi *et al.*, 1995). The greatest level of LTR-driven expression in EC cells from a retroviral vector combined use of the MPSV LTR, $tRNA^{Glu}$ PBS, and deletion of the upstream negative control region (Challita *et al.*, 1995).

In most cases the MLV LTR is functional in haematopoietic cells (Correll *et al.*, 1994), although there are some reports of inactivation (Challita and Kohn, 1994). Most notably, long-term LTR-driven expression of adenosine deaminase in modified lymphocytes or haematopoietic stem cells in human gene therapy subjects has recently been reported (Blaese *et al.*, 1995; Bordignon *et al.*, 1995). Several of the mutations described previously that relieve repression in EC cells have been incorporated into vectors for use in haematopoietic cells. Thus, incorporating the MPSV LTR or the B2 PBS mutation into the vector MFG gives improved gene expression in all haematopoietic lineages of reconstituted mice (Riviere *et al.*, 1995). The combined use of enhancer and PBS mutations also improves expression in primitive murine haematopoietic cells *in vitro* (Baum *et al.*, 1995).

In many of the vectors that utilize the LTR to express the gene of interest, the cDNA is encoded in a transcript that begins at the natural viral cap site and contains a long sequence 5′ of the coding region. This includes the 5′ part of *gag* which overlaps the φ^+ packaging sequence (Bender *et al.*, 1987). The resultant RNA may not be optimal for expression because translation can initiate at the upstream *gag* initiation codon and other intervening ATG codons may inhibit efficient translation of the cDNA coding region. Because of this some vectors possess mutations that disrupt initiation of *gag* synthesis. Additionally, the widely used MFG vector retains the splice donor site and positions the splice acceptor site used for generating the *env* mRNA upstream of the insert (Dranoff *et al.*, 1993). This vector design is superior to that involving the LTR and internal promoters in two gene constructs, both in terms of viral titer and level of expression in transduced cells (Byun *et al.*, 1996). As an alternative strategy for improving protein expression by avoiding long sequences 5′ of the coding region, the cDNA can be inserted into the R region of the LTR, close to the retroviral promoter but upstream of the polyadenylation site (Adam *et al.*, 1995). Because R region mutations are not copied from the 3′ to the 5′ LTR, such inserts in R must be made in both LTRs of the vector, unlike those in U3. This resulted in enhanced protein expression in one case, but reduced viral titer.

2.2.3. Tissue-Specific Expression

The MLV LTR is functional in a wide range of mammalian cell types, but mutation of transcription factor binding sites within the viral enhancer can modify transcriptional specificity (Speck *et al.*, 1990). Replacement of U3 sequences with those derived from other related murine retroviruses results in chimeric LTRs displaying various transcriptional specificities (Baum *et al.*, 1995; Couture *et al.*, 1994). Nonretroviral sequences can also be used to modify LTR function. Thus, replacement of the viral enhancer with that of a polyoma mutant selected to grow in EC cells yielded a hybrid LTR functional in these cells (Valerio *et al.*, 1989). The strength of the LTR is also improved severalfold by adding the CMV-IE enhancer upstream of the viral enhancer (Wollenberg *et al.*, 1994).

However, when restricted specificity of the cDNA expression in the transduced target cells is required, tissue-specific heterologous promoters must be used. As noted previously, promoter interference is a problem if the vector also contains a functional LTR. An alternative to deleting viral enhancer function (see section 2.2.1) (Figure 3F) is using exogenous enhancers and promoters within U3 (Figure 3G). Adding the muscle creatine kinase enhancer between the viral enhancer and promoter resulted in differentiation-specific expression in myogenic cells but was not entirely tissue-specific because it failed to block constitutive LTR function in some cells (Ferrari *et al.*, 1995). Incorporating lymphoid-specific enhancers failed to modify specificity of expression (Moore *et al.*, 1991). However, replacing the viral enhancer with the tyrosinase enhancer and promoter enabled specific expression in melanoma cells (Vile *et al.*, 1995). It seems likely that the optimal vectors will also avoid the use of an additional promoter for selectable marker expression, but it is not clear whether it will be possible ultimately to incorporate all of the control sequences necessary to faithfully reproduce tissue-specificity and expression level of a given gene. These include intron sequences that necessitate a reverse orientation vector design. This has been most carefully studied for globin gene expression, where internal insertion of part of the β-globin locus control region and the β-globin gene gives an expression level which does not entirely depend copy number (Sadelain *et al.*, 1995). This implies that the retroviral backbone and/or integration site still exert some effect.

2.2.4. Long-Term Expression *in Vivo*

Sustained expression in retrovirus-modified cells *in vivo* cannot always be predicted on the basis of *in vitro* experiments. For example, fibroblasts are attractive targets for modification to synthesise systemic products. However, although mice transplanted with a collagen matrix dermal graft of primary fibroblasts, modified to produce clotting factor IX, showed high initial serum levels of factor IX, this was of short duration and fell to baseline within one month (Palmer *et al.*, 1989). The same result was obtained whether expression was driven from the LTR or from internal SV40 or CMV-IE promoters, all of which maintained high levels of expression *in vitro.* Similarly, adenosine deaminase expression from the LTR in fibroblasts was undetectable within one month after transplantation into syngeneic rats (Palmer *et al.*, 1991). In this experiment the modified cells persist for more than eight months but when reestablished *in vitro* expression of both ADA and the neo^R gene was shut off despite the presence of the vector DNA. The nature of the suggested transcriptional block is unknown because expression could not be reactivated in the presence of 5-azacytidine. No immune response to the foreign protein was detected. Furthermore, an identical vector is functional for ADA expression in modified mouse bone marrow cells (Kaleko *et al.*, 1990) and in vascular smooth muscle cells grafted in the carotid artery (Lynch *et al.*, 1992) more than six months following transplantation.

This problem of *in vivo* expression has been solved empirically for a number of tissue grafts. Long-term expression of β-galactosidase was achieved in transplanted mouse embryo fibroblasts modified with a vector for expression from an internal dihydrofolate reductase promoter but not from the CMV-IE promoter (Scharfmann *et al.*, 1991). Similar problems were observed in grafted myoblasts, where inactivation of expression of factor IX from the CMV-IE promoter is prevented by including the cell-specific muscle creatine kinase enhancer. However, this enhancer cannot prevent inactivation when the α-globin promoter is used (Dai *et al.*, 1992). Sustained *in vivo* expression from modified fibroblasts implanted as synthetic organoids has been achieved using an internal phosphoglycerate kinase promoter (Moullier *et al.*, 1993, 1995; Naffakh *et al.*, 1995). More recently, long-term *in vivo* expression of human growth hormone driven from the the LTR has been obtained in rat fibroblasts using a bicistronic vector in which the neo^R gene is expressed by internal ribosomal entry rather than from a second promoter (Chen *et al.*, 1995).

Hepatocytes modified *in vitro* to express low-density lipoprotein receptor from a β-actin promoter, transplanted in the rabbit model for familial hypercholesterolaemia, maintained expression *in vivo* (Chowdhury *et al.*, 1991). A similar experiment in dogs to express α_1-antitrypsin (AAT) from the CMV-IE promoter resulted in loss of serum protein by one month, although the cells survived and no immune response was detected (Kay *et al.*, 1992), analogous to the transcriptional shut-off observed for fibroblasts. A series of constructs employing different liver-specific promoters to express AAT was used for *in vivo* transduction of hepatocytes. This demonstrated that promoter choice significantly affects expression levels but that this correlates poorly with expression *in vivo* (Hafenrichter *et al.*, 1994).

Thus, there is a complex interplay, as yet poorly understood, between vector design, promoter use, and target cell to obtain sustained expression *in vivo*. The examples discussed previously suggest that the use of tissue-specific or housekeeping sequences for expression and/or simplified vectors that possess a single transcriptional unit are most likely to result in sustained expression *in vivo*.

2.2.5. Infection of Nondividing Cells

The foregoing discussion has focused on the development of recombinant replication-defective vectors based on murine C-type retroviruses. Recently, the potential for similarly exploiting foamy viruses and lentiviruses has been addressed. The high natural titers, large genome size, and wide host range of foamy viruses are potential advantages for vector development. A human foamy virus vector in which *env* is replaced by a reporter gene can be complemented by cotransfection with a plasmid that expresses *env* to generate a replication-deficient vector capable of stable integration (Russell and Miller, 1996). Such vectors infect non-dividing cells more efficiently than MLV vectors but still show preferential transduction of proliferating cells (Bieniasz *et al.*, 1995; Russell and Miller, 1996). The ability of HIV efficiently to infect nondividing cells (Lewis *et al.*, 1992) makes this virus particularly attractive for development as a vector. Systems based solely on HIV components can transduce $CD4^+$ cells (Poznansky *et al.*, 1991; Shimada *et al.*, 1991), but the host range of HIV can be extended by pseudotyping (Landau *et al.*, 1991). A packaging construct whose expression is driven by the CMV-IE enhancer/promoter in place of the 5′ LTR, replacement of the 3′ LTR with SV40 polyadenylation sequences, and deletion of the packaging signal complements the MLV amphotropic envelope or VSV-G for transferring a vector containing the HIV packaging signal (Naldini *et al.*, 1996). In contrast to MLV-based vectors, such vectors can stably transduce nondividing cells and nonproliferating monocyte-derived macrophages *in vitro*. Additionally, *in vivo* transduction of terminally differentiated neurones is possible. Such vectors offer great potential for gene transfer to quiescent cells, such as neurones or haematopoietic stem cells. However, for safety, vectors based on nonhuman lentiviruses are more appropriate for human gene therapy.

3. THE PACKAGING CELL

To package the retroviral vector in a virion, it must be expressed in a cell which provides the necessary retroviral proteins. These include structural proteins of the viral core encoded by the *gag* gene, enzymes necessary for viral replication encoded by the *pol* gene, and the viral envelope proteins encoded by the *env* gene. The vector genome consists of two copies of full-length mRNA contained within the viral core. Viruses bud from the plasma membrane and so acquire a lipid bilayer, surrounding the core, which contains the envelope proteins.

3.1. Viral Proteins

Two polyproteins, the gag and gag-pol precursors, are synthesized from the unspliced RNA of MLV, initiating at the same internal AUG which is preceded by an IRES (Berlioz and Darlix, 1995; Vagner *et al.*, 1995). Both polyproteins are necessary to form virions (Felsenstein and Goff, 1988). A second glycosylated *gag* product initiates at an upstream CUG. This is necessary for efficient retroviral spread *in vivo*, but is dispensable for a single round of infection (Corbin *et al.*, 1994). The gag-pol polyprotein is generated by partial read through of the *gag* stop codon, directed by a cellular suppressor tRNA (Panganiban, 1988). The gag and gag-pol polyproteins are myristylated and thus membrane associated, which is necessary for budding of virions (Gottlinger *et al.*, 1989). A sequence in the HIV and RSV gag proteins, the L-domain, located in the C-terminus of the HIV precursor (Gottlinger *et al.*, 1991) or the N-terminus of the RSV precursor (Willis *et al.*, 1994), is essential for virion budding. A similar sequence is yet to be identified in MLV. Following budding of immature virions, the protease domain at the N-terminus of the pol region cleaves the polyprotein precursors to form the mature virion (see later). Retroviral RNA and envelope proteins do not have to be incorporated for the mature core structure to form.

3.1.1. Gag Proteins

The 15-kDa matrix (MA) protein, cleaved from the N-terminus of gag, sits in the virion between the viral protein core and the plasma membrane-derived lipid envelope (Figure 4). It contains the myristyl group and other membrane attachment signals (Zhou *et al.*, 1994), which are necessary to direct correct virion assembly. In D-type retroviruses, which assemble in the cytoplasm then move to the plasma membrane, MA directs the nascent virion from one site to the other (Rhee and Hunter, 1990). MLV assembly is less complex because virions assemble directly at

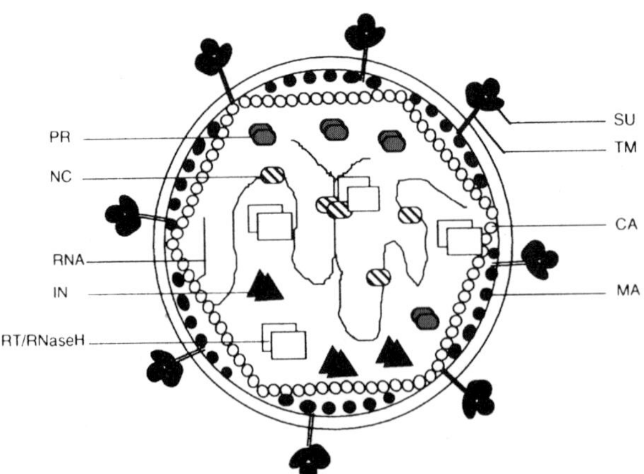

FIGURE 4. Schematic illustration of retroviral particle. The retroviral particle is enveloped by a lipid bilayer derived from the host cell in which the viral envelope is inserted, comprising surface (SU) and transmembrane (TM) domains. The matrix (MA) protein is beneath the membrane and within this the capsid (CA). Within the core are the dimeric RNA genome and other products of the *gag* and *pol* genes, including the nucleocapsid (NC), protease (PR), reverse transcriptase (RT)/RNaseH, and integrase (IN) proteins.

the plasma membrane. For some retroviruses, for example, HIV, there is evidence for sequence specific interaction between MA and the cytoplasmic tail of the envelope transmembrane (TM) protein which is necessary for envelope incorporation (Freed and Martin, 1996; Zhou *et al.*, 1994). However, there is no evidence for a similar stringent requirement for TM/MA interaction in MLV. MA may have additional function(s) in viral infectivity. This has been best described for HIV, where a nuclear localization signal (nls) in MA participates in virion core nuclear entry in nondividing cells (von-Schwedler *et al.*, 1994). MA is plasma-membrane-targeted during HIV assembly, then tyrosine phosphorylation of MA by a cell-encoded, virion-associated kinase redirects MA to the nucleus and promotes its attachment to the viral core via IN (Gallay *et al.*, 1995a,b). MLV can integrate only when the nuclear envelope breaks down during mitosis (Roe *et al.*, 1993), and so infection is restricted to dividing cells (Miller *et al.*, 1990). However, a simple substitution of MLV MA by HIV MA does not allow infection of nondividing cells (Deminie and Emerman, 1994) probably because the vpr protein of HIV is also necessary for efficient nuclear entry (Gallay *et al.*, 1996). A second block to retroviral infection at the level of completing reverse transcription is also found in truly resting (G0) cells probably caused by limiting nucleotide triphosphate levels (Goulaouic *et al.*, 1994).

Three further proteins are encoded by the *gag* region of MLV. Adjacent to MA is p12, the function of which is unknown, then the 30 kDa capsid (CA) protein, and finally the 10-kDa NC protein, which is involved in viral RNA packaging into virions (see section 2.1.2) (Figure 4). CA is the major structural protein of the viral core. Assembly of core-like structures is observed when the gag precursor is expressed in bacteria (Klikova *et al.*, 1995). Assembly efficiency is increased by the presence of RNA (Campbell and Vogt, 1995). A stretch of sequence similarity, the major homology region (MHR), is shared between retroviral CA proteins. Mutations in this region result in either a severe phenotype, where gag precursor assembly and gag-pol precursor incorporation are disrupted, or a mild phenotype, where noninfectious particles are produced (Craven *et al.*, 1995; Srinivasakumar *et al.*, 1995; Strambio-de-Castillia and Hunter, 1992). This demonstrates a role of CA in infection. There is some evidence that CA remains associated with the viral genome until integration into the target cell DNA (Bowerman *et al.*, 1989), and MLV susceptibilty of different mouse strains has identified a cellular locus, Fv, which interacts with CA at a postentry step during infection (Best *et al.*, 1996).

3.1.2. Pol Proteins

Mutational inactivation of the 14-kDa protease (PR) encoded by the 5′ end of *pol* in most retroviruses results in producing immature viral particles which are not infectious. PR cleaves both the gag precursor and the gag-pol precursor polyproteins. The protease itself constitutes a domain of the latter. When expressed as recombinant proteins, retroviral proteases correctly process gag precursors (Debouck *et al.*, 1987; Kotler *et al.*, 1988). The recently determined crystal structures of HIV and RSV proteases have provided a model for the mechanism of PR activation during virion formation. The retroviral enzymes are aspartic proteases, related to cellular aspartic proteases. However, the latter contain two structurally homologous domains whereas the retroviral protease is a monomer (Wlodawer *et al.*, 1989). This implies that the retroviral protease domains must dimerize to be active, which probably occurs when the precursor protein is assembled into virions via dimerization in the NC region (Zybarth and Carter, 1995). PR activation may start within the assembling virion (Kaplan *et al.*, 1994), although most polyprotein precursor cleavage occurs after budding. Creation of artificially linked dimer retroviral proteases results in premature precursor cleavage and inhibits virion formation (Krausslich, 1991). Following virus budding, in addition to processing the gag and gag-pol precursors, PR removes a small fragment from the cytoplasmic tail of the TM envelope protein (Rein *et al.*, 1994). The cleaved TM is fusogenic, so this mechanism prevents envelope-induced fusion of virus producing cells and allows fusion of infecting viruses.

The *pol* region additionally encodes RT/RNaseH and IN. The mechanism of proviral DNA synthesis by the RT and RNaseH enzymes was described in section 2.1.2 (see Figure 2). These two activities are carried out by a single 80-kDa protein in MLV, which probably homodimerizes to function (Telesnitsky and Goff, 1993a). Both activities are essential for viral replication. However, mutations in the two domains can complement *in trans* in phenotypically mixed virions to synthesise viral DNA (Telesnitsky and Goff, 1993b). RT is inactive in the gag-pol protein precursor. Therefore, reverse transcription starts in the virion but is completed only within the target cell (Trono, 1992). Structures for HIV and MLV RT and HIV RNaseH have been determined (Davies *et al.*, 1991; Georgiadis *et al.*, 1995; Kohlstaedt *et al.*, 1992) as has that for the catalytic domain of IN (Bujacz *et al.*, 1995), which is also cleaved from the gag-pol precursor to form a separate protein.

The 46-kDa IN is structurally a dimer and is known to multimerize for function (Engelman *et al.*, 1993; van-Gent *et al.*, 1993). It is essential for MLV replication (Donehower and Varmus, 1984) and is responsible for integrating the proviral DNA into target cell chromatin. The terminal base pairs and some adjacent sequences within the 13-bp inverted repeat at the 5′ end of U3 and the 3′ end of U5 are necessary for recognizing and cleaving the integration precursor by the MLV integrase (IN)(Murphy *et al.*, 1993). Studies of IN function have been facilitated by *in vitro* integration assays of proviral-like substrates into nonspecific target DNA, which can be catalyzed by recombinant IN in the absence of ATP (Brown *et al.*, 1987). These have demonstrated that IN recognizes the termini of linear proviral DNA (Krogstad and Champoux, 1990), then creates nicks two nucleotides from the 3′OH ends (Ishimoto *et al.*, 1991). Target DNA is also nicked on both strands, four nucleotides apart in the case of MLV IN (Dotan *et al.*, 1995). For MLV subsequent strand transfer and repair results in the loss of the terminal two bp of viral DNA and the duplication of four bp of host DNA flanking the integrated provirus. The concerted cleavage and integration of both ends of a linear substrate does not proceed efficiently *in vitro*, and some cellular functions which enhance integration have been identified (Bouille *et al.*, 1995; Kalpana *et al.*, 1994). Retroviral INs contain a conserved core catalytic site (Kulkovsky *et al.*, 1992). Some flanking regions are dispensable for *in vitro* reactions but necessary for viral infectivity

(Wiskerchen and Muesing, 1995). Retroviral integration into the target cell genome is not completely random (Shih *et al.*, 1988). Preferential sites may be directed by the local nucleosomal structure, the presence of cellular site-specific DNA proteins (Pryciak and Varmus, 1992), DNA methylation (Kitamura *et al.*, 1992), and the viral machinery itself (Pryciak and Varmus, 1992). The observation that only one daughter cell inherits the provirus after cell division indicates that integration occurs in postreplication DNA (Hajihosseini *et al.*, 1993). Attachment of a sequence-specific DNA binding domain to IN can target integration *in vitro* (Bushman, 1994; Katz *et al.*, 1996), but this remains to be achieved *in vivo*.

3.1.3. The Viral Envelope

The MLV envelope is synthesized as a precursor in the plasma membrane of the packaging cell. It is subsequently cleaved by a cellular protease to yield gp70 surface (SU) and p15E transmembrane (TM) subunits, which remain noncovalently associated. Cleavage is necessary to produce an infectious envelope (Sithanandam and Rapp, 1988). Viral env proteins are preferentially incorporated in the budding virion, but although the process excludes most other cell surface proteins, the viral envelope also contains other proteins abundant in the plasma membrane (Suomalainen and Garoff, 1994). Both SU and TM regions are involved in envelope multimerization. The mature envelope probably forms a tetramer (Li *et al.*, 1996; Pinter and Fleissner, 1979; Tucker *et al.*, 1991). The N-terminal region of SU is responsible for receptor binding (Battini *et al.*, 1992, 1995). Four strains of MLV with different receptor tropisms have been identified. The ecotropic envelope directs infection via EcoR/CAT1, a rodent amino acid transporter (Albritton *et al.*, 1989), the amphotropic envelope recognizes Ram-1, a phosphate transporter widely expressed on mammalian cells (Kavanaugh *et al.*, 1994; Miller *et al.*, 1994), the xenotropic envelope recognizes an unidentified receptor on nonrodent cells, and the 10A1 envelope recognises both Ram-1 and Galvr-1 (Miller and Miller, 1994) (see later). Packaging cells that express the first two of these envelopes are available (see section 3.2). In addition, it is possible to complement MLV cores with further C-type viral envelopes, so that packaging cells expressing MLV *gag-pol* genes and envelopes from gibbon ape leukaemia virus (GALV) (Miller *et al.*, 1991) and feline RD114 envelope (Cosset *et al.*, 1995a) have also been produced. The GALV envelope recognizes Galvr-1, a further phosphate transporter homologous to Ram-1 (O'Hara *et al.*, 1990), and the RD114 receptor is an unidentified locus on human chromosome 19 (Sommerfelt *et al.*, 1990).

This range of different envelopes allows the potential selection of an appropriate packaging cell for the species and cell lineage to be infected (Porter *et al.*, 1996). However, viral entry is not entirely controlled at the level of receptor expression. For example, the ecotropic MLV receptor requires a cofactor to permit viral entry (Wang *et al.*, 1991). There also may be specific postreceptor blocks to viral infection. Several strategies have been used to modify retroviral envelope proteins to target entry via new cell suface receptors. Small regions of SU responsible for avian leukosis virus receptor interaction have been replaced with RGD-containing peptides, which allows infection via integrins but with very low efficiency (Valesesia-

Wittman *et al.*, 1994). The MLV SU tolerates insertions of entire protein domains encoding single chain antibodies (Russell *et al.*, 1993) or peptide growth factors at its N-terminus (Cosset *et al.*, 1995b). Such envelopes are efficiently folded and incorporated into virions. When a retroviral SU receptor binding fragment is inserted at this position, efficient targeting is achieved (Valesia-Wittmann *et al.*, 1996). However, attempts to retarget retroviral infection to novel surface molecules, for example, MHC class I (Marin *et al.*, 1996), have resulted in efficient viral attachment but low titers. This probably reflects lack of an appropriate conformational change to allow fusion (see later) after binding by such modified envelopes. Several studies have also replaced the N-terminal receptor binding domain of SU with either peptide growth factors (Han *et al.*, 1995; Kasahara *et al.*, 1994), single chain antibodies (Somia *et al.*, 1995), or part of the CD4 molecule (Matano *et al.*, 1995). These chimeric envelopes can retarget infection, but they need to be coexpressed with wild-type envelope, and titers are not reproducibly high.

A flexible proline-rich hinge region separates the N-terminal receptor binding domain of SU from the C-terminal domain which interacts with TM. Multiple intramolecular disulphide bonds in the N-terminal and C-terminal domains maintain these as more rigid structures (Linder *et al.*, 1994). Mutations in the hinge of SU and in TM affect the ability of the envelope to trigger membrane fusion (Andersen, 1994; Ragheb and Anderson, 1994). The crystal structure of TM reveals many similarities to the crystal structure of the fusion peptide of influenza haemagglutinin (HA) (Fass *et al.*, 1996). As described in section 3.1.2, the cytoplasmic tail of TM must be cleaved during virion maturation to generate a fusion-competent envelope. It seems likely that a subsequent conformational change in the envelope, after SU binding to receptor, then allows TM-mediated fusion. Most C-type viral envelopes, except ecotropic MLV, fuse at neutral rather than acidic pH, suggesting that this occurs at the cell surface rather than in the endosomal pathway (McClure *et al.*, 1990). The region that directs endosomal fusion of ecotropic MLV lies in the C-terminus of SU (Nussbaum *et al.*, 1993).

The MLV envelope is glycosylated with both N- and O-linked sugars (Pinter and Honnen, 1988). Single mutations in five of seven N-linked glycosylation sites do not affect envelope function. One produces a temperature-sensitive phenotype, and one abolishes envelope incorporation (Felkner and Roth, 1992). The nature of the producer cell directs the precise sugar structures present on the envelope. For example, retroviruses produced in human cells lack terminal α(1–3)galactosyl sugars because the enzyme α(1–3)galactosyl transferase is not present in humans (Takeuchi *et al.*, 1996). This allows the production of retroviruses resistant to inactivation resulting from the binding of anti-α(1–3)galactosyl antibodies in human serum (Cosset *et al.*, 1995a). This will be important for *in vivo* gene delivery applications where exposure to human serum occurs.

3.2. Packaging Cell Lines

Packaging cell lines, into which vector sequences must be introduced to produce recombinant retroviral vectors, express viral proteins from plasmid constructs which lack the portion of φ^+ upstream of the *gag* protein start codon (Figure 1). Until recently they have all been derived from NIH3T3 cells. The first packaging cell lines, such as φ2 (Mann *et al.*, 1983) and φAM (Cone and Mulligan, 1984), contained a single stably integrated plasmid consisting of the ecotropic Moloney-MLV provirus or a derivative containing 4070A amphotropic envelope sequences, with a 351 base-pair deletion of this φ deletion. These transfer the packaging genome to target cells because the φ deletion reduces packaging efficiency only by 10^3 (Mann and Baltimore, 1985), and could also produce replication-competent virus (RCV) after a single recombination of packaging genome with vector (Otto *et al.*, 1994; Scarpa *et al.*, 1991). In the "second generation" amphotropic packaging cell PA317, the 3′ LTR and polypurine tract necessary for initiating +ve strand DNA synthesis were additionally replaced with an SV40 polyadenylation sequence (Miller and Buttimore, 1986). This modification reduces the occurrence of RCV because two recombination events between genome and vector are required. Additionally, part of the 5′ LTR necessary for integration was deleted in a further safeguard against inadvertent transfer of the construct. "Third-generation" lines, such as the ecotropic envelope expressing GP + E86 (Markowitz *et al.*, 1988b) and φCRE (Danos and Mulligan, 1988), or the amphotropic GP + envAm12 (Markowitz *et al.*, 1988a) and φCRIP (Danos and Mulligan, 1988), which are currently widely used, supply *gag-pol* and *env* genes on separate stably integrated expression plasmids, both of which lack φ and the 3′ LTR (the so-called "split-packaging" strategy; Figure 5) and require multiple recombinations to generate RCV. Further modifications to minimize the extent and sequence homology of overlappring regions between the individual helper plasmids and the vector, as in the Babe vector/ΩE packaging cell system, should still further reduce the probability of recombination (Morgenstern and Land, 1990). RCV-free virus stocks, however, may still transfer individual packaging functions at low frequency (Kozak and Kabat, 1990). This is undesirable because a proportion of infected cells will express viral proteins and has been reduced in the newer FLYA13 cells by removing further viral sequences from the packaging constructs (Cosset *et al.*, 1995a). Although many improvements have been made on the original systems, packaging cell optimization is still at an early stage and further strategies for improving viral protein expression remain open. Thus, the Ampli-GPE system uses episomal amplification of plasmids that contain bovine papilloma virus sequences (Takahara *et al.*, 1992), FLYA13 cells employ a strategy for reinitiating translation for selectable marker expression (Cosset *et al.*, 1995a), and ProPak-A uses the strong CMV IE promoter (Rigg *et al.*, 1996) to achieve high levels of *gag-pol* and *env* gene expression. The latter two packaging cells are based on human HT1080 and 293 cells, respectively. Table I lists the currently available packaging cells for murine C-type retroviruses.

The sensitivity of a virus to inactivation in the presence of human serum may be a consideration in some instances of gene therapy application of retroviral vectors which may influence choice of packaging cells. This can be overcome by producing virus in cells lacking α(1–3)galactosyl transferase activity, such as the newer human cell-based packaging cells (Cosset *et al.*, 1995a; Rigg *et al.*, 1996), or by using derivatives of murine packaging cells in which expression of this epitope is down-regulated (Rother *et al.*, 1995).

Table I
Packaging Cell Systems

Packaging cell line	Parental cell line	Nature of packaging constructs	Drug resistance	Tropism/ envelope	Reference
A. Retroviral envelope packaging cell systems					
ψ2	3T3	LTR,ψ^-,*gag-pol*,*env*,LTR	gpt	Ecotropic	Mann *et al.*, 1983
ψAM	3T3	LTR,ψ^-,*gag-pol*,4070A*env*,LTR	gpt	Amphotropic	Cone and Mulligan, 1984
PA12	3T3tk^-	LTR,ψ^-,*gag-pol*,4070A*env*,LTR	HSV-TK	Amphotropic	Miller *et al.*, 1985[a]
PE501	3T3tk^-	LTR,ψ^-,*gag-pol*,*env*,ppt^-,SV40pA	HSV-TK	Ecotropic	Miller and Rosman, 1989[b]
PA317	3T3tk^-	LTR,ψ^-,*gag-pol*,4070A*env*,ppt^-,SV40pA	HSV-TK	Amphotropic	Miller and Buttimore, 1986
Clone 32	3T3	mMT-I,SD^-,ψ^-,*gag-pol*,*env*,LTR mMT-I,SD^-,ψ^-,*env*,LTR	neo	Ecotropic	Bosselman *et al.*, 1987[c]
ψCRE	3T3	LTR,ψ^-,*gag-pol*,*env*(x),SV40pA LTR,ψ^-,*gag-pol*(x),*env*,SV40pA	hygro gpt	Ecotropic	Danos and Mulligan, 1988
ψCRIP	3T3	LTR,ψ^-,*gag-pol*,*env*(x),SV40pA LTR,ψ^-,*gag-pol*(x),4070A*env*,SV40pA	hygro gpt	Amphotropic	Danos and Mulligan, 1988
GP+E−86	3T3	LTR,ψ^-,*gag-pol* LTR,ψ^-,*env*	gpt	Ecotropic	Markowitz *et al.*, 1988b
GP+envAm12	3T3	LTR,ψ^-,*gag-pol* LTR,ψ^-,4070A*env*	gpt hygro	Amphotropic	Markowitz *et al.*, 1988a
ΩE	3T3	LTR($U5^-$),SD^-,ψ^-,*gag-pol*,SV40pA LTR($U5^-$),SD^-,ψ^-,*env*,SV40pA	gpt	Ecotropic	Morgenstern and Land, 1990
PG13	3T3tk^-	LTR,ψ^-,*gag-pol*,SV40pA LTR,ψ^-,$GALV_{Seato}$*env*,SV40pA	HSV-TK dhfr	GALV	Miller *et al.*, 1991
AmpliGPE	3T3	mMT-I,SD^-,ψ^-,*gag-pol*,β-globinpA,BPV mMT-I,SD^-,ψ^-,*env*,β-globinpA,BPV	neo	Ecotropic	Takahara *et al.*, 1992
FLYA13	HT1080	LTR,ψ^-,*gag-pol*,SV40pA LTR,ψ^-,4070A*env*,SV40pA	bsr phleo	Amphotropic	Cosset *et al.*, 1995a

FLYRD18	HT1080	LTR,ψ^-,*gag-pol*,SV40pA LTR,ψ^-,RD114$_{SC3C}$*env*,SV40pA	bsr phleo	RD114	Cosset *et al.*, 1995a
ProPak-A	293	CMV-IE,SD$^-$,ψ^-,*gag-pol*,SV40pA CMV-IE,SD$^-$,y$^-$,4070A*env*,SV40pA	puro hygro	Amphotropic	Rigg *et al.*, 1996
B. VSV-G pseudotrype packaging cell systems					
	293	CMV-IE,SD$^-$,ψ^-,*gag-pol*,SV40pA CMV-IE,VSV-G,βglobinpA (transient transfection)	dhfr	Pantropic	Yee *et al.*, 1994
GP7c−tTA−G10	3T3tk$^-$	SV40early,SD$^-$,ψ^-,*gag-pol*,SV40pA CMV-IE,tet^R/VP16,SV40pA (tet^0)$_7$-CMV$_{minimal}$,VSV-G,SV40pA	hygro puro HSV-TK	Pantropic	Yang *et al.*, 1995
293GP/tTAER/G	293	CMV-IE,SD$^-$,ψ^-,*gag-pol*,SV40pA CMV-IE,tet^R/VP16/ER,βglobinpA (tet^0)$_7$-CMV$_{minimal}$,VSV-G,SV40pA	dhfr hygro puro	Pantropic	Chen *et al.*, 1996

[a]gpt, [b]HSV-TK, [c]neo, [d]hygro, [e]dhfr, [f]bsr, [g]phleo, [h]puro; drug resistance marker genes xanthine-guanine phosphoribosyl transferase, herpes simplex virus thymidine kinase, neomycin phosphotransferase, hygromycin B phosphotransferase, dihydrofolate reductase, blastic din S deaminase, bleomycin (phleomycin) binding protein, puromycin N-acetyl transferase.
[i]4070A*env*: envelope from amphotropic MLV strain 4070.
[j]ppt: polypurine tract.
[k]SV40pA: β-globinpA; polyadenylation signal from SV40 virus or β-globin gene.
[l]mMT-I: murine metallothionein I promoter.
[m]SD: retroviral splice donor site.
[n]*env*(x), *gag-pol*(x): *env*, *gag-pol* gene sequences present but mutated to prevent expression.
[o]GALV$_{Seato}$*env*, RD114$_{SC3C}$*env*: envelope from gibbon ape leukaemia virus strain Seato or RD114 virus strain SC3C.
[p]BPV: bovine papilloma virus sequences for episomal maintenance.
[q]CMV-IE: cytomegalovirus immediate-early promoter.
[r]SV40 early: SV40 virus early promoter.
[s]tet^R/VP16: tetracycline transactivator: fusion of tet repressor and activation domain of herpes simplex virus virion protein 16, active in absence of tetracycline.
[t](tet^0)$_7$-CMV$_{minimal}$: minimal cytomegalovirus promoter linked to seven tandem tetracycline repressor binding sites.
[u]tet^R/VP16/ER: fusion of hormone binding domain of estrogen receptor to tet^R/VP16, requiring presence of estrogen for activation in absence of tetracycline.

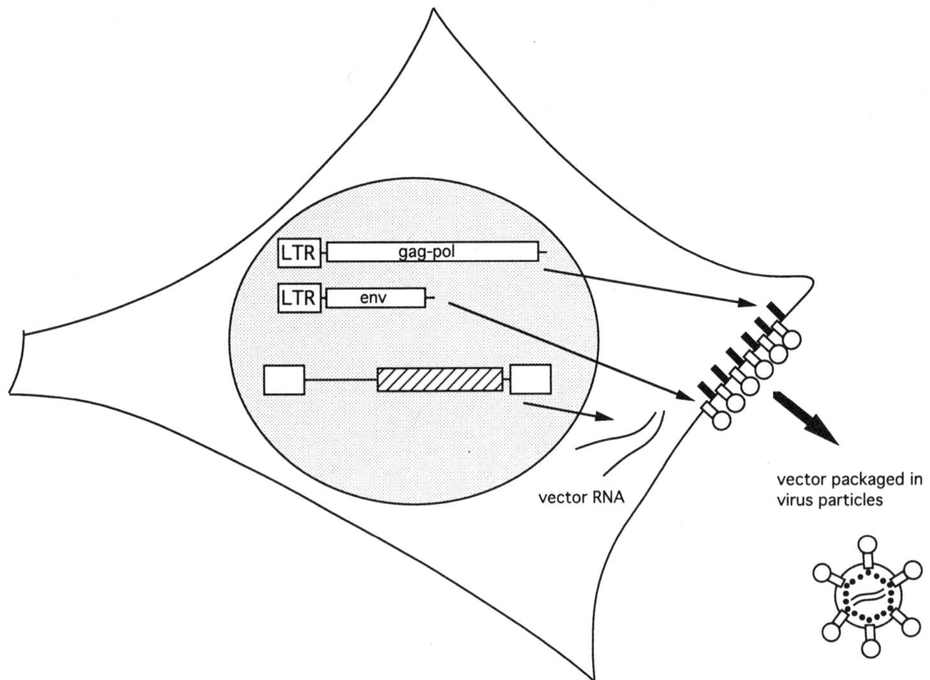

FIGURE 5. Retroviral vector packaging cell. The "split packaging" strategy for constructing a packaging cell is illustrated. Separately transfected constructs drive expression of the *gag-pol* and *env* genes. Signals involved in replication and packaging but unnecessary for expression of these genes are deleted to prevent transmission of the packaging functions and to minimize recombination with vector sequences. After transfection of the vector construct, the derived mRNA is packaged as a recombinant viral particle.

3.2.1. Envelope Pseudotyping

The widely used third-generation packaging cells referred to previously are available for producing recombinant retroviruses that bear MLV envelopes with either an ecotropic or amphotropic host range. Additionally, the cell lines PG13 and FLYRD18 (analogous to FLYA13) are available for producing viruses pseudotyped with the envelopes of the retroviruses GALV (Miller *et al.*, 1991) and RD114 (Cosset *et al.*, 1995a). Like the amphotropic envelope, these alternatives also have wide tropisms, but their envelopes utilize different cell surface receptors which may offer advantages for some applications (Bauer *et al.*, 1995; Bunnell *et al.*, 1995; Porter *et al.*, 1996). The RD114 envelope used in the human FLYRD18 packaging cells is particularly resistant to serum inactivation (Takeuchi *et al.*, 1994). Recently, a system has been developed for pseudotyping retroviral constructs with the envelope of vesicular stomatitis virus (VSV). The advantages of such vectors are that the broad host range of VSV allows generating "pantropic" vectors, and the VSV envelope permits concentrating virions by ultracentrifugation (Burns *et al.*, 1993), a technique which is problematic with retroviral envelopes because the noncovalently associated SU protein detaches from the virion. Expression of the VSV-G protein alone is sufficient to pseudotype retroviral core particles (Emi *et al.*, 1991) but establishing stable packaging cell lines has not been trivial because of the toxicity of continued expression of this protein in mammalian cells. The initial method involved encoding VSV-G within the retroviral vector (Burns *et al.*, 1993). A more generally applicable version involves stable introduction of the vector into 293 cells expressing *gag-pol* and transient virus harvest after transfecting a construct for high expression of VSV-G (Yee *et al.*, 1994). In addition to infecting mammalian cells, such pseudotyped vectors have been used to infect cells of vertebrate and invertebrate organisms outside of the tropism of any of the retroviral envelopes. More recently, stable packaging cells, in which expression of VSV-G is inducible upon tetracycline withdrawal (Yang *et al.*, 1995) and estrogen induction (Chen *et al.*, 1996) have been described. Table I includes available packaging systems for pseudotyped murine C-type retroviruses.

3.2.2. Replication-Competent Virus

As alluded to previously, great consideration to the possibilities for producing RCV has been given during the development of retroviral packaging systems. The initial packaging cells, such as φ2 and PA317, generate RCV following single recombination between regions of homology in the vector and plasmids encoding packaging functions (Otto *et al.*, 1994; Scarpa *et al.*, 1991). This readily occurs if multiple rounds of infection are encouraged, for example, by using the "ping-pong" method to enhance viral titers by cocultivating packaging cells (Muenchau *et al.*, 1990). Packaging systems based on the "split packaging" strategy are safer because they require multiple recombinations to generate RCV. The first detection of RCV in such a packaging cell (GP + envAm-12) was reported only recently, despite the wide usage of this cell line (Chong and Vile, 1996). The significance of the presence of RCV in retroviral vector preparations is illustrated by the induction of T cell lymphoma in rhesus monkeys after gene transfer to bone marrow cells with RCV-contaminated stocks (Donahue *et al.*, 1992). Although murine amphotropic RCV is not pathogenic in rhesus monkeys after intravenous injection or implantation of virus-producing autologous cells (Cornetta *et al.*, 1990) a chronic infection arose in these animals, perhaps related to their immunosuppression, leading to transformation by insertional mutagenesis (Vanin *et al.*, 1994). RCV may occur following vector/packaging plasmid recombination and also after recombination with endogenous mink cell focus-forming sequences present in murine packaging cells.

3.2.3. Endogenous Retroviral Sequences

In addition to the production of RCV, a further safety consideration is the packaging of endogenous retroviral sequences expressed in the packaging cell lines.

Mouse cells express the endogenous VL30 sequence at high levels, so virus from packaging cell lines based on NIH3T3 cells contains equivalent amounts of vector and VL30 sequences (Scadden *et al.*, 1990). The extensive analysis of RCV transfer in the rhesus monkey experiment referred to previously also revealed the transfer of several other murine endogenous elements (Purcell *et al.*, 1996). The human cell lines used to make FLYA13/RD18 and ProPak-A cells are not known to express any endogenous viral genomes which can be packaged (Cosset *et al.*, 1995a; Rigg *et al.*, 1996). However, use of human cells to prepare clinical reagents may not be ideal because there would presumably be no barrier to transmitting any as yet unknown human viruses.

3.2.4. Transient Packaging Systems

For retroviral applications where a large batch of high titer, safety-tested virus is desirable, the stable transfection of a packaging cell line with vector plasmid remains the best approach. However, this is time-consuming because many individual clones must be selected and assessed for viral titer to obtain the best producer cell. An alternative, which is suitable for producing small batches of virus, is to use virus harvested after transient transfection. This may be of particular value for viruses that encode toxic products not suitable for producing stable transfectants but is also convenient when rapid comparison of different vectors is required. Transient transfection of vector plasmids into the packaging cell lines described previously generally results in low titer virus, so a number of systems have been developed that are more suited to transient virus production. The first such system involved cotransfection of helper and vector plasmids bearing SV40 origins of replication into COS-7 cells (Landau and Littman, 1992). BOSC-23 is a stably transfected packaging cell, based on 293T cells, which uses the same helper plasmids as φCRE and the high transfection efficiencies attainable with these cells to yield high titers of ecotropic virus following transient transfection of vector (Pear *et al.*, 1993). An amphotropic version, CAK8 (or BING), is available (ATCC 11554-CRL) although unpublished. Because these cells express SV40 T antigen, the presence of an SV40 origin of replication on the vector plasmid should enhance transient vector RNA expression. Two other systems also exploit the high transfection efficiencies attainable with 293 cells and require cotransfection of helper and vector plasmids (Finer *et al.*, 1994; Soneoka *et al.*, 1995). Both utilize the strong CMV IE enhancer/promoter to express helper functions and vector, which can be enhanced further by including SV40 origins and using 293T cells (Soneoka *et al.*, 1995).

4. REFERENCES

Adam, M., 1988, Identification of a signal in a murine retrovirus that is sufficient for packaging of non retroviral RNA into virions, *J. Virol.* **62:**3802–3806.

Adam, M., Osborne, W., and Miller, A., 1995, R-region cDNA inserts in retroviral vectors are compatible with virus replication and high-level protein synthesis from the insert, *Hum. Gene. Ther.* **6:**1169–1176.

Akgun, E., Ziegler, M., and Grez, M., 1991, Determinants of retrovirus gene expression in embryonal carcinoma cells, *J. Virol.* **65:**382–388.

Albritton, L., Tseng, L., Scadden, D., and Cunningham, J., 1989, A putative murine ecotropic retrovirus receptor gene encodes a multiple membrane-spanning protein and confers susceptibility to virus infection, *Cell* **57:**659–666.

Allain, B., Lapadat-Tapolsky, M., Berlioz, C., and Darlix, J., 1994, Transactivation of the minus-strand DNA transfer by nucleocapsid protein during reverse transcription of the retroviral genome, *EMBO J.* **13:**973–981.

Andersen, K., 1994, A domain of murine retrovirus surface protein gp70 mediates cell fusion, as shown in a novel SC-1 cell fusion system, *J. Virol.* **68:**3175–3182.

Aran, J., Gottesman, M., and Pastan, I., 1994, Drug-selected coexpression of human glucocerebrosidase and P-glycoprotein using a bicistronic vector, *Proc. Natl. Acad. Sci. USA* **91:**3176–3180.

Artelt, P., Grannemann, R., Stocking, C., Friel, J., Bartsch, J., and Hauser, H., 1991, The prokaryotic neomycin-resistance-encoding gene acts as a transcriptional silencer in eukaryotic cells, *Gene* **99:**249–254.

Barat, C., Lullien, V., Schatz, O., Keith, G., Nugeyre, M., Gruninger-Leitch, F., Barre-Sinoussi, F., LeGrice, S., and Darlix, J., 1989, HIV-1 reverse transcriptase specifically interacts with the anticodon domain of its cognate primer tRNA, *EMBO J.* **8:**3279–3285.

Barklis, E., Mulligan, R., and Jaenisch, R., 1986, Chromosomal position or virus mutation permits retrovirus expression in embryonal carcinoma cells, *Cell* **47:**391–399.

Battini, J., Danos, O., and Heard, J., 1995, Receptor-binding domain of murine leukaemia virus envelope glycoproteins, *J. Virol.* **69:**713–719.

Battini, J., Heard, J., and Danos, O., 1992, Receptor choice determinants in the envelope glycoproteins of amphotropic, xenotropic, and polytropic murine leukemia viruses, *J. Virol.* **66:**1468–1475.

Bauer, T., Miller, A., and Hickstein, D., 1995, Improved transfer of the leukocyte integrin CD18 subunit into hematopoietic cell lines by using retroviral vectors having a gibbon ape leukemia virus envelope, *Blood* **86:**2379–2387.

Baum, C., Hegewisch Becker, S., Eckert, H., Stocking, C., and Ostertag, W., 1995, Novel retroviral vectors for efficient expression of the multidrug resistance (mdr-1) gene in early hematopoietic cells, *J. Virol.* **69:**7541–7547.

Bender, M., Palmer, T., Gelinas, R., and Miller, A., 1987, Evidence that the packaging signal of Moloney murine leukemia virus extends into the gag region, *J. Virol.* **61:**1639–1646.

Benz, E., Wydro, R., Nadal-Ginard, B., and Dino, D., 1980, Moloney murine sarcoma proviral DNA is a transcriptional unit, *Nature* **288:**665–669.

Berlioz, C., and Darlix, J.-L., 1995, An internal ribosomal entry mechanism promotes translation of murine leukaemia virus gag polyprotein precursors, *J. Virol.* **69:**2214–2222.

Best, S., Tissier, P. L., Towers, G., and Stoye, J., 1996, Positional cloning of the mouse retrovirus restriction element Fv1, *Nature* **382:**826–829.

Bieniasz, P., Weiss, R., and McClure, M., 1995, Cell cycle dependence of foamy retrovirus infection, *J. Virol.* **69:**7295–7299.

Blaese, R., Culver, K., Miller, A., Carter, C., Fleisher, T., Clerici, M., Shearer, G., Chang, L., Chiang, Y., Tolstoshev, P., Greenblatt, J., Rosenberg, S., Klein, H., Berger, M., Mullen, C., Ramsey, W., Muul, L., Morgan, R., and Anderson, W., 1995, T lymphocyte-directed gene therapy for ADA- SCID: Initial trial results after 4 years, *Science* **270:**475–480.

Bordignon, C., Notarangelo, L., Nobili, N., Ferrari, G., Casorati, G., Panina, P., Mazzolari, E., Maggioni, D., Rossi, C., Servida, P., Ugazio, A., and Mavilio, F., 1995, Gene therapy in peripheral blood lymphocytes and bone marrow for ADA- immunodeficient patients, *Science* **270:**470–475.

Bouille, P., Subra, F., Goulaouic, H., Carteau, S., and Auclair, C., 1995, Impairment of Moloney murine leukaemia virus integration in a cell line underexpressing DNA topoisomerase II, *Cancer Res.* **55:**3211–3217.

Bosselman. R. A., Hsu, R.-Y., Bruszewski, J., Hu, S., Martin, F., and Nicolson, N., 1987, Replication-defective chimeric helper proviruses and factors affecting generation of competent virus: Expression of Moloney murine leukemia virus structural genes via the metallothionein promoter, *Mol. Cell Biol.* **7:**1797–1806.

Bowerman, B., Brown, P., Bishop, J., and Varmus, H., 1989, A nucleoprotein complex mediates the integration of retroviral DNA, *Genes Dev.* **3:**469–478.

Brown, P., Bowerman, B., Varmus, H., and Bishop, J., 1987, Correct integration of retroviral DNA in vitro, *Cell* **49:**347–356.

Bujacz, G., Jaskolski, M., Alexandratos, J., Wlodawer, A., Merkel, G., Katz, R., and Skalka, A., 1995, High-resolution structure of the catalytic domain of avian sarcoma virus integrase, *J. Mol. Biol.* **253:**333–346.

Bunnell, B., Muul, L., Donahue, R., Blaese, R., and Morgan, R., 1995, High efficiency retroviral-mediated gene transfer into human and nonhuman primate peripheral blood lymphocytes, *Proc. Natl. Acad. Sci. USA* **90:**8033–8037.

Burns, J., Friedmann, T., Driever, W., Burrascano, M., and Yee, J., 1993, VSV-G pseudotyped retroviral vectors: concentration to very high titer and efficient gene transfer into mammalian and nonmammalian cells, *Proc. Natl. Acad. Sci. USA* **90:**8033–8037.

Bushman, F., 1994, Tethering HIV-1 integrase to a DNA site directs integration to nearby sequences, *Proc. Natl. Acad. Sci. USA* **91:**9233–9237.

Byun, J., Kim, S.-H., Kim, J., Yu, S. S., Robbins, P., Yim, J., and Kim, S., 1996, Analysis of the relative level of gene expression from different retroviral vectors used for gene therapy, *Gene Ther.* **3:**780–788.

Campbell, S., and Vogt, V., 1995, Self-assembly in vitro of purified CA-NC proteins from RSV and HIV-1, *J. Virol.* **69:**6487–6499.

Cepko, C., Roberts, B., and Mulligan, R., 1984, Construction and applications of a highly transmissible murine retrovirus shuttle vector, *Cell* **37:**1053–1062.

Challita, P.-M., and Kohn, D., 1994, Lack of expression from a retroviral vector after transduction of murine hematopoietic stem cells is associated with methylation in vivo, *Proc. Natl. Acad. Sci. USA* **91:**2567–2571.

Challita, P.-M., Skelton, D., El-Khoueiry, A., Yu, X.-J., Einberg, K., and Kohn, D., 1995, Multiple modifications in cis elements of the long terminal repeat of retroviral vectors lead to increased expression and decreased DNA methylation in embryonic carcinoma cells, *J. Virol.* **69:**748–755.

Chen, B., Hwang, L., and Chen, D., 1993, Characterisation of a bicistronic retroviral vector composed of the swine vesicular disease virus internal ribosome entry site, *J. Virol.* **67:**2142–2148.

Chen, B.-F., Chang, W.-C., Chen, S.-T., Chen, D.-S., and Hwang, L.-H., 1995, Long-term expression of the biologically active growth hormone in genetically modified fibroblasts after implantation into a hypophysectomized rat, *Hum. Gene Ther.* **6:**917–926.

Chen, S.-T., Iida, A., Guo, L., Friedmann, T., and Yee, J.-K., 1996, Generation of packaging cell lines for pseudotyped retroviral vectors of the G protein of vesicular stomatitis virus by using a modified tetracycline inducible system, *Proc. Natl. Acad. Sci. USA* **93:**10057–10062.

Cherrington, J., and Ganem, D., 1992, Regulation of polyadenylation in HIV; contribution of promoter proximity and upstream sequences, *EMBO J.* **11:**1513–1524.

Chong, H., and Vile, R., 1996, Replication-competent retrovirus produced by a "split-function" third generation amphotropic packaging cell line, *Gene Ther.* **3:**624–629.

Chowdhury, J., Grossman, M., Gupta, S., Chowdhury, N., Baker, J., and Wilson, J., 1991, Long-term improvement of hypercholesterolemia after ex vivo gene therapy in LDLR-deficient rabbits, *Science* **254:**1802–1805.

Cone, R., and Mulligan, R., 1984, High-efficiency gene transfer into mammalian cells: Generation of helper-free recombinant retrovirus with broad mammalian host-range, *Proc. Acad. Natl. Sci. USA* **81:**6349–6353.

Cone, R., Weber-Benarous, A., Baorto, D., and Mulligan, R., 1987, Regulated expression of a complete human beta-globin gene encoded by a transmissible retrovirus vector, *Mol. Cell. Biol.* **7:**887–897.

Corbin, A., Prats, A., Darlix, J.-L., and Sitbon, M., 1994, A nonstructural gag-encoded glycoprotein is necessary for efficient spreading and pathogenesis of murine leukaemia virus, *J. Virol.* **68:**3857–3867.

Cornetta, K., Moen, R., Culver, K., Morgan, R., McLachlin, J., Sturm, S., Selegue, J., London, W., Blaese, R., and Anderson, W., 1990, Amphotropic murine leukemia retrovirus is not an acute pathogen for primates, *Hum. Gene Ther.* **1:**15–30.

Correll, P., Colclla, S., and Karlsson, S., 1994, Retroviral vector design for long-term expression in murine hematopoietic cells in vivo, *Blood* **84:**18112–1822.

Cosset, F., Takeuchi, Y., Battini, J., Weiss, R., and Collins, M., 1995a, High titre packaging cells producing recombinant retroviruses resistant to human serum, *J. Virol.* **69:**7430–7436.

Cosset, F.-L., Morling, F., Takeuchi, Y., Weiss, R., Collins, M., and Russell, S., 1995b, Retroviral retargeting by envelopes expressing an N-terminal binding domain, *J. Virol.* **69:**7430–7436.

Couture, L., Mullen, C., and Morgan, R., 1994, Retroviral vector containing chimaeric promoter/enhancer elements exhibit cell-type-specific gene expression, *Hum. Gene Ther.* **5:**667–677.

Craven, R., Leure-duPree, A., Weldon, R., and Wills, J., 1995, Genetic analysis of the major homology region of the RSV gag protein, *J. Virol.* **69:**4213–4227.

Dai, Y., Roman, M., Naviaux, R., and Verma, I., 1992, Gene therapy via primary myoblasts: Long-term expression of factor IX protein following transplantation in vivo, *Proc. Natl. Acad. Sci. USA* **89:**10892–10895.

Danos, O., and Mulligan, R., 1988, Safe and efficient generation of recombinant retroviruses with amphotropic and ecotropic host ranges, *Proc. Natl. Acad. Sci. USA* **85:**6460–6464.

Davies, J., Hostomska, Z., Hostomsky, Z., Jordan, S., and Matthews, D., 1991, Crystal structure of the ribonuclease H domain of HIV-1 reverse transcriptase, *Science* **252:**88–95.

Debouck, C., Gorniak, J., Strickler, J., Meek, T., Metcalf, B., and Rosenberg, M., 1987, HIV protease expressed in *E. coli* exhibits autoprocessing and specific maturation of the gag precursor, *Proc. Natl. Acad. Sci. USA* **84:**8903–8906.

Deminie, C., and Emerman, M., 1994, Functional exchange of an oncoretrovirus and a lentivirus matrix protein, *J. Virol.* **68:**4442–4449.

Donahue, R., Kessler, S., Bodine, D., McDonagh, K., Dunbar, C., Goodman, S., Agricola, B., Byrne, E., Raffeld, M., Moen, R., Bacher, J., Zsebo, K., and Nienhuis, A., 1992, Helper virus induced T cell lymphoma in nonhuman primates after retroviral mediated gene transfer, *J. Exp. Med.* **176:**1125–1135.

Donehower, L., and Varmus, H., 1984, A mutant murine leukaemia virus with a single missense codon in pol is defective in a function affecting integration, *Proc. Natl. Acad. Sci. USA* **81:**6461–6465.

Dotan, I., Scottoline, B., Heuer, T., and Brown, P., 1995, Characterization of recombinant murine leukaemia virus integrase, *J. Virol.* **69:**456–468.

Dougherty, J., and Temin, H., 1987, A promoterless retroviral vector indicates that there are sequences in U3 required for 3′ RNA processing, *Proc. Natl. Acad. Sci. USA* **84:**1197–1201.

Dranoff, G., Jaffee, E., Lazenby, A., Golumbek, P., Levitsky, H., Brose, K., Jackson, V., Hamada, H., Pardoll, D., and Mulligan, R., 1993, Vaccination with irradiated tumor cells engineered to secrete murine granulocyte-macrophage colony-stimulating factor stimulates potent, specific, and long-lasting anti-tumor immunity, *Proc. Natl. Acad. Sci. USA* **90:**3539–3543.

Emerman, M., and Temin, H., 1984, Genes with promoters in retrovirus vectors can be independently suppressed by an epigenetic mechanism, *Cell* **39:**459–467.

Emerman, M., and Temin, H., 1986, Comparison of promoter suppression in avian and murine retrovirus vectors, *Nucleic Acids Res.* **14:**9381–9396.

Emi, N., Friedmann, T., and Yee, J., 1991, Pseudotype formation of murine leukaemia virus with the G protein of vesicular stomatitis virus, *J. Virol.* **65:**1202–1207.

Engelman, A., Bushman, F., and Craigie, R., 1993, Identification of discrete functional domains of HIV-1 integrase and their organization within an active multimeric complex, *EMBO J.* **12:**3269–3275.

Fass, D., Harrison, S., and Kim, P., 1996, Retrovirus envelope domain at 1.7A resolution, *Nat. Struct. Biol.* **3:**465–469.

Felkner, R., and Roth, M., 1992, Mutational analysis of the N-linked glycosylation sites of the SU envelope protein of Moloney murine leukaemia virus, *J. Virol.* **66:**4258–4264.

Felsenstein, K., and Goff, S., 1988, Expression of the gag-pol fusion protein of Moloney murine leukaemia virus without gag protein does not induce virion formation or proteolytic processing, *J. Virol.* **62:**2179–2182.

Ferrari, G., Salvatori, G., Rossi, C., Cossu, G., and Mavilio, F., 1995, A retrovirus vector containing a muscle-specific enhancer drives gene expression only in differentiated muscle fibers, *Hum. Gene Ther.* **6:**733–742.

Finer, M., Dull, T., Qin, L., Farson, D., and Roberts, M., 1994, kat: A high-efficiency retroviral transduction system for primary human T lymphocytes, *Blood* **83:**43–50.

Flanagan, J., Becker, K., Ennist, D., Gleason, S., Driggers, P., Levi, B.-Z., Appella, E., and Ozato, K., 1991, Cloning of a negative transcription factor that binds to the upstream conserved region of Moloney murine leukemia virus, *Mol. Cell. Biol.* **12:**38–44.

Freed, E., and Martin, M., 1996, Domains of the HIV-1 matrix and gp41 cytoplasmic tail required for envelope incorporation into virions, *J. Virol.* **70:**341–351.

Gallay, P., Stitt, V., Mundy, C., Oettinger, M., and Trono, D., 1996, Role of the karyopherin pathway in HIV-1 nuclear import, *J. Virol.* **70:**1027–1032.

Gallay, P., Swingler, S., Aitken, C., and Trono, D., 1995a, HIV-1 infection of nondividing cells: C-terminal phosphorylation of the viral matrix protein is a key regulator, *Cell* **80:**379–388.

Gallay, P., Swingler, S., Song, J., Bushman, F., and Trono, D., 1995b, HIV nuclear import is governed by the phosphotyrosine-mediated binding of matrix to the core domain of integrase, *Cell* **83:**569–576.

Georgiadis, M., Jessen, S., Ogata, C., Telesnitsky, A., and Goff, S., 1995, Mechanistic implications from the structure of a catalytic fragment of Moloney murine leukaemia virus reverse transcriptase, *Structure* **3:**879–892.

Ghattas, I., Sanes, J., and Majors, J., 1991, The encephalomyocarditis virus internal ribosome entry site allow efficient coexpression of two genes from a recombinant provirus in cultured cells and embryos, *Mol. Cell. Biol.* **11:**5848–5859.

Gorman, C., Rigby, P., and Lane, D., 1985, Negative regulation of viral enhancers in undifferentiated embryonic stem cells, *Cell* **42:**519–526.

Gottlinger, H., Dorfman, T., Sodroski, J., and Haseltine, W., 1991, Effect of mutations affecting the p6 gag protein on human immunodeficiency virus particle release, *Proc. Natl. Acad. Sci. USA* **88:**3195–3199.

Gottlinger, H., Sodroski, J., and Haseltine, W., 1989, Role of capsid precursor processing and myristoylation in morphogenisis and infectivity of human immunodeficiency virus type 1, *Proc. Natl. Acad. Sci. USA* **86:**5781–5785.

Goulaouic, H., Subra, F., Mouscadet, J., Carteau, S., and Auclair, C., 1994, Exogenous nucleosides promote the completion of MoMLV DNA synthesis in G0-arrested Balb c/3T3 fibroblasts, *Virology* **200:**87–97.

Grez, M., Akgun, E., Hilberg, F., and Ostertag, W., 1990, Embryonic stem cell virus, a recombinant murine retrovirus with expression in embryonic stem cells, *Proc. Natl. Acad. Sci. USA* **87:**9202–9206.

Grez, M., Zornig, M., Nowock, J., and Ziegler, M., 1991, A single point mutation activates the Moloney murine leukemia virus long terminal repeat in embryonal carcinoma cells, *J. Virol.* **65:**4691–4698.

Hafenrichter, D., Wu, X., Rettinger, S., Kennedy, S., Flye, M., and Ponder, K., 1994, Quantitative evaluation of liver-specific promoters from retroviral vectors after in vivo transduction of hepatocytes, *Blood* **84:**3394–3404.

Hajihosseini, M., Iavachev, L., and Price, J., 1993, Evidence that retroviruses integrate into post-replication host DNA, *EMBO J.* **12:**4969–4974.

Han, X., Kasahara, N., and Kan, Y., 1995, Ligand-directed retroviral targeting of human breast cancer cells, *Proc. Natl. Acad. Sci. USA* **92:**9747–9751.

Hantzopoulos, P., Sullenger, B., Ungers, G., and Gilboa, E., 1989, Improved gene expression upon transfer of the adenosine deaminase minigene outside the transciptional unit of a retroviral vector, *Proc. Natl. Acad. Sci. USA* **86:**3519–3523.

Housset, V., De-Rocquigny, H., Roques, B., and Darlix, J., 1993, Basic amino acids flanking the zinc finger of Moloney murine leukaemia virus nucleocapsid protein NCp10 are critical for virus infectivity, *J. Virol.* **67:**2537–2545.

Ishimoto, L., Halperin, M., and Champoux, J., 1991, Moloney murine leukaemia virus IN protein from disrupted virions binds and specifically cleaves its target sequence in vitro, *Virology* **180:**527–534.

Kaleko, M., Garcia, J., Osborne, W., and Miller, A., 1990, Expression of human adenosine deaminase in mice after transplantation of genetically-modified bone marrow, *Blood* **8:**1733–1741.

Kalpana, G., Marmon, S., Wang, W., Crabtree, G., and Goff, S., 1994, Binding and stimulation of HIV-1 integrase by a human homolog of yeast transcription factor SNF5, *Science* **266:**2002–2006.

Kaplan, A., Manchester, M., and Swanstrom, R., 1994, The activity of the protease of HIV-1 is initiated at the membrane of infected cells before the release of viral proteins and is required for release to occur with maximum efficiency, *J. Virol.* **68:**6782–6786.

Kasahara, N., Dozy, A., and Kan, Y., 1994, Tissue-specific targeting of retroviral vectors through ligand-receptor interactions, *Science* **266:**1373–1376.

Katz, R., Merkel, G., and Skalka, A., 1996, Targeting of retroviral integrase by fusion to a heterologous DNA binding domain: In vitro activities and incorporation of a fusion protein into viral particles, *Virology* **217:**178–190.

Kavanaugh, M., Miller, D., Zhang, W., Law, W., Kozak, S., Kabat, D., and Miller, A., 1994, Cell-surface receptors for gibbon ape leukemia virus and amphotropic murine retrovirus are inducible sodium-dependent phosphate symporters, *Proc. Natl. Acad. Sci. USA* **91:**7071–7075.

Kay, M., Baley, P., Rothenberg, S., Leland, F., Fleming, L., Ponder, K., Liu, T.-J., Finegold, M., Darlington, G., Pokorny, W., and Woo, S., 1992, Expression of human alpha-1-antitrypsin in dogs after autologous transplantation of retroviral transduced hepatocytes, *Proc. Natl. Acad. Sci. USA* **89:**89–93.

Kempler, G., Freitag, B., Berwin, B., Nanassy, O., and Barklis, E., 1993, Characterisation of the Moloney murine leukemia virus stem cell-specific repressor binding site, *Virology* **193:**690–699.

Kitamura, Y., Lee, Y., and Coffin, J., 1992, Nonrandom integration of retroviral DNA in vitro: Effect of CpG methylation, *Proc. Natl. Acad. Sci. USA* **89:**5532–5536.

Klikova, M., Rhee, S., Hunter, E., and Ruml, T., 1995, Efficient in vivo and in vitro assembly of retroviral capsids from gag precursor proteins expressed in bacteria, *J. Virol.* **69:**1093–1098.

Koeberl, D., Halbert, C., Krumm, A., and Miller, A., 1995, Sequences within the coding regions of clotting factor VIII and CFTR block transcriptional elongation, *Hum. Gene Ther.* **6:**469–479.

Kohlstaedt, L., Wang, J., Friedman, J., Rice, P., and Steitz, T., 1992, Crystal structure at 3.5Å resolution of HIV-1 reverse transcriptase complexed with an inhibitor, *Science* **256:**1783–1790.

Kotler, M., Katz, R., and Skalka, A., 1988, Activity of avian retroviral protease expressed in *E. coli, J. Virol.* **62:**2696–2700.

Kozak, S. L., and Kabat, D., 1990, Ping-pong amplification of retroviral vector achieves high-level gene expression: Human growth hormone production, *J. Virol.* **64:**3500–3800.

Krausslich, H., 1991, HIV proteinase dimer as component of the viral polyprotein prevents particle assembly and viral infectivity, *Proc. Natl. Acad. Sci. USA* **88:**3213–3217.

Krogstad, P., and Champoux, J., 1990, Sequence-specific binding of DNA by the Moloney murine leukaemia virus integrase protein, *J. Virol.* **64:**2796–2801.

Kulkovsky, J., Jones, K., Katz, R., Mack, J., and Skalka, A., 1992, Resisues critical for retroviral integrative recombination in a region that is highly conserved among retroviral/retrotransposon integrases and bacterial insertion sequence transposases, *Mol. Cell. Biol.* **12:**2331–2338.

Landau, N., and Littman, D., 1992, Packaging system for rapid production of murine leukemia virus vectors with variable tropism, *J. Virol.* **66:**5110–5113.

Landau, N., Page, K., and Littman, D., 1991, Pseudotyping with human T-cell leukemia virus type I broadens the human immunodeficiency virus host range, *J. Virol.* **65:**162–169.

Lewis, P., Hensel, M., and Emerman, M., 1992, Human immunodeficiency virus infection of cells arrested in the cell cycle, *EMBO J.* **11:**3053–3058.

Li, X., McDermott, B., Yuan, B., and Goff, S., 1996, Homomeric interactions between transmembrane proteins of Moloney murine leukaemia virus, *J. Virol.* **70:**1266–1270.

Linder, M., Wenzel, V., Linder, D., and Stirm, S., 1994, Structural elements in glycoprotein 70 from polytropic Friend mink cell focus-inducing virus and glycoprotein 71 from ecotropic Friend murine leukaemia virus, as defined by disulfide-bonding pattern and limited proteolysis, *J. Virol.* **68:**5133–5141.

Linney, E., Davis, B., Overhauser, J., Chao, E., and Fan, H., 1984, Non-function of a Moloney murine leukaemia virus regulatory sequence in F9 embryonal carcinoma cells, *Nature* **308:**470–472.

Lobel, L., and Goff, S., 1985, Reverse transcription of retroviral genomes: Mutations in the terminal repeat sequences, *J. Virol.* **53:**447–455.

Lund, A., Duch, M., Lovmand, J., Jorgensen, P., and Pedersen, F., 1993, Mutated primer binding sites interacting with different tRNAs allow efficient murine leukaemia virus replication, *J. Virol.* **67:**7125–7130.

Lynch, C., Clowes, M., Osborne, W., Clowes, A., and Miller, A., 1992, Long-term expression of human adenosine deaminase in vascular smooth muscle cells of rats: A model for gene therapy, *Proc. Natl. Acad. Sci. USA* **89:**1138–1142.

Mann, R., and Baltimore, D., 1985, Varying the position of a retrovirus packaging sequence results in the encapsidation of both unspliced and spliced RNAs, *J. Virol.* **54:**401–407.

Mann, R., Mulligan, R., and Baltimore, D., 1983, Construction of a retrovirus packaging mutant and its use to produce helper-free defective retrovirus, *Cell* **33:**153–159.

Marin, M., Noel, D., Valesia-Wittman, S., Brockly, F., Etienne-Julan, M., Russell, S., Cosset, F., and Piechaczyk, M., 1996, Targeted infection of human cells via major histocompatibility complex class I molecules by Moloney murine leukaemia virus-derived viruses displaying single-chain antibody fragment-envelope fusion proteins, *J. Virol.* **70:**2957–2962.

Markowitz, D., Goff, S., and Bank, A., 1988a, Construction and use of a safe and efficient amphotropic packaging cell line, *Virology* **167:**400–406.

Markowitz, D., Goff, S., and Bank, A., 1988b, A safe packaging line for gene transfer: Separating viral genes on two different plasmids, *J. Virol.* **82:**1120–1124.

Matano, T., Odawara, T., Iwamoto, A., and Yoshikura, H., 1995, Targeted infection of a retrovirus bearing a CD4-Env chimera into human cells expressing HIV-1, *J. Gen. Virol.* **76:**3165–3169.

McClure, M., Sommerfelt, M., Marsh, M., and Weiss, R., 1990, The pH independence of mammalian retrovirus infection, *J. Gen. Virol.* **71:**767–773.

Meric, C., and Goff, S., 1989, Characterisation of Moloney murine leukaemia virus mutants with single-amino-acid substitutions in the Cys-His box of the nucleocapsid protein, *J. Virol.* **63:**1558–1568.

Miller, A., Garcia, J., Suhr, N. V., Lynch, C., Wilson, C., and Eiden, M., 1991, Construction and properties of retrovirus packaging cells based on gibbon ape leukemia virus, *J. Virol.* **65:**2220–2224.

Miller, A. D., and Buttimore, C., 1986, Redesign of retrovirus packaging cell lines to avoid recombination leading to helper virus production, *Mol. Cell. Biol.* **6:**2895–2902.

Miller, D., Adam, M., and Miller, A., 1990, Gene transfer by retrovirus vectors occurs only in cells that are actively replicating at the time of infection, *Mol. Cell. Biol.* **10:**4239–4242.

Miller, D., Edwards, R., and Miller, A., 1994, Cloning of the cellular receptor for amphotropic murine retroviruses reveals homology to that for gibbon ape leukemia virus, *Proc. Natl. Acad. Sci. USA* **91:**78–82.

Miller, D., and Miller, A., 1994, A family of retroviruses that utilise related phosphate transporters for cell entry, *J. Virol.* **68:**8270–8276.

Moore, K., Scarpa, M., Kooyer, S., Utter, A., Caskey, C., and Belmont, J., 1991, Evaluation of lymphoid-specific enhancer addition or substitution in a basic retrovirus vector, *Hum. Gene Ther.* **2:**307–315.

Morgan, R., Couture, L., Elroy-Stein, O., Ragheb, J., Moss, B., and Anderson, W., 1992, Retroviral vectors containing putative internal ribnosome entry sites: Development of a polycistronic gene transfer system and applications to gene therapy, *Nucleic Acids Res.* **20:**1293–1299.

Morgenstern, J., and Land, H., 1990, Advanced mammalian gene transfer: High titre retroviral vectors with multiple drug selection markers and a complementary helper-free packaging cell line, *Nucleic Acids Res.* **18:**3587–3596.

Moullier, P., Bohl, D., Cardoso, J., Heard, J., and Danos, O., 1995, Long-term delivery of a lysosomal enzyme by genetically modified fibroblasts in dogs, *Nat. Medicine* **1:**353–357.

Moullier, P., Bohl, D., Heard, J., and Danos, O., 1993, Correction of lysosomal storage in the liver and spleen of MPS VII mice by implantation of genetically modified skin fibroblasts, *Nat. Genet.* **4:**154–159.

Muenchau, D. D., Freeman, S. M., Cornetta, K., Zwiebel, J. A., and Anderson, W. F., 1990, Analysis of retroviral packaging lines for generation of replication-competent virus, *Virology* **176:**262–265.

Murphy, J., De-Los-Santos, T., and Goff, S., 1993, Mutational analysis of the sequences at the termini of the Moloney murine leukemia virus DNA required for integration, *Virology* **195:**432–440.

Murphy, J., and Goff, S., 1989, Construction and analysis of deletion mutants in the U5 region of Moloney murine leukaemia virus: Effects on RNA packaging and reverse transcription, *J. Virol.* **63:**319–327.

Naffakh, N., Henri, A., Villeval, J., Rouyer-Fessard, P., Moullier, P., Blumenfeld, N., Danos, O., Vainchenker, W., Heard, J., and Beuzard, Y., 1995, Sustained delivery of erythropoietin in mice by genetically modified skin fibroblasts, *Proc. Natl. Acad. Sci. USA* **92:**3194–3198.

Nakajima, K., Ikenaka, K., Nakahira, K., Morita, N., and Mikoshiba, K., 1993, An improved retroviral vector for assaying promoter activity, *FEBS Lett.* **315:**129–133.

Naldini, L., Blomer, U., Gallay, P., Ory, D., Mulligan, R., Gage, F., Verma, I., and Trono, D., 1996, In vivo gene delivery and stable transduction of nondividing cells by a lentiviral vector, *Science* **272:**263–267.

Nussbaum, O., Roop, A., and Anderson, W., 1993, Sequences determining the pH dependence of viral entry are distinct from the host range-determining region of the murine ecotropic and amphotropic retrovirus envelope proteins, *J. Virol.* **67:**7402–7405.

O'Hara, B., Johann, S., Klinger, H., Blair, D., Rubinson, H., Dunn, K., Sass, P., Vitek, S., and Robbins, T., 1990, Characterisation of the human gene conferring sensitivity to infection by gibbon ape leukemia virus, *Cell Growth Diff.* **1:**119–127.

Oliff, A., Signorelli, K., and Collins, L., 1984, The envelope gene and LTR sequences contribute to the pathogenic phenotype of helper independent Friend viruses, *J. Virol.* **51:**788–794.

Otto, E., Jones-Trower, A., Vanin, E., Stambaugh, K., Mueller, S., Anderson, W., and McGarrity, G., 1994, Characterisation of a replication-competent retrovirus resulting from the recombination of packaging and vector sequences, *Hum. Gene Ther.* **5:**567–575.

Palmer, T., Rosman, G., Osborne, W., and Miller, A., 1991, Genetically modified skin fibroblasts persist long after transplantation but gradually inactivate introduced genes, *Proc. Natl. Acad. Sci. USA* **88:**1330–1334.

Palmer, T., Thompson, A., and Miller, A., 1989, Production of human factor IX in animals by genetically modified skin fibroblasts: Potential therapy for hemophilia B, *Blood* **73:**438–445.

Panganiban, A., 1988, Retroviral gag gene amber codon suppression is caused by an intrinsic cis-acting component of the viral mRNA, *J. Virol.* **62:**3574–3580.

Panganiban, A., and Fiore, D., 1988, Ordered interstrand and intrastrand DNA transfer during reverse transcriptase, *Science* **241:**1064–1069.

Pear, W., Nolan, G., Scott, M., and Baltimore, D., 1993, Production of high titer helper-free retroviruses by transient transfection, *Proc. Natl. Acad. Sci. USA* **90:**8392–8396.

Peterson, R., Kempler, G., and Barklis, E., 1991, A stem cell-specific silencer in the primer-binding site of a retrovirus, *Mol. Cell. Biol.* **11:**1214–1221.

Pinter, A., and Fleissner, E., 1979, Structural studies of retroviruses: Characterisation of oligomeric complexes of murine and feline leukaemia virus envelope and core components, *J. Virol.* **30:**157–165.

Pinter, A., and Honnen, W., 1988, O-linked glycosylation of retroviral envelope gene products, *J. Virol.* **62:**1016–1021.

Porter, C., Collins, M., Tailor, C., Parkar, M., Cosset, F., Weiss, R., and Takeuchi, Y., 1996, Comparison of efficiency of infection of human gene therapy target cells via four different retroviral receptors, *Hum. Gene Ther.* **7:**913–919.

Poznansky, M., Lever, A., Bergeron, L., Haseltine, W., and Sodroski, J., 1991, Gene transfer into human lymphocytes by a defective human immunodeficiency virus type I vector, *J. Virol.* **65:**532–536.

Prats, A., Roy, C., Wang, P., Erard, M., Housset, V., Gabus, C., Paoletti, C., and Darlix, J., 1990, Cis elements and trans-acting factors involved in dimer formation of murine leukaemia virus RNA, *J. Virol.* **64:**774–783.

Prince, V., and Rigby, P., 1991, Derivatives of Moloney murine sarcoma virus capable of being transcribed in embryonal carcinoma stem cells have gained a functional Sp1 binding site, *J. Virol.* **65:**1803–1811.

Pryciak, P., and Varmus, H., 1992, Nucleosomes, DNA-binding proteins and DNA sequence modulate retroviral integration target site selection, *Cell* **69:**769–780.

Purcell, D., Broscius, C., Vanin, E., Buckler, C., Nienhuis, A., and Martin, M., 1996, An array of murine leukemia virus-related elements is transmitted and expressed in a primate recipient of retroviral gene transfer, *J. Virol.* **70:**887–897.

Ragheb, J., and Anderson, W., 1994, Uncoupled expression of Moloney murine leukaemia virus envelope polypeptides SU and TM: A functional analysis of the role of TM domains in viral entry, *J. Virol.* **68:**3207–3219.

Rattray, A., and Champoux, J., 1989, Plus-strand priming by Moloney murine leukaemia virus. The sequence features important for cleavage by RNase H, *J. Mol. Biol.* **208:**445–456.

Rein, A., Mirro, J., Haynes, J., Ernst, S., and Nagashima, K., 1994, Function of the cytoplasmic domain of a retroviral transmembrane protein: p15E-p2E cleavage activates the membrane fusion capability of the murine leukemia virus env protein, *J. Virol.* **68:**1773–1781.

Rhee, S., and Hunter, E., 1990, A single amino acid substitution within the matrix protein of a type D retrovirus converts its morphogenesis to that of a type C retrovirus, *Cell* **63:**77–86.

Rigg, R., Chen, J., Dando, J., Forestell, S., Plavec, I., and Bohnlein, E., 1996, A novel human amphotropic packaging cell line: High titer, complement resistance and improved safety, *Virology* **218:**290–295.

Riviere, I., Brose, K., and Mulligan, R., 1995, Effects of retroviral vector design on expression of human adenosine deaminase in murine bone marrow transplant recipients engrafted with genetically modified cells, *Proc. Natl. Acad. Sci. USA* **92:**6733–6736.

Roe, T., Reynolds, T., Yu, G., and Brown, P., 1993, Integration of murine leukemia virus DNA depends on mitosis, *EMBO J.* **12:**2099–2108.

Rother, R., Fodor, W., Springhorn, J., Birks, C., Setter, E., Sandrin, M., Squinto, S., and Rollins, S., 1995, A novel mechanism of retrovirus inactivation in human serum mediated by anti-α-galactosyl natural antibody, *J. Exp. Med.* **182:**1345–1355.

Russell, D., and Miller, A., 1996, Foamy virus vectors, *J. Virol.* **70:**217–222.

Russell, S. J., Hawkins, R. E., and Winter, G., 1993, Retroviral vectors displaying functional antibody fragments, *Nucleic Acids Res.* **21:**1081–1085.

Sadelain, M., Wang, C., Antoniou, M., Grosveld, F., and Mulligan, R., 1995, Generation of a high-titer retroviral vector capable of expressing high levels of the human beta-globin gene, *Proc. Natl. Acad. Sci. USA* **92:**6728–6732.

Scadden, D., Fuller, B., and Cunningham, J., 1990, Human cells infected with retrovirus vectors acquire an endogenous murine provirus, *J. Virol.* **64:**424–427.

Scarpa, M., Cournoyer, D., Muzny, D. M., Moore, K. A., Belmont, J. W., and Caskey, C. T., 1991, Characterization of recombinant helper retroviruses from Moloney-based vectors in ecotropic and amphotropic packaging cell lines, *Virology* **180:**849–852.

Scharfmann, R., Axelrod, J., and Verma, I., 1991, Long-term in vivo expression of retrovirus-mediated gene transfer in mouse fibroblast implants, *Proc. Natl. Acad. Sci. USA* **88:**4626–4630.

Schultz, S., Whiting, S., and Champoux, J., 1995, Cleavage specificities of Moloney murine leukaemia virus RNase H implicated in the second strand transfer during reverse transcription, *J. Biol. Chem.* **270:**24135–24145.

Shih, C., Stoye, J., and Coffin, J., 1988, Highly prefered targets for retrovirus integration, *Cell* **53:**531–537.

Shimada, T., Fujii, H., Mitsuya, H., and Nienhuis, A., 1991, Targeted and highly efficient gene transfer into CD4+ cells by a recombinant human immunodeficiency virus retroviral vector, *J. Clin. Invest.* **88:**1043–1047.

Sithanandam, G., and Rapp, U., 1988, A single point mutation in the envelope gene is responsible for replication and XC fusion deficiency of the endogenous ecotropic C3H/He murine leukaemia virus and for its repair in culture, *J. Virol.* **62:**932–943.

Somia, N., Zoppe, M., and Verma, I., 1995, Generation of targeted retroviral vectors by using single-chain variable fragment: An approach to in vivo gene therapy, *Proc. Natl. Acad. Sci. USA* **92:**7570–7574.

Sommerfelt, M., Williams, B., McKnight, A., Goodfellow, P., and Weiss, R., 1990, Localisation of the receptor gene for type D simian retroviruses on human chromosome 19, *J. Virol.* **64:**6214–6220.

Soneoka, Y., Cannon, P., Ramsdale, E., Griffiths, J., Romano, G., Kingsman, S., and Kingsman, A., 1995, A transient three-plasmid expression system for the production of high titer retroviral vectors, *Nucleic Acid Res.* **23:**628–633.

Sorge, J., and Hughes, S., 1982, Polypurine tract adjacent to the U3 region of the Rous sarcoma virus genome provides a cis-acting function, *J. Virol.* **43:**482–488.

Speck, N., and Baltimore, D., 1987, Six distinct nuclear factors interact with the 75-base-pair repeat of the Moloney murine leukemia virus enhancer, *Mol. Cell. Biol.* **7:**1101–1110.

Speck, N., Renjifo, B., and Hopkins, N., 1990, Point mutations in the Moloney murine leukemia virus enhancer identify a lymphoid-specific viral core motif and 1,3-phorbol myristate acetate-inducible element, *J. Virol.* **64:**543–550.

Srinivasakumar, N., Hammarskjold, M., and Rekosh, D., 1995, Characterisation of deletion mutations in the capsid region of HIV-1 that affect particle formation and gag-pol precursor incorporation, *J. Virol.* **69:**6106–6114.

Stocking, C., Kollek, R., Bergholz, U., and Ostertag, W., 1986, Point mutations in the U3 region of the LTR of Moloney murine leukaemia virus determine the disease specificity of the myeloproliferative sarcoma virus, *Virology* **153:**145–149.

Strambio-de-Castillia, C., and Hunter, E., 1992, Mutational analysis of the major homology region of Mason Pfizer monkey virus by use of saturation mutagenesis, *J. Virol.* **66:**7021–7032.

Stuhlmann, H., Jaenisch, R., and Mulligan, R., 1989, Transfer of a mutant dihydrofolate reductase gene into pre- and postimplantation mouse embryos by a replication-competent retrovirus vector, *J. Virol.* **63:**4857–4865.

Suomalainen, M., and Garoff, H., 1994, Incorporation of homologous and heterologous proteins into the envelope of Moloney murine leukemia virus, *J. Virol.* **68:**4879–4889.

Swain, A., and Coffin, J., 1989, Polyadenylation at correct sites in genome RNA is not required for retrovirus replication or genome encapsidation, *J. Virol.* **63:**3301–3306.

Takahara, Y., Hamada, K., and Housman, D., 1992, A new retrovirus packaging cell for gene transfer constructed from amplified long terminal repeat-free chimeric proviral genes, *J. Virol.* **66:**3725–3732.

Takeuchi, Y., Cosset, F., Lachmann, P., Okada, H., Weiss, R., and Collins, M., 1994, Type C retrovirus inactivation by human complement is determined by both the viral genome and producer cell, *J. Virol.* **68:**8001–8007.

Takeuchi, Y., Porter, C., Strahan, K., Preece, A., Gustafsson, K., Cosset, F.-L., Weiss, R., and Collins, M., 1996, Sensitization of cells and retroviruses to human serum by α(1–3) galactosyltransferase, *Nature* **379:**85–88.

Takeuchi, Y., Simpson, G., Vile, R., Weiss, R., and Collins, M., 1992, Retroviral pseudotypes produced by rescue of Moloney murine leukemia virus vector by C-type, but not D-type, retroviruses, *Virology* **186:**792–794.

Tanese, N., Telesnitsky, A., and Goff, S., 1991, Abortive reverse transcription by mutants of Moloney murine leukaemia virus deficient in the reverse transcriptase-associated RNase H function, *J. Virol.* **65:**4387–4397.

Telesnitsky, A., and Goff, S., 1993a, RNase H domain mutations affect the interaction between Moloney murine leukaemia virus reverse transcriptase and its primer-template, *Proc. Natl. Acad. Sci. USA* **90:**1276–1280.

Telesnitsky, A., and Goff, S., 1993b, Two defective forms of reverse transcriptase can complement to restore retroviral infectivity, *EMBO J.* **12:**4433–4438.

Torrent, C., Gabus, C., and Darlix, J., 1994, A small and efficient dimerization/packaging signal of rat VL 30 RNA and its use in murine leukaemia virus-VL30-derived vectors for gene transfer, *J. Virol.* **68:**661–667.

Trono, D., 1992, Partial reverse transcripts in virions from human immunodeficiency and murine leukaemia viruses, *J. Virol.* **66:**4893–4900.

Tucker, S., Srinivas, R., and Compans, R., 1991, Molecular domains involved in oligomerisation of the Friend murine leukaemia virus envelope, *Virology* **185:**710–720.

Vagner, S., Waysbort, A., Marenda, M., Gensac, M.-C., Amalric, F., and Prats, A.-C., 1995, Alternative translation initiation of the Moloney murine leukemia virus mRNA controlled by internal ribosome entry involving the p57/PTB splicing factor, *J. Biol. Chem.* **270:**20376–20383.

Valerio, D., Einerhand, M., Wamsley, P., Bakx, T., Li, C., and Verma, I., 1989, Retrovirus-mediated gene transfer into embryonal carcinoma and haematopoietic stem cells: Expression from a hybrid long terminal repeat, *Gene* **84:**419–427.

Valesesia-Wittman, S., Drynda, A., Deleage, G., Aumailley, M., Heard, J., Verdier, G., and Cosset, F., 1994, Modifications in the binding domain of avian retrovirus envelope protein to redirect the host range of retroviral vectors, *J. Virol.* **68:**4609–4619.

Valesia-Wittmann, S., Morling, F., Nilson, B., Russell, S., and Cossett, F., 1996, Improvement of retroviral retargeting by using amino acid spacers between an additional binding domain and the N terminus of Moloney murine leukaemia virus SU, *J. Virol.* **70:**2059–2064.

van-Gent, D., Vink, C., Groeneger, A., and Plasterk, R., 1993, Complementation between HIV integrase proteins mutated in different domains, *EMBO J.* **12:**3261–3267.

Vanin, E. F., Kaloss, M., Broscius, C., and Nienhuis, A. W., 1994, Characterization of replication-competent retroviruses from nonhuman primates with virus-induced T-cell lymphomas and observations regarding the mechanism of oncogenesis, *J. Virol.* **68:**4241–4250.

Vile, R., Diaz, R., Miller, N., Mitchell, S., Tuszyanski, A., and Russell, S., 1995, Tissue-specific gene expression from Mo-MLV retroviral vectors with hybrid LTRs containing the murine tyrosinase enhancer/promoter, *Virology* **214:**307–313.

Vogt, M., Haggblom, C., Swift, S., and Haas, M., 1985, Envelope gene and long terminal repeat determine the different biological properties of Rauscher, Friend and Moloney mink cell focus-forming viruses, *J. Virol.* **55:**184–192.

von-Schwedler, U., Kornbluth, R., and Trono, D., 1994, The nuclear localization signal of the matrix protein of HIV-1 allows the establishment of infection in macrophages and quiescent T lymphocytes, *Proc. Natl. Acad. Sci. USA* **91:**6992–6996.

Wang, H., Paul, R., Burgeson, R., Keene, D., and Kabat, D., 1991, Plasma membrane receptors for ecotropic murine retroviruses require a limiting accessory factor, *J. Virol.* **65:**6468–6477.

Waters, L., Mullin, B., Bailiff, E., and Popp, R., 1980, Differential association of transfer RNAs with the genomes of murine, feline and primate retroviruses, *Biochim. Biophys. Acta* **608:**112–126.

Willis, J., Cameron, C., Wilson, C., Xiang, Y., Bennett, R., and Leis, J., 1994, An assembly domain of the Rous sarcoma virus gag protein required late in budding, *J. Virol.* **68:**6605–6618.

Wiskerchen, M., and Muesing, M., 1995, HIV-1 integrase: Effects of mutations on viral ability to integrate, direct viral gene expression from unintegrated viral DNA templates and sustain viral propagation in primary cells, *J. Virol.* **69:**376–386.

Wlodawer, A., Miller, M., Jaskolski, M., Sathyanarayana, B., Baldwin, E., Weber, I., Selk, L., Clawson, L., Schneider, J., and Kent, S., 1989, Conserved folding in retroviral proteases: Crystal structure of a synthetic HIV-1 protease, *Science* **245:**616–621.

Wollenberg, C. v. d., Hoeben, R., Ormondt, H. v., and Eb, A. v. d., 1994, Insertion of the human cytomegalovirus enhancer into a myeloproliferative sarcoma virus long terminal repeat creates a high-expression retroviral vector, *Gene* **144:**237–241.

Yamauchi, M., Freitag, B., Khan, C., Berwin, B., and Barklis, E., 1995, Stem cell factor binding to retrovirus primer binding site silencers, *J. Virol.* **69:**1142–1149.

Yang, Y., Vanin, E., Whitt, M., Fornerod, M., Zwart, R., Schneiderman, R., Grosveld, G., and Nienhuis, A., 1995, Inducible, high-level production of infectious murine leukemia retroviral vector particles pseudotyped with vesicular stomatitis virus G envelope protein, *Hum. Gene Ther.* **6:**1203–1213.

Yee, J., Miyanohara, A., LaPorte, P., Bouic, K., Burns, J., and Friedmann, T., 1994, A general method for the generation of high-titre, pantropic retroviral vectors: Highly efficient infection of primary hepatocytes, *Proc. Natl. Acad. Sci. USA* **91:**9564–9568.

Yee, J.-K., Moores, J., Jolly, D., Wolff, J., Respess, J., and Friedmann, T., 1987, Gene expression from transcriptionally disabled retroviral vector, *Proc. Natl. Acad. Sci. USA* **84:**5197–5201.

Yu, S.-F., von-Ruden, T., Kantoff, P., Garber, C., Seiberg, M., Ruther, U. anderson, W., Wagner, E., and Gilboa, E., 1986, Self-inactivating retroviral vectors designed for transfer of whole genes into mammalian cells, *Proc. Natl. Acad. Sci. USA* **83:**3194–3198.

Zhou, W., Parent, L., Wills, J., and Resh, M., 1994, Identification of a membrane-binding domain within the amino-terminal region of HIV-1 gag protein which interacts with acidic phospholipids, *J. Virol.* **68:**2556–2569.

Zitvogel, L., Tahara, H., Cai, Q., Storkus, W., Muller, G., Wolf, S., Gately, M., Robbins, P., and Lotze, M., 1994, Construction and characterisation of retroviral vectors expressing biologically active interleukin-12, *Hum. Gene Ther.* **5:**1493–1506.

Zybarth, G., and Carter, C., 1995, Domains upstream of the protease in HIV-1 gag-pol influence PR autoprocessing, *J. Virol.* **69:**3878–3884.

Chapter 4

Parvoviral Vectors for Human Hematopoietic Gene Therapy

Arun Srivastava

1. INTRODUCTION

The concept of treating human diseases by introducing normal alleles of genes into appropriate target cells is a clinical milestone (Anderson, 1995). Although a number of physical and chemical methods for gene transfer have been developed, viruses have generally proven much more efficient in transferring genetic material into cells. Indeed, viral vectors based on retroviruses and adenoviruses have already been employed in a number of clinical trials (Crystal, *et al.*, 1994; Rosenberg *et al.*, 1990; Zabner *et al.*, 1993). Although initial results with retroviral vectors have been encouraging (Blaese *et al.*, 1995; Bordignon *et al.*, 1995; Grossman *et al.*, 1994) their use in nonhuman primate studies have been reported to lead to malignancy (Donahue *et al.*, 1992), and the efficacy of adenoviral vectors has been questioned (Knowles *et al.*, 1995), Because retroviruses and most of the DNA-containing viruses are the etiologic agents of, or are intimately associated with, malignant disorders (Tooze, 1981; Weiss *et al.*, 1984), the search for an alternative viral vector continues (Hodgson, 1995; Miller and Vile, 1995). Parvoviruses, which are among the smallest of the DNA-containing viruses that infect a wide variety of vertebrates (Siegl *et al.*, 1985), remain the only group of viruses that have thus far not been associated with malignant disease (Cotmore and Tattersall, 1987; Pattison, 1988). In fact, parvoviruses possess antitumor properties (Cukor *et al.*, 1975; Mayor *et al.*,

Arun Srivastava Departments of Microbiology and Immunology and Medicine, Walther Oncology Center, Indiana University School of Medicine, and Walther Cancer Institute, Indianapolis, Indiana 46202-5120.

Blood Cell Biochemistry, Volume 8: Hematopoiesis and Gene Therapy, edited by Fairbairn and Testa. Kluwer Academic/Plenum Publishers, New York, 1999.

1973; Ostrove *et al.*, 1981). One of the members of the *Parvoviridae* family, the adeno-associated virus 2 (AAV), has gained significant attention primarily because AAV is a nonpathogenic human parvovirus (Blacklow, 1988), and the wild-type (wt) AAV genome establishes a latent infection in human cells where the viral genome integrates into the chromosomal DNA in a site-specific manner (Kotin *et al.*, 1989, 1990, 1991, 1992; Samulski *et al.*, 1991). Although several reviews on AAV vectors have been published (Berns and Linden, 1995; Carter, 1993; Flotte and Carter, 1995; Kotin, 1994; Muzyczka, 1992; Samulski, 1993; Srivastava, 1994; Srivastava *et al.*, 1996; Xiao *et al.*, 1993), this article highlights salient features of parvoviruses in general and outlines a number of advantages that support the potential use of parvovirus vectors in human gene therapy.

2. LIFE CYCLE OF HUMAN PARVOVIRUSES

The general features of the two parvoviruses of human origin, AAV and parvovirus B19, that have been studied extensively (Berns and Bohenzky, 1987; Brown *et al.*, 1994), are summarized in Figure 1. Whereas AAV is a nonpathogenic virus, parvovirus B19 is now known to be a common human pathogen. Approximately 90% of the human population is sero-positive for AAV, whereas approximately 60% of humans have been exposed to B19. AAV requires coinfection with a helper virus, such as adenovirus, herpesvirus, or vaccinia virus, for optimal replication (Berns, 1990), but in the absence of a helper virus, the AAV genome establishes a latent infection (Berns and Linden, 1995; Cheung *et al.*, 1980). B19, on the other hand, is an autonomously replicating virus with a remarkable tropism for the human erythroid progenitor cells (Ozawa *et al.*, 1986, 1987; Schwarz *et al.*, 1992; Srivastava and Lu, 1988; Takahashi *et al.*, 1990; Yaegashi *et al.*, 1989). The genomes

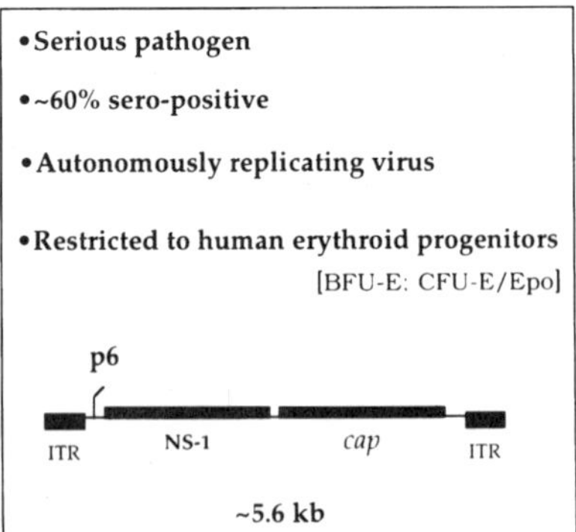

FIGURE 1. Salient features of parvoviruses of human origin. AAV, discovered in 1965 as a contaminant of adenovirus preparations, is a nonpathogenic human parvovirus. Parvovirus B19, discovered serendipitously in 1975 in sera of asymptomatic blood donors, is the etiologic agent of a number of human clinical disorders. The genomic organization of each of the viruses is also depicted and detailed in the text.

of both viruses have been molecularly cloned (Cotmore and Tattersall, 1984; Laughlin *et al.*, 1983; Samulski *et al.*, 1982; Shade *et al.*, 1986), which has greatly facilitated genetic analyses of these parvoviruses (Srivastava *et al.*, 1989, 1990; Hermonat *et al.*, 1984).

2.1. Infection and Host Cell Receptors

The life cycle of AAV is schematically depicted in Figure 2. In the presence of a helper virus, such as adenovirus, AAV undergoes a lytic infection (A). In the absence of a helper virus, wt AAV establishes a latent infection (B). In view of the broad host range of AAV that transcends species barriers (Muzyczka, 1992), it was generally believed that infection by AAV was mediated by a mechanism akin to phagocytosis. However, it now appears that AAV infection involves cell surface heparan sulfate proteoglycan (HSPG) as a receptor (Summerford and Samulski, 1998), and, in addition, the involvement of human fibroblast growth factor receptor 1 (FGFR1) has been implicated as a coreceptor in mediating successful infection of human cells by AAV (Mah *et al.*, 1998; Qing *et al.*, 1999; Srivastava *et al.*, 1995). The availability of this information should facilitate further studies on the virus–host cell interactions. The identification and characterization of the receptor as well as the

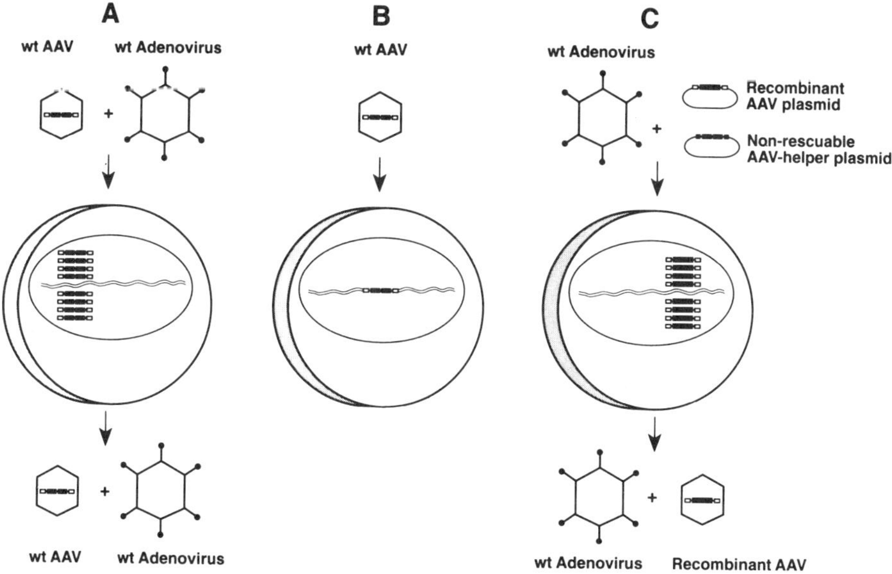

FIGURE 2. Life cycle of the wt AAV and generation of the recombinant AAV. In the presence of a helper virus, the wt AAV undergoes a lytic infection (A), but in the absence of a helper virus the wt AAV establishes a latent infection, and the proviral genome integrates into the chromosomal DNA in a site-specific manner (B). The recombinant AAV is generated by cotransfecting a plasmid that contains the gene of interest between the AAV-ITRs (open boxes) and a plasmid that contains the wt AAV coding sequences between the adenovirus-ITRs (closed boxes) in adenovirus-infected human cells (C). The recombinant AAV can be physically separated from the wt adenovirus by centrifugation on CsCl density gradients (Srivastava, 1994).

coreceptor for AAV also has important implications in the potential use of AAV-based vectors in human gene therapy.

It has been suggested that the target-cell specificity for B19 infection is mediated by the erythrocyte P antigen (Brown *et al.*, 1993). However, a number of nonerythroid cells that express this receptor are nonpermissive for B19 replication (Brown *et al.*, 1994; Cooling *et al.*, 1995; Rouger *et al.*, 1987; Srivastava *et al.*, 1990). In addition, the P antigen is expressed in high quantities in mature erythrocytes (Marcus *et al.*, 1981) but not on erythroid progenitors (BFU-E and CFU-E) or proerythroblasts (von dem Borne *et al.*, 1986). Numerous studies have identified erythroid progenitors as B19 target cells, so it is difficult to reconcile how P antigen alone might mediate successful infection by B19 because mature erythrocytes lack nuclei and B19 infection of these cells would be nonproductive. The globoside (glycosphingolipid) nature of the B19 receptor, nonetheless, makes it less amenable to further genetic analyses.

2.2. DNA Replication and Gene Expression

Because of the single-stranded nature of the parvoviral DNA genome, at least one round of DNA synthesis must precede prior to initiation of viral gene expression. The palindromic nature of the viral inverted terminal repeats (ITRs) means these are primers for viral DNA replication, which utilizes the host cell DNA polymerases. The original model for replication of linear, single-stranded DNA suggested by Cavalier-Smith (1974) and all available data on AAV DNA replication share remarkable similarities (Srivastava, 1987). Two AAV sequences are required for viral DNA replication. The first is the viral *rep* gene, which encodes four nonstructural proteins that are synthesized from a single open reading frame by using alternate promoters and by mRNA splicing (Srivastava *et al.*, 1983). The second is the viral origin of DNA replication which consists of a 145-nucleotide inverted terminal repeat (ITR) sequence (Lusby *et al.*, 1980). Two of the viral Rep proteins (Rep78 and Rep68) are site-specific and strand-specific endonucleases that specifically bind to and cleave at the terminal resolution site (trs) within the AAV-ITRs (Ashktorab and Srivastava, 1989; Im and Muzyczka, 1989, 1990, 1992; Snyder *et al.*, 1990). AAV genomes with mutations in the *rep* gene are defective for viral DNA replication (Hermonat *et al.*, 1984; Owens and Carter, 1992; Tratschin *et al.*, 1984). The terminal 125 nucleotides form a palindrome that can fold back on itself to form a T-shaped hairpin (HP) structure. The terminal HP is used as a primer for initiating viral DNA replication (Berns and Bohenzky, 1987; Lusby *et al.*, 1980; Muzyczka, 1992; Srivastava, 1987). Previous *in vivo* and *in vitro* studies have demonstrated that the intact ITRs are required in *cis* for AAV DNA replication and for rescue or excision from prokaryotic plasmids (Gottlieb and Muzyczka, 1988; Hong *et al.*, 1992, 1994; Ni *et al.*, 1994; Samulski *et al.*, 1982, 1983; Senapathy *et al.*, 1984). The ITR also contains a stretch of 20-nucleotides, designated the D-sequence, which is not involved in the hairpin formation. Recently, Wang *et al* (1995a, 1996b) provided experimental evidence to suggest that the D-sequence may be the packaging signal for AAV. Furthermore, although previous studies have shown that the AAV-Rep proteins specifically interact with the AAV-ITRs that are present in a cruciform structure (Ashktorab and Srivastava, 1989; Im and Muzyczka, 1989), and catalyze replication and resolution of the viral genome (Im and Muzyczka, 1990, 1992), the existence of a hitherto unknown cellular protein(s) that specifically interacts with the D-sequence has also been demonstrated (Wang *et al.*, 1996b). It is highly likely that this cellular protein is specifically recruited by AAV to ensure efficient replication and encapsidation of the viral genomes (Wang *et al.*, 1996b).

Much less is currently known about the biochemistry of B19 DNA replication. In contrast to the AAV-ITRs, the B19-ITRs are much more structurally complex (Deiss *et al.*, 1990). It is generally believed that B19-ITRs are also utilized as primers for viral DNA synthesis. Because of approximately 52% similarity and 30% identity at the amino acid level between AAV Rep and B19 nonstructural (NS-1) proteins, it stands to reason that the basic underlying mechanism of B19 DNA replication parallels that of AAV.

The AAV genome contains three distinct promoters at map units 5 (p5), 19 (p19), and 40 (p40), respectively (Srivastava *et al.*, 1983). Expression of the viral *rep* gene is under the control of the p5 and p19 promoters, whereas expression of the viral capsid genes is controlled by the p40 promoter. Little expression from any of the AAV promoters occurs in the absence of a helper virus (Berns and Linden, 1995). Several early gene products of adenovirus have been implicated in regulating AAV gene expression (Berns and Bohenzky, 1987). In the absence of a helper virus, the AAV Rep proteins appear to down-regulate expression from the viral promoters because all viral promoters contain the putative Rep-binding sites (RBS) (McCarty *et al.*, 1994a,b). The p5 promoter also contains two binding sites for the host cell transcription factor YY1, and the adenovirus E1A protein relieves the YY1-mediated negative regulation of expression from the p5 promoter (Shi *et al.*, 1991).

The expression of the B19 genes is somewhat unique. In contrast to all other parvoviral genomes, the B19 genome contains a single promoter at map unit 6 (p6) that controls the expression of the viral NS-1 and the capsid proteins (Ozawa *et al.*, 1987). Although the viral genomes contain a putative promoter at map unit 44 (p44), expression from which can be transactivated *in vitro* by coinfection with adenovirus in nonpermissive cells (Ponnazhagan *et al.*, 1995c), this promoter is nonfunctional under a natural infection of primary human erythroid progenitor cells by B19 (Ozawa *et al.*, 1987).

2.3. Viral Assembly

Following viral DNA replication and capsid protein synthesis, progeny virions are assembled in infected cell nuclei. Although it is believed that this poorly understood process is spontaneous and, recent studies from two laboratories have begun to examine AAV assembly in some detail (Hölscher *et al.*, 1994, 1995; Prasad and Trempe, 1995; Wistuba *et al.*, 1995). In addition, Wang *et al.* (1996b) identified the packaging signal for the AAV genome, and studies by Kube *et al.* (1997) revealed that the viral Rep proteins are also encapsidated in mature progeny virions. Because productive replication of the helper virus leads to a lytic response, the role of AAV in this process is not entirely clear (Berns and Linden, 1995).

Little, if any, information is available on the assembly mechanism of B19 progeny virions during a natural infection (Brown *et al.*, 1994), but autonomous viral replication results in selective loss of erythroid progenitor cells (Ozawa *et al.*, 1986, 1987; Srivastava and Lu, 1988), which is consistent with the cytolytic nature of parvoviruses in general (Cotmore and Tattersall, 1987).

2.4. Proviral Integration, Rescue, and Replication

In the absence of coinfection with a helper virus, the wt AAV genome establishes a latent infection and integrates into the host chromosomal DNA in a site-specific manner (Kotin and Berns, 1989; Kotin *et al.*, 1990, 1991; Samulski *et al.*, 1991). Upon superinfection with a helper virus, the proviral genome undergoes rescue, followed by replication much the same way as during a lytic infection (Berns and Hauswirth, 1979; Berns and Linden, 1995).

Latent infection by B19, on the other hand, has been difficult to document experimentally. Although it is believed that autonomously replicating parvoviruses generally do not establish a latent infection (Cotmore and Tattersall, 1987), numerous clinical studies documenting persistent B19-infection (Frickhofen and Young, 1989; Gahr *et al.*, 1991; Kurtzman *et al.*, 1988, 1989; Pont *et al.*, 1992; Weiland *et al.*, 1989) strongly suggest that B19 might establish a latent infection by a hitherto unknown mechanism (S. Z. Zhou and A. Srivastava, unpublished results).

3. RECOMBINANT PARVOVIRAL VECTORS

The nonpathogenic nature of AAV, coupled with the site-specificity of integration of the viral genome, has garnered sufficient enthusiasm to develop AAV as an alternative to the more commonly used retrovirus- and adenovirus-based vectors. The revelation that B19 possesses a remarkable tissue tropism further suggests the possibility of developing parvovirus-based vectors for erythroid cell delivery and/or expression of therapeutic genes (Srivastava *et al.*, 1989; Srivastava, 1994; Ponnazhagan *et al.*, 1998).

3.1. Construction Strategies

The overall strategy to construct recombinant AAV vectors is depicted in Figure 2 (C). Briefly, a gene of interest is molecularly cloned in the Xba I sites engineered near the two AAV-ITRs in a bacterial plasmid, p*Sub*201 (Samulski *et al.*, 1987). This plasmid is cotransfected into adenovirus-infected human cells with a helper plasmid, pAAV/Ad (Samulski *et al.*, 1989), that contains the entire AAV coding sequences, but lacks the AAV-ITRs and contains the adenovirus-ITRs at the Xba I sites instead. As a result, the AAV genome cannot undergo rescue and replication but provides all AAV gene products *in trans*. In earlier studies, AAV DNA sequences containing insertions that were too large to be packaged into progeny virions were used as helper plasmids (Hermonat and Muzyczka, 1984). However, because of extensive DNA sequence homology in the ITR sequences between the recombinant and the helper plasmids, replication-competent wt AAV was generated (McLaughlin *et al.*, 1988). Although p*Sub*201-based recombinant and pAAV/Ad helper plasmid sequences lack obvious sequence homology, low levels of wt AAV contamination in some preparations of highly purified recombinant AAV stocks have been detected (Flotte *et al.*, 1995; Kube *et al.*, 1997). Recent studies suggest that non-homologous recombination between the recombinant and the helper plasmids to lead to the generation of wt AAV (Wang *et al.*, 1998). Thus, for clinical use, it is desirable to develop alternative means to generate recombinant AAV stocks that are completely free of wt AAV and adenovirus.

3.2. Rescue and Packaging Cell Lines

Several investigators have reported the development of AAV rescue and packaging cell lines that can be induced to express the viral proteins (Hölscher *et al.*, 1994, 1995; Luhovy *et al.*, 1996; Ponnazhagan *et al.*, 1995a; Tamayose *et al.*, 1996; Yang *et al.*, 1994). Further refinements of these systems are likely to yield viral titers significantly higher than those produced by the conventional two-plasmid cotransfection method (Samulski *et al.*, 1989).

In an attempt to develop additional parvovirus-based vectors in which the recombinant genome is encapsidated inside the B19 capsid, a number of substitution constructs have been made in which the AAV-*cap* gene sequences were replaced by the B19-*cap* gene sequences under the control of a variety of promoters, such as AAVp5, B19p6, and the CMV promoters. Although the viral titers are low, the progeny virions selectively transduce primary human erythroid progenitor cells (S. Ponnazhagan, P. Mukherjee, and A. Srivastava, unpublished results). Thus, B19-mediated targeted delivery of therapeutic genes to primitive erythroid progenitors in the human hematopoietic system may be feasible.

3.3. High-Titer Vector Stocks and Viral Purification

One of the major limitations in utilizing AAV vectors for human gene therapy has been the relative difficulty in generating large quantities of high-titer vector stocks. A number of investigators have attempted to circumvent some of the problems by a variety of means. For example, Ponnazhagan *et al.* (1995a) described the following three strategies: (1) eliminating the need for two-plasmid cotransfection by inserting the AAV *rep* and *cap* gene sequences in the same recombinant AAV plasmid; (2) developing helper plasmids that can rescue and replicate but are unable to become packaged; and (3) Developing an AAV-*rep* cell line in which high levels of Rep proteins can be induced after adenovirus infection. Additional refinements in transfection protocols and subsequent purification of progeny virions on sucrose cushion and CsCl density gradients have also facilitated the generation of recombinant viral titers ranging between 10^{11}–10^{12} particles/ml (Kube *et al.*, 1996). Using NB324K cells and dl309 mutant adenovirus, Maxwell *et al.* (1995) also increased the yield of recombinant AAV. Flotte *et al.* (1995) described an improved method of obtaining titers in the range of 10^{11}/ml by using the HIV-LTR promoter to drive the expression of the AAV-*rep* genes and by using cell lines containing rescuable recombinant AAV genomes. Whereas Mamounas *et al.* (1995) utilized the adenovirus-polylysine DNA complex system to increase viral titers by two orders of magnitude over the conventional method, Chiorini *et al.* (1995) described a method utilizing an SV40 replicon to amplify the AAV structural genes in COS cells that yields 60-fold higher viral titers compared with that from a nonreplicating helper plasmid. The development of a "semi-packaging" (Luhovy *et al.*, 1996) and AAV packaging cell lines (Tamayose *et al.*, 1996) purporting to yield transducing viral titers ranging between 10^6-10^8/ml has also been reported recently. Finally, Colosi *et al.* (1995) devised a novel means of generating high-titer (10^{11}–10^{12} particles/ml) recombinant AAV in the absence of coinfection by adenovirus. Thus, it is clear that in time the availability of high-titer, clinical-grade recombinant AAV will cease to be a limitation.

3.4. Defective-Interfering Particles

It is well known that during a natural infection with wt AAV, defective-interfering (DI) particles are generated (Hauswirth and Berns, 1977). It has been estimated that the DI to infectious particle ratio for wt AAV ranges between 20–100 (Muzyczka, 1992). It is intriguing that the same ratio for recombinant AAV is as high as 10^6 (Russell *et al.*, 1995). In an attempt to gain an insight into this problem, Wang *et al.* (1996a) reexamined rescue and replication of the wt AAV genome from recombinant plasmids in adenovirus-infected human cells because in contrast to infection with wt AAV, the recombinant AAV genome must first be rescued from a plasmid. The resolution of the AAV-ITRs is a key step during viral DNA rescue and replication. Previous studies have demonstrated that the viral *rep* gene products (Rep78 and Rep68) bind specifically to the cruciform structures of the AAV-ITRs (Ashktorab and Srivastava, 1989; Im and Muzyczka, 1989). The Rep proteins also possess a site-specific and strand-specific endonuclease activity which specifically cleaves at the terminal resolution site (trs) within the ITR sequences (Im and Muzyczka, 1990, 1992; Snyder *et al.*, 1990). Both the secondary structural element of the ITR and a specific sequence at the trs are required for recognition and cleavage by the Rep proteins (Snyder *et al.*, 1993). However, recent *in vitro* studies have shown that the purified Rep68 protein binds to the ITR and also to some linear DNA sequences, such as the A-sequence, and the AAVp5, AAVp19, and the AAVp40 promoter sequences (McCarty *et al.*, 1994a,b). Although it is believed that the RBS in AAVp5 promoter is involved in *rep* gene expression (Kÿostio *et al.*, 1995) and AAV DNA integration (Giraud *et al.*, 1995), Rep-mediated binding to these sequences followed by cleavage in adenovirus-infected human cells has been detected (Wang *et al.*, 1996a). Thus, the existence of additional putative "trs-like" sequences in the AAV genome, other than those present within the ITRs, that are utilized in the Rep-mediated cleavage of the viral genome during a natural AAV infection has been shown. Because Rep-mediated cleavage could be abolished following deletion of the RBS that, as previously shown, binds the AAV Rep proteins *in vitro* (McCarty *et al.*, 1994a,b), these results provide further evidence that the "trs-like" sites near the AAV promoter sequences also constitute binding sites for the AAV Rep proteins *in vivo* (Wang *et al.*, 1996a). Recent studies also revealed that wt AAV genomes that have containing only one ITR sequence can be packaged into progeny virions (Wang *et al.*, 1996b). Thus, it is becoming clear how naturally occurring DI AAV particles are generated and why only one out of 20–100 wt AAV particles is infectious. Therefore, it seems plausible, that by deliberately deleting the putative RBS in the recombinant AAV genomes without altering the coding sequences, the extent of generation of DI particles might be significantly diminished.

4. PARVOVIRUS-MEDIATED TRANSDUCTION AND EXPRESSION OF GENES

A number of investigators have utilized the AAV-based vector system to successfully transduce and obtain short- and long-term expression of a variety of reporter genes *in vitro* and *in vivo* (Berns and Linden, 1995; Flotte and Carter, 1995; Kotin, 1994; Muzyczka, 1992; Srivastava, 1994). Table I lists all potentially therap-

Table I
AAV-Mediated Transduction of Potentially Therapeutic Genes

Genes	References
Antisense α-globin	Ponnazhagan *et al.*, 1994*a*
Antisense HIV[a]	Chatterjee *et al.*, 1992
B7-2[b]	Chiorini *et al.*, 1995
β-globin	Dixit *et al.*, 1991; Einerhand *et al.*, 1995; Zhou *et al.*, 1996
CFTR[c]	Egan *et al.*, 1992; Flotte *et al.*, 1993a,b
FAC-C[d]	Walsh *et al.*, 1993
Flt-3[e]	Broxmeyer *et al.*, 1995
FR[f]	Sun *et al.*, 1995
γ-globin	Walsh *et al.*, 1992; Miller *et al.*, 1994; Ponnazhagan *et al.*, 1997
GM-CSF[g]	Luo *et al.*, 1995
IL-2[h]	Philip *et al.*, 1994
NADPH-oxidase	Thrasher *et al.*, 1995
Neuropeptide Y	We *et al.*, 1994
TH[i]	Kaplitt *et al.*, 1994
TH[j]	Su *et al.*, 1996

[a] Human immunodeficiency virus-1.
[b] T cell costimulatory protein.
[c] Cystic fibrosis transmembrane conductance regulator.
[d] Fanconi's anemia-complementation group C.
[e] Ligand for Flt-3/Flk-2 tyrosine kinase receptor.
[f] Folate receptor.
[g] Granulocyte-macrophage colony-stimulating factor.
[h] Interleukin-2.
[i] Tyrosine hydroxylase.
[j] Thymidine kinase.

eutic gene sequences that have been transduced using this vector system. However, there has been some debate whether or not AAV transduces nondividing cells (Alexander *et al.*, 1994; Kaplitt *et al.*, 1994; Podsakoff *et al.*, 1994b; Russell *et al.*, 1994). Although it is clear that DNA-damaging agents can greatly increase AAV-mediated transduction (Alexander *et al.*, 1994, 1996), the lack of efficient transduction of some cells by AAV may also be a consequence of the need for the recombinant AAV genome to undergo second-strand DNA synthesis (Ferrari *et al.*, 1996; Fisher *et al.*, 1996). Thus, it appears that the efficiency of transduction may be cell type-specific (Ponnazhagan *et al.*, 1995c, 1996b,d), and studies are warranted to further examine this issue.

4.1. Nature of the Proviral Genome

Previous studies by Kotin *et al* (1989, 1990, 1991, 1992), and Samulski *et al.* (1991) established that the wt AAV genome integrates specifically on human chromosome 19q13.3-qter with very high frequency in established human cell lines. Previous studies with wt AAV also revealed that integrated proviral genome is almost always present in linear, tandem repeats (Giraud *et al.*, 1994, 1995). However, the site-specificity of integration of recombinant AAV vectors has not been documented (Goodman *et al.*, 1994; Ponnazhagan *et al.*, 1996a; Xiao *et al.*, 1993). Furthermore, recent studies by Afione *et al.* (1996) suggest that in a rhesus macaque model system *in vivo*, the recombinant AAV vector sequences persist in an episomal form for up to three months. Interestingly, however, using murine bone marrow primary and secondary transplant model systems, the sustained presence of and expression from, the recombinant proviral genomes in hematopoietic cells approximately one year posttransplantation have been documented (Podsakoff *et al.*, 1994a; Ponnazhagan *et al.*, 1995b, 1996c). These studies strongly suggest that successful transduction of the pluripotent hematopoietic stem cell, and by inference, stable integration of the proviral genome into host chromosomal DNA, does indeed occur. Again, although further studies are clearly warranted, these observations underscore the need to critically evaluate the interaction of recombinant AAV with each specific cell type being transduced.

4.2. Site Specificity of Integration

Although wt AAV is nonpathogenic, the general concept that the recombinant AAV vectors are also nonpathogenic and capable of site-specific delivery of therapeutic genes has not been rigorously examined. Ponnazhagan *et al.* (1996a) have attempted to examine the underlying molecular basis of the site-specific integration of the AAV genome in human cells. In these studies, the integration patterns of recombinant AAV genomes that lack one or both of the viral coding sequences were examined. Four recombinant AAV genomes were constructed containing (1) the genes for resistance to tetracycline (Tc^R) and the herpesvirus thymidine kinase (TK) promoter-driven gene for resistance to neomycin (*neo*^{R}; vTc.Neo), (2) the genes for resistance to ampicillin (Ap^R) and TK-*neo*^{R} (vAp.Neo), (3) the genes for AAV replication (*rep*) and TK-*neo*^{R} (vRep.Neo), or (4) the AAV capsid (*cap*) genes and TK-*neo*^{R} (vCap.Neo). The integration pattern of each of the recombinant AAV genomes in individual clonal isolates of human cells analyzed on Southern blots using a *neo*-specific DNA probe was distinctly different. In addition, in none of the clones examined was the proviral genome covalently linked to the previously described AAV right-junction (Rt.Jn.) human chromosomal DNA fragment (Kotin and Berns, 1989), the putative specific site of integration for the wt AAV genome. Furthermore, whereas a 276-bp DNA fragment was readily amplified by polymerase chain reaction (PCR) from each of these clones, using a *neo*-specific primer-pair, no amplified DNA product was obtained using a *neo*- and Rt.Jn. primer-pair under identical conditions. The pattern of integration of these recombinant AAV genomes was heterogeneous when cells were transduced at a multiplicity of infection (moi) of 1 (~.010100 physical particles). Furthermore, the putative site(s) of integration of each of these recombinant AAV genomes was distinctly different from that characterized for the wt AAV genome in cells transduced at an moi of 250 (~2,500 particles) (Kotin and Berns, 1989). Ponnazhagan *et al.* (1996a) also examined the putative role of the viral coding sequences in site-specific integration. For example, previous studies have indicated that the AAV-*rep* gene sequences mediate site-specific integration (Chiorini *et al.*, 1994; Giraud *et al.*, 1994, 1995; Weitzman *et al.*, 1994). However, at low moi, targeted integration of recombinant AAV genomes containing the AAV-*rep* gene in *cis* was not detected in several different clones that were analyzed. No functional activity of the transduced viral *rep* gene was detected in any of the clones examined, most likely because of deletions and/or rearrangements in these sequences upon integration or after application of a selective pressure. Interestingly, however, the integration pattern of recombinant AAV genomes in clones containing a functional *rep* gene was also heterogeneous. Similarly, heterogeneity in the integration patterns of the recombinant AAV genomes containing the viral *cap* gene sequences in *cis* was also observed. The transduced viral *cap* gene sequences, however, remained unaltered. Hence, it is clear that the site(s) of integration of the recombinant AAV genomes is different from that reported for the wild-type AAV (Ponnazhagan *et al.*, 1996a). Similar observations have been made using recombinant AAV genomes in established and primary human hematopoietic cells (Goodman *et al.*, 1994; Walsh *et al.*, 1992). Fluorescent *in situ* hybridization (FISH) analyses further revealed the lack of integration of the recombinant AAV into human chromosome 19, even in the presence of a functional *rep* gene. For example, none of the Rep-positive clones transduced with the vRep.Neo vector showed recombinant AAV integration in the long arm of chromosome 19 (Ponnazhagan *et al.*, 1996a). These data are consistent with previous studies documenting the lack of site-specific integration of recombinant AAV genomes into human chromosome 19 (Kearns *et al.*, 1996; Xiao *et al.*, 1993) and suggest that in the absence of optimal levels of expression of the Rep proteins recombinant AAV genomes integrate at sites that are different from those characterized for the wt AAV genome. However, Kube *et al.* (1997) showed that AAV Rep proteins are encapsidated in highly purified mature progeny virions. Whether the AAV-encapsidated Rep proteins at high moi play a role in *trans* in site-specific integration of the viral genome on human chromosome 19 remains to be investigated. In this context, it is noteworthy that the wt AAV genome integrates on chromosome 17 in

HeLa cells (Walz and Schlehofer, 1992), but in these studies cells were infected twice with AAV at an moi of 10. However, because normal human diploid cells are the most likely recipients for AAV-mediated gene therapy, now it is important to systematically investigate the molecular interaction of recombinant AAV with human cells in general and diploid cells in particular (Srivastava, 1994; Zhou *et al.*, 1993, 1994).

4.3. Tissue Specificity of Gene Expression

Previous studies have established that two key components are required for successful replication of the human parvoviral genome. These include the viral ITR sequences that serve as the origin of DNA replication (Lusby *et al.*, 1980; Srivastava, 1987), and the viral nonstructural (NS) proteins, called Rep for AAV and NS-1 for B19 (Shade *et al.*, 1986; Srivastava *et al.*, 1983). In AAV, expression of the major Rep proteins occurs from the p5 promoter (Hermonat *et al.*, 1984), whereas in B19 the NS-1 gene is expressed from the p6 promoter (Ozawa *et al.*, 1987). Previous studies also established that the cloned wt AAV genome undergoes DNA replication in human cells in the presence of a helper virus (Nahreini and Srivastava, 1989, 1992; Samulski *et al.*, 1982, 1983). However, the cloned B19 genome is not infectious because of deletions in its ITR sequences (Shade *et al.*, 1986). Srivastava *et al.* (1989) previously reported constructing a recombinant AAV-B19 genome in which the B19-ITRs were replaced by the AAV-ITRs. This hybrid virus was biologically indistinguishable from wt B19 and demonstrated autonomous replication in and cytotoxicity to human erythroid progenitor cells (Srivastava *et al.*, 1989, 1990). Because the remarkable features of these two parvoviruses were combined into the AAV-B19 hybrid virus, it led to the speculation that such a hybrid vector might prove useful for high-efficiency transduction of primary human hematopoietic progenitor cells (Srivastava *et al.*, 1989). Based on these results, a recombinant AAV-B19 hybrid vector has been developed and the construction of this is shown schematically in Figure 3. Using a number of reporter gene constructs in this hybrid vector, expression from the B19p6 promoter has not been detected in nonerythroid cells under nonselective conditions of recombinant virus infections (Ponnazhagan *et al.*, 1995c; 1996d).

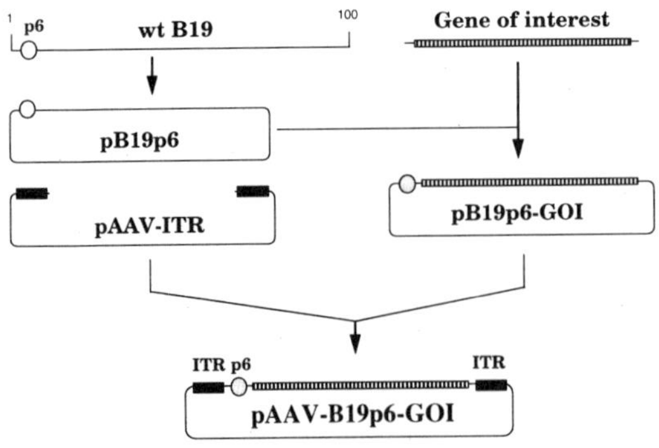

FIGURE 3. Construction strategy for generating recombinant AAV-B19 hybrid vectors. Parvovirus B19 promoter at map unit 6 (shaded circle), molecularly cloned in a bacterial plasmid, was ligated upstream of the gene of interest (hatched box) and subsequently inserted between the AAV-ITRs (closed boxes) by the standard techniques of molecular cloning described by Sambrook *et al.* (1989).

To further establish the erythroid cell specificity of expression from the B19p6 promoter, a novel AAV genome has been constructed in which only the authentic promoter at map unit 5 (AAVp5) has been replaced by the B19p6 promoter (Figure 4). Although the wt AAV requires a helper virus for its optimal replication, it was hypothesized that insertion of the B19p6 promoter in a recombinant AAV would permit autonomous viral replication, but only in primary human erythroid progenitor cells. The B19p6AAV hybrid genomes could be readily packaged into mature AAV virions that underwent successful replication in KB cells, but only in the presence of adenovirus (Wang *et al.*, 1995b). Thus, rescue, replication, and packaging of the B19p6AAV genome were indistinguishable from those of the wt AAV in KB cells (Nahreini and Srivastava, 1989). These results also indicated that the extent of rescue and replication of the recombinant B19p6AAV genome in the presence of adenovirus is nearly identical to that of the wt AAV genome from the plasmid p*Sub*201, suggesting that the B19p6 promoter is transactivated by adenovirus, similarly to the AAVp5 promoter (Samulski *et al.*, 1982, 1983). No rescue and replication occurred in the absence of adenovirus-infection (Wang *et al.*, 1995b). Since parvovirus B19 replicates autonomously in human hematopoietic cells, it was next examined whether the recombinant B19p6AAV virions autonomously replicate in normal human bone marrow cells. Equivalent stocks of the vB19p6AAV and the wt AAV were used separately to infect low-density human bone marrow (LDBM) cells in the presence of erythropoietin (Epo). Whereas no replication of wt AAV was detected, either in the absence or the presence of adenovirus (Wang *et al.*, 1995b),

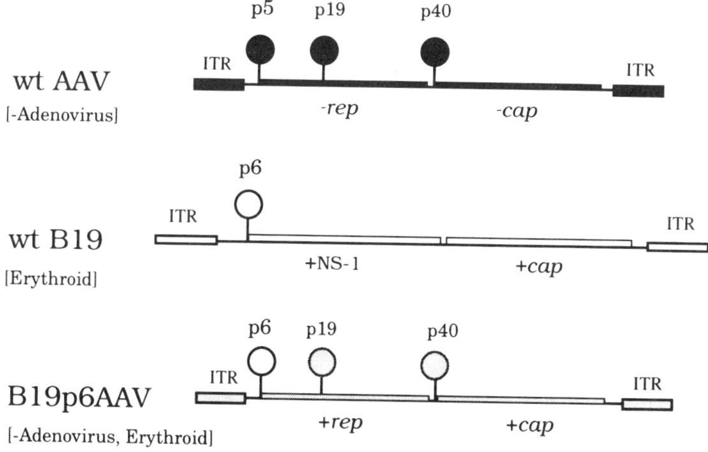

FIGURE 4. Schematic organizational representation of the wt AAV, wt B19, and recombinant B19p6AAV genomes. Expression of the AAV *rep* and the *cap* gene sequences from the three promoters (closed circles) in the viral genome does not occur in the absence of adenovirus, and a result, the wt AAV fails to replicate. Expression of the B19 NS-1 and *cap* genes under the control of the viral promoter at map unit 6 (open circle), on the other hand, occurs in human hematopoietic cells during erythroid differentiation, and as a result, the wt B19 autonomously replicates. When the AAVp5 promoter is replaced by the B19p6 promoter in the AAV genome, expression of the wt AAV *rep* and *cap* genes from this promoter occurs in human erythroid cells, and consequently, the recombinant B19p6AAV autonomously replicates (Wang *et al.*, 1995b).

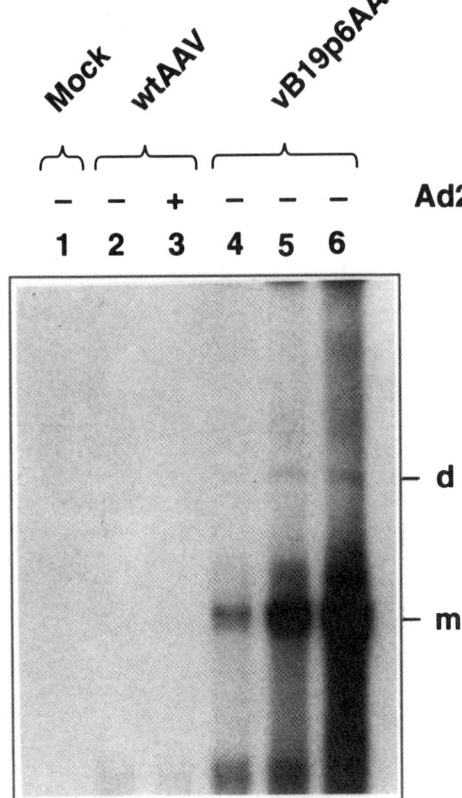

FIGURE 5. Southern blot analysis of replication of the recombinant vB19p6AAV in normal human bone marrow cells. Low-density bone marrow cells were mock-infected (lane 1), infected with wt AAV in the absence (lane 2) or the presence (lane 3) of adenovirus, or infected with purified vB19p6AAV (lanes 4–6) in the presence of erythropoietin. Recombinant viral stocks were generated as previously described (Nahreini *et al.*, 1993). Low M_r DNA samples were isolated by the method described by Hirt (1967), 72 hr (lanes 1–3 and 6), 24 hrs (lane 4), and 48 hrs (lane 5) postinfection, and analyzed on Southern blots (Southern, 1975) using a ^{32}P-labeled AAV DNA probe. m and d denote monomeric and dimeric replicative viral DNA intermediates, respectively (Wang *et al.*, 1995b).

vB19p6AAV underwent successful, autonomous replication in LDBM cells, as evidenced by the presence of the characteristic monomeric (m) and dimeric (d) replicative DNA intermediates on a Southern blot (Figure 5). The kinetics of autonomous replication of the recombinant B19p6AAV virions is remarkably similar to that of the wt parvovirus B19 (Munshi *et al.*, 1993; Ozawa *et al.*, 1986, 1987; Srivastava *et al.*, 1989, 1990, 1992). These results indicate that the B19p6 promoter sequence is necessary to confer autonomous replication-competence on AAV in primary human hematopoietic progenitor cells.

It has previously been shown that the parvovirus B19 selectively inhibits colony formation by erythroid progenitor cells in human bone marrow (Ozawa *et al.*, 1986, 1987; Srivastava and Lu, 1988, Srivastava *et al.*, 1989, 1990). AAV, on the other hand, infects myeloid and erythroid hematopoietic progenitors cells (Zhou *et al.*, 1993, 1994). Hematopoietic progenitor cell assays (colony-forming unit—granulocyte-macrophage, CFU-GM; burst-forming unit—erythroid, BFU-E) were carried out following mock infection or infections with the wt AAV or the vB19p6AAV virions under identical conditions (Moritz *et al.*, 1994; Yoder *et al.*, 1993). These results are shown in Figure 6. Whereas CFU-GM colony formation is not affected, infection with the vB19p6AAV virions significantly reduces BFU-E

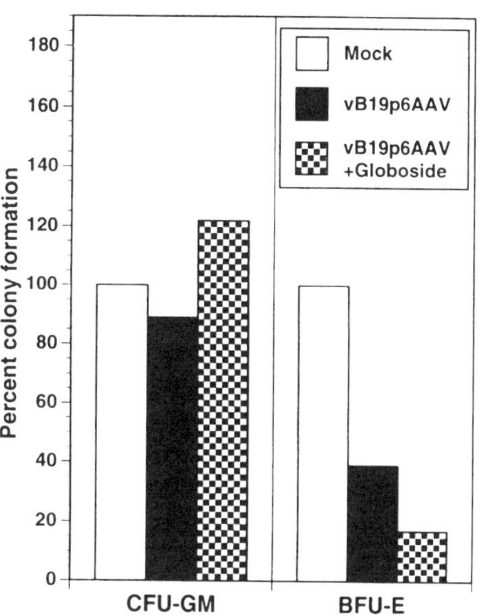

FIGURE 6. Effect of vB19p6AAV infection on primary human hematopoietic progenitor cells. Low-density human bone marrow cells were mock-infected (open bars) or infected with purified recombinant vB19p6AAV either with no treatment (closed bars) or pretreated (checkered bars) with 100µg/ml of globoside. Equivalent numbers of cells were analyzed in clonogenic assays for the frequency of colony-forming unit—granulocyte/macrophage (CFU-GM) and burst-forming unit—erythroid (BFU-E) progenitor-derived colonies, as previously described (Wang *et al.*, 1995b).

colony formation in hematopoietic progenitor cell assays. Furthermore, pretreatment of the recombinant vB19p6AAV with a large excess of globoside had no effect indicating that the putative receptor for AAV is distinct from the erythrocyte P antigen. Under identical conditions, wt AAV had no effect on CFU-GM and BFU-E colony formation (Wang *et al.*, 1995b). These results indicate that the B19p6 promoter is sufficient to impart erythroid-cell tropism to AAV in primary human hematopoietic progenitor cells. This simple substitution is necessary and sufficient to convert the otherwise noninfectious AAV to undergo successful, autonomous replication in the erythroid lineage in primary human hematopoietic progenitor cells. Thus, expression from the B19p6 promoter is erythroid-cell-specific and plays a crucial role in the post P antigen erythroid cell-tropism of parvovirus B19. These observations further distinguish the putative cellular receptors that mediate successful infection of human cells by AAV and B19, respectively (Ponnazhagan *et al.*, 1995c, 1996d; Wang *et al.*, 1995b).

4.4. Gene Therapy of Human Hemoglobinopathies

In the hope of exploiting the erythroid-cell specificity of expression from the B19p6 promoter, the potential of gene therapy of human hemoglobinopathies mediated by the recombinant AAV-B19 hybrid vector has been contemplated (Wang *et al.*, 1995b; Zhou *et al.*, 1996). For example, sickle-cell anemia and β-thalassemia are among the most well-characterized human hemoglobinopathies (Stamatoyannopoulos and Nienhuis, 1994), and because the molecular defects in these diseases are known and can potentially be corrected by introduction of normal alleles of the human β-globin gene, gene therapy of these diseases appears possible (Walsh *et al.*, 1993). Although retrovirus-based vectors have been developed and

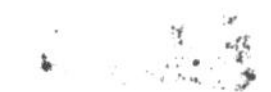

shown to stably transduce a normal human β-globin gene into murine and human hematopoietic progenitor cells (Bender *et al.*, 1988, 1989; Cone *et al.*, 1987; Dzierzak *et al.*, 1988; Karlsson *et al.*, 1987, 1988; Miller *et al.*, 1988), the low-level expression of the transduced gene in these cells limits the utility of these vectors in human gene therapy. Furthermore, although a strong erythroid-cell-specific enhancer, the locus control region (LCR) that flanks the human globin gene cluster, induces expression of the transduced globin genes *in vitro* and *in vivo* (Chang *et al.*, 1992; Novak *et al.*, 1990; Tuan *et al.*, 1989), efforts to develop retroviral vectors in which the structural integrity of the LCR is intact have become successful only recently (Leboulch *et al.*, 1994; Plavec *et al.*, 1993).

Zhou *et al.* (1996) described the construction of recombinant AAV vectors containing a normal human β-globin gene marked with a 4-bp Cla I linker, TK-*neo*^{R}

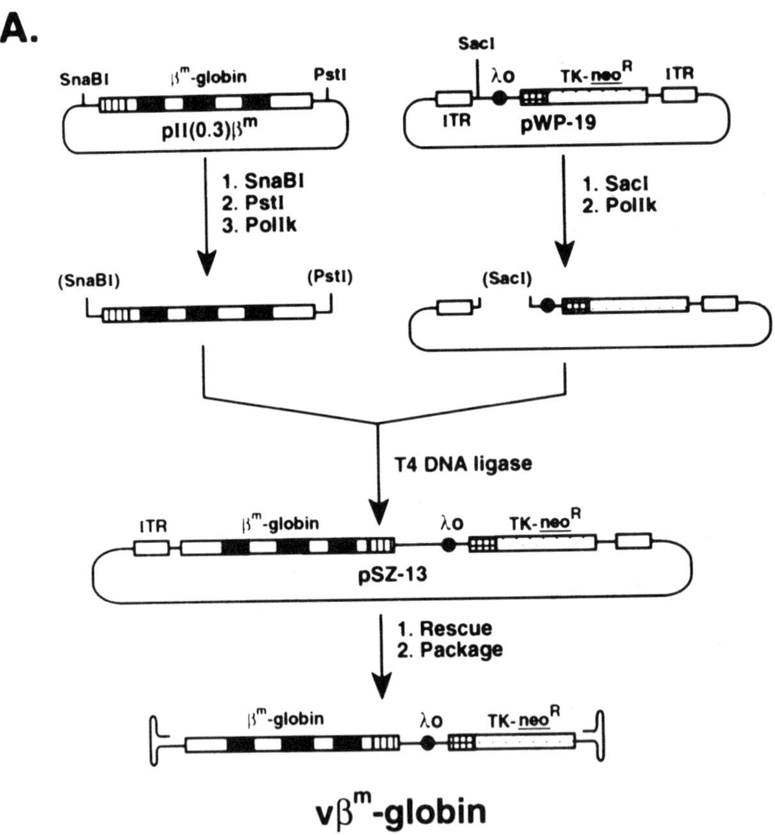

FIGURE 7. Strategy for constructing the recombinant AAV-β-globin plasmids and virions. Recombinant AAV genomes containing the genomic copy of a mutationally marked human β-globin gene and a gene for resistance to neomycin (*neo*^{R}) driven by the herpesvirus thymidine kinase promoter (vβ^m-globin; A), as well as that containing the HS-2 enhancer element (vHS2-β^m-globin; B) were constructed and were packaged into recombinant progeny AAV, as previously described (Zhou *et al.*, 1996).

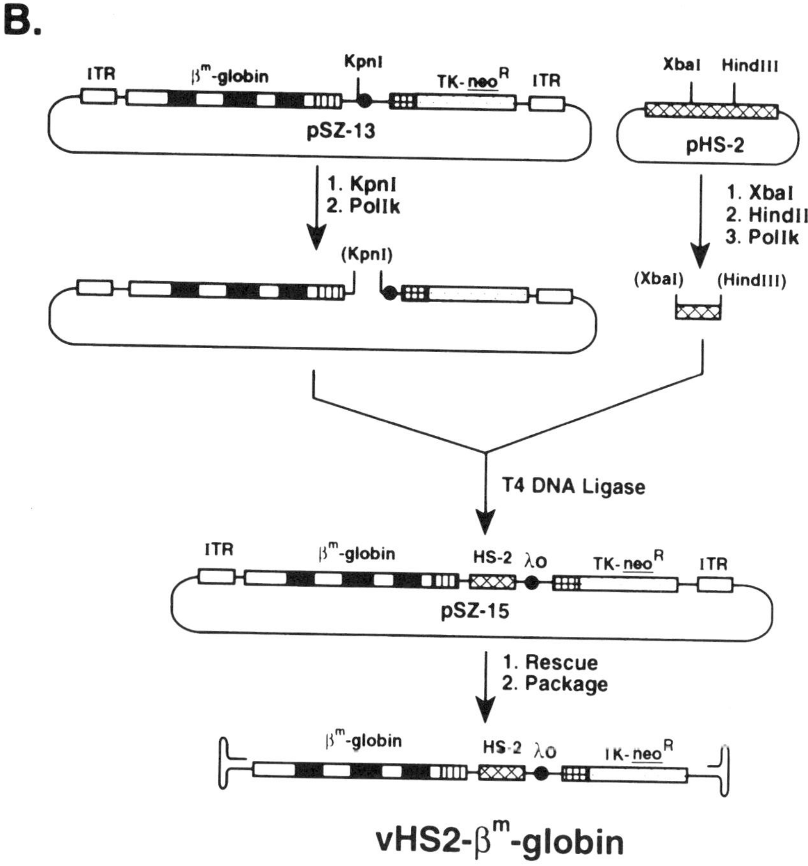

FIGURE 7. (*continued*)

(vβ^m-globin), and vectors containing an upstream DNase I-hypersensitive site 2 (HS-2) from the locus control region (LCR) of the human β-globin gene cluster (vHS2-β^m-globin). The construction strategies are depicted in Figure 7. An additional vector, in which the unmarked β-globin promoter was replaced by the B19p6 promoter, was also constructed (vHS2-B19p6-β-globin). These recombinant virions were used to infect a human erythroleukemia cell line (K562) or a nonerythroid human nasopharyngeal carcinoma cell line (KB) followed by selection with G418 and Southern blot analyses to indicate stable integration of the recombinant viral genome in these cells (Zhou *et al.*, 1996). Additional restriction mapping suggested that the integration *per se* does not lead to structural rearrangements in the recombinant viral genomes. K562 cells offer a useful system for expression analysis of the transduced β-globin gene because these cells do not normally express the endogenous β-globin gene (Charnay and Maniatis, 1983). RNase protection assays were carried out to detect whether transcription of the transduced gene occurs in these cells. Because the transduced β-globin gene is marked by a 4-bp insertion at the Cap site, an antisense RNA probe is expected to hybridize to RNA transcripts derived from this gene and produce a 136-nt protected fragment following digestion with RNases. These data are presented in Figure 8. As can be seen, whereas no protected fragment was detected in mock-infected cells (lane 1), cells infected with the vTK-Neo virions lacking the β-globin gene (lane 2), or those infected with the vβ^{m}-globin virions (lane 3), a protected fragment of 136-nt was clearly detected in cells infected with the vHS2-β^{m}-globin virions (lane 4). These data strongly suggest that the HS-2 enhancer element is required in *cis* to obtain high-level expression of the transduced β-globin gene. Because the β-globin gene used in the vHS2-B19p6-β-globin construct did not contain the 4-bp Cla I linker, the protected fragment could not be detected by RNase protection assays (lane 5). However, subsequent studies have clearly established that expression from this promoter, in the context of a parvoviral genome, does not occur in established human cell lines (Ponnazhagan *et al.*, 1995c; 1996d). However, erythroid-cell-specific expression of the transduced β-globin in K562, but not in KB cells has also been observed (Zhou *et al.*, 1996). These studies indicate that it is indeed feasible to obtain AAV-mediated transduction and erythroid-cell-specific expression of human globin genes.

In addition to the potential benefit to patients with sickle-cell anemia, transfer and expression of a normal human β-globin gene is also likely to ameliorate clinical symptoms of β-thalassemia, often a fatal disease. Although in β-thalassemia, which

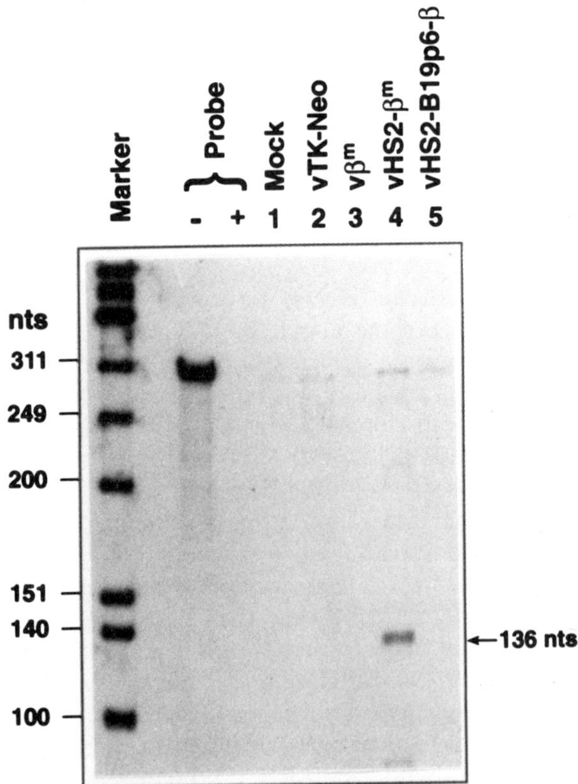

FIGURE 8. Expression of the transduced β-globin gene in K562 cells. Total cellular RNA samples isolated from mock-infected (lane 1) or infected either with the vTK-Neo virus (lane 2), vβ^{m}-globin virus (lane 3), vHS2-β^{m}-globin virus (lane 4), or the vHS2-B19p6-β-globin virus (lane 5) were analyzed by RNase protection assays. ^{32}P-labeled Hinf 1-cleaved ϕX174 DNA fragments were coelectrophoresed to serve as size markers (lane Marker). A 286-nt uniformly labeled β-globin-specific RNA probe (lanes Probe) untreated (−) or treated (+) with RNases was also electrophoresed. A 136-nt protected RNA fragment (arrow) indicates expression of the transduced β^{m}-globin gene (Zhou *et al.*, 1996).

is characterized by defective β-globin production, a mechanism to deliver a functional β-globin gene would be a preferred form of treatment, a second line of therapeutic measures which could ameliorate the severity of this disease would be to suppress the accumulation of excessive levels of the α-globin chains in red blood cells. Therefore, the potential usefulness of the AAV-based vectors to suppress the excess production of the human α-globin gene has also been investigated because in the homozygous condition β-thalassemia is also characterized by accumulation of excessive free α-globin chains which results in premature death of erythroid progenitor cells before they reach the reticulocyte stage. A mechanism that could control the excess production of free α-globin chains would be expected to largely benefit in ameliorating the clinical severity of this disease. For this purpose, recombinant AAV vectors have been generated that contain the human α-globin gene sequences in antisense orientation driven by the herpesvirus thymidine kinase (TK) promoter, the SV40 early gene promoter, and the human α-globin gene promoter, respectively, as well as a bacterial gene for resistance to neomycin (*neo*^{R}) as a selectable marker (Ponnazhagan *et al.*, 1994a). The overall strategy for constructing the three different recombinant AAV plasmids is illustrated in Figure 9. These recombinant virions were used to infect K562 cells, which express high levels of α-globin mRNA. Clonal populations of *neo*^{R} cells were obtained following selection with G418. Total genomic DNA samples isolated from these cells were analyzed on Southern blots to document stable integration of the transduced *neo* and α-globin genes (Ponnazhagan *et al.*, 1994a). Total cellular RNA samples isolated from mock-infected and the recombinant virus-infected cultures were also analyzed by Northern blots to determine whether the transduced antisense α-globin sequences modulate the levels of expression of the constitutively expressed α-globin gene in K562 cells. These results are shown in Figure 10. It is evident that when a *neo*-specific DNA is used as probe (Panel A), no hybridization is detected in mock-infected K562 cells (lane 1), whereas the probe detected specific RNA transcripts in the three recombinant virus-infected cultures (lanes 2–4). The sizes of the transcripts correspond to their respective genomes. When the same blot is probed with an α-globin probe (Panel B), mock-infected (lane 1) and vTKp-globin-α virus-infected (lane 2) K562 show abundant expression of the endogenous α-globin gene. However, cell populations transduced with vSV40p-globin-α (lane 3) and vαp-globin-α (lane 4) virions show a clear suppression of expression of the endogenous gene. Densitometric analyses of the hybridization signals revealed that the extent of this suppression is approximately 29% with vSV40p-globin-α and 91% with vαp-globin-α recombinant virions referred to the levels of β-actin mRNA (Panel C). These levels also correspond well with ethidium bromide-induced fluorescent intensities of 28s and 18s ribosomal RNA bands in these cell populations (Panel D). Expression of the *neo*-specific RNA transcripts is significantly lower with the TK promoter than with the SV40 promoter (Panel A) indicating the relative inefficiency of the TK promoter function compared with that of the SV40 promoter in K562 cells. The strategy employed was based on suppressing the augmented α-globin levels at the transcriptional stage by producing antisense α-globin RNA sequences mediated by AAV. Significantly inhibited expression of the endogenous α-globin gene in K562 cells was observed upon infection with recombinant AAV virions

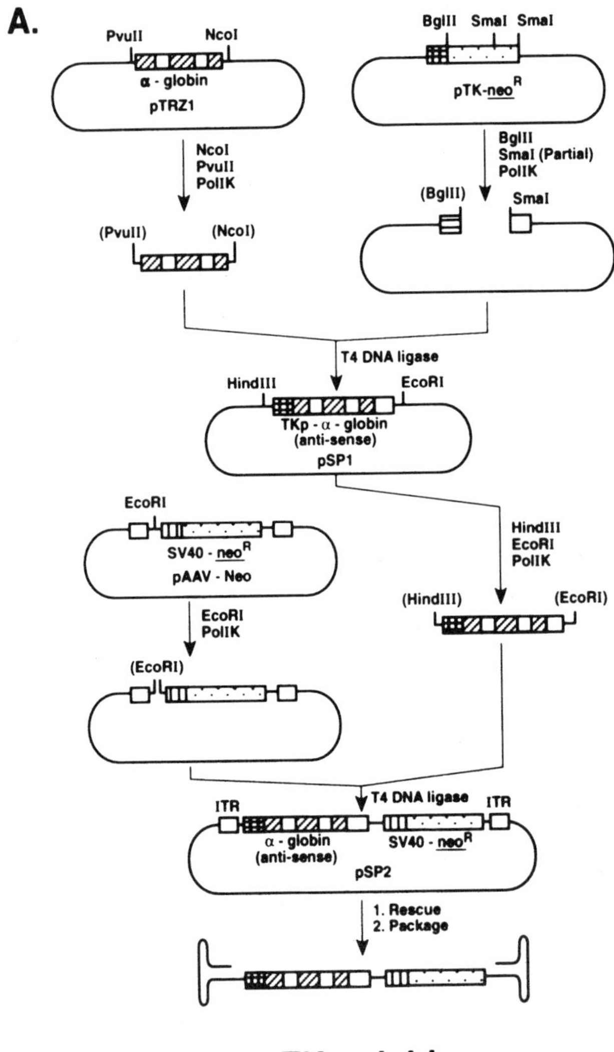

FIGURE 9. Strategy of constructing antisense human α-globin gene-containing recombinant AAV plasmids and virions. The overall strategy for constructing the recombinant AAV genomes containing antisense α-globin sequences driven by the TK promoter (vTKp-globin-α; A), the SV40 promoter (vSV40p-globin-α; B), and the α-globin promoter (vαp-globin-α; C) is depicted. Recombinant virus stocks were generated, as previously described (Ponnazhagan *et al.*, 1994a).

harboring the antisense human α-globin DNA sequences driven either by the SV40 early promoter or the human α-globin gene promoter. Thus, the AAV-based vector system may prove useful in the potential gene therapy of human hemoglobinopathies in general and β-thalassemia in particular.

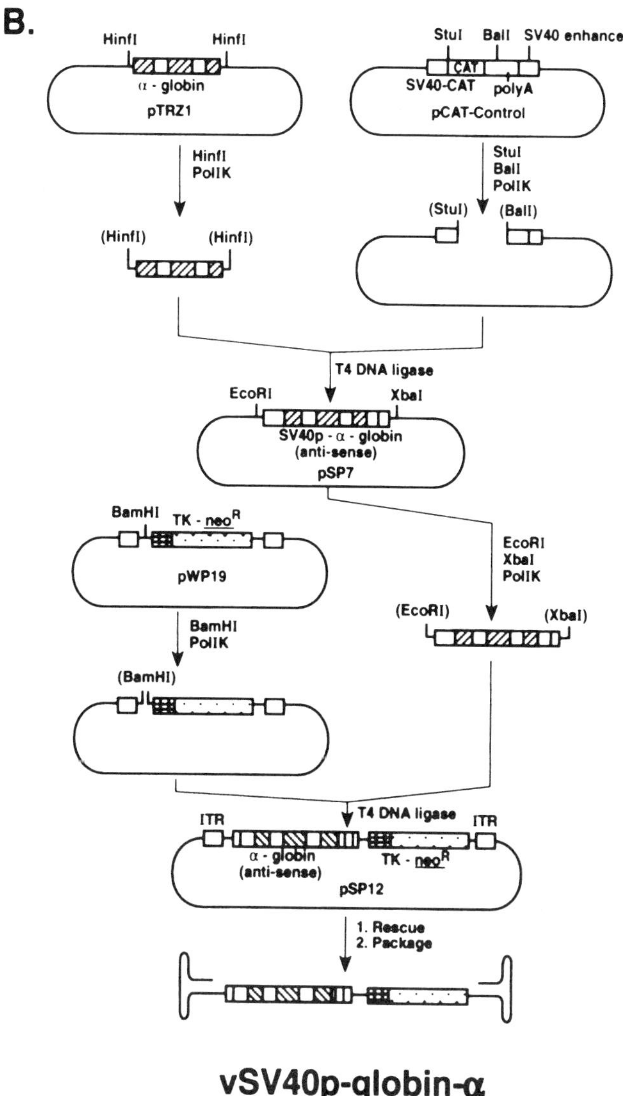

FIGURE 9. *(continued)*

Although a high-level of suppression of expression of the endogenous α-globin gene in clonal populations of relatively homogeneous K562 cells is readily obtained, it may be undesirable to completely block the expression of the required basal amounts of the endogenous α-globin gene in primary human hematopoietic cells by overproducing the antisense α-globin RNA transcripts. However, given the heterogeneous nature of the primary human hematopoietic cells, this is unlikely to be the case. Efforts are currently underway to deliver a normal allele of the β-globin gene

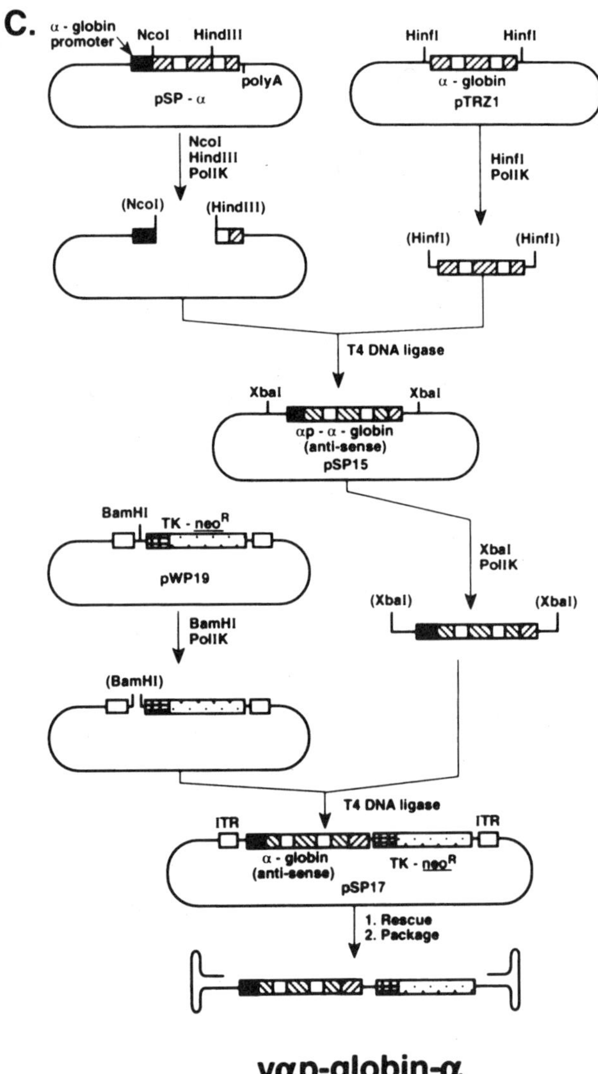

FIGURE 9. *(continued)*

and the antisense α-globin sequences contained within the same chimeric AAV vector (C. Kurpad and A. Srivastava, unpublished results). Whether this strategy with primary cultures will prove effective *in vitro* remains to be determined. It also remains to be ascertained whether this treatment will be safe and efficacious in an animal model *in vivo* before it is used in human gene therapy. This form of gene transfer using antisense RNA production may, nonetheless, prove useful for treating a wide variety of diseases that are characterized by undesirable overexpression of endogenous genes or genes from infectious agents.

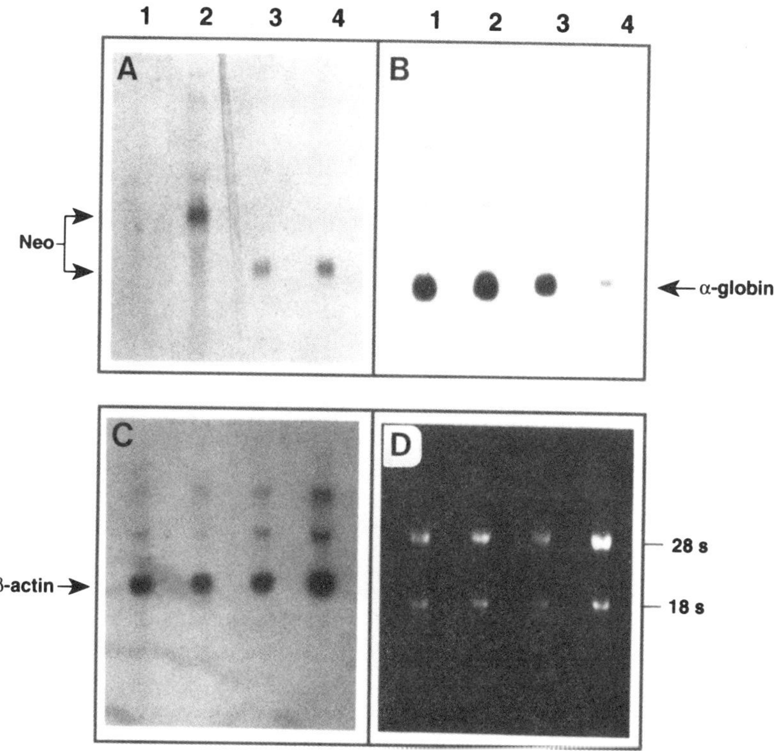

FIGURE 10. Expression of the endogenous human α-globin gene in K562 cells. Total RNA samples isolated from mock-infected (lane 1), vTKp-globin-α virus-infected (lane 2), vSV40p-globin-α virus-infected (lane 3), and vαp-globin-α virus-infected (lane 4) K562 cells were analyzed on Northern blots using the following DNA probes: *neo* (A), α-globin (B), and β-actin (C). Ethidium bromide-induced fluorescence of 28s and 18s ribosomal RNAs is also shown (D). Gene expression was quantitated by densitometry (Ponnazhagan *et al.*, 1994a).

5. ADVANTAGES AND DISADVANTAGES OF PARVOVIRUS VECTORS

In contrast to retroviruses and all other DNA-containing viruses, parvoviruses remain the only group of viruses that have not been associated to date with any malignant disease, and in fact, possess anti-tumor properties. Specifically, the nonpathogenic nature of AAV, and the remarkable tissue-tropism of B19, make these viruses extremely attractive for developing vectors for human gene therapy. The following brief account attests to the fact that the advantages far outnumber the disadvantages of the parvovirus-based vector system for human gene therapy.

5.1. Size Limitation

Perhaps, one of the main limitations of the parvovirus vectors is the size of a DNA sequence that can be packaged into mature virions. However, this vector should be useful for packaging most cDNA copies of therapeutic genes.

5.2. Large-Scale Production

It is increasingly clear that the problem of large-scale, commercial production of high-titer recombinant AAV vectors is not as insurmountable as initially perceived. Although low-levels of contamination with wt AAV in some of the recombinant vectors have been observed, it is not entirely clear how critical this problem will be for gene therapy. The stability of parvoviruses between pH 3.0 and 9.0, resistance to lipid solvents, and resistance to heat inactivation at 56°C should, nonetheless, contribute to global application of gene therapy with these vectors.

5.3. Host Range

With the sole exception to date of human megakaryocytic leukemia cells (Ponnazhagan *et al.*, 1996d), AAV thus far has an extremely broad host range that transcends species barriers (Muzyczka, 1992). The ability of AAV to transduce nondividing cells and that of B19 to selectively infect human erythroid cells, coupled with the potential nonrandom integration of the proviral genome in human cells, are also desirable features. Vector mobilization is a finite possibility but is unlikely because simultaneous infections by wt AAV and adenovirus would be required and that rescue of the integrated proviral genome occurs only in approximately 30% of transduced cells, at least *in vitro* (McLaughlin *et al.*, 1988). On the other hand, superinfection immunity by AAV has not been observed, at least *ex vivo* (Lebkowski *et al.*, 1988). In contrast to the clinical application of retrovirus vectors, which are of murine origin, both AAV and B19 are human viruses and therefore may be physiologically more relevant for human gene therapy.

5.4. Safety and Efficacy

In contrast to adenovirus-based vectors, none of the wt AAV genes is present in most recombinant vectors. Thus, the possibility of an adverse immune response to these vectors *in vivo* is greatly diminished (Ponnazhagan *et al.*, 1996b). However, because a great majority of the population is sero-positive for human parvoviruses, successful transduction of human cells *in vivo* would be challenging, if not insurmountable. Recent *in vivo* studies with animal models documenting long-term expression of AAV-mediated transduced genes (Chatterjee *et al.*, 1995; Flotte *et al.*, 1993a,b; Kaplitt *et al.*, 1994; Ponnazhagan *et al.*, 1996c), argue in favor of utilizing the parvovirus-based vector system in human gene therapy.

6. SUMMARY AND CONCLUSIONS

From the foregoing discussion it is clear that although a number of issues related to the parvovirus-based vectors still need to be resolved, this unique vector system can be a safe and effective alternative to the more commonly used retrovirus- and adenovirus-based vectors in human gene therapy. It is evident that extensive studies on AAV vectors are currently underway in a number of laboratories. Our own efforts have focused on developing AAV-B19 hybrid vectors (Srivastava *et al.*, 1996). We anticipate that these vectors will prove useful in gene therapy of human hemoglobinopathies in general and sickle-cell anemia and β-thalassemia in particular.

7. FUTURE PROSPECTS

Detailed characterization of parvoviral interaction with primary human cells will undoubtedly yield new and useful information applicable in further developing parvovirus-based vectors. Understanding the molecular mechanisms underlying viral assembly, viral entry into target cells, stability of integration, and sustained expression of transduced genes will also be critical in realizing the full potential of this vector system. And finally, in addition to potential treatment of human hemoglobinopathies, the AAV-based vector system promises to lead to gene therapy of a variety of clinical human disorders, both genetic and acquired.

ACKNOWLEDGMENTS. I thank Drs. Kenneth I. Berns, Hal E. Broxmeyer, David A. Williams, and Mervin C. Yoder for their encouragement and support. I also thank Drs. Richard J. Samulski, George Stamatoyannopoulos, Peter J. Tattersall, and Tim M. Townes for their kind gifts of recombinant plasmids and the past and present members of my laboratory for helpful discussions.

The research in the author's laboratory was supported in part by grants from the National Institutes of Health (Public Health Service grants AI-26323, HL-48342, HL-53586, HL-58881, and DK-49218, Centers of Excellence in Molecular Hematology), Phi Beta Psi Sorority, and an Established Investigator Award from the American Heart Association.

8. REFERENCES

Afione, S. A., Conrad, C. K., Kearns, W. G., Chunduru, S., Adams, R., Reynolds, T. C., Guggino, W. G., Cutting, G. R., Carter, B. J., and Flotte, T. R., 1996, In vivo model of adeno-associated virus vector persistence and rescue, *J. Virol.* **70:**3235–3241.

Alexander, I. A., Russell, D. W., and Miller, A. D., 1994, DNA-damaging agents greatly increase the transduction of nondividing cells by adeno-associated virus vectors, *J. Virol.* **68:**8282–8287.

Alexander, I. A., Russell, D. W., Spence, A. M., and Miller, A. D., 1996, Effects of gamma irradiation on the transduction of dividing and nondividing cells in brain and muscle of rats by adeno-associated virus vectors, *Hum. Gene Ther.* **7:**841–850.

Anderson, W. F., 1995, Gene therapy, *Sci. Am.* **273:**124–128.

Ashktorab, H., and Srivastava, A., 1989, Identification of nuclear proteins that specifically interact with adeno-associated virus type 2 inverted terminal repeat hairpin DNA, *J. Virol.* **63:**3034–3039.

Bender, M. A., Gelinas, R. E., and Miller, A. D., 1989, A majority of mice show long-term expression of a human β-globin gene into hematopoietic stem cells, *Mol. Cell. Biol.* **9:**1426–1434. Retroviral-mediated transfer of genomic globin genes leads to regulated production of RNA.

Bender, M. A., Miller, A. D., and Gelinas, R. E., 1988, Expression of the human β-globin gene after retroviral transfer into murine erythroleukemia cells and human BFU-E cells, *Mol. Cell. Biol.* **8:**1725–1735.

Berns, K. I., 1990, Parvovirus replication, *Microbiol. Rev.* **54:**316–329.

Berns, K. I., and Bohenzky, R. A., 1987, Adeno-associated viruses: An update, *Adv. Virus Res.* **32:**243–306.

Berns, K. I., and Hauswirth, W. W., 1979, Adeno-associated viruses, *Adv. Virus Res.* **25:**407–449.

Berns, K. I., and Linden, R. M., 1995, The cryptic life style of adeno-associated virus, *BioEssays* **17:**237–245.

Blacklow, N. R., 1988, in *Parvoviruses and Human Disease*, CRC Press, Boca Raton.

Blaese, R. M., Culver, K. W., Miller, A. D., Carter, C. S., Fleisher, T., Clerici, M., Shearer, G., Chang, L., Chiang, Y., Tolstoshev, P., Greenblatt, J. J., Rosenberg, S. A., Klein, H., Berger, M., Mullen, C. A., Ramsey, W. J., Muul, L., Morgan, R. A., and Anderson, W. F., 1995, T lymphocyte-directed gene therapy for ADA⁻ SCID: Initial trial results after 4 years, *Science* **270:**475–480.

Bordignon, C., Notarangelo, L. G., Nobili, N., Ferrari, G., Casorati, G., Panina, P., Mazzolari, E., Maggioni, D., Rossi, C., Servida, P., Ugazio, A. G., and Mavilio, F., 1995, Gene therapy in peripheral blood lymphocytes and bone marrow for ADA⁻ immunodeficient patients, *Science* **270:**470–475.

Brown, K. E., Anderson, S. M., and Young, N. S., 1993, Erythrocyte P antigen: Cellular receptor for B19 parvovirus, *Science* **262:**114–117.

Brown, K. E., Young, N. S., and Liu, J. M., 1994, Molecular, cellular and clinical aspects of parvovirus B19 infection, *Crit. Rev. Oncol. Hematol.* **16:**1–31.

Broxmeyer, H. E., Cooper, S., Etienne-Julan, M., Wang, X.-S., Ponnazhagan, S., Braun, S., Lu, L., and Srivastava, A., 1995, Cord blood transplantation and the potential for gene therapy: Gene transduction using a recombinant adeno-associated viral vector, *Ann. NY Acad. Sci.* **770:**105–115.

Carter, B. J., 1993, Adeno-associated virus vectors, *Curr. Opinion Biotechnol.* **3:**533–539.

Cavalier-Smith, T., 1974, Palindromic base sequences and replication of eukaryotic chromosome ends, *Nature* **350:**467–470.

Chang, J. C., Liu, D., and Kan, Y. W., 1992, A 36 base pair core sequence of locus control region enhances retrovirally transferred human β-globin gene expression, *Proc. Natl. Acad. Sci. USA* **89:**3107–3110.

Charnay, P., and Maniatis, T., 1983, Transcriptional regulation of globin gene expression in the human erythroid cell line K562, *Science* **220:**1281–1283.

Chatterjee, S., Johnson, P. R., and Wong, K. K., 1992, Dual-target inhibition of HIV-1 by means of an adeno-associated virus antisense vector, *Science* **258:**1485–1488.

Chatterjee, S., Lu, D., Podsakoff, G., and Wong, K. K., 1995, Strategies for efficient gene transfer into hematopoietic cells: The use of adeno-associated virus vectors in gene therapy, *Ann. NY Acad. Sci.* **770:**79–90.

Cheung, A. K. M., Hoggan, M. D., Hauswirth, W. W., and Berns, K. I., 1980, Integration of the adeno-associated virus genome into cellular DNA latently infected human Detroit 6 cells, *J. Virol.* **33:**739–748.

Chiorini, J. A., Wendtner, C. M., Urcelay, E., Safer, B., Hallek, M., and Kotin, R. M., 1995, High-efficiency transfer of the T cell co-stimulatory molecule B7-2 to lymphoid cells using high-titer recombinant adeno-associated virus vectors, *Hum. Gene Ther.* **6:**1531–1541.

Colosi, P., Elliger, S., Elliger, C., and Kurtzman. G., 1995, AAV vectors can be efficiently produced without helper virus, *Blood* **10:**627a.

Cone, R. D., Weber-Benarous, A., Baorto, D., and Mulligan, R. C., 1987, Regulated expression of a complete human β-globin gene encoded by a transmissible retrovirus vector, *Mol. Cell. Biol.* **7:**887–897.

Cooling, L. L. W., Koerner, T. A. W., and Naides, S. J., 1995, Multiple glycosphingolipids determine the tissue tropism of parvovirus B19, *J. Inf. Dis.* **172:**1198–1205.

Cotmore, S. F., and Tattersall, P. J., 1984, Characterization and molecular cloning of a human parvovirus genome, *Science* **226:**1161–1165.

Cotmore, S. F., and Tattersall, P. J., 1987, The autonomously replicating parvoviruses of vertebrates, *Adv. Virus Res.* **33:**91–174.

Crystal, R. G., McElvaney, N. G., Rosenfeld, M. A., Chu, C. S., Mastrangeli, A., Hay, J. G., Brody, S. L., Jaffe, H. A., Eissa, N. T., and Danel, C., 1994, Administration of an adenovirus containing the human *CFTR* cDNA to the respiratory tract of individuals with apticfibrosis, *Nature Genet.* **270:**404–410.

Cukor, G., Blacklow, N. R., Kibrick, S., and Swan, I. C., 1975, Effect of adeno-associated virus on cancer expression by herpesvirus-transformed hamster cells, *J. Natl. Cancer Inst.* **55:**957–959.

Deiss, V., Tratschin, J.-D., Weitz, M., and Siegl, G., 1990, Cloning of the human parvovirus B19 genome and structural analysis of its palindromic termini, *Virology* **175:**247–254.

Dixit, M., Webb, M. S., Smart, W. C., and Ohi, S., 1991, Construction and expression of a recombinant adeno-associated virus that harbors a human β-globin-encoding cDNA, *Gene* **104:**253–257.

Donahue, R. E., Kessler, S. W., Bodine, D., McDonagh, K., Dunbar, C., Goodman, S., Agricola, B., Byrne, E., Raffeld, M., Moen, R., Bacher, J., Zsebo, K. M., and Nienhuis, A. W., 1992, Helper virus induced T cell lymphoma in non-human primates after retroviral mediated gene transfer, *J. Exp. Med.* **176:**1125–1135.

Dzierzak, E. A., Papayannopoulou, T., and Mulligan, R. C., 1988, Lineage-specific expression of a human β-globin in murine bone marrow transplant recipients reconstituted with retrovirus-transduced stem cells, *Nature* **331:**35–41.

Egan, M., Flotte, T. R., Afione, S., Solow, R., Zeitlin, P. L., Carter, B. J., and Guggino, W. G., 1992, Defective regulation of outwardly rectifying Cl⁻ channels by protein kinase A corrected by insertion of CFTR, *Nature* **358:**581–584.

Einerhand, M. P. W., Antoniou, M., Zolotukhin, S., Muzyczka, N., Berns, K. I., Grosveld, F., and Valerio, D., 1995, Regulated high-level human beta-globin gene expression in erythroid cells following recombinant adeno-associated virus-mediated gene transfer, *Gene Ther.* **2:**336–343.

Ferrari, F. K., Samulski, T., Shenk, T., and Samulski, R. J., 1996, Second-strand synthesis is a rate-limiting step for efficient transduction by recombinant adeno-associated virus vectors, *J. Virol.* **70:**3227–3234.

Fisher, K. J., Gao, G.-P., Weitzman, M. D., DeMatteo, R., Burda, J. F., and Wilson, J. M., 1996, Transduction with recombinant adeno-associated virus for gene therapy is limited by leading-strand synthesis, *J. Virol.* **70:**520–532.

Flotte, T. R., Afione, S. A., Conrad, C., McGrath, S. A., Solow, R., Oka, H., Zeitlin, P., Guggino, W., and Carter, B. J., 1993a, Stable in vivo expression of the cystic fibrosis transmembrane conductance regulator with an adeno-associated virus vector, *Proc. Natl. Acad. Sci. USA* **90:**10613–10617.

Flotte, T. R., Afione, S. A., Solow, R., Drumm, M. L., Markakis, D., Guggino, W. B., Zeitlin, P., and Carter, B. J., 1993b, Expression of the cystic fibrosis transmembrane conductance regulator from a novel adeno-associated virus promoter, *J. Biol. Chem.* **268:**3781–3790.

Flotte, T. R., Barraza-Oritz, X., Solow, R., Afione, S. A., Carter, B. J., and Guggino, W. B., 1995, An improved system for packaging recombinant adeno-associated virus vectors capable of in vivo transduction, *Gene Ther.* **2:**29–37.

Flotte, T. R., and Carter, B. J., 1995, Adeno-associated virus vectors for gene therapy, *Gene Ther.* **2:**357–362.

Frickhofen, N., and Young, N. S., 1989, Persistent parvovirus B19 infections in humans, *Microb. Pathog.* **7:**319–327.

Gahr, M., Pekrun, A., and Eilfert, H., 1991, Persistence of parvovirus B19-DNA in blood of a child with severe combined immunodeficiency associated with chronic pure red cell aplasia, *Eur. J. Pediatr.* **150:**470–472.

Giraud, C., Winocour, E., and Berns, K. I., 1994, Site-specific integration by adeno-associated virus is directed by a cellular DNA sequence, *Proc. Natl. Acad. Sci. USA* **91:**10039–10043.

Giraud. C., Winocour, E., and Berns, K. I., 1995, Recombinant junctions formed by site-specific integration of adeno-associated virus into an episome, *J. Virol.* **69:**6917–6924.

Goodman, S., Xiao, X., Donahue, R. E., Moulton, A., Miller, J., Walsh, C., Young, N. S., Samulski, R. J., and Nienhuis, A. W., 1994, Recombinant adeno-associated virus mediated gene transfer into hematopoietic progenitor cells, *Blood* **84:**1492–1500.

Gottlieb, J., and Muzyczka, N., 1988, In vitro excision of adeno-associated virus DNA from recombinant plasmids: Isolation of an enzyme fraction from HeLa cells that cleaves DNA at poly(G) sequences, *Mol. Cell. Biol.* **6:**2513–2522.

Grossman, M., Raper, S. E., Kozarsky, K., Stein, E. A., Engelhardt, J. F., Muller, D., Lupien, P. J., and Wilson, J. M., 1994, Successful ex vivo gene therapy directed to liver in a patient with familial hypercholesterolaemia, *Nat. Genet.* **6:**335–341.

Hauswirth, W. W., and Berns, K. I., 1979, Adeno-associated virus DNA replication: Nonunit length molecules, *Virology* **93:**57–68.

Hermonat, P. L., Labow, M. A., Wright, R., Berns, K. I., Muzyczka, N., 1984, Genetics of adeno-associated virus: Isolation and preliminary characterization of adeno-associated virus type 2 mutants, *J. Virol.* **51:**329–339.

Hermonat, P. L., and Muzyczka, N., 1984, Use of adeno-associated virus as a mammalian DNA cloning vector: Transduction of neomycin resistance into mammalian tissue culture cells, *Proc. Natl. Acad. Sci. USA* **81:**6466–6470.

Hirt, B., 1967, Selective extraction of polyoma DNA from infected mouse cultures, *J. Mol. Biol.* **26:**365–369.

Hodgson, C. P., 1995, The vector void in gene therapy, *Bio/Technol.* **13:**222–225.

Hölscher, C., Hörer, M., Kleinschmidt, J. A., Zentgraf, H., Bürkle, A., and Heilbronn, R., 1994, Cell lines inducibly expressing the adeno-associated virus (AAV) *rep* gene: Requirements for productive replication of *rep*-negative AAV mutants, *J. Virol.* **68:**7169–7177.

Hölscher, C., Kleinschmidt, J. A., and Bürkle, A., 1995, High-level expression of adeno-associated virus (AAV) Rep78 protein is sufficient for infectious-particle formation by a *rep*-negative AAV mutant, *J. Virol.* **69:**6880–6885.

Hong, G., Ward, P., and Berns, K. I., 1992, In vitro replication of adeno-associated virus DNA, *Proc. Natl. Acad. Sci. USA* **89:**4673–4677.

Hong, G., Ward, P., and Berns, K. I., 1994, Intermediates of adeno-associated virus DNA replication in vitro, *J. Virol.* **68:**2011–2015.

Im, D.-S., and Muzyczka, N., 1989, Factors that bind to adeno-associated virus terminal repeats, *J. Virol.* **63:**3095–3104.

Im, D.-S., and Muzyczka, N., 1990, The AAV origin binding protein Rep68 is an ATP-dependent site-specific endonuclease with DNA helicase activity, *Cell* **61:**447–457.

Im, D.-S., and Muzyczka, N., 1992, Partial purification of adeno-associated virus Rep78, Rep52, and Rep40 proteins and their biochemical characterization, *J. Virol.* **66:**1119–1128.

Kaplitt, M. G., Leone, P., Samulski, R. J., Xiao, X., Pfaff, D. W., O'Malley, K. L., and During, M. J., 1994, Long-term gene expression and phenotypic correction using adeno-associated virus vectors in the mammalian brain, *Nat. Genet.* **8:**148–153.

Karlsson, S., Bodine, D. M., Perry, L., Papayannopoulou, T., and Nienhuis, A. W., 1988, Expression of the human β-globin gene following retroviral-mediated multipotential hematopoietic progenitors of mice, *Proc. Natl. Acad. Sci. USA* **85:**6062–6066.

Karlsson, S., Papayannopoulou, T., Schweiger, S. G., Stamatoyannopoulos, G., and Nienhuis, A. W., 1987, Retroviral-mediated transfer of genomic globin genes leads to regulated production of RNA and protein, *Proc. Natl. Acad. Sci. USA* **84:**2411–2415.

Kearns, W. G., Afione, S. A., Fulmer, S. B., Pang, M. G., Erikson, D., Egan, M., Landrum, M., Flotte, T. R., and Cutting, G. R., 1996, Recombinant adeno-associated virus (AAV-CFTR) vectors do not integrate in a site-specific fashion in an immortalized epithelial cell line, *Gene Ther.*, in press.

Knowles, M. R., Hohneker, K. W., Zhou, Z., Olsen, J. C., Noah, T. L., Hu, P.-C., Leigh, M. W., Engelhardt, J. F., Edwards, L. J., Jones, K. R., Grossman, M., Wilson, J. M., Johnson, L. G., and Boucher, R. C., 1995, A controlled study of adenoviral vector-mediated gene transfer in the nasal epithelium of patients with cystic fibrosis, *N. Engl. J. Med.* **333:**823–831.

Kotin, R. M., 1994, Prospects for the use of adeno-associated virus as a vector for human gene therapy, *Hum. Gene Ther.* **5:**793–801.

Kotin, R. M., and Berns, K. I., 1989, Organization of adeno-associated virus DNA in latently infected Detroit 6 cells, *Virology* **170:**460–467.

Kotin, R. M., Linden, R. M., and Berns, K. I., 1992, Characterization of a preferred site on human chromosome 19q for integration of adeno-associated virus DNA by non-homologous recombination, *EMBO J.* **11:**5071–5078.

Kotin, R. M., Menninger, J. C., Ward, D. C., Berns, K. I., 1991, Mapping and direct visualization of a region-specific viral DNA integration site on chromosome 19q13-qter, *Genomics* **10:**831–834.

Kotin, R. M., Siniscalco, M., Samulski, R. J., Zhu, X., Hunter, L., Laughlin, C. A., McLaughlin, S., Muzyczka, N., Rocchi, M., and Berns, K. I., 1990, Site-specific integration by adeno-associated virus, *Proc. Natl. Acad. Sci. USA* **87:**2211–2215.

Kube, D. M., Ponnazhagan, S., and Srivastava, A., 1997, Encapsidation of adeno-associated virus type 2 Rep proteins in wild type and recombinant progeny virions: Rep-mediated growth inhibition of primary human cells, *J. Virol.* **71:**7361–7371.

Kurtzman G. J., Cohen, B., Meyers, P., Amunullah, A., and Young, N. S., 1988, Persistent B19 parvovirus infection as a cause of severe chronic anaemia in children with acute lymphocytic leukaemia, *Lancet* **ii:**1159–1162.

Kurtzman, G. J., Frickhofen, N., Kimball, J., Jenkins, D. W., Nienhuis, A. W., and Young, N. S., 1989, Pure red-cell aplasia of 10 years' duration due to persistent parvovirus B19 infection and its cure with immunoglobulin therapy, *N. Engl. J. Med.* **321:**519–523.

Kÿostio, S. R. M., Wonderling, R. S., and Owens, R. A., 1995, Negative regulation of the adeno-associated virus (AAV) p5 promoter involves both the p5 rep binding site and the consensus ATP-binding motif of the AAV rep68 protein, *J. Virol.* **69:**6787–6796.

Labow, M. A., and Berns, K. I., 1988, The adeno-associated virus rep gene inhibits replication of an adeno-associated virus/simian virus 40 hybrid genome in cos-7 cells, *J. Virol.* **62:**1705–1712.

Laughlin, C. A., Tratschin, J.-D., Coon, H., and Carter, B. J., 1983. Cloning of infectious adeno-associated virus genomes in bacterial plasmids, *Gene* **23:**65–73.

Lebkowski, J. S., McNally, M. M., Okarma, T. B., and Lerch, L. B., 1988, Adeno-associated virus: A vector system for efficient introduction of DNA into a variety of mammalian cell types, *Mol. Cell. Biol.* **8:**3988–3996.

Leboulch, P., Huang, G. M. S., Humphries, R. K., Oh, Y. H., Eaves, C. J., Tuan, D. Y. H., and London, I. M., 1994, Mutagenesis of retroviral vectors transducing human β-globin gene and β-globin locus control region derivatives results in stable transmission of an active transcriptional structure, *EMBO J.* **13:**3065–3076.

Luhovy, M., McCune, S., Dong, J. Y., Prchal, J. F., Townes, T. M., and Prchal, J. T., 1996, Stable transduction of recombinant adeno-associated virus into hematopoietic stem cells from normal and sickle cell patients, *Biol. Blood Marrow Transplant* **2:**24–30.

Luo, F., Zhou, S. Z., Cooper, S., Munshi, N. C., Boswell, H. S., Broxmeyer, H. E., and Srivastava, A., 1995, Adeno-associated virus 2-mediated gene transfer and functional expression of the human granulocyte-macrophage colony-stimulating factor, *Exp. Hematol.* **23:**1261–1267.

Lusby, E., Fife, K. H., and Berns, K. I., 1980, Nucleotide sequence of the inverted terminal repetition in adeno-associated virus DNA, *J. Virol.* **34:**402–409.

Mah, C., Qing, K. Y., Khuntirat, B., Ponnazhagan, S., Wang, X.-S., Kube, D. M., Yoder, M. C., and Srivastava, A., 1998, Adeno-associated virust type 2-mediated gene transter: Role of epidermal growth factor receptor protein tyrosine kinase in transgene expression, *J. Virol.* **72:**9835–9843.

Mamounas, M., Leavitt, M., Yu, M., and Wong-Staal, F., 1995, Increased titer of recombinant AAV vectors by gene transfer with adenovirus coupled to DNA-polylysine complexes, *Gene Ther.* **2:**429–432.

Marcus, D. M., Kundu, S. K., and Suzuki, A., 1981, The P blood group system: Recent progress in immunochemistry and genetics, *Sem. Hematol.* **18:**63–71.

Mayor, H. D., Houlditch, G. S., and Mumford, D. M., 1973, Influence of adeno-associated satellite virus on adenovirus-induced tumors in hamsters, *Nat. New Biol.* **241:**44–46.

Maxwell, F., Harrison, G., and Maxwell, I. H., Improved methods for production of recombinant AAV and determination of infectious titer, *VIth Parvovirus Workshop,* Montpellier, France, 1995, p. 72.

McCarty, D. M., Pereira, D. J., Zolotukhin, I., Zhou, X., Ryan, J. H., and Muzyczka, N., 1994a, Identification of linear DNA sequences that specifically bind the adeno-associated virus rep protein, *J. Virol.* **68:**4988–4997.

McCarty, D. M., Ryan, J. H., Zolotukhin, I., Zhou, X., and Muzyczka, N., 1994b. Interaction of the adeno-associated virus rep protein with a sequence within the palindrome of the viral terminal repeat, *J. Virol.* **68:**4998–5006.

McLaughlin, S. K., Collis, P., Hermonat, P. L., and Muzyczka, N., 1988, Adeno-associated virus general transduction vectors: Analysis of proviral structures, *J. Virol.* **62:**1963–1973.

Miller, A. D., Bender, M. A., Harris, E. A. S., Kalecko, M., and Gelinas, R. E., 1988, Design of retrovirus vector for transfer and expression of the human β-globin gene, *J. Virol.* **62:**4337–4345.

Miller, J. L., Donahue, R. E., Sellers, S. E., Samulski, R. J., Young, N. S., and Nienhuis, A. W., 1994, Recombinant adeno-associated virus (rAAV)-mediated expression of human γ-globin gene in human progenitor-derived erythroid cells, *Proc. Natl. Acad. Sci. USA* **91:**10183–10187.

Miller, N., and Vile, R., 1995, Targeted vectors for gene therapy, *FASEB J.* **9:**190–199.

Moritz, T., Patel, V. K., and Williams, D. A., 1994, Bone marrow extracellular matrix molecules improve gene transfer into human hematopoietic cells via retroviral vectors, *J. Clin. Invest.* **93:**1451–1457.

Munshi, N. C., Zhou, S. Z., Woody, M. J., Morgan, D. A., and Srivastava, A., 1993, Successful replication of parvovirus B19 in the human megakaryocytic leukemia cell line MB-02, *J. Virol.* **67:**562–566.

Muzyczka, N., 1992, Use of adeno-associated virus as a general transduction vector for mammalian cells, *Curr. Top. Microbiol. Immunol.* **158:**97–129.

Nahreini, P., and Srivastava, A., 1989, Rescue and replication of the adeno-associated virus 2 genome in mortal and immortal human cells, *Intervirology* **30:**74–85.

Nahreini, P., and Srivastava, A., 1992, Rescue of the adeno-associated virus 2 genome correlates with alterations in DNA-modifying enzymes in human cells, *Intervirology* **33:**109–115.

Nahreini, P., Woody, M. J., Zhou, S. Z., and Srivastava, A., 1993, Versatile adeno-associated virus 2-based vectors for constructing recombinant virions, *Gene* **124:**257–262.

Ni, T.-H., Zhou, X.-H., McCarty, D. M., Zolotukhin, I., and Muzyczka, N., 1994, In vitro replication of adeno-associated virus DNA, *J. Virol.* **68:**1128–1138.

Novak, U., Harris, E., Forrester, W., Groudine, M., and Gelinas, R. E., 1990, High-level β-globin expression after retroviral transfer of locus activation region-containing human β-globin gene derivatives into murine erythroleukemia cells, *Proc. Natl. Acad. Sci. USA* **87:**3386–3390.

Ostrove, J. M., Duckworth, D. H., and Berns, K. I., 1981, Inhibition of adenovirus-transformed cell oncogenicity by adeno-associated virus, *Virology* **113:**521–533.

Owens, R. A., and Carter, B. J., 1992, In vitro resolution of adeno-associated virus DNA hairpin termini by wild-type Rep protein is inhibited by a dominant-negative mutant of Rep, *J. Virol.* **66:**1236–1240.

Ozawa, K., Kurtzman, G. J., and Young, N. S., 1986, Replication of the B19 parvovirus in human bone marrow cultures, *Science* **233:**883–886.

Ozawa, K., Kurtzman, G. J., and Young, N. S., 1987, Productive infection by B19 parvovirus of human erythroid bone marrow cells *in vitro*, *Blood* **70:**384–391.

Pattison, J. R., 1988, in *Parvovirus and Human Disease*, CRC Press, Boca Raton.

Philip, R., Brunette, E., Kilinski, L., Murugesh, D., McNally, M. A., Ucar, K., Rosenblatt, J., Okarma, T. B., and Lebkowski, J. S., 1994, Efficient and sustained gene expression in primary T lymphocytes and primary and cultured tumor cells mediated by adeno-associated virus plasmid DNA complexed to cationic liposomes, *Mol. Cell. Biol.* **14:**2411–2418.

Plavec, I., Papayannopoulou, T., Maury, C., and Meyer, F., 1993, A human β-globin gene fused to the human β-globin locus control region is expressed at high levels in erythroid cells of mice engrafted with retrovirus transduced hematopoietic stem cells, *Blood* **81:**1384–1392.

Podsakoff, G., Shaughnessy, E. A., Lu, D., Wong, K. K., and Chatterjee, S., 1994a, Long term in vivo reconstitution with murine marrow cells transduced with an adeno-associated virus vector, *Blood* **84:**256a.

Podsakoff, G., Wong, K. K., and Chatterjee, S., 1994b, Stable and efficient gene transfer into nondividing cells by adeno-associated virus (AAV)-based vectors, *J. Virol.* **68:**5656–5666.

Ponnazhagan, S., Erikson, D., Kearns, W. G., Zhou, S. Z., Nahreini, P., Wang, X.-S., and Srivastava, A., 1997a, Lack of site-specific integration of the recombinant adeno-associated virus genomes in human cells, *Hum. Gene Ther.* **8:**275–284.

Ponnazhagan, S., Mukherjee, P., Yoder, M. C., Wang, X.-S., Zhou, S. Z., Kaplan, J., Wadsworth, S., and Srivastava, A., 1996b, Adeno-associated mediated gene transfer *in vivo*: Organ tropism and expression of transduced sequences in mice, *Gene* **190:**203–210.

Ponnazhagan, S., Nallari, M. L., and Srivastava, A., 1994a, Suppression of human α-globin gene expression mediated by the recombinant adeno-associated virus 2-based antisense vectors, *J. Exp. Med.* **179:**733–738.

Ponnazhagan, S., Wang, X.-S., Kang, L. Y., Woody, M. J., Nallari, M. L., Munshi, N. C., Zhou, S. Z., and Srivastava, A., 1994b, Transduction of human hematopoietic cells by the adeno-associated virus 2 vectors is receptor-mediated, *Blood* **84:**742a.

Ponnazhagan, S., Wang, X.-S., and Srivastava, A., 1995a, Alternative strategies for generating recombinant AAV vectors, *VIth Parvovirus Workshop,* Montpellier, France, p. 71.

Ponnazhagan, S., Wang, X.-S., Srivastava, A., and Yoder, M. C., 1995b, Adeno-associated virus 2-mediated gene transfer and expression in murine hematopoietic progenitor cells in vivo, *Blood* **86:**240a.

Ponnazhagan, S., Wang, X.-S., Woody, M. J., Luo, F., Kang, L. Y., Nallari, M. L., Munshi, N. C., Zhou, S. Z., and Srivastava, A., 1996d, Differential expression in human cells from the p6 promoter of human parvovirus B19 following plasmid transfection and recombinant adeno-associated virus 2 (AAV) infection: Human megakaryocytic leukaemia cells are non-permissive for AAV infection, *J. Gen. Virol.* 77:1111–1112.

Ponnazhagan, S., Woody, M. J., Wang, X.-S., Zhou, S. Z., and Srivastava, A., 1995c, Transcriptional transactivation of parvovirus B19 promoters in nonpermissive human cells by adenovirus type 2, *J. Virol.* **69:**8096–8101.

Ponnazhagam, S., Yoder, M. C., and Srivastava, A., 1997, Adeno-associated virus type 2-mediated transduction of murine repopulating ability and sustained expression of a human globin gene *in vivo*, *J. Virol.* **71:**3098–3104.

Ponnazhagan, S., Weigel, K. A., Raikwar, S. R., Mukherjee, P., Yoder, M. C., and Srivastava, A., 1998, Recombinant human parvovirus B19 vectors: Erythroid cell-specific delivery and expression of transduced genes, *J. Virol.* **72:**5224–5230.

Pont, J., Puchhammer-Stockl, E., and Chott, A., 1992, Recurrent granulocytic aplasia as clinical presentation of a persistent parvovirus B19 infection, *Br. J. Haematol.* **80:**160–165.

Prasad, K.-M. R., and Trempe, J. P., 1995, The adeno-associated virus Rep78 protein is covalently linked to viral DNA in a preformed virion, *Virology* **214:**360–370.

Qing, K. Y., Mah, C., Hansen, J., Zhou, S. Z., Pwarki, V. J., and Srivastava, A., 1999, Human fibroblast growth factor receptor 1 is a co-receptor for infection with adeno-associated virus 2, *Nature Med.* in press.

Rosenberg, S. A., Abersold, P., Cornetta, K., Kasid, A., Morgan, R. A., Moen, R., Karson, E. M., Lotze, M. T., Yang, J. C., Topalian, S. L., Merino, M. J., Culver, K., Miller, A. D., Blaese, R. M., and Anderson, W. F., 1990, Oene transfer into humans: Immunotherapy of patients with advanced melanoma, using tumor-infiltrating lymphocytes modified by retroviral gene transduction, *N. Engl. J. Med.* **323:**570–577.

Rouger, P., Gane, P., and Salmon, C., 1987, Tissue distribution of H, Lewis and P antigens shown by a panel of 18 monoclonal antibodies, *Rev. Fr. Trans. Immunohematol.* **30:**699–708.

Russell, D. W., Miller, A. D., and Alexander, I. E., 1994, Adeno-associated virus vectors preferentially transduce cells in S phase, *Proc. Natl. Acad. Sci. USA* **91:**8915–8919.

Russell, D. W., Alexander, I. E., and Miller, A. D., 1995, DNA synthesis and topoisomerase inhibitors increase transduction by adeno-associated virus vectors, *Proc. Natl. Acad. Sci. USA* **92:**5719–5723.

Sambrook, J., Fritsch, E. F., and Maniatis, T., 1989. in *Molecular Cloning: A Laboratory Manual.* Cold Spring Harbor Laboratory Press, Cold Spring Harbor, NY, pp. 1.53–1.110.

Samulski, R. J., 1993, Adeno-associated virus: Integration at a specific chromosomal locus, *Curr. Opinion Genet. Dev.* **3:**74–80.

Samulski, R. J., Berns, K. I., Tan, M., and Muzyczka, N., 1982, Cloning of adeno-associated virus into pBR322: Rescue of intact virus from the recombinant plasmid in human cells, *Proc. Natl. Acad. Sci. USA* **79:**2077–2081.

Samulski, R. J., Chang, L.-S., and Shenk, T., 1987, A recombinant plasmid from which an infectious adeno-associated virus genome can be excised in vitro and its use to study viral replication, *J. Virol.* **61:**3096–3101.

Samulski, R. J., Chang, L.-S., and Shenk, T., 1989, Helper-free stocks of recombinant adeno-associated viruses: Normal integration does not require viral gene expression, *J. Virol.* **63:**3822–3828.

Samulski, R. J., Srivastava, A., Berns, K. I., and Muzyczka, N., 1983, Rescue of adeno-associated virus from recombinant plasmids: Gene correction within the terminal repeats of AAV, *Cell* **33:**135–143.

Samulski, R. J., Zhu, X., Xiao, X., Brook, J., Houseman, D. E., Epstein, N., and Hunter, L. A., 1991, Targeted integration of adeno-associated virus (AAV) into human chromosome 19, *EMBO J.* **10:**3941–3950.

Schwarz, T. F., Serke, S., Hottentrager, B., von Brunn, A., Baurmann, H., Kirsch, A., Stolz, W., Hunn, D., Deinhardt, F., and Roggendrof, M., 1992, Replication of parvovirus B19 in hematopoietic progenitor cells generated in vitro from normal human peripheral blood, *J. Virol.* **67:**562–566.

Senapathy, P., Tratschin, J.-D., and Carter, B. J., 1984, Replication of adeno-associated virus DNA. Complementation of naturally occurring rep$^-$ mutants by a wild-type genome or an ori$^-$ mutant and correction of terminal palindrome deletions, *J. Mol. Biol.* **179:**1–20.

Shade, R. O., Blundell, M. C., Cotmore, S. F., Tattersall, P. J., and Astell, C. R., 1986, Nucleotide sequence and genome organization of human parvovirus B19 isolated from the serum of a child during aplastic crisis, *J. Virol.* **58:**921–936.

Shi, Y., Seto, E., Chang, L.-S., and Shenk, T., 1991, Transcriptional repression by YY1, a human GLI-Kruppel-related protein, and relief of repression by adenovirus E1A protein, *Cell* **67:**377–388.

Siegl, G., Bates, R. C., Berns, K. I., Carter, B. J., Kelly, D. C., Kurstak, E., and Tattersall, P., 1985, Characteristics and taxonomy of parvoviridae, *Intervirology* **23:**61–73.

Snyder, R. O., Im, D.-S., Ni, T.-H., Xiao, X., Samulski, R. J., and Muzyczka, N., 1993, Features of the adeno-associated virus origin involved in substrate recognition by the viral Rep protein, *J. Virol.* **67:**6096–6104.

Snyder, R. O., Samulski, R. J., and Muzyczka, N., 1990, In vitro resolution of covalently joined AAV chromosome ends, *Cell* **60:**105–113.

Southern, E. M., 1975, Detection of specific sequences among DNA fragments separated by gel electrophoresis, *J. Mol. Biol.* **98:**503–517.

Srivastava, A., 1987, Replication of the adeno-associated virus DNA termini in vitro, *Intervirology* **27:**138–147.

Srivastava, A., 1994, Parvovirus-based vectors for human gene therapy, *Blood Cells* **20:**531–538.

Srivastava, A., Bruno, E., Briddell, R., Cooper, R., Srivastava, C. H., van Besien, K., and Hoffman, R., 1990, Parvovirus B19-induced perturbation of human megakaryocytopoiesis in vitro, *Blood* **76:**1997–2004.

Srivastava, A., and Lu, L., 1988, Replication of B19 parvovirus in highly enriched hematopoietic progenitor cells from normal human bone marrow, *J. Virol.* **62:**3059–3063.

Srivastava, A., Lusby, E. W., and Berns, K. I., 1983, Nucleotide sequence and organization of the adeno-associated virus 2 genome, *J. Virol.* **45:**555–564.

Srivastava, A., Wang, X.-S., Ponnazhagan, S., Zhou, S. Z., and Yoder, M. C., Parvovirus-based vectors for human gene therapy, *VIth Parvovirus Workshop*, Montpellier, France, 1995, p. 29.

Srivastava, A., Wang, X.-S., Ponnazhagan, S., Zhou, S. Z., and Yoder, M. C., 1996, Adeno-associated virus 2-mediated transduction and erythroid lineage-specific expression in human hematopoietic progenitor cells, *Curr. Top. Microbiol. Immunol.* **218:**93–117.

Srivastava, C. H., Samulski, R. J., Lu, L., Larsen, S. H., and Srivastava, A., 1989, Construction of a recombinant human parvovirus B19: Adeno-associated virus 2 (AAV) DNA inverted terminal repeats are functional in an AAV-B19 hybrid virus, *Proc. Natl. Acad. Sci. USA* **86:**8078–8082.

Srivastava, C. H., Zhou, S. Z., Munshi, N. C., and Srivastava, A., 1992, Parvovirus B19 replication in human umbilical cord blood cells, *Virology* **189:**456–461.

Stamatoyannopoulos, G., and Nienhuis, A. W., 1994, in *The Molecular Basis of Blood Diseases* W. B. Saunders, Philadelphia, pp. 107–155.

Su, H., Chang, J. C., Xu, S. M., and Kan, Y. W., 1996, Selective killing of AFP-positive hepatocellular carcinoma cells by adeno-associated virus transfer of the herpes simplex virus thymidine kinase gene, *Hum. Gene Ther.* **7:**463–470.

Sun, X.-L., Murphy, B. R., Li, Q. J., Gullapalli, S., Mackins, J., Jayaram, H. N., Srivastava, A., and Antony, A. C., 1995, Transduction of folate receptor cDNA into cervical carcinoma cells using recombinant adeno-associated virions delays cell proliferation in vivo, *J. Clin. Invest.* **96:**1535–1547.

Takahashi, T., Ozawa, K., Takahashi, K., Asano, S., and Takaku, F., 1990, Susceptibility of human erythropoietic cells to B19 parvovirus in vitro increases with differentiation, *Blood* **75:**603–610.

Tamayose, K., Hirai, Y., and Shimada, T., 1996, A new strategy for large-scale preparation of high-titer recombinant adeno-associated virus vectors by using sulfonated cellulose column chromatography, *Hum. Gene Ther.* **7:**507–513.

Thrasher, A. J., de Alwis, M., Casimir, C. M., Kinnon, C., Page, K., Lebkowski, J., Segal, A. W., and Levinsky, R. J., 1995, Functional reconstitution of the NADPH-oxidase by adeno-associated virus gene transfer, *Blood* **86:**761–765.

Tooze, J., 1981, in *DNA Tumor Viruses*, Cold Spring Harbor Press, Cold Spring Harbor New York.

Tratschin, J.-D., Miller, I. L., and Carter, B. J., 1984, Genetic analysis of adeno-associated virus: Properties of deletion mutants constructed in vitro and evidence for an adeno-associated virus replication function, *J. Virol.* **51:**611–619.

Tuan, D. Y. H., Solomon, W. B., London, I. M., and Lee, D. P., 1989, An erythroid specific, development stage-independent enhancer far upstream of the human "β-like globin" genes, *Proc. Natl. Acad. Sci. USA* **86:**2554–2559.

von dem Borne, A. E. G. K., Bos, M. J. E., Joustra-Maas, N., Tromp, J. F., van Wijngaarden-du Bois, R., and Tetteroo, P. A. T., 1986, A murine monoclonal IgM antibody specific blood group P antigen (globoside), *Br. J. Haematol.* **63:**35–46.

Walsh, C. E., Liu, J. M., Miller, J. L., Nienhuis, A. W., and Samulski, R. J., 1993, Gene therapy for human hemoglobinopathies, *Proc. Soc. Exp. Biol. Med.* **204:**289–300.

Walsh, C. E., Liu, J. M., Xiao, X., Young, N. S., Nienhuis, A. W., and Samulski, R. J., 1992, Regulated high level expression of a human γ-globin gene introduced into erythroid cells by an adeno-associated virus vector, *Proc. Natl. Acad. Sci. USA* **89:**7257–7261.

Walsh, C. E., Nienhuis, A. W., Samulski, R. J., Brown, M. G., Miller, J. L., Young, N. S., and Liu, J. M., 1994, Phenotypic correction of Fanconi anemia in human hematopoietic cells with a recombinant adeno-associated virus vector, *J. Clin. Invest.* **94:**1440–1448.

Walz, C., and Schlehofer, J., 1992, Modification of some biological properties of HeLa cells containing adeno-associated virus DNA integrated into chromosome 17, *J. Virol.* **66:**2990–3002.

Wang, X. S., Khuntirat, B., Qing, K. Y., Ponnazhagan, S., Kube, D. M., Zhou, S. Z., Dwarki, V. J., and Srivastava, A., 1998, Characterization of wild-type adeno-associated virus type 2-like particles generated during recombinant viral vector production and strategies for their elimination, *J. Virol.* **72:**5472–5480.

Wang, X.-S., Ponnazhagan, S., and Srivastava, A., 1995a, Rescue and replication signals of the adeno-associated virus 2 genome, *J. Mol. Biol.* **250:**573–580.

Wang, X.-S., Ponnazhagan, S., and Srivastava, A., 1996b, Rescue and replication of adeno-associated virus type 2 genome as well as vector DNA sequences from recombinant plasmids containing deletions in the viral inverted terminal repeats: Selective encapsidation of the viral genomes in progeny virions, *J. Virol.* **70:**1668–1677.

Wang, X.-S., and Srivastava, A., 1997a, A novel terminal resolution-like site in the adeno-associated virus type 2 genome. *J. Virol.* **71:**1140–1146.

Wang, X.-S., Yoder, M. C., Zhou, S. Z., and Srivastava, A., 1995b, Parvovirus B19 promoter at map unit 6 confers replication competence and erythroid specificity to adeno-associated virus 2 in primary human hematopoietic progenitor cells, *Proc. Natl. Acad. Sci. USA* **92:**12416–12420.

Weiland, H. T., Salimans, M. M., Fibbe, W. E., Kluin, P. M., and Cohen, B. J., 1989, Prolonged parvovirus B19 infection with severe anaemia in a bone marrow transplant patient, *Br. J. Haematol.* **71:**300.

Weiss, R. N., Teich, N., Varmus, H. E., and Coffin, J. M., 1984, in *RNA Tumor Viruses*, Cold Spring Harbor Press, Cold Spring Harbor, New York.

Weitzman, M. D., Kÿostio, S. R. M., Kotin, R. M., and Owens, R. A., 1994, Adeno-associated virus (AAV) Rep proteins mediate complex formation between AAV DNA and its integration site in human DNA, *Proc. Natl. Acad. Sci. USA* **91:**5808–5812.

Wistuba, A., Weger, S., Kern, A., and Kleinschmidt, J. A., 1995, Intermediates of adeno-associated virus type 2 assembly: Identification of soluble complexes containing Rep and Cap proteins, *J. Virol.* **69:**5311–5319.

Wu, P., Ziska, D., Bonell, M. A., Grouzmann, E., Millard, W. J., and Meyer, E. M., 1994, Differential neuropeptide Y gene expression in post-mitotic versus dividing neuroblastoma cells driven by an adeno-associated virus vector, *Brain Res. Mol. Brain Res.* **24:**27–33.

Xiao, X., deVlaminck, W., and Monahan, J., 1993, Adeno-associated virus (AAV) vectors for gene transfer, *Adv. Drug Delivery Rev.* **12:**201–215.

Yang, Q., Kadam, A., and Trempe, J. P., 1994, Characterization of cell lines that inducibly express the adeno-associated virus Rep proteins, *J. Virol.* **68:**4847–4856.

Yaegashi, N., Shiraishi, Y., Takeshita, T., Nakamura, M., Yajima, A., and Sugamura, K., 1989, Propagation of human parvovirus B19 in primary culture of erythroid lineage cells derived from fetal liver, *J. Virol.* **63:**2422–2426.

Yoder, M. C., Du, X.-X., and Williams, D. A., 1993, High proliferative potential colony-forming cell heterogeneity identified using counterflow centrifugal elutriation, *Blood* **82:**385–391.

Zabner, J., Couture, L. A., Gregory, R. J., Graham, S. M., Smith, A. E., and Welsh, M. J., 1993, Adenovirus-mediated gene transfer transiently corrects the chloride transport defect in nasal epithelia of patients with cystic fibrosis, *Cell* **75:**207–216.

Zhou, S. Z., Broxmeyer, H. E., Cooper, S., Harrington, M. A., and Srivastava, A., 1993, Adeno-associated virus 2-mediated gene transfer in murine hematopoietic progenitor cells, *Exp. Hematol.* **21:**928–933.

Zhou, S. Z., Cooper, S., Kang, L. Y., Ruggieri, L., Heimfeld, S., Srivastava, A., and Broxmeyer, H. E., 1994, Adeno-associated virus 2-mediated high efficiency gene transfer into immature and mature subsets of hematopoietic progenitor cells in human umbilical cord blood, *J. Exp. Med.* **179:**1867–1875.

Zhou, S. Z., Li, Q., Stamatoyannopoulos, G., and Srivastava, A., 1996, Adeno-associated virus 2-mediated transduction and erythroid cell-specific expression of a human β-globin gene, *Gene Ther.* **3:**223–229.

Chapter 5

Nonviral Methods for Gene Transfer

A. Djeha and L. S. Lashford

1. INTRODUCTION

Nucleic acids have acquired considerable significance as clinical reagents in genetic diseases. In genetic approaches to human disease, genes are introduced into cells to synthesize therapeutically active products which may in turn influence the clinical progression of the disease. Successful gene therapy requires identifying an appropriate therapeutic gene and also developing delivery systems through which genes are efficiently transferred to the desired cell type. One approach is to use viruses which, through evolutionary pressures, have been selected to introduce genes successfully into mammalian cells. This is manifested by the development of sophisticated and highly specific mechanisms which facilitate viral cell binding to target cells, cellular entry, and survival, followed by rapid intracellular liberation of the viral contents and subsequent replication of the virus genome. Rapid progress in understanding the mechanisms of viral infection of cells has inspired the development of gene delivery systems that emulate many functions of viruses. However, the safety of any therapy is of paramount importance. The ideal agents for gene therapy are those which are unlikely to infect cells outside the target tissue and are also nontoxic and unable to induce a host immune response. Many viral vectors in clinical use have been chosen because they are efficient and relatively stable in gene transfer. However, there are significant concerns regarding the safety of virally

A. Djeha CRC Department of Experimental Haematology, Paterson Institute for Cancer Research, Manchester M20 4BX, United Kingdom. **L. S. Lashford** Paterson Institute for Cancer Research, Christie Hospital (NHS) Trust, Manchester M20 4BX, United Kingdom.

Blood Cell Biochemistry, Volume 8: Hematopoiesis and Gene Therapy, edited by Fairbairn and Testa. Kluwer Academic/Plenum Publishers, New York, 1999.

mediated gene transfer. The report of a breakout of a replication-competent retrovirus in a producer cell line that is widely considered among the safest used in clinical trials has sent a strong warning signal (Chong and Vile, 1996).

Consequently, increasing interest is shown in designing flexible, specific, and safe, nonviral methods for gene transfer. In all of these methods DNA must cross multiple subcellular barriers to reach the site of gene expression within the nucleus. It is proposed that artificially created vectors are safer than those based on viral systems, but because all new pharmacological agents are potentially toxic, this risk needs to be carefully and systematically evaluated. Presently, the major theoretical limiting factor to using nonviral systems for gene therapy is the short-term persistence and expression of transferred genes. For therapeutic applications which require permanent reconstitution of a functional gene, repeated administrations are currently required to ensure continuous gene expression.

However, when the concept of gene therapy is broadened to include transient cellular events as therapeutic endpoints, the issue of stable gene expression is irrelevant. These may include inducing beneficial and desirable cytotoxic or immunomodulatory activities mediated by hormones, growth factors, or proteins, which are synthesized only under specific conditions. In these situations nonvirally mediated techniques may be particularly attractive because these systems mediate episomal, transient expression.

Furthermore, nonviral gene therapy readily lends itself to manufacturing scale-up and quality control, which are required if gene transfer technology is to be applied on a wide clinical scale.

This chapter focuses on the attributes of nonviral gene delivery systems and their potential for human gene therapy. The properties of each of these are evaluated for efficiency in transferring functional genes into cells both *in vitro* and *in vivo*.

2. PLASMID DNA-BASED METHODS

2.1. Physical Methods

Several physical methods for transferring DNA into mammalian cells have been developed, based on applying a nonphysiologic force to perturb the cell membrane. The efficiencies of these techniques vary considerably. Some cells respond better to one approach than to others.

2.1.1. Electroporation

Electroporation is a simple method for gene introduction and is useful for a wide variety of cell types (Potter, 1988). This technique involves applying a voltage across a cell, which results in the indiscriminate formation of physical pores in the cell membrane and an increase in the conductance for a short period of time, which permits the uptake of DNA by candidate mechanisms, such as electrical drift, electrosmosis, or diffusion. The many critical parameters and conditions that need to be optimized include the electric field strength, frequency, shape of the pulse, cell concentration and the electroporation medium (Yang *et al.*, 1995).

Electroporation causes cell stress and a substantial loss of viability (Neil and Zimmermann, 1993) and a correlation has been found between the fraction of cells killed and the efficiency of transfecting the surviving cells (Andreason and Evans, 1989). Therefore, the efficiency of this method is limited by the high incidence of cell death at the electric field strength required to introduce large molecules of nucleic acid. It has been reported that an improvement in the viability of electropermeabilized cells, reflected in enhanced exogenous gene expression, is obtained when bipolar electrical pulses are used instead of a single pulse (Tekle *et al.*, 1991). Another disadvantage of this method is the low frequency of gene delivery. However, it has been suggested that electroporation is superior to lipofection and other traditional transfection methods, such as dimethylaminoethy (DEAE)-dextran and calcium phosphate precipitation, in for expression frequency and morphological changes (Chu *et al.*, 1987; Puchalski and Fahl, 1992).

There are several reports on the effectiveness of electroporation for introducing genes into various cell types, even cells that are normally refractory to other transfection protocols. Thus, successful transfection has been achieved in mouse (Jelinek *et al.*, 1988; Narayanan *et al.*, 1986, 1989) and human haemopoietic stem and progenitor cells (Toneguzzo and Keating, 1986) and in human bone marrow stromal cells (Keating *et al.*, 1990). It has been suggested that the applicability of electroporation for gene delivery into hematopoietic stem cells may be enhanced by expanding these using growth factors (Takahashi *et al.*, 1992).

2.1.2. Jet Injection

Jet injection of DNA in solution as an alternative method to needle injection is a further technique that can be used to transfer naked DNA into mammalian cells (Furth *et al.*, 1992). The technique involves injecting small volumes of soluble, naked DNA by propelling the solution under pressure with sufficient force to travel into the target tissue. Various tissues of sheep have been successfully transfected with DNA using this injection method, resulting in minimal morbidity to surrounding tissues (Furth *et al.*, 1995). As with particle bombardment, this technology is potentially useful for genetic immunization, because a low level of gene expression is often sufficient to achieve an immunological response (Davis *et al.*, 1994).

2.1.3. Particle Bombardment

Particle bombardment, initially developed to introduce DNA into plant cells and tissues, has evolved into a useful tool for gene transfer into various somatic tissues *in situ* (Williams *et al.*, 1991). The basic principle of this technique is accelerating DNA coated onto heavy tungsten or gold micoparticles at high velocity (300–600 m/s) using a gas pressure pulse, an explosive, or an electric discharge device to penetrate into target cells or animals (Christou, 1995). It is not known what size of intact DNA can be delivered by this method, but a potential problem is that this procedure may shear large DNA molecules. However, this method is effective in transferring DNA *in vivo*, and *ex vivo*, and high levels of transgene activity have been obtained in the skin and liver tissues of rats, mice (Williams *et al.*, 1991; Yang *et al.*, 1990), rabbits, and monkeys (Cheng *et al.*, 1993). Comparative studies have found that this method is superior to dimethylaminoethyl-dextran, electroporation, and lipofection (Heiser, 1994). The most important parameters that affect the efficiency of DNA uptake and expression by particle bombardment are the DNA loading of the microparticle, the size of the particle, the particle velocity, and bombardment conditions, such as the target distance (Klein *et al.*, 1992). This technique has been used mainly as an alternative method for genetic vaccination by introducting an antigen-encoding expression vector into T-cells *in vitro* (Hui *et al.*, 1994; Zarozinski *et al.*, 1995) or *in situ* in the skin and muscle of mice (Eisenbraun *et al.*, 1993, Lai *et al.*, 1995). This technique has also been used for cytokine and immunotherapy of cancer *via* transfection of tumor cells with a plasmid DNA encoding an antibody-cytokine fusion protein (Nicolet *et al.*, 1995).

All of these physical systems of DNA transfer are only suitable for transient gene expression because there is no mechanism for integrating the DNA into the host chromosome. Moreover, expression levels are low unless genes are coupled with viral promoters which function in a broad range of tissues. The importance of the choice of promoter for gene transfer has been demonstrated by directly administering naked DNA into muscle by particle bombardment. In a comparative study where skin, liver, and muscle were bombarded with different plasmids containing a reporter gene under the regulatory control of various viral and mammalian gene promoters, tissue preferences for gene expression were observed (Cheng *et al.*, 1993). Moreover, the same authors noted differences in promoter preference within the same cell type located in two different anatomical places, for example, muscle cells in the panniculus cornices of the dermis differ in regulating gene expression compared to abdominal muscle cells. This suggests that other physiological factors need to be evaluated in gene therapy experiments to devise an effective strategy.

2.2. Direct Injection of Naked DNA

The possibility of detecting gene expression by directly injecting naked DNA into animal tissues was initially demonstrated by Dubensky and co-workers (1984), who showed that calcium phosphate precipitated plasmid DNA injected into the liver or spleen of mice is expressed at detectable levels. Similar results were obtained when precipitated DNA was injected intraperitoneally into newborn rats (Benvenisty and Reshef, 1986). The evidence to date suggests that DNA itself exhibits no apparent toxicity in animals. However, it has been reported that a synergistic effect of DNA with cationic lipids contributed to cationic lipid-DNA complex-induced hemolysis (van der Woude, 1995). Repetitive intramuscular injections of naked DNA induce anti-DNA antibodies in nonhuman primates (Jiao *et al.*, 1992).

Successful direct injection of naked DNA-mediated transgene expression is not strictly confined to striated muscle fibers. It has been reported that naked plasmid DNA administered by various routes is expressed at significant levels in a variety of tissues *in vivo*. Intratracheal administration of DNA resulted in gene expression in mouse airways (Meyer *et al*., 1995). In the thyroid gland, levels of expression comparable to those obtained in muscle have been reported (Sikes *et al*., 1994). Repetitive intrahepatic injections of DNA in isotonic solutions resulted in uptake and significant transient gene expression within confined areas of the liver of animals treated with dexamethasone (Hickman *et al*., 1994; Malone *et al*., 1994). Transient foreign gene expression has also been achieved following intra-articular (Yovandich *et al*., 1995) and intradermal (Hengge *et al*., 1995) injections within the joint and skin respectively. A single intravenous injection of plasmid DNA containing the human tissue kallikrein gene into spontaneously hypertensive rats produced a sustained reduction in blood pressure for six weeks (Wang *et al*., 1995). Intravascular delivery of naked DNA has been reported following intraportal injection in hypertonic solutions, and expression has been detected throughout the entire liver. This was an improvement over interstitial delivery, which was much less efficient with limited distribution (Budker *et al*., 1996). Naked DNA injected intracerebrally into the mouse brain produces uptake and expression of a reporter gene and is more consistent than cationic lipid-mediated DNA expression (Schwartz *et al*., 1996). Tracheal insufflation of plasmid DNA resulted in efficient transfection of the lungs in rats (Tsan *et al*., 1995). Successful gene delivery into rat stomach after injecting plasmid DNA into the submucosa has been reported (Takehara *et al*., 1996), and arterial gene transfer and expression using naked plasmid DNA applied to a standard angioplasty catheter balloon coated with hydrogel was achieved in rabbits (Riessen *et al*., 1993).

Muscle has been identified as very permissive tissue for *in vivo* delivery of naked DNA, compared to other tissues (Wolff *et al*., 1990), and can take up and express DNA in solution or in the form of precipitates, although the latter has achieved higher levels of expression (Wolff *et al*., 1991). In mature skeletal muscle, plasmid DNA is superior to viral vectors for direct gene transfer (Davis *et al*., 1993a). Direct cardiac injection of plasmid DNA also mediates uptake and expression in the heart muscle of rats (Acsadi *et al*., 1991b; Lin *et al*., 1990). In view of these encouraging observations, transfer of DNA into skeletal and cardiac muscle has been the subject of considerable scrutiny. Unfortunately, only a small proportion of the muscle fibers (1–2%) is transfected (Davis *et al*., 1993a), and the distribution of fibers expressing the foreign gene are limited mainly to the injection site (Wolff *et al*., 1990). Multiple injections at different sites resulted in reporter gene expression in several fibers in the vicinity of each injection site and at relatively low levels (Davis and Jasmin, 1993). Connective tissue surrounding the myocytes significantly limits DNA distribution through the interstitial space of the muscle reducing the number of transfected myofibres (Jiao *et al*., 1992). Additionally, the technique of needle injection affects the efficiency of plasmid DNA transfer. For example, longitudinal, parallel injections to the myofibres yield higher levels of reporter gene expression compared to perpendicular injections (Levy *et al*., 1996), and it is likely that the wide variability in the level of expression after injection of a given amount of DNA into the muscle arises from variation in injection techniques. It is likely that some of the DNA enters *via* the lesions produced in myocytes by the needle (Hickman *et al*., 1994; Malone *et al*., 1994). However, the discordant responses in different tissues, and the observation that expression is not entirely limited to the injection site within the muscle mass suggest a more fundamental mechanism. The interconnected structure of muscle cells may be one explanation. It has been hypothesized that some DNA enters through the T-tubule system, which provides contact between myocytes and the interstitial space (Kitsis *et al.*, 1991; Wolff *et al.*, 1992) and is present in both skeletal and cardiac muscles. In addition, potocytosis through specific interactions between the DNA and caveolae has also been proposed as a mechanism of DNA uptake by muscle cells (Wolff *et al.*, 1992). Preinjection of sucrose before direct transfer significantly reduces the variability and increases the level and distribution of transgene expression (Davis *et al.*, 1993c).

Another factor observed which may aid expression is that injecting naked DNA into regenerating skeletal muscles leads to levels of gene expression relatively higher than in normal muscles (Davis *et al.*, 1994; Vitadello *et al.*, 1994). The same observation was reported for young mice compared to older animals and males as opposed to females (Wells and Goldspink, 1992). It has also been reported that agents that cause proliferative damage, such as snake venom and bupivicaine, have a similar effect (Danko *et al.*, 1994).

Despite the local nature of exogenous gene delivery in the muscle, most reports have shown that the expression persists for a relatively prolonged time compared with other types of tissue, for example, up to two months in skeletal muscle (Wolff *et al.*, 1990) and two weeks in cardiac muscle (Acsadi *et al.*, 1991b). This may be explained by a greater ability to retain intact DNA, which is detected in muscle for much longer periods of time than any other tissue. The DNA administered to the muscle acts as a "stock" to supply either ongoing transfection or transcription. There has been no report of any evidence of integration into the host genomic DNA. Indeed, it has been demonstrated that plasmid DNA is found in a free, circular form in murine skeletal muscle without integration into the chromosomal DNA and is probably maintained and repaired episomally like genomic DNA (Nabel *et al.*, 1990; Wolff *et al.*, 1990). In addition, it has been hypothesized that plasmid diffusion in the myofibers is a likely explanation for the lag time to peak expression (Levy *et al.*, 1996).

As with particle bombardment, direct intramuscular (Davis *et al.*, 1993b; Manthorpe *et al.*, 1993) or intradermal (Raz *et al.*, 1994) injection of DNA forms the base of a broad approach for generating a DNA-mediated immunization. This consists of the inducing an immune response to an antigen transiently expressed *in vivo* by the transferred gene. This technique has been used to elicit humoral immune responses in animals against several viral agents, including human immunodeficiency virus in mice and monkeys (Wang *et al.*, 1993), bovine herpes virus 1 in mice and cattle (Cox *et al.*, 1993), hepatitis B virus in mice (Davis *et al.*, 1993b; Michel *et al.*, 1995), hepatitis C virus in mice (Major *et al.*, 1995), influenza virus in chicken (Robinson *et al.*, 1993) and rabies in mice (Xiang *et al.*, 1994). Hepatitis B virus envelope proteins have been used to induce highly specific and potent cytotoxic responses in mice after intratumoral DNA injection (Davis *et al.*, 1995; Ulmer *et al.*, 1993; Xiang *et al.*, 1994). A humoral and cellular response has also been reported against the malarial circumsporozoite protein expressed in mice (Sedegah *et al.*,

1994). It is proposed that both the transfected skeletal muscle fibers and antigen-presenting cells, such as dendritic cells, participate in priming cytotoxic T-lymphocytes to elicit this cellular response.

Direct DNA injection offers vaccine applications and also can be considered for specific therapeutic applications. Expression of human dystrophin was induced in myofibers of the *mdx* mouse, a model of Duchenne muscular dystrophy, after intramuscular injection of plasmid DNA (Acsadi *et al.*, 1991a; Danko *et al.*, 1993). However, this approach is limited by the volume of muscle mass to be transduced, the number of muscle groups, and the need for sustained gene expression over the lifetime of an individual. Another potential therapeutic role for direct gene transfer, in addition to treatment of primary myopathies, is to provide systemic delivery of nonmuscular, secreted recombinant proteins for treating other inherited disorders. Once again, this approach is best suited to conditions where relatively transient expression of protein is a useful therapeutic end point. Proof of this principle has been demonstrated for the clotting factor in mice (Baru *et al.*, 1995) and apolipoprotein-E in a hereditary cholesterolemic rat model (Fazio *et al.*, 1994). Other applications under investigation include antitumoral therapy (Vile and Hart, 1994) and cellular modulation via the production of cytokines in the skin (Hengge *et al.*, 1995). Intramuscular injection of plasmid DNA containing a cDNA encoding cytokine transforming growth factor-β (TGF-β) effectively ameliorate experimentally induced colitis in rats (Giladi *et al.*, 1995).

Although direct instillation of DNA into tissues confers some degree of localized specificity, tissues are composed of many cell types including stromal elements, endothelial cells and the predominant tissue cell type. When exquisite tissue specificity is required, perhaps to elicit a cytokine response, then it is logical to include an effective tissue-specific promoter and other regulatory elements which control gene expression at a cellular level. It is possible to direct exogenous gene expression to normal and neoplastic melanocytes *in vitro* and *in vivo* by using the melanocyte-specific, tyrosinase promoter (Vile and Hart, 1993). This approach has been extended to obtain tissue-specific expression of a suicide gene in squamous cell lung cancer under the control of human surfactant protein A gene transcriptional regulatory sequences (Smith *et al.*, 1994). This strategy may also be useful for switching genes either "on" or "off." By coinjecting rat cardiac and skeletal muscles with reporter genes linked to the cardiac-α myosin heavy-chain promoter, Kitsis *et al.* (1991) demonstrated that the heart can be transfected *in vivo* and that the directly injected vector is active and hormonally regulated in heart but not in skeletal muscle.

3. ARTIFICIAL SELF-ASSEMBLING SYSTEMS

3.1. Lipid-Mediated Gene Delivery Methods

3.1.1. Liposomes

The methods of DNA transfer described previously (sections 2.1–2.3) concentrated on systems which largely apply to a regional approach to gene therapy.

Liposomal gene delivery has been explored because it holds the promise of systemic gene delivery. Lipid vesicle technology has been exploited in devising phospholipid vesicles to be used as carriers for gene delivery both *in vitro* and *in vivo* (Fraley *et al.*, 1981; Soriano *et al.*, 1983; Walther *et al.*, 1988; Wang and Huang, 1987b). Molecules which have both hydrophilic and hydrophobic regions (amphipathic) form enclosed unilamellar vesicles and are called "liposomes." Liposomes contain integrated pairs of monolayers inside which all of the hydrophobic regions are shielded from interaction with water. They are composed predominantly of an amphipathic molecule such as phosphatidylethanolamine (PE), which cannot form a stable bilayer until mixed with a lipid, such as cholesterol. These liposomes have a net negative surface charge which confers resistance to nonspecific aggregation. It is thought that nucleic acid encapsulated in liposomes is protected against eukaryotic degradation, probably because of the limited permeability of these vesicles. It has been shown that liposome-encapsulated DNA maintains 70% of the transfection activity even in the presence of 40% serum, whereas DNA complexed to cationic lipids almost completely loses its activity in the presence of 5% serum (Mizuguchi *et al.*, 1996). Endocytosis is the principal means by which most liposome formulations enter cells (Straubinger *et al.*, 1983). However, a small proportion of liposomes fuse with cell membranes and evade the endosomal pathway. Small liposomes (~50 nm) are more effective than larger liposomes (~140 nm) in delivering the human α1-antitrypsin gene to parenchymal cells of the liver of mice because of their easier access to hepatocytes through the liver synaptia (Aliño *et al.*, 1993, 1994, 1996).

Gene delivery using liposomes has been demonstrated in many tissues *in vivo* including the liver (Aliño *et al.*, 1994; Leibiger *et al.*, 1990; Nicolau *et al.*, 1983), the hair follicles of mice after topical application of a reporter gene entrapped in liposomes (Li and Hoffman, 1995), and in the rodent colonic epithelium (Westbrook *et al.*, 1994).

Expression of genes introduced by endocytosed liposomes is limited by the trapping and rapid degradation of the DNA in endosomal compartments. One approach to improving the efficiency of gene delivery mediated by liposomes is the including of selected pharmacological agents that enhance DNA uptake and expression. Treating mice with the antimalarial drug chloroquine and other lysosomotropic agents, such as colchicine, before injecting the human factor IX gene DNA encapsulated in liposomes significantly increases the level of human factor IX in the plasma of the animals (Baru *et al.*, 1995). Lysosomotropic agents act by increasing the endosomal pH and thus inhibiting the activity of degradative enzymes. Amphiphilic peptides, such as the cyclic peptide gramicidin S, and short-chain phospholipids, such as dicaprylphosphatidylcholine, both of which disrupt cell membranes, can be useful effectors to facilitate DNA entry into cells (Legendre and Supersaxo, 1995).

Some viruses enter cells *via* the cell vesicle system. However, these possess specific mechanisms to facilitate escape from endosomes and permit their genetic material to reach the nucleus allowing the viral life cycle to proceed. One approach to overcoming the problem of endosomal entrapment of liposome-encapsulated DNA is exploiting the components of viruses that possess an endosomal destabilizing capacity. The construction of fusogenic liposomes by complexing UV-irradiated Sendi viruses or recombinant viral envelope proteins has led to increased cellular binding and fusogenic activity, and these liposomes bypass the endosomal pathway and deliver their content directly into the cytoplasm of the cell, resulting in a marked increase in mediating efficient gene expression. These so called "virosomes" have been successfully used to transfect cells and move more efficiently than cationic lipid-DNA complexes, both *in vitro* (Morishita *et al.*, 1993) and *in vivo* (Mizuguchi *et al.*, 1996; Nakamura *et al.*, 1996). Sendai virosomes fuse with cultured neurones more efficiently than pure liposomes (de Fiebre *et al.*, 1993; Wu *et al.*, 1995). Virosomes have also been successfully used to mediate efficient gene delivery and expression in various tissues and organs. These include the liver (Kaneda *et al.*, 1989a,b; Kato *et al.*, 1991a,b), the vascular wall (Dzau *et al.*, 1993), the kidney (Tomita *et al.*, 1992), neurones (Wu *et al.*, 1996) and the myocardium after coronary infusion of liposome-encapsulated DNA (Sawa *et al.*, 1995).

The interaction of liposomes with cells is enhanced in the presence of some ligands coupled to the vesicular membrane. Liposomes may be coupled to various ligands enabling the construction of DNA vehicles targeted at specific cell populations. The fate of liposomes taken up by receptor-mediated endocytosis is determined by the fate of the cell surface molecule to which they bind and also by the cell type and the target molecule. Augmented gene delivery has been achieved by using targeted liposomes, such as immunoliposomes (Wang and Huang, 1987a, 1989). Immunoliposomes containing an antibody to a cell-surface antigen of rat glial cells mediated expression of a reporter gene specifically into these cells *in vitro* (Holmberg *et al.*, 1994) and after administration into the brain and the spinal cord *in vivo* (Geisert *et al.*, 1995). Liposomes encapsulating a reporter gene have also been specifically targeted at hepatocytes by incorporating an asialoglycoprotein, which targets the receptors present on these cells (Hara *et al.*, 1995).

Moreover, the efficiency of gene transfer is enhanced by condensing the plasmid DNA with a nonhistone, nuclear, highly mobile protein (Kaneda *et al.*, 1989a; Kato *et al.*, 1991b) or with spermine (Tikchonenko *et al.*, 1988) before encapsulation within the liposome. These nuclear proteins increase the efficiency of nuclear translocation because of the nuclear localization signals (NLS) which are specific motifs, rich in basic amino acids, such as lysine, and are recognized by the nuclear importing machinery of the cell.

Vector design is as important as proper liposome formulation in generating a functional vehicle that mediates successful exogenous gene transfer in the appropriate tissue. Thierry *et al.* (1995) looked at the systemic biodistribution of a reporter gene administered intravenously in mice by using a liposomal delivery system and demonstrated that the cytomegalovirus (CMV) promoter mediates higher levels of expression in spleen than in lung compared to the Rous sarcoma virus (RSV) promoter. The same authors showed that a human papovavirus-derived vector, an episomally replicative vector, produces long-term systemic gene expression as long as three months. This vector consists of an origin of replication and a gene coding for the protein that binds to the origin. Such a plasmid reaches a stable unintegrated copy number and allows extrachromosomal maintenance of the exogenous DNA in the target cell and redistribution of copies to daughter cells. Moreover, it has been reported that modification to other nongene regulatory elements of a reporter gene plasmid vector backbone, such as the polyadenylation and transcriptional termination sequences, results in increased expression levels when injected into mice muscle (Hartikka *et al.*, 1996).

3.1.2. Cationic Lipids

Cationic lipids have contributed to the development of a standard transfection technique which has been used successfully with a variety of cell types *in vitro* and *in vivo.* Several cationic lipid reagents, such as Lipofectin, Lipofect Amine and Transfect Ace, are available commercially and are currently used in many laboratories. Many others are being developed. Comparative studies have shown that cationic lipid-mediated gene delivery is much more efficient than plasmid DNA on its own and that the mechanism of gene transfer also differs (Liu *et al.*, 1995). Cationic lipids also mediate higher gene uptake and expression compared to pure liposomes (Legendre and Szoka, 1992).

1,2-Dioleyoxypropyl-3-trimethyl ammonium bromide (DOTMA) is the conventional cationic lipid that has been widely used since the pioneering work of Felgner and coworkers (1987). Combining this lipid with neutral lipids, such as dioleoylphosphatidylethanolamine (DOPE) or cholesterol, which possess membrane-destabilizing properties, produces DNA complexes with high transfection ability. Comparative studies have identified the combination of 1,2-dimyristyloxypropyl-*N*,*N*-dimethyl-hydroxyethyl ammonium (DMRIE) and DOPE as the most efficient cationic lipid for gene transfer *in vitro* and *in vivo* (Fasbender *et al.*, 1995; Felgner *et al.*, 1994). This lipid has been proposed for clinical trials in patients with cystic fibrosis (Hart *et al.*, 1995b), melanoma (Nabel *et al.*, 1994), renal carcinoma (Vogelzang *et al.*, 1994), and hepatic metastases of colorectal carcinoma (Rubin *et al.*, 1994).

The mechanisms of lipid-DNA interaction and the structural features of the resulting complexes are still largely unclear. Unlike liposomes, in which the DNA molecules are encapsulated within unilamellar vesicles, it has been thought that the cationic lipid molecules interact electrostatically with DNA *via* their positively charged head groups causing the DNA to collapse into condensed particles (Ghirlando *et al.*, 1992). However, it has been demonstrated that cationic lipid binding does not lead to DNA condensation and that an excess of lipid in terms of charge leads to entrapping the DNA molecules between the lamellae in clusters of aggregated multilamellar structures (Reimer *et al.*, 1995). Another model has also been proposed where both phenomena are involved sequentially, namely lipid-DNA fusion followed by condensation of the DNA molecules when a critical cationic lipid concentration is reached (Gershon *et al.*, 1993).

Formulations are of great importance because these will almost certainly determine the efficacy of the cationic lipid-DNA complexes in mediating DNA transfer (Felgner *et al.*, 1995). Wide variations in the charge ratio of DNA to lipid in the complex have been reported, depending on the lipid type used and the formulation conditions. It has been widely reported that optimal *in vitro* gene delivery with cationic lipids requires an excess of positive charge with respect to the DNA anionic phosphate backbone to enable the positively charged lipid-DNA complex to interact spontaneously with the anionic sialic acid residues on the cell membrane. However, it is also reported that electrically neutral lipopolyamine-DNA complex particles mediate good transfection levels (Remy *et al.*, 1995).

The efficiency of cationic lipid-mediated transfection varies for different cell types (Farhood *et al.*, 1992; Gao and Huang, 1991; Zabner *et al.*, 1995). The choice of cationic lipid incorporated into the DNA complex offers some level of tissue targeting *in vivo* (Jarnagin *et al.*, 1992; Zhu *et al.*, 1993). This may result from selective interactions of individual cationic lipids with specific cell types. The population of cationic lipid-DNA complex particles is heterogenous in size and shape (Mahato *et al.*, 1995). However, each complex is ordered in a regular multilamellar pattern with periodicity of approximately 3.2–4.5 nm (Zabner *et al.*, 1995). It has been thought for some time that cationic lipid-mediated gene transfer is accomplished by direct entry of the complex into the cytoplasm of the cell by fusion with biological membranes (Felgner *et al.*, 1987; Smith *et al.*, 1993). However, there is mounting evidence that the major mechanism of entry of cationic lipid-DNA complexes is endocytosis (Felgner *et al.*, 1994; Zabner *et al.*, 1995). It has also been suggested that cationic lipids participate in preventing the delivery of DNA to lysosomes, thus augmenting the chance of endosomal escape into the cytosol (Wattiaux *et al.*, 1995).

In some tissues, such as the lung, most of the widely available cationic lipids poorly enhance DNA expression above that obtained with naked DNA (Felgner *et al.*, 1995). Hybrid cationic lipids which incorporate nonlipid cations, such as polylysine (Vitiello *et al.*, 1996; Zhou *et al.*, 1991; Zhou and Huang, 1994), polylysine-antibody conjugates (Trubetskoy *et al.*, 1992a), and polyamine (Behr *et al.*, 1989; Remy *et al.*, 1994, 1995) have been successfully used to increase expression of foreign genes. Polylysine and protamine enhance the transfection efficiency of several types of cationic lipids by dramatically reducing the particle size of the complex (Gao and Huang, 1996). It has been observed that administering the anticancer drugs cisplatin (Son and Huang, 1994), nitrogen mustard, and taxol (Son and Huang, 1996) to *in vivo* transfected ovarian carcinoma cells using cationic lipids leads to elevated gene expression. The efficiency of transfection mediated by cationic lipids is also enhanced by using "adenosomes," cationic lipids that contain adenoviral components which promote endosomal escape (Zhou *et al.*, 1995). A targeted molecular transfection system based on lipopolyamine-DNA particles with galactosyl residues has been developed to specifically transfect hepatocytes (Remy *et al.*, 1995). However, in a extensive study of the mechanisms of DNA uptake mediated by cationic lipids, Zabner *et al.* (1995) demonstrated that the major reason for the inefficiency of cationic lipid-based methods is not the ability to deliver DNA inside the cells, because most of the DNA is taken up, but its translocation to the nucleus. Inclusion of an SV40 nuclear localization signal into cationic lipid-adenovirus-DNA particles results in significantly enhanced gene transfer in rabbit muscle (Raja-Walia *et al.*, 1995). However, it has also been reported that incorporating a nuclear localization peptide in a cationic lipid-DNA complex significantly enhances the effect on an already efficient system (Remy *et al.*, 1995).

Cationic lipids are being extensively investigated as potential vehicles for gene transfer *in vivo*. Because they are not biodegradable, the toxicity of the majority of cationic lipids, is one of the major drawbacks to their successful use for gene delivery. A vigorous inflammatory response to DMRIE and *N*-(1-(2,3-dioleoyloxy)propyl)-*N*,*N*,*N*-trimethylammoniummethylsulphate (DOTAP), which was associated with tissue damage at the injection site, has been reported (Raz *et al.*, 1994). However, many improved reagents have been developed which have minimal toxicity. A DNA complex formulation with DMRIE:DOPE, which has been used successfully to induce an antitumor response in mice, is very well tolerated by the experimental animals and shows no toxicity (San *et al.*, 1993). Encouraging results of a cationic lipid-based clinical gene therapy trial of cystic fibrosis have been reported, and no adverse clinical effects or abnormal immunological or histological changes to the target tissue were seen (Caplen *et al.*, 1995). Some cationic lipids are poorly immunogenic (Farhood *et al.*, 1994), and repeated intravenous injections or aerosol administration of cationic lipid-DNA complexes had no adverse effects on several histological and physiological properties of the lung (Canonico *et al.*, 1994).

Direct intravenous injection of plasmid DNA complexed to cationic lipids in mice resulted in the transferred gene being detected in multiple tissues. It has been reported that intravenous injection of genes complexed with cationic lipids leads to expression in large numbers of cells located primarily within the vascular compartment (Zhu *et al.*, 1993). Transient exogenous gene expression was detected in the lung after intravenous injection (Brigham *et al.*, 1989) and when administered as a small-particle aerosol (Schwarz *et al.*, 1996). The lung is more susceptible to gene transfer mediated by cationic lipids than most other tissues. It has been reported that instillation (Hyde *et al.*, 1993; Logan *et al.*, 1995) or nebulization (Alton *et al.*, 1993) of a cationic lipid-DNA complex containing the cystic fibrosis transductance regulator (CFTR) gene into a mouse model showed transgene expression and correction of a range of ion transport abnormalities. Now clinical trials using cationic liposome-mediated DNA transfer have been initiated, and encouraging results from a cystic fibrosis clinical trial have been reported (Caplen *et al.*, 1995). Expression is enhanced through improved vector design for intravenous gene delivery by varying several components of the DNA vector, such as promoters and intron sequences. It has been reported that after intravenous injection of DNA complexed to cationic lipids, expression could be targeted to specific tissues and cell types, depending on the promoter used (Zhu *et al.*, 1993). Intravenous injection of a CMV-based expression vector into mice transfects nearly every tissue examined (Liu *et al.*, 1995). Systemic delivery of plasmids encoding mouse granulocyte-macrophage colony-stimulating factor (GM-CSF) and human granulocyte colony-stimulating factor (G-CSF) using cationic lipids produces high levels of these growth factors in the circulation of mice (Liu *et al.*, 1995).

The route of administration may be chosen to enhance targeting, and site-specific expression is achieved by direct administration *in vivo*. The majority of splenic and lymph node-derived T lymphocytes have been transfected by intraperitoneal injection of cationic lipid-DNA complexes into mice (Philip *et al.*, 1993, 1994). Cationic lipids have also been used to deliver and mediate DNA expression in arteries by using a catheter (Nabel *et al.*, 1990; Shi *et al.*, 1994). Direct injection of lipospermine-based DNA complexes leads to uptake and expression in the newborn mouse brain (Schwartz *et al.*, 1995) and in the caudal putamen of the brain of adult mice (Ono *et al.*, 1990; Roessler and Davidson, 1994). In addition, direct injection of plasmid DNA, which contains the tyrosine hydroxylase gene, into the brain of a rat model for Parkinson's disease, results in intracerebral expression of the gene and improved rotational behavior of the animal (Cao *et al.*, 1995). Moreover, cationic lipid complexes have been used to mediate transfection in ocular tissue *in vivo* (Jones *et al.*, 1994), and mouse fetuses have been transfected *in utero* after injecting cationic lipid-DNA complexes intravenously into pregnant mice (Tsukamoto *et al.*, 1995).

Cationic lipid-mediated gene transfer has an anticancer therapeutic potential (Cooper, 1996). Immunotherapy of colon adenocarcinoma and fibrosarcoma has been achieved in mice by intratumoral injections of cationic lipid-DNA complexes containing the murine I *H*-2K gene (Plautz *et al.*, 1993). The human major histocompatibility protein HLA-B7 gene was introduced into subcutaneous melanoma tumors of HLA-B7-negative patients by direct gene transfer using cationic lipid-DNA complexes (Nabel *et al.*, 1993). HLA-B7 protein were detected within all injected tumors and immune responses to HLA-B7 autologous tumors were detected. However, the therapeutic success of this trial was minimal. Cationic lipid-mediated delivery of the wild-type p53 gene produces significant antitumor effects in nude mice bearing human tumors lacking p53 expression (Lesoon Wood *et al.*, 1995). Cationic lipid-mediated gene transfer has also been used in cytokine gene therapy of tumors (Schmidt *et al.*, 1995b). Following injection of cationic lipid-DNA complexes containing the IL-4 gene into melanoma tumors *in vivo* (Missol *et al.*, 1995) or the IL-2 gene into lung tumor xenografts (Egilmez *et al.*, 1996), regression of these tumors has been observed because of a cytokine-mediated cytotoxic response.

3.2. Ligand-Mediated Gene Delivery Methods

Molecular conjugate-based methods for DNA delivery have become one of the major approaches to nonviral gene therapy. Receptor-mediated gene transfer relies on the physiological and highly efficient endogenous pathway that eukaryotic cells utilize to internalize macromolecules. The concept of ligand-directed gene transfer was first introduced by Cheng *et al.* (1983) who described a method for linking α-2-macroglobin to DNA to achieve ligand-directed gene transfer. The procedure consists of attaching a molecule that has a DNA-binding function and is designed to condense the expression vector with a cell-specific ligand. This potentially generates a delivery vehicle that is capable of cell-specific targeting both *in vitro* and *in vivo*.

The polycation moiety and ligand are usually conjugated by covalent cross-linking using bifunctional reagents (Cotten *et al.*, 1993a; McKee *et al.*, 1994). However, other coupling strategies have been successfully employed, such as nonenzymatic reductive glycosylation of polylysine (Martinez-Fong *et al.*, 1994) and a biotin-streptavidin bridge between polylysine and the ligand (Schoeman *et al.*, 1995; Schwarzenberger *et al.*, 1996).

Although the assembly of various components of the synthetic delivery system appears uncomplicated, it is in fact of crucial importance because failure in any of the mixing steps generates an inefficient or even ineffective product. The phosphate backbone of the DNA molecule is highly negatively charged which confers a rodlike shape in aqueous solution on the nucleic acid polymer. Condensation and charge neutralization are required for this long polyanionic molecule to cross an intact cytoplasmic membrane. The addition of the DNA-binding moiety to DNA results in electroneutrality, which in turn produces extensive compaction and eventually precipitation, unless the concentration of DNA is minimized (Cotten *et al.*, 1993a). The DNA complex should be condensed to a particle size that is sufficiently small to allow entry into the endocytic pit, the first step in the endocytosis pathway. Many studies have identified a size-function relationship and thus the expression level of reporter genes targeted at various cell types correlates with the formation of highly condensed, small, isolated spheres or toroids of DNA which can be visualized by electron microscopy (Perales *et al.*, 1994a; Wagner *et al.*, 1991a). Consequently, careful titration of the optimum DNA to polylysine charge ratio is needed to enable the formation of particles that mediate successful transfection. The degree of compaction of the DNA determines its resistance to nuclease degradation. Highly condensed forms of DNA are more resistant to nuclease digestion (Baeza *et al.*, 1987), and thus may contribute to DNA survival and subsequent expression *in vivo* (Chiou *et al.*, 1994). The physical characteristics of the cationic polymers, the mode of binding, and the dynamics of their interaction with DNA determine the colloidal properties and stability of the resulting complex. The quality of the DNA, especially the presence of contaminating endotoxins in the plasmid preparation, plays a crucial role in the efficiency of transfection. The purity of plasmid DNA preparations is of paramount importance for successful transfection to primary cells because impurities, such as bacterial lipopolysaccharides, are highly toxic to cells (Cotten *et al.*, 1994a).

Because the properties of the DNA complex are also strongly influenced by the formulation conditions, these should be carefully optimized and standardized to produce a complex of the desired qualities. Various methods have been used to generate soluble DNA condensates suitable for endocytosis-mediated gene transfer. The conjugation method used originally by Wu and coworkers is based on adding both polylysinated ligands and DNA in a high salt solution (>2 M NaCl) followed by a stepwise dilution to near physiological ionic strength (Findeis *et al.*, 1994). The method used by Birnstiel and colleagues (Cotten *et al.*, 1993a), however, relies on gradually and slowly adding the polycationic moiety-ligand to a diluted DNA solution in a fixed salt concentration (150 mM NaCl). This method of complex formation generates a toroid-like structure of 80–100 nm in diameter that mediates efficient transfection *in vitro* (Wagner et el., 1991a). A new method has been reported which generates an even smaller particle size complex (10–12 nm diameter) that targets cells both *in vitro* and *in vivo* (Ferkol *et al.*, 1995, 1996b; Perales *et al.*, 1994b). In this method the cationic polymer is added to a highly concentrated solution of DNA which forms insoluble aggregates. Then the solution is cleared by an upward titration of its ionic strength to achieve a soluble complex solution in which the complex has the required properties at a fairly high ionic strength (0.5–1 M NaCl).

The size of the cationic polymer influences the ionic strength at which the DNA condenses and profoundly affects the size of the DNA complex formed. High molecular weight polylysine, for instance, produces large heterogenous complexes

120–300 nm in diameter. In contrast, small polylysine molecules generate smaller complexes that are more uniformly distributed (20–30 nm diameter; Wolfert and Seymour, 1996). DNA sequence and size may also influence the formation of the ligand-DNA complex (Perales *et al.*, 1994b). Nonetheless, very large plasmid DNA (48 kb) is condensed by transferrin-polylysine conjugates and may be successfully delivered to cells *in vitro* (Cotten at al., 1992). This demonstrates the flexibility, in terms of size of the DNA construct, that ligand-mediated gene delivery methods possess for alleviating any size constraints in using large exogenous genes and allowing the inclusion of appropriate complex regulatory sequences, such as locus control regions (LCR). In principle, an exogenous mammalian artificial chromosome that contains a centromere, telomeres, one or more origins of replication, and enough DNA sequences to drive and control expression of the gene of interest, as suggested by Huxley (1994), could be delivered by this method. However, the basic research must elucidate the feasibility of this strategy before it yields strong prospects of achieving this goal.

The condensing agent used very strongly influences the physical characteristics of the DNA complex. Several polycationic compounds that bind DNA have been used for coupling with the ligand. These include synthetic polypeptides, such as polylysine, the most used polycation. Other high-affinity DNA binding proteins and peptides, such as protamine, which are arginine-rich strong basic proteins (Wagner *et al.*, 1991a) and the nuclear proteins histones and their derivative peptides (Böttger *et al.*, 1988; Chen *et al.*, 1994) have also been used to link a ligand of interest to DNA. Other alternative strategies of binding DNA to the relevant ligand include the use of DNA intercalating agents such as *bis*-acridine (Haensler and Szoka, 1993b) and ethidium dimers (Wagner *et al.*, 1991b), or streptavidin-labeled ligand that binds to biotinylated DNA (Plank *et al.*, 1994) as DNA binding moieties. However these systems, which do not use electrostatic interaction with the DNA, could be limited by the difficulties of achieving proper DNA condensation. Moreover, it has been reported that an alternative technique of generating antibody-DNA complexes by covalently coupling the antibody directly to plasmid DNA by using benzoquinone mediates successful transfections both *in vitro* and *in vivo* (Poncet *et al.*, 1996).

New synthetic cationic polymers called "Starburst Dendrimers" or polyamidoamine (PAMAM) have been developed to transfer genetic material into cells (Haensler and Szoka, 1993a). Dendrimers are tree-like, three-dimensional, spheroidal, cationic polymers that are unprecedentedly regular in structure and have highly predictable numbers of positively charged surfaces and diameters. These structures interact on a charge basis with DNA, and unlike other polycationic polymers, nontargeted DNA complexes of these molecules transfect a variety of cells. Most probably because they bind phospholipids on the cell membrane and trigger endocytosis. *In vivo* transfection of lung tissues has been achieved after endobronchial administration of dendrimer-DNA complexes to rats (Backer, personal communication).

Several ligands have been exploited for selectively targeting cells that possess complementary receptors and achieve efficient internalization of ligand-DNA complexes. The nature of the ligand's specificity for the receptor, affinity, and efficiency of internalization are considerably important for the delivery of exogenous genes. The most extensively analyzed ligands in mediating exogenous gene transfer into a variety of cell types are the asialoglycoproteins (Grasso and Wu, 1994) and transferrin (Wagner *et al.*, 1994). Effective gene delivery using ligand-mediated endocytosis was first described by Wu and Wu (1987). This was achieved by complexing polylysinated asialoorosomucoid, a ligand that binds specifically to asialoglycoprotein receptors present on hepatocytes, to DNA. Hepatocytes and hepatoma cells has been successfully transfected *in vitro* (Wu and Wu, 1988a) and *in vivo* (Wu and Wu, 1988b; Wu *et al.*, 1989) by using these molecular conjugates. Transferrin, the iron transport protein which is a ligand that is recycled back and forth to the cell surface through a receptor-mediated endocytosis pathway, is very effective in targeting various cell types *in vitro* (Wagner *et al.*, 1990; Zenke *et al.*, 1990) and *in vivo* (Gao *et al.*, 1993).

Some cell-surface receptors, such as transferrin are shared between a variety of cell types and could compromise the ability to achieve tissue or cell-specific gene transfer. Alternatively, antibodies could be used because they fulfil many of the features of a suitable ligand, target highly restricted cell-specific surface antigens, have high affinity for their epitopes and possibly trigger internalization more efficiently by cross-linking epitope sites. An anti-CD3 and an anti-CD5 monoclonal antibody have been successfully used to specifically transfect primary peripheral blood lymphocytes (Buschle *et al.*, 1995) and a human T-cell line *in vitro* (Merwin *et al.*, 1995), respectively. A monoclonal antibody to a specific tumor cell-surface cryptantigen, Tn, has also been employed to mediate specific expression in malignant T-cells (Thurnher *et al.*, 1994). Additionally, an immunoglobulin G targeting the Fc receptor on alveolar macrophages has been successfully used to transfect these cells *in vitro* (Rojanasakul *et al.*, 1994). A specific binding fragment of an antibody which binds to an epitope on the surface of the target cell an also be used. The Fab fragment of antibodies to the polymeric immunoglobulin receptor have also been used to specifically and efficiently transfect tracheal epithelial cells *in vitro* (Ferkol *et al.*, 1993) and *in vivo* (Ferkol *et al.*, 1995, 1996a).

An alternative approach is using lectins for which there is a cognate carbohydrate structure on the cell surface. Various lectins conjugated to polylysine or histone and complexed to DNA that contains a reporter gene and subsequently administered to airway epithelial cells (Yin and Cheng, 1994) and peripheral blood monocyte-derived macrophages (Erbacher *et al.*, 1996; Ferkol *et al.*, 1996b) have successfully transfect these tissues. Other potential ligands include a malarial protein (Ding *et al.*, 1995), a naturally occurring molecule such as the hormone insulin (Huckett *et al.*, 1990), both of which bind specifically to hepatocytes, and surfactant-associated protein A (Ross *et al.*, 1995) and surfactant protein B (Baatz *et al.*, 1994) have been used as ligands to target epithelial airway cells. Small peptides resembling naturally occurring integrin ligands have also been tried (Hart *et al.*, 1995a).

Despite the fact that molecular conjugate-DNA complexes possess an efficient mechanism to achieve cellular internalization, the efficacy of these vectors has been idiosyncratic. As with liposomes and other physical methods of gene transfer, a major factor in determining the expression level of the gene transferred into target cells involves the survival and delivery of the exogenous DNA to the nucleus. It has been shown that chloroquine treatment increases gene expression by inhibiting the lysosomal degradation of internalized DNA (Cotten *et al.*, 1990; Erbacher *et al.*, 1996). The drug colchicine, which disrupts microtubule formation, prolongs exogenous gene expression mediated by an asialoglycoprotein-DNA conjugate in the liver of rats (Chowdhury *et al.*, 1996). Some cationic polymers have a lysosomal buffering capacity that protects DNA from degradation. DNA complexes with polyethyleneimine (PEI), a branched polymer, mediate very efficiently *in vitro* and *in vivo* gene transfer without the need for any enhancing agent (Boussif *et al.*, 1995).

As with liposomes, viruses that enter cells by endocytosis and which possess an endosomal destabilizing capacity have been used as enhancing agents. The most extensively used viral enhancing agent for ligand-mediated gene transfer is the human adenovirus Type 5 (Curiel, 1994). Simultaneously adding DNA complexes and intact capsids of replication-defective adenovirus dramatically augments the efficiency of ligand-mediated gene transfer and expression in a dose-dependent manner (Curiel *et al.*, 1991; Seth *et al.*, 1994; Wagner *et al.*, 1992b; Wu *et al.*, 1994). Adenovirus can be made replication-defective, while it maintains its entry and membrane disruption functions by irradiation with short waves UV (Cotten *et al.*, 1992) or by psoralen treatment (Cotten *et al.*, 1994b). Once adenoviral particles bind to cells *via* their specific fiber capsid proteins, the particles are cointernalized within endosomes together with the ligand-DNA complex *via* clathrin-coated pits. Acidification of the endocytic vesicle triggers a conformational change in the virus capsid penton base protein, which in turn, causes disruptive interaction of the hydrophobic domains of the protein with the endosomal membrane, releasing its content into the cytosol.

Adenovirus and DNA contained in the same complex are more efficient at mediating gene delivers than when viral particles are added in a free form. Replication-defective adenovirus particles incorporated into a asialoorosomucoid-polylysine-DNA complex gives transfection efficiencies of virtually 100% in a hepatoma cell line *in vitro* (Fisher and Wilson, 1994). The adenovirus particle could be directly coupled to polylysine by chemical modification *via* glutamyl and lysyl residues of the virus (Cristiano *et al.*, 1993; Curiel *et al.*, 1991; Wagner *et al.*, 1992b) or *via* carbohydrate residues on adenovirus fiber (Wu *et al.*, 1994). Alternatively, adenovirus can be linked to polylysine by an antibody bridge *via* a heterologous hexon protein of the viral capsid (Curiel *et al.*, 1992) or biotinylated to link to polylysine via streptavidin (Wagner *et al.*, 1992b). It has been shown that a targeted adenovirus is generated by genetically engineering the fusion of a peptide ligand with the fiber protein of the viral capsid (Michael *et al.*, 1995). It has also been demonstrated that apart from its ability to disrupt vesicular membranes, the adenovirus *per se* augments the rate of endocytosis because the capsid interacts with its cell-surface receptor (Curiel, 1994). Autologous rabbit jugular vein segments have been successfully transfected *ex vivo* by using adenovirus-transferrin-polylysine-DNA complexes (Kupfer *et al.*, 1994). When adenovirus-polylysine-DNA complexes are administered to isolated human kidneys under the conditions of organ preservation, appreciable levels of gene expression are detected predominantly in proximal tubular epithelial cells (Ziegler *et al.*, 1996). The conjugated adenovirus complexed to DNA has also been used to deliver plasmid DNA to hepatocytes

(Cristiano *et al.*, 1993) and human B-cells *in vitro* (Curiel *et al.*, 1994). Many unsuccessful attempts have been made to incorporate single viral components instead of the full capsid into the DNA complex.

In an attempt to use safer viral capsids, chicken adenovirus particles have been used as endosomal disruptive agents because these are defective in mammalian cells. This resulted in a massive improvement in receptor-mediated gene transfer (Cotten *et al.*, 1993b). It has been reported that human rhinovirus (Zauner *et al.*, 1995) and polyoma virus (Forstová *et al.*, 1995) also enhance the efficiency of gene transfer.

Alternative strategies to enhance ligand-mediated gene transfer and expression have used hemagglutinin-derived sequences with fusogenic activity. The synthetic influenza virus peptides significantly improve the efficiency of reporter gene expression in various cell types when used either as part of a transferrin-polylysine-DNA complex (Plank *et al.*, 1994; Wagner *et al.*, 1992a) and polyaminoamine-DNA complexes (Haesler and Szoka, 1993a) or when added together with lactosylated-polylysine-DNA complexes to cultured cells (Midoux *et al.*, 1993). It is thought that endosomal acidification triggers the peptide to adopt an α-helical conformation which penetrates the endosomal membrane and disrupts it. When perfringolysin O, a sulfydryl-activated bacterial membrane protein, is incorporated into a DNA complex through a biotin-streptavidin link as an endosomal disruptive agent, it enhances efficient gene delivery and expression in murine myoblasts *in vitro* (Gottschalk *et al.*, 1995).

Efficient translocation of the DNA to the nucleus is a necessary step in successful exogenous gene expression. As with liposomes, agents that facilitate the migration of foreign DNA into the nucleus and consequently augment its translation have been used as enhancing agents. Histone H1, H3, and H4 and protamine have been incorporated into a transferrin-DNA complex resulting in elevated expression of the transferred gene (Wagner *et al.*, 1991a). Similar results have been obtained when galactosylated histone H1 was used as part of the DNA complex (Chen *et al.*, 1994).

Despite the many problems facing the application of ligand-mediated gene delivery systems *in vivo*, there are numerous reports documenting successful expression mediated by this method. There are concerns that the gene delivery agents or the therapeutic gene products themselves might exhibit immunogenicity, and thus the immunologic properties of the DNA complex must be carefully assessed. Repetitive administrations of a glycoprotein-polylysine-DNA (Stankovics *et al.*, 1994) and antibody-polylysine-DNA complexes (Ferkol *et al.*, 1996a) provoked a humoral response to the complex resulting in reduced efficiency of subsequent gene transfer. Additionally, many studies have reported that there is no correlation between results obtained *in vivo* and *in vitro* when using the same DNA vehicle formulated under the same conditions. This highlights the need for a systematic approach to formulation which should be tailored especially to each experimental setting. There are many potential factors which may account for the differences in results obtained in synthetic media as opposed to physiological milieu which are quite different in their composition and texture. The stability of the DNA complex in the blood, for instance, almost certainly determines its lifetime and thereby the fate of DNA administered intravenously. A DNA ligand must be stable in the blood long enough to be taken up and internalized by the appropriate cells. It is known that DNA complexes are very unstable and suffer from rapid clearance by the reticuloendothelial system. Moreover, in a comparative study, Plank *et al.* (1996) found that, unlike cationic lipids, various synthetic polycationic molecules, including high molecular weight polylysine, polyethyleneimine, and PAMAM, strongly activate the complement system and that complement activation by their respective DNA complexes depends on the charge ratio. The same authors demonstrated that coating DNA complexes with polyethyleneglycol (PEG), a hydrophilic steric stabilizer, minimizes complement activation. Incidentally, most successful intravenous transfections employing polylysine-DNA complexes described below had a polycation to DNA charge ratio slightly less than 1.

Despite these problems, liver cells have been successfully targeted *in vivo* by using a galactose-terminal asialoglycoprotein-polylysine-DNA complex (Wu and Wu, 1988b) or a glycopeptide-polylysine-DNA complex (Merwin *et al.*, 1994) and prolonged expression is obtained *in vivo* when partial hepatectomy is performed after transfection (Chowdhury *et al.*, 1993). Similar results have been obtained when galactosylated polylysine conjugates, complexed to DNA under high ionic strength conditions, were injected in the caudal cava vein of rats (Perales *et al.*, 1994a). Hepatic receptor-mediated gene delivery may offer a valuable therapeutic tool in treating many diseases of this vital organ. Amelioration of hypercholesterolemia (Wilson *et al.*, 1992) and analbuminemia (Wu *et al.*, 1991) has been achieved by targeting the liver with a DNA complex that contains the low-density lipoprotein receptor gene and the albumin gene in the relevant animal model, respectively. Intravenous administration of an asialoglycoprotein-polylysine-DNA complex that contains the defective gene responsible for methylmalonic acidemia defect elevated the enzyme to therapeutic levels (Stankovics *et al.*, 1994).

The lung is another tissue that has been targeted *in vivo* by molecular conjugates. Direct *in vivo* gene transfer to airway epithelium by instillation of a polylysinated-transferrin-DNA complex achieved exogenous gene expression for up to one week (Gao *et al.*, 1993). Mouse endothelial lung cells have been successfully targeted *in vivo* using a DNA complex containing an antibody to the cell-surface protein thrombomodulin (Trubetskoy *et al.*, 1992b).

Finally, it has been demonstrated that ligand-mediated gene transfer could have an anticancer therapeutic potential. The diphtheria toxin gene was delivered to a SCID mouse model for B-cell lymphoma using adenovirus polylysine conjugates, and protection against the tumor was observed (Cook *et al.*, 1994). Tumor cells have also been successfully targeted using the folate receptor, which is abundantly present on these cells (Gottschalk *et al.*, 1994). Stable antitumor immunization has been achieved after transferrin conjugates enhanced by adenovirus mediated gene transfer of IL-2 into tumor cells (Maass *et al.*, 1995a,b; Schmidt *et al.*, 1995a).

Each individual method of nonviral gene transfer described previously has its own advantages and may be suitable in a particular part of the body. However, new approaches may incorporate aspects of more than one system to generate superior gene delivery agents that can be used to deliver DNA to specific targets. The difficult challenge to develop efficient, synthetic vectors for gene therapy faces enormous constraints. Although, some promising products have entered the clinic, this field is still very much in an experimental stage. Studies to better understand the basic mechanisms of action of each nonviral method of gene transfer will help in the further developing and optimizing these techniques toward the ultimate goal of making these systems very efficient in achieving safe genetic modifications of cells and tissues.

4. REFERENCES

Acsadi, G., Dickson, G., Love, D. R., Jani, A., Walsh, F. S., Gurusinghe, A., Wolff, J. A., and Davies, K. E., 1991a, Human dystrophin expression in mdx mice after intramuscular injection of DNA constructs, *Nature* **352:**815–818.

Acsadi, G., Jiao, S. S., Jani, A., Duke, D., Williams, P., Chong, W., and Wolff, J. A., 1991b, Direct gene transfer and expression into rat heart *in vivo*, *New Biol.* **3:**71–81.

Aliño, S. F., Bobadilla, M., Garcia Sanz, M., Lejarreta, M., Unda, F., and Hilario, E., 1993, *In vivo* delivery of human alpha 1-antitrypsin gene to mouse hepatocytes by liposomes, *Biochem. Biophys. Res. Commun.* **192:**174–181.

Aliño, S. F., Crespo, J., Bobadilla, M., Lejarreta, M., Blaya, C., and Crespo, A., 1994, Expression of human alpha 1-antitrypsin in mouse after *in vivo* gene transfer to hepatocytes by small liposomes, *Biochem. Biophys. Res. Commun.* **204:**1023–1030.

Aliño, S. F., Mobadilla, M., Crespo, J., and Lejarreta, M., 1996, Human 1 antitrypsin gene transfer to *in vivo* mouse hepatocytes, *Hum. Gene Ther.* **7:**531–536.

Alton, E. W., Middleton, P. G., Caplen, N. J., Smith, S. N., Steel, D. M., Munkonge, F. M., Jeffery, P. K., Geddes, D. M., Hart, S. L., Williamson, R., *et al.*, 1993, Non-invasive liposome-mediated gene delivery can correct the ion transport defect in cystic fibrosis mutant mice, *Nat. Genet.* **5:**135–142.

Andreason, G. L., and Evans, G. A., 1989, Optimization of electroporation for transfection of mammalian cell lines, *Anal. Biochem.* **180:**269–275.

Baatz, J. E., Bruno, M. D., Ciraolo, P. J., Glasser, S. W., Stripp, B. R., Smyth, K. L., and Korfhagen, T. R., 1994, Utilization of modified surfactant-associated protein B for delivery of DNA to airway cells in culture, *Proc. Natl. Acad. Sci. USA* **91:**2547–2551.

Baeza, I., Gariglio, P., Rangel, L. M., Chavez, P., Cervantes, L., Arguello, C., Wong, C., and Montanez, C., 1987, Electron microscopy and biochemical properties of polyamine-compacted DNA, *Biochemistry* **26:**6387–6392.

Baru, M., Axelrod, J. H., and Nur, I., 1995, Liposome-encapsulated DNA-mediated gene transfer and synthesis of human factor IX in mice, *Gene* **161:**143–150.

Behr, J. P., Demeneix, B., Loeffler, J. P., and Perez Mutul, J., 1989, Efficient gene transfer into mammalian primary endocrine cells with lipopolyamine-coated DNA, *Proc. Natl. Acad. Sci. USA* **86:**6982–6986.

Benvenisty, N., and Reshef, L., 1986, Direct introduction of genes into rats and expression of the genes, *Proc. Natl. Acad. Sci. USA* **83:**9551–9555.

Böttger, M., Vogel, F., Platzer, M., Kiessling, U., Grade, K., and Strauss, M., 1988, Condensation of vector DNA by the chromosomal protein HMG1 results in efficient transfection, *Biochim. Biophys. Acta* **950:**221–228.

Boussif, O., Lezoulc'h, F., Zanta, M. A., Schermann, D., Demeneix, B., and Behr, J. P., 1995, A versatile vector for gene and oligonucleotide transfer into cells in culture and *in vivo*: Polyethylenimine, *Proc. Natl. Acad. Sci. USA* **92:**7297–7301.

Brigham, K. L., Meyrick, B., Christman, B., Magnuson, M., King, G., and Berry, L. C., Jr., 1989, *In vivo* transfection of murine lungs with a functioning prokaryotic gene using a liposome vehicle, *Am. J. Med. Sci.* **298:**278–281.

Budker, V., Zhang, G., Knechtle, S., and Wolff, J. A., 1996, Naked DNA delivered intraportally expresses efficiently in hepatocytes, *Gene Ther.* **3:**593–598.

Buschle, M., Cotten, M., Kirlappos, H., Mechtler, K., Schaffner, G., Zauner, W., Birnstiel, M. L., and Wagner, E., 1995, Receptor-mediated gene transfer into human T lymphocytes via binding of DNA/CD3 antibody particles to the CD3 T cell receptor complex, *Hum. Gene Ther.* **6:**753–761.

Canonico, A. E., Plitman, J. D., Conary, J. T., Meyrick, B. O., and Brigham, K. L., 1994, No lung toxicity after repeated aerosol or intravenous delivery of plasmid-cationic liposome complexes, *J. Appl. Physiol.* **77:**415–419.

Cao, L., Zheng, Z. C., Zhao, Y. C., Jiang, Z. H., Liu, Z. G., Chen, S. D., Zhou, C. F., and Liu, X. Y., 1995, Gene therapy of Parkinson disease model rat by direct injection of plasmid DNA-lipofectin complex, *Hum. Gene Ther.* **6:**1497–1501.

Caplen, N. J., Alton, E. W., Middleton, P. G., Dorin, J. R., Stevenson, B. J., Gao, X., Durham, S. R., Jeffery, P. K., Hodson, M. E., Coutelle, C., *et. al.*, 1995, Liposome-mediated CFTR gene transfer to the nasal epithelium of patients with cystic fibrosis, *Nat. Med.* **1:**39–46.

Chen, J., Stickles, R. J., and Daichendt, K. A., 1994, Galactosylated histone-mediated gene transfer and expression, *Hum. Gene Ther.* **5:**429–435.

Cheng, S., Merlino, G. T., and Pastan, I. H., 1983, A versatile method for the coupling of protein to DNA: Synthesis of alpha 2-macroglobulin-DNA conjugates, *Nucleic Acids Res.* **11:**659–669.

Cheng, L., Ziegelhoffer, P. R., and Yang, N. S., 1993, *In vivo* promoter activity and transgene expression in mammalian somatic tissues evaluated by using particle bombardment, *Proc. Natl. Acad. Sci. USA* **90:**4455–4459.

Chiou, H. C., Tangco, M. V., Levine, S. M., Robertson, D., Kormis, K., Wu, C. H., and Wu, G. Y., 1994, Enhanced resistance to nuclease degradation of nucleic acids complexed to asialoglycoprotein-polylysine carriers, *Nucleic. Acids. Res.* **22:**5439–5446.

Chong, H., and Vile, R. G., 1996, Replication-competent retrovirus produced by a 'split-function' third generation amphotropic packaging cell line, *Gene Ther.* **3:**624–629.

Chowdhury, N. R., Wu, C. H., Wu, G. Y., Yerneni, P. C., Bommineni, V. R., and Chowdhury, J. R., 1993, Fate of DNA targeted to the liver by asialoglycoprotein receptor-mediated endocytosis *in vivo*. Prolonged persistence in cytoplasmic vesicles after partial hepatectomy, *J. Biol. Chem.* **268:**11265–11271.

Chowdhury, N. R., Hays, R. M., Bommineni, V. R., Franki, N., Chowdhury, J. R., Wu, C. H., and Wu, G. Y., 1996, Microtubular disruption prolongs the expression of human bilirubinuridinediphospho-glucuronate-glucuronosyltransferase-1 gene transferred into Gunn rat livers, *J. Biol. Chem.* **271:**2341–2346.

Christou, P., 1995, Particle bombardment, *Methods Cell. Biol.* **50:**375–382.

Chu, G., Hayakawa, H., and Berg, P., 1987, Electroporation for the efficient transfection of mammalian cells with DNA, *Nucleic Acids Res.* **15:**1311–1326.

Cook, D. R., Maxwell, I. H., Glode, L. M., Maxwell, F., Stevens, J. O., Purner, M. B., Wagner, E., Curiel, D. T., and Curiel, T. J., 1994, Gene therapy for B-cell lymphoma in a SCID mouse model using an immunoglobulin-regulated diphtheria toxin gene delivered by a novel adenovirus-polylysine conjugate, *Cancer Biother.* **9:**131–141.

Cooper, M. J., 1996, Noninfectious gene transfer and expression systems for cancer gene therapy, *Semin. Oncol.* **23:**172–187.

Cotten, M., Langle Rouault, F., Kirlappos, H., Wagner, E., Mechtler, K., Zenke, M., Beug, H., and Birnstiel, M. L., 1990, Transferrin-polycation-mediated introduction of DNA into human leukemic cells: Stimulation by agents that affect the survival of transfected DNA or modulate transferrin receptor levels, *Proc. Natl. Acad. Sci. USA* **87:**4033–4037.

Cotten, M., Wagner, E., Zatloukal, K., Phillips, S., Curiel, D. T., and Birnstiel, M. L., 1992, High-efficiency receptor-mediated delivery of small and large (48 kilobase gene constructs using the endosome-disruption activity of defective or chemically inactivated adenovirus particles, *Proc. Natl. Acad. Sci. USA* **89:**6094–6098.

Cotten, M., Wagner, E., and Birnstiel, M. L., 1993a, Receptor-mediated transport of DNA into eukaryotic cells, *Methods Enzymol.* **217:**618–644.

Cotten, M., Wagner, E., Zatloukal, K., and Birnstiel, M. L., 1993b, Chicken adenovirus (CELO virus) particles augment receptor-mediated DNA delivery to mammalian cells and yield exceptional levels of stable transformants, *J. Virol.* **67:**3777–3785.

Cotten, M., Baker, A., Saltik, M., Wagner, E., and Buschle, M., 1994a, Lipopolysaccharide is a frequent contaminant of plasmid DNA preparations and can be toxic to primary human cells in the presence of adenovirus, *Gene Ther.* **1:**239–246.

Cotten, M., Saltik, M., Kursa, M., Wagner, E., Maass, G., and Birnstiel, M. L., 1994b, Psoralen treatment of adenovirus particles eliminates virus replication and transcription while maintaining the endosomolytic activity of the virus capsid, *Virology* **205:**254–261.

Cox, G. J., Zamb, T. J., and Babiuk, L. A., 1993, Bovine herpesvirus 1: Immune responses in mice and cattle injected with plasmid DNA, *J. Virol.* **67:**5664–5667.

Cristiano, R. J., Smith, L. C., Kay, M. A., Brinkley, B. R., and Woo, S. L., 1993, Hepatic gene therapy: Efficient gene delivery and expression in primary hepatocytes utilizing a conjugated adenovirus-DNA complex, *Proc. Natl. Acad. Sci. USA* **90:**11548–11552.

Curiel, D. T., Agarwal, S., Wagner, E., and Cotten, M., 1991, Adenovirus enhancement of transferrin-polylysine-mediated gene delivery, *Proc. Natl. Acad. Sci. USA* **88:**8850–8854.

Curiel, D. T., Wagner, E., Cotten, M., Birnstiel, M. L., Agarwal, S., Li, C. M., Loechel, S., and Hu, P. C., 1992, High-efficiency gene transfer mediated by adenovirus coupled to DNA-polylysine complexes, *Hum. Gene Ther.* **3:**147–154.

Curiel, D. T., 1994, High-efficiency gene transfer mediated by adenovirus-polylysine-DNA complexes, *Ann. NY Acad. Sci.* **716:**36–56; discussion 56–38.

Curiel, T. J., Cook, D. R., Bogedain, C., Jilg, W., Harrison, G. S., Cotten, M., Curiel, D. T., and Wagner, E., 1994, Efficient foreign gene expression in Epstein–Barr virus-transformed human B-cells, *Virology* **198:**577–585.

Danko, I., Fritz, J. D., Latendresse, J. S., Herweijer, H., Schultz, E., and Wolff, J. A., 1993, Dystrophin expression improves myofiber survival in mdx muscle following intramuscular plasmid DNA injection, *Hum. Mol. Genet.* **2:**2055–2061.

Danko, I., Fritz, J. D., Jiao, S., Hogan, K., Latendresse, J. S., and Wolff, J. A., 1994, Pharmacological enhancement of *in vivo* foreign gene expression in muscle, *Gene Ther.* **1:**114–121.

Davis, H. L., and Jasmin, B. J., 1993, Direct gene transfer into mouse diaphragm, *FEBS Lett.* **333:**146–150.

Davis, H. L., Demeneix, B. A., Quantin, B., Coulombe, J., and Whalen, R. G., 1993a, Plasmid DNA is superior to viral vectors for direct gene transfer into adult mouse skeletal muscle, *Hum. Gene Ther.* **4:**733–740.

Davis, H. L., Michel, M. L., and Whalen, R. G., 1993b, DNA-based immunization induces continuous secretion of hepatitis B surface antigen and high levels of circulating antibody, *Hum. Mol. Genet.* **2:**1847–1851.

Davis, H. L., Whalen, R. G., and Demeneix, B. A., 1993c, Direct gene transfer into skeletal muscle *in vivo*: Factors affecting efficiency of transfer and stability of expression, *Hum. Gene Ther.* **4:**151–159.

Davis, H. L., Michel, M. L., Mancini, M., Schleef, M., and Whalen, R. G., 1994, Direct gene transfer in skeletal muscle: Plasmid DNA-based immunization against the hepatitis B virus surface antigen, *Vaccine* **12:**1503–1509.

Davis, H. L., Schirmbeck, R., Reimann, J., and Whalen, R. G., 1995, DNA-mediated immunization in mice induces a potent MHC class I-restricted cytotoxic T lymphocyte response to the hepatitis B envelope protein, *Hum. Gene Ther.* **6:**1447–1456.

Ding, Z. M., Cristiano, R. J., Roth, J. A., Takacs, B., and Kuo, M. T., 1995, Malarial circumsporozoite protein is a novel gene delivery vehicle to primary hepatocyte cultures and cultured cells, *J. Biol. Chem.* **270:**3667–3676.

Dubensky, T. W., Campbell, B. A., and Villarreal, L. P., 1984, Direct transfection of viral and plasmid DNA into the liver or spleen of mice, *Proc. Natl. Acad. Sci. USA* **81:**7529–7533.

Dzau, V. J., Morishita, R., and Gibbons, G. H., 1993, Gene therapy for cardiovascular disease, *Trends Biotechnol.* **11:**205–210.

Egilmez, N. K., Cuenca, R., Yokota, S. J., Sorgi, F., and Bankert, R. B., 1996, *In vivo* cytokine gene therapy of human tumor xenogrates in SCID mice by liposome-mediated DNA delivery, *Gene Ther.* **3:**607–614.

Eisenbraun, M. D., Fuller, D. H., and Haynes, J. R., 1993, Examination of parameters affecting the elicitation of humoral immune responses by particle bombardment-mediated genetic immunization, *DNA Cell. Biol.* **12:**791–797.

Erbacher, P., Bousser, M. T., Raimond, J., Monsigny, M., Midoux, P., and Roche, A. C., 1996, Gene transfer by DNA/glycosylated polylysine complexes into human blood monocyte-derived macrophages, *Hum. Gene Ther.* **7:**721–729.

Farhood, H., Bottega, R., Epand, R. M., and Huang, L., 1992, Effect of cationic cholesterol derivatives on gene transfer and protein kinase C activity, *Biochim. Biophys. Acta.* **1111:**239–246.

Farhood, H., Gao, X., Son, K., Yang, Y. Y., Lazo, J. S., Huang, L., Barsoum, J., Bottega, R., and Epand, R. M., 1994, Cationic liposomes for direct gene transfer in therapy of cancer and other diseases, *Ann. NY Acad. Sci.* **716:**23–34.

Fasbender, A. J., Zabner, J., and Welsh, M. J., 1995, Optimization of cationic lipid-mediated gene transfer to airway epithelia, *Am. J. Physiol.* **269:**L45–51.

Fazio, V. M., Fazio, S., Rinaldi, M., Catani, M. V., Zotti, S., Ciafre, S. A., Seripa, D., Ricci, G., and Farace, M. G., 1994, Accumulation of human apolipoprotein-E in rat plasma after *in vivo* intramuscular injection of naked DNA, *Biochem. Biophys. Res. Commun.* **200:**298–305.

Felgner, P. L., Gadek, T. R., Holm, M., Roman, R., Chan, H. W., Wenz, M., Northrop, J. P., Ringold, G. M., and Danielsen, M., 1987, Lipofection: A highly efficient, lipid-mediated DNA-transfection procedure, *Proc. Natl. Acad. Sci. USA* **84:**7413–7417.

Felgner, J. H., Kumar, R., Sridhar, C. N., Wheeler, C. J., Tsai, Y. J., Border, R., Ramsey, P., Martin, M., and Felgner, P. L., 1994, Enhanced gene delivery and mechanism studies with a novel series of cationic lipid formulations, *J. Biol. Chem.* **269:**2550–2561.

Felgner, P. L., Tsai, Y. J., Sukhu, L., Wheeler, C. J., Manthorpe, M., Marshall, J., and Cheng, S. H., 1995, Improved cationic lipid formulations for *in vivo* gene therapy, *Ann. NY Acad. Sci.* **772:**126–139.

Ferkol, T., Kaetzel, C. S., and Davis, P. B., 1993, Gene transfer into respiratory epithelial cells by targeting the polymeric immunoglobulin receptor, *J. Clin. Invest.* **92:**2394–2400.

Ferkol, T., Perales, J. C., Eckman, E., Kaetzel, C. S., Hanson, R. W., and Davis, P. B., 1995, Gene transfer into the airway epithelium of animals by targeting the polymeric immunoglobulin receptor, *J. Clin. Invest.* **95:**493–502.

Ferkol, T., Pellicena-Palle, A., Eckman, E., Perales, J. C., Trzaska, T., Tosi, M., Redline, R., and Davis, P. B., 1996a, Immunologic responses to gene transfer into mice via the polymeric immunoglobulin receptor, *Gene Ther.* **3:**669–678.

Ferkol, T., Perales, J. C., Mularo, F., and Hanson, R. W., 1996b, Receptor-mediated gene transfer into macrophages, *Proc. Natl. Acad. Sci. USA* **93:**101–105.

de Fiebre, C. M., Bryant, S. O., Notabartolo, D., Wu, P., and Meyer, E. M., 1993, Fusogenic properties of Sendai virosome envelopes in rat brain preparations, *Neurochem. Res.* **18:**1089–1094.

Findeis, M. A., Wu, C. H., and Wu, G. Y., 1994, Ligand-based carrier systems for delivery of DNA to hepatocytes, *Methods Enzymol.* **247:**341–351.

Fisher, K. J., and Wilson, J. M., 1994, Biochemical and functional analysis of an adenovirus-based ligand complex for gene transfer, *Biochem. J.* **299:**49–58.

Forstová, J., Krauzewicz, N., Sandig, V., Elliot, J., Plaková, Z., Strauss, M., and Griffin, B. E., 1995, Polyoma virus as efficient carriers of heterologous DNA into mammalian cells, *Hum. Gene Ther.* **6:**297–306.

Fraley, R., Straubinger, R. M., Rule, G., Springer, E. L., and Papahadjopoulos, D., 1981, Liposome-mediated delivery of deoxyribonucleic acid to cells: Enhanced efficiency of delivery related to lipid composition and incubation conditions, *Biochemistry* **20:**6978–6987.

Furth, P. A., Shamay, A., Wall, R. J., and Hennighausen, L., 1992, Gene transfer into somatic tissues by jet injection, *Anal. Biochem.* **205:**365–368.

Furth, P. A., Kerr, D., and Wall, R., 1995, Gene transfer by jet injection into differentiated tissues of living animals and in organ culture, *Mol. Biotechnol.* **4:**121–127.

Gao, L., Wagner, E., Cotten, M., Agarwal, S., Harris, C., Romer, M., Miller, L., Hu, P. C., and Curiel, D., 1993, Direct *in vivo* gene transfer to airway epithelium employing adenovirus-polylysine-DNA complexes, *Hum. Gene Ther.* **4:**17–24.

Gao, X., and Huang, L., 1991, A novel cationic liposome reagent for efficient transfection of mammalian cells, *Biochem. Biophys. Res. Commun.* **179:**280–285.

Gao, X., and Huang, L., 1996, Potentiation of cationic liposome-mediated gene delivery by polycations, *Biochemistry* **35:**1027–1036.

Geisert, E. E., Jr., Del Mar, N. A., Owens, J. L., and Holmberg, E. G., 1995, Transfecting neurons and glia in the rat using pH-sensitive immunoliposomes, *Neurosci. Lett.* **184:**40–43.

Gershon, H., Ghirlando, R., Guttman, S. B., and Minsky, A., 1993, Mode of formation and structural features of DNA-cationic liposome complexes used for transfection, *Biochemistry* **32:**7143–7151.

Ghirlando, R., Wachtel, E. J., Arad, T., and Minsky, A., 1992, DNA packaging induced by micellar aggregates: A novel *in vitro* DNA condensation system, *Biochemistry* **31:**7110–7119.

Giladi, E., Raz, E., Karmeli, F., Okon, E., and Rachmilewitz, D., 1995, Transforming growth factor-beta gene therapy ameliorates experimental colitis in rats, *Eur. J. Gastroenterol. Hepatol.* **7:**341–347.

Gottschalk, S., Cristiano, R. J., Smith, L. C., and Woo, S. L., 1994, Folate receptor mediated DNA delivery into tumor cells: Potosomal disruption results in enhanced gene expression, *Gene Ther.* **1:**185–191.

Gottschalk, S., Tweten, R. K., Smith, L. C., and Woo, S. L., 1995, Efficient gene delivery and expression in mammalian cells using DNA coupled with perfringolysin O, *Gene Ther.* **2:**498–503.

Grasso, A. W., and Wu, G. Y., 1994, Therapeutic implications of delivery and expression of foreign genes in hepatocytes, *Adv. Pharmacol.* **28:**169–192.

Haensler, J., and Szoka, F. C., Jr., 1993a, Polyamidoamine cascade polymers mediate efficient transfection of cells in culture, *Bioconjugate Chem.* **4:**372–379.

Haensler, J., and Szoka, F. C., Jr., 1993b, Synthesis and characterization of a trigalactosylated bisacridine compound to target DNA to hepatocytes, *Bioconjugate Chem.* **4:**85–93.

Hara, T., Aramaki, Y., Takada, S., Koike, K., and Tsuchiya, S., 1995, Receptor-mediated transfer of pSV2CAT DNA to a human hepatoblastoma cell line HepG2 using asialofetuin-labeled cationic liposomes, *Gene* **159:**167–174.

Hart, S. L., Harbottle, R. P., Cooper, R., Miller, A., Williamson, R., and Coutelle, C., 1995a, Gene delivery and expression mediated by an integrin-binding peptide, *Gene Ther.* **2:**552–554.

Hart, S. L., Mayall, E., Stern, M., Munkonge, F. M., Frost, A., Huang, L., Vasilliou, M., Williamson, R., Alton, E. W., and Coutelle, C., 1995b, The introduction of two silent mutations into a CFTR cDNA construct allows improved detection of exogenous mRNA in gene transfer experiments, *Hum. Mol. Genet.* **4:**1597–1602.

Hartikka, J., Sawdey, M., Cornefert-Jensen, F., Margalith, M., Barnhart, K., Nolasco, M., Vahlsing, H. L., Meek, J., Marquet, M., Hobart, P., Norman, J., and Manthorpe, M., 1996, An improved plasmid DNA expression vector for direct injection into skeletal muscle, *Hum. Gene Ther.* **7:**1205–1217.

Heiser, W. C., 1994, Gene transfer into mammalian cells by particle bombardment, *Anal. Biochem.* **217:**185–196.

Hengge, U. R., Chan, E. F., Foster, R. A., Walker, P. S., and Vogel, J. C., 1995, Cytokine gene expression in epidermis with biological effects following injection of naked DNA, *Nat. Genet.* **10:**161–166.

Hickman, M. A., Malone, R. W., Lehmann Bruinsma, K., Sih, T. R., Knoell, D., Szoka, F. C., Walzem, R., Carlson, D. M., and Powell, J. S., 1994, Gene expression following direct injection of DNA into liver, *Hum. Gene Ther.* **5:**1477–1483.

Holmberg, E. G., Reuer, Q. R., Geisert, E. E., and Owens, J. L., 1994, Delivery of plasmid DNA to glial cells using pH-sensitive immunoliposomes, *Biochem. Biophys. Res. Commun.* **201:**888–893.

Huckett, B., Ariatti, M., and Hawtrey, A. O., 1990, Evidence for targeted gene transfer by receptor-mediated endocytosis. Stable expression following insulin-directed entry of NEO into HepG2 cells, *Biochem. Pharmacol.* **40:**253–263.

Hui, K. M., Sabapathy, T. K., Oei, A. A., and Chia, T. F., 1994, Generation of allo-reactive cytotoxic T lymphocytes by particle bombardment-mediated gene transfer, *J. Immunol. Methods* **171:**147–155.

Huxley, C., 1994, Mammalian artificial chromosomes: A new tool for gene therapy, *Gene Ther.* **1:**7–12.

Hyde, S. C., Gill, D. R., Higgins, C. F., Trezise, A. E., MacVinish, L. J., Cuthbert, A. W., Ratcliff, R., Evans, M. J., and Colledge, W. H., 1993, Correction of the ion transport defect in cystic fibrosis transgenic mice by gene therapy, *Nature* **362:**250–255.

Jarnagin, W. R., Debs, R. J., Wang, S. S., and Bissell, D. M., 1992, Cationic lipid-mediated transfection of liver cells in primary culture, *Nucleic Acids Res.* **20:**4205–4211.

Jelinek, J., Kleibl, K., Dexter, T. M., and Margison, G. P., 1988, Transfection of murine multi-potent haemopoietic stem cells with an *E. coli* DNA alkyltransferase gene confers resistance to the toxic effects of alkylating agents, *Carcinogenesis* **9:**81–87.

Jiao, S., Williams, P., Berg, R. K., Hodgeman, B. A., Liu, L., Repetto, G., and Wolff, J. A., 1992, Direct gene transfer into nonhuman primate myofibers *in vivo*, *Hum. Gene Ther.* **3:**21–33.

Jones, S. E., McHugh, J. D., Jomary, C., Shallal, A., and Neal, M. J., 1994, Assessment of liposomal transfection of ocular tissues *in vivo*, *Gene Ther.* **1**(Suppl 1)**:**S61.

Kaneda, Y., Iwai, K., and Uchida, T., 1989a, Increased expression of DNA cointroduced with nuclear protein in adult rat liver, *Science* **243:**375–378.

Kaneda, Y., Iwai, K., and Uchida, T., 1989b, Introduction and expression of the human insulin gene in adult rat liver, *J. Biol. Chem.* **264:**12126–12129.

Kato, K., Kaneda, Y., Sakurai, M., Nakanishi, M., and Okada, Y., 1991a, Direct injection of hepatitis B virus DNA into liver induced hepatitis in adult rats, *J. Biol. Chem.* **266:**22071–22074.

Kato, K., Nakanishi, M., Kaneda, Y., Uchida, T., and Okada, Y., 1991b, Expression of hepatitis B virus surface antigen in adult rat liver. Co-introduction of DNA and nuclear protein by a simplified liposome method, *J. Biol. Chem.* **266:**3361–3364.

Keating, A., Horsfall, W., Hawley, R. G., and Toneguzzo, F., 1990, Effect of different promoters on expression of genes introduced into hematopoietic and marrow stromal cells by electroporation, *Exp. Hematol.* **18:**99–102.

Keating, A., and Toneguzzo, F., 1990, Gene transfer by electroporation: A model for gene therapy, *Prog. Clin. Biol. Res.* **333:**491–498.

Kitsis, R. N., Buttrick, P. M., McNally, E. M., Kaplan, M. L., and Leinwand, , L. A., 1991, Hormonal modulation of gene injected into rat heart *in vivo*, *Proc. Natl. Acad. Sci. USA* **88:**4138–4142.

Klein, T. M., Arentzen, R., Lewis, P. A., and Fitzpatrick McElligott, S., 1992, Transformation of microbes, plants and animals by particle bombardment, *Biotechnol. NY* **10:**286–291.

Kupfer, J. M., Ruan, X. M., Liu, G., Matloff, J., Forrester, J., and Choux, A., 1994, High efficiency gene transfer to autologous rabbit jugular vein grafts using adenovirus-transferrin/polylysine-DNA complexes, *Hum. Gene Ther.* **5:**1437–1443.

Lai, W. C., Bennett, M., Johnston, S. A., Barry, M. A., and Pakes, S. P., 1995, Protection against *Mycoplasma pulmonis* infection by genetic vaccination, *DNA Cell Biol.* **14:**643–651.

Legendre, J. Y., and Szoka, F. C., Jr., 1992, Delivery of plasmid DNA into mammalian cell lines using pH-sensitive liposomes: Comparison with cationic liposomes, *Pharm. Res.* **9:**1235–1242.

Legendre, J. Y., and Supersaxo, A., 1995, Short-chain phospholipids enhance amphipathic peptide-mediated gene transfer, *Biochem. Biophys. Res. Commun.* **217:**179–185.

Leibiger, I., Leibiger, B., Sarrach, D., Walther, R., and Zuhlke, H., 1990, Genetic manipulation of rat hepatocytes *in vivo*. Implications for a therapy model of type-1 diabetes, *Biomed. Biochim. Acta* **49:**1193–1200.

Lesoon Wood, L. A., Kim, W. H., Kleinman, H. K., Weintraub, B. D., and Mixson, A. J., 1995, Systemic gene therapy with p53 reduces growth and metastases of a malignant human breast cancer in nude mice, *Hum. Gene Ther.* **6:**395–405.

Levy, M. Y., Barron, L. G., Meyer, K. B., and Szoka, F. C., 1996, Characterization of plasmid DNA transfer into mouse skeletal muscle: Evaluation of uptake mechanism, expression and secretion of gene products into blood, *Gene Ther.* **3:**201–211.

Li, L., and Hoffman, R. M., 1995, The feasibility of targeted selective gene therapy of the hair follicle, *Nat. Med.* **1:**705–706.

Lin, H., Parmacek, M. S., Morle, G., Bolling, S., and Leiden, J. M., 1990, Expression of recombinant genes in myocardium *in vivo* after direct injection of DNA, *Circulation* **82:**2217–2221.

Liu, Y., Liggitt, D., Zhong, W., Tu, G., Gaensler, K., and Debs, R., 1995, Cationic liposome-mediated intravenous gene delivery, *J. Biol. Chem.* **270:**24864–24870.

Logan, J. J., Bebok, Z., Walker, L. C., Peng, S., Felgner, P. L., Siegal, G. P., Frizzell, R. A., Dong, J., Howard, M., Matalon, A., *et al.*, 1995, Cationic lipids for reporter gene and CFTR transfer to rat pulmonary epithelium, *Gene Ther.* **2:**38–49.

Maass, G., Schweighoffer, T., Berger, M., Schmidt, W., Herbst, E., Zatloukal, K., Buschle, M., and Birnstiel, M. L., 1995a, Tumor vaccines: Effects and fate of IL-2 transfected murine melanoma cells *in vivo*, *Int. J. Immunopharmacol.* **17:**65–73.

Maass, G., Schmidt, W., Berger, M., Schilcher, F., Koszik, F., Schneeberger, A., Stingl, G., Birnstiel, M. L., and Schweighoffer, T., 1995b, Priming of tumor-specific T cells in the draining lymph nodes after immunization with interleukin 2-secreting tumor cells: Three consecutive stages may be required for successful tumor vaccination, *Proc. Natl. Acad. Sci. USA* **92:**5540–5544.

Mahato, R. I., Kawabata, K., Nomura, T., Takakura, Y., and Hashida, M., 1995, Physicochemical and pharmacokinetic characteristics of plasmid DNA/cationic liposome complexes, *J. Pharm. Sci.* **84:**1267–1271.

Major, M. E., Vitvitski, L., Mink, M. A., Schleef, M., Whalen, R. G., Trepo, C., and Inchauspe, G., 1995, DNA-based immunization with chimeric vectors for the induction of immune responses against the hepatitis C virus nucleocapsid, *J. Virol.* **69:**5798–5805.

Malone, R. W., Hickman, M. A., Lehmann Bruinsma, K., Sih, T. R., Walzem, R., Carlson, D. M., and Powell, J. S., 1994, Dexamethasone enhancement of gene expression after direct hepatic DNA injection, *J. Biol. Chem.* **269:**29903–29907.

Manthorpe, M., Cornefert Jensen, F., Hartikka, J., Felgner, J., Rundell, A., Margalith, M., and Dwarki, V., 1993, Gene therapy by intramuscular injection of plasmid DNA: Studies on firefly luciferase gene expression in mice, *Hum. Gene Ther.* **4:**419–431.

Martinez Fong, D., Mullersman, J. E., Purchio, A. F., Armendariz Borunda, J., and Martinez Hernandez, A., 1994, Nonenzymatic glycosylation of poly-l-lysine: A new tool for targeted gene delivery, *Hepatology* **20:**1602–1608.

McKee, T. D., DeRome, M. E., Wu, G. Y., and Findeis, M. A., 1994, Preparation of asialoorosomucoid-polylysine conjugates, *Bioconjugate Chem.* **5:**306–311.

Merwin, J. R., Noell, G. S., Thomas, W. L., Chiou, H. C., DeRome, M. E., McKee, T. D., Spitalny, G. L., and Findeis, M. A., 1994, Targeted delivery of DNA using YEE(GalNAcAH)3, a synthetic glycopeptide ligand for the asialoglycoprotein receptor, *Bioconjugate Chem.* **5:**612–620.

Merwin, J. R., Carmichael, E. P., Noell, G. S., DeRome, M. E., Thomas, W. L., Robert, N., Spitalny, G., and Chiou, H. C., 1995, CD5-mediated specific delivery of DNA to T lymphocytes: Compartmentalization augmented by adenovirus, *J. Immunol. Methods* **186:**257–266.

Meyer, K. B., Thompson, M. M., Levy, M. Y., Barron, L. G., and Szoka, F. C., Jr., 1995, Intratracheal gene delivery to the mouse airway: Characterization of plasmid DNA expression and pharmacokinetics, *Gene Ther.* **2:**450–460.

Michael, S. I., Hong, J. S., Curiel, D. T., and Engler, J. A., 1995, Addition of a short peptide ligand to the adenovirus fiber protein, *Gene Ther.* **2:**660–668.

Michel, M. L., Davis, H. L., Schleef, M., Mancini, M., Tiollais, P., and Whalen, R. G., 1995, DNA-mediated immunization to the hepatitis B surface antigen in mice: Aspects of the humoral response mimic hepatitis B viral infection in humans, *Proc. Natl. Acad. Sci. USA* **92:**5307–5311.

Midoux, P., Mendes, C., Legrand, A., Raimond, J., Mayer, R., Monsigny, M., and Roche, A. C., 1993, Specific gene transfer mediated by lactosylated poly-L-lysine into hepatoma cells, *Nucleic Acids Res.* **21:**871–878.

Missol, E., Sochanik, A., and Szala, S., 1995, Introduction of murine Il-4 gene into B16(F10) melanoma tumors by direct gene transfer with DNA-liposome complexes, *Cancer Lett.* **97:**189–193.

Mizuguchi, H., Nakagawa, T., Nakanishi, M., Imazu, S., Nakagawa, S., and Mayumi, T., 1996, Efficient gene transfer into mammalian cells using fusogenic liposome, *Biochem. Biophys. Res. Commun.* **218:**402–407.

Morishita, R., Gibbons, G. H., Kaneda, Y., Ogihara, T., and Dzau, V. J., 1993, Novel *in vitro* gene transfer method for study of local modulators in vascular smooth muscle cells, *Hypertension* **21:**894–899.

Nabel, E. G., Plautz, G., and Nabel, G. J., 1990, Site-specific gene expression *in vivo* by direct gene transfer into the arterial wall, *Science* **249:**1285–1288.

Nabel, G. J., Nabel, E. G., Yang, Z. Y., Fox, B. A., Plautz, G. E., Gao, X., Huang, L., Shu, S., Gordon, D., and Chang, A. E., 1993, Direct gene transfer with DNA-liposome complexes in melanoma: Expression, biologic activity, and lack of toxicity in humans, *Proc. Natl. Acad. Sci. USA* **90:**11307–11311.

Nabel, G. J., Chang, A. E., Nabel, E. G., Plautz, G. E., Ensminger, W., Fox, B. A., Felgner, P., Shu, S., and Cho, K., 1994, Immunotherapy for cancer by direct gene transfer into tumors, *Hum. Gene Ther.* **5:**57–77.

Nakamura, N., Horibe, S., Matsumoto, N., Tomita, T., Natsuume, T., Kaneda, Y., Shino, K., and Ochi, T., 1996, Transient introduction of a foreign gene into healing rat patellar ligament, *J. Clin. Invest.* **97:**226–231.

Narayanan, R., Jastreboff, M. M., Chiu, C. F., and Bertino, J. R., 1986, *In vivo* expression of a nonselected gene transferred into murine hematopoietic stem cells by electroporation, *Biochem. Biophys. Res. Commun.* **141:**1018–1024.

Narayanan, R., Tare, N. S., Benjamin, W. R., and Gubler, U., 1989, A sensitive technique to monitor gene transfer and expression in bone marrow stem cells, *Exp. Hematol.* **17:**832–835.

Neil, G. A., and Zimmermann, U., 1993, Electroinjection, *Methods Enzymol.* **221:**339–361.

Nicolau, C., Le Pape, A., Soriano, P., Fargette, F., and Juhel, M. F., 1983, *In vivo* expression of rat insulin after intravenous administration of the liposome-entrapped gene for rat insulin I, *Proc. Natl. Acad. Sci. USA* **80:**1068–1072.

Nicolet, C. M., Burkholder, J. K., Gan, J., Culp, J., Kashmiri, S. V., Schlom, J., Yang, N. S., and Sondel, P. M., 1995, Expression of a tumor-reactive antibody-interleukin 2 fusion protein after *in vivo* particle-mediated gene delivery, *Cancer Gene Ther.* **2:**161–170.

Ono, T., Fujino, Y., Tsuchiya, T., and Tsuda, M., 1990, Plasmid DNAs directly injected into mouse brain with lipofectin can be incorporated and expressed by brain cells, *Neurosci. Lett.* **117:**259–263.

Perales, J. C., Ferkol, T., Beegen, H., Ratnoff, O. D., and Hanson, R. W., 1994a, Gene transfer *in vivo*: Sustained expression and regulation of genes introduced into the liver by receptor-targeted uptake, *Proc. Natl. Acad. Sci. USA* **91:**4086–4090.

Perales, J. C., Ferkol, T., Molas, M., and Hanson, R. W., 1994b, An evaluation of receptor-mediated gene transfer using synthetic DNA-ligand complexes, *Eur. J. Biochem.* **226:**255–266.

Philip, R., Liggitt, D., Philip, M., Dazin, P., and Debs, R., 1993, *In vivo* gene delivery. Efficient transfection of T lymphocytes in adult mice, *J. Biol. Chem.* **268:**16087–16090.

Philip, R., Brunette, E., Kilinski, L., Murugesh, D., McNally, M. A., Ucar, K., Rosenblatt, J., Okarma, T. B., and Lebkowski, J. S., 1994, Efficient and sustained gene expression in primary T lymphocytes and primary and cultured tumor cells mediated by adeno-associated virus plasmid DNA complexed to cationic liposomes, *Mol. Cell. Biol.* **14:**2411–2418.

Plank, C., Oberhauser, B., Mechtler, K., Koch, C., and Wagner, E., 1994, The influence of endosome-disruptive peptides on gene transfer using synthetic virus-like gene transfer systems, *J. Biol. Chem.* **269:**12918–12924.

Plank, C., Mechtler, K., Szoka, F. C., Jr., and Wagner, E., 1996, Activation of the complement system by synthetic DNA complexes: A potential barrier for intravenous gene delivery, *Hum. Gene Ther.* **7:**1437–1446.

Plautz, G. E., Yang, Z. Y., Wu, B. Y., Gao, X., Huang, L., and Nabel, G. J., 1993, Immunotherapy of malignancy by in vivo gene transfer into tumors, *Proc. Natl. Acad. Sci. USA* **90:**4645–4659.

Poncet, P., Panczak, A., Goupy, C., Gustafsson, K., Blanpied, C., Chavanel, G, Hirsch, R., and Hirsch, F, 1996, Antifection: An antibody-mediated method to introduce genes into lymphoid cells *in vitro* and *in vivo*, *Gene Ther.* **3:**731–738.

Potter, H., 1988, Electroporation in biology: Methods, applications, and instrumentation, *Anal. Biochem.* **174:**361–373.

Potter, C. G., Tan, C. C., and Ratcliffe, P. J., 1991, Quantification of ^{32}P-labeled samples in gel fragments using the flat-bed liquid scintillation counter, *Anal. Biochem.* **197:**121–124.

Puchalski, R. B., and Fahl, W. E., 1992, Gene transfer by electroporation, lipofection, and DEAE-dextran transfection: Compatibility with cell-sorting by flow cytometry, *Cytometry* **13:**23–30.

Raja-Walia, R., Webber, J., Naftilan, J., Chapman, G. D., and Naftilan, A. J., 1995, Enhancement of liposome-mediated gene transfer into vascular tissue by replication-deficient adenovirus, *Gene Ther.* **2:**521–530.

Raz, E., Carson, D. A., Parker, S. E., Parr, T. B., Abai, A. M., Aichinger, G., Gromkowski, S. H., Singh, M., Lew, D., Yankauckas, M. A., *et al.*, 1994, Intradermal gene immunization: The possible role of DNA uptake in the induction of cellular immunity to viruses, *Proc. Natl. Acad. Sci. USA* **91:**9519–9523.

Reimer, D. L., Zhang, Y., Kong, S., Wheeler, J. J., Graham, R. W., and Bally, M. B., 1995, Formation of novel hydrophobic complexes between cationic lipids and plasmid DNA, *Biochemistry* **34:**12877–12883.

Remy, J. S., Sirlin, C., Vierling, P., and Behr, J. P., 1994, Gene transfer with a series of lipophilic DNA-binding molecules, *Bioconjugate Chem.* **5:**647–654.

Remy, J. S., Kichler, A., Mordvinov, V., Schuber, F., and Behr, J. P., 1995, Targeted gene transfer into hepatoma cells with lipopolyamine-condensed DNA particles presenting galactose ligands: A stage toward artificial viruses, *Proc. Natl. Acad. Sci. USA* **92:**1744–1748.

Riessen, R., Rahimizadeh, H., Blessing, E., Takeshita, S., Barry, J. J., and Isner, J. M., 1993, Arterial gene transfer using pure DNA applied directly to a hydrogel-coated angioplasty balloon, *Hum. Gene Ther.* **4:**749–758.

Robinson, H. L., Hunt, L. A., and Webster, R. G., 1993, Protection against a lethal influenza virus challenge by immunization with a haemagglutinin-expressing plasmid DNA, *Vaccine* **11:**957–960.

Roessler, B. J., and Davidson, B. L., 1994, Direct plasmid mediated transfection of adult murine brain cells *in vivo* using cationic liposomes, *Neurosci. Lett.* **167:**5–10.

Rojanasakul, Y., Wang, L. Y., Malanga, C. J., Ma, J. K., and Liaw, J., 1994, Targeted gene delivery to alveolar macrophages via Fc receptor-mediated endocytosis, *Pharm. Res.* **11:**1731–1736.

Ross, G. F., Morris, R. E., Ciraolo, G., Huelsman, K., Bruno, M., Whitsett, J. A., Baatz, J. E., and Korfhagen, T. R., 1995, Surfactant protein A-polylysine conjugates for delivery of DNA to airway cells in culture, *Hum. Gene Ther.* **6:**31–40.

Rubin, J., Charboneau, J. W., Reading, C., and Kovach, J. S., 1994, Phase I study of immunotherapy of hepatic metastases of colorectal carcinoma by direct gene transfer, *Hum. Gene Ther.* **5:**1385–1399.

San, H., Yang, Z. Y., Pompili, V. J., Jaffe, M. L., Plautz, G. E., Xu, L., Felgner, J. H., Wheeler, C. J., Felgner, P. L., Gao, X., *et al.*, 1993, Safety and short-term toxicity of a novel cationic lipid formulation for human gene therapy, *Hum. Gene Ther.* **4:**781–788.

Sawa, Y., Suzuki, K., Bai, H. Z., Shirakura, R., Morishita, R., Kaneda, Y., and Matsuda, H., 1995, Efficiency of *in vivo* gene transfection into transplanted rat heart by coronary infusion of HVJ liposome, *Circulation* **92:**II479–482.

Schmidt, W., Schweighoffer, T., Herbst, E., Maass, G., Berger, M., Schilcher, F., Schaffner, G., and Birnstiel, M. L., 1995a, Cancer vaccines: The interleukin-2 dosage effect, *Proc. Natl. Acad. Sci. USA* **92:**4711–4714.

Schmidt Wolf, G. D., and Schmidt Wolf, I. G., 1995b, Cytokines and gene therapy, *Immunol. Today* **16:**173–175.

Schoeman, R., Joubert, D., Ariatti, M., and Hawtrey, A. O., 1995, Further studies on targeted DNA transfer to cells using a highly efficient delivery system of biotinylated transferrin and biotinylated polylysine complexed to streptavidin, *J. Drug Target.* **2:**509–516.

Schwarz, L. A., Johnson, J. L., Black, M., Cheng, S. H., Hogan, M. E., and Waldrep, J. C., 1996, Delivery of DNA-cationic liposome complexes by small-particle aerosol, *Hum. Gene Ther.* **7:**731–741.

Schwartz, P., Benoist, C., Abdallah, B., Scherman, D., Behr, J-P., and Demeneix, B. A., 1995, Lipospermine-based gene transfer into the newborn mouse brain is optimized by a low lipospermine DNA charge ratio, *Hum. Gene Ther.* **6:**1515–1524.

Schwartz, P., Benoist, C., Abdallah, B., Ragara, R., Hassan, J-P., Scherman, D., and Demeneix, B. A., 1996, Gene transfer by naked DNA into adult mouse brain, *Gene Ther.* **3:**405–411.

Schwarzenberger, P., Spence, S. E., Gooya, J. M., Michiel, D., Curiel, D. T., Ruscetti, F. W., and Keller, J. R., 1996, Targeted gene transfer to human hematopoietic progenitor cell lines through the c-kit receptor, *Blood* **87:**472–478.

Sedegah, M., Hedstrom, R., Hobart, P., and Hoffman, S. L., 1994, Protection against malaria by immunization with plasmid DNA encoding circumsporozoite protein, *Proc. Natl. Acad. Sci. USA* **91:**9866–9870.

Seth, P., Rosenfeld, M., Higginbotham, J., and Crystal, R. G., 1994, Mechanism of enhancement of DNA expression consequent to cointernalization of a replication-deficient adenovirus and unmodified plasmid DNA, *J. Virol.* **68:**933–940.

Shi, Y., Fard, A., Vermani, P., and Zalewski, A., 1994, Transgene expression in the coronary circulation: Transcatheter gene delivery, *Gene Ther.* **1:**408–414.

Sikes, M. L., O'Malley B. W., Jr., Finegold, M. J., and Ledley, F. D., 1994, *In vivo* gene transfer into rabbit thyroid follicular cells by direct DNA injection, *Hum. Gene Ther.* **5:**837–844.

Smith, J. G., Walzem, R. L., and German, J. B., 1993, Liposomes as agents of DNA transfer, *Biochim. Biophys. Acta* **1154:**327–340.

Smith, M. J., Rousculp, M. D., Goldsmith, K. T., Curiel, D. T., and Garver, R. I., Jr., 1994, Surfactant protein A-directed toxin gene kills lung cancer cells *in vitro*, *Hum. Gene Ther.* **5:**29–35.

Son, K., and Huang, L., 1994, Exposure of human ovarian carcinoma to cisplatin transiently sensitizes the tumor cells for liposome-mediated gene transfer, *Proc. Natl. Acad. Sci. USA* **91:**12669–12672.

Son, K., and Huang, L., 1996, Factors influencing the drug sensitlization of human tumor cells for *in situ*. lipofection, *Gene Ther.* **3:**630–634.

Soriano, P., Dijkstra, J., Legrand, A., Spanjer, H., Londos Gagliardi, D., Roerdink, F., Scherphof, G., and Nicolau, C., 1983, Targeted and nontargeted liposomes for *in vivo* transfer to rat liver cells of a plasmid containing the preproinsulin I gene, *Proc. Natl. Acad. Sci. USA* **80:**7128–7131.

Stankovics, J., Crane, A. M., Andrews, E., Wu, C. H., Wu, G. Y., and Ledley, F. D., 1994, Overexpression of human methylmalonyl CoA mutase in mice after *in vivo* gene transfer with asialoglycoprotein/polylysine/DNA complexes, *Hum. Gene Ther.* **5:**1095–1104.

Straubinger, R. M., Hong, K., Friend, D. S., and Papahadjopoulos, D., 1983, Endocytosis of liposomes and intracellular fate of encapsulated molecules: Encounter with a low pH compartment after internalization in coated vesicles, *Cell* **32:**1069–1079.

Takahashi, M., Furukawa, T., Tanaka, I., Nikkuni, K., Aoki, A., Kishi, K., Koike, T., Moriyama, Y., and Shibata, A., 1992, Gene introduction into granulocyte-macrophage progenitor cells by electroporation: The relationship between introduction efficiency and the proportion of cells in S-phase, *Leukemia Res.* **16:**761–767.

Takehara, T., Hayashi, N., Yamamoto, M., Miyamoto, Y., Fusamoto, H., and Kameda, T., 1996, *In vivo* gene transfer and expression in rat stomach by submucosal injection of plasmid DNA, *Hum. Gene Ther.* **7:**589–593.

Tekle, E., Astumian, R. D., and Chock, P. B., 1991, Electroporation by using bipolar oscillating electric field: An improved method for DNA transfection of NIH 3T3 cells, *Proc. Natl. Acad. Sci. USA* **88:**4230–4234.

Thierry, A. R., Lunardi Iskandar, Y., Bryant, J. L., Rabinovich, P., Gallo, R. C., and Mahan, L. C., 1995, Systemic gene therapy: Biodistribution and long-term expression of a transgene in mice, *Proc. Natl. Acad. Sci. USA* **92:**9742–9746.

Thurnher, M., Wagner, E., Clausen, H., Mechtler, K., Rusconi, S., Dinter, A., Birnstiel, M. L., Berger, E. G., and Cotten, M., 1994, Carbohydrate receptor-mediated gene transfer to human T leukaemic cells, *Glycobiology* **4:**429–435.

Tikchonenko, T. I., Glushakova, S. E., Kislina, O. S., Grodnitskaya, N. A., Manykin, A. A., and Naroditsky, B. S., 1988, Transfer of condensed viral DNA into eukaryotic cells using proteoliposomes, *Gene* **63:**321–330.

Tomita, N., Higaki, J., Morishita, R., Kato, K., Mikami, H., Kaneda, Y., and Ogihara, T., 1992, Direct *in vivo* gene introduction into rat kidney, *Biochem. Biophys. Res. Commun.* **186:**129–134.

Toneguzzo, F., and Keating, A., 1986, Stable expression of selectable genes introduced into human hematopoietic stem cells by electric field-mediated DNA transfer, *Proc. Natl. Acad. Sci. USA* **83:**3496–3499.

Trubetskoy, V. S., Torchilin, V. P., Kennel, S., and Huang, L., 1992a, Cationic liposomes enhance targeted delivery and expression of exogenous DNA mediated by N-terminal modified poly(L-lysine)-antibody conjugate in mouse lung endothelial cells, *Biochim. Biophys. Acta* **1131:**311–313.

Trubetskoy, V. S., Torchilin, V. P., Kennel, S. J., and Huang, L., 1992b, Use of N-terminal modified poly(L-lysine)-antibody conjugate as a carrier for targeted gene delivery in mouse lung endothelial cells, *Bioconjugate Chem.* **3:**323–327.

Tsan, M. F., White, J. E., and Shepard, B., 1995, Lung-specific direct *in vivo* gene transfer with recombinant plasmid DNA, *Am. J. Physiol.* **268:**L1052–1056.

Tsukamoto, M., Ochiya, T., Yoshida, S., Sugimura, T., and Terada, M., 1995, Gene transfer and expression in progeny after intravenous DNA injection into pregnant mice, *Nat. Genet.* **9:**243–248.

Ulmer, J. B., Donnelly, J. J., Parker, S. E., Rhodes, G. H., Felgner, P. L., Dwarki, V. J., Gromkowski, S. H., Deck, R. R., DeWitt, C. M., Friedman, A., *et al.*, 1993, Heterologous protection against influenza by injection of DNA encoding a viral protein, *Science* **259:**1745–1749.

Vile, R. G., and Hart, I. R., 1993, *In vitro* and *in vivo* targeting of gene expression to melanoma cells, *Cancer Res.* **53:**962–967.

Vile, R. G., and Hart, I. R., 1994, Targeting of cytokine gene expression to malignant melanoma cells using tissue specific promoter sequences, *Ann. Oncol.* **5**(Suppl. 4)**:**59–65.

Vitadello, M., Schiaffino, M. V., Picard, A., Scarpa, M., and Schiaffino, S., 1994, Gene transfer in regenerating muscle, *Hum. Gene Ther.* **5:**11–18.

Vitiello, L., Chonn, A., Wasserman, J. D., Duff, C., and Worton, R. G., 1996, Condensation of plasmid DNA with polylysine improves liposome-mediated gene transfer into established and primary muscle cells, *Gene Ther.* **3:**396–404.

Vogelzang, N. J., Lestingi, T. M., Sudakoff, G., and Kradjian, S. A., 1994, Phase I study of immunotherapy of metastatic renal cell carcinoma by direct gene transfer into metastatic lesions, *Hum. Gene Ther.* **5:**1357–1370.

Wagner, E., Zenke, M., Cotten, M., Beug, H., and Birnstiel, M. L., 1990, Transferrin-polycation conjugates as carriers for DNA uptake into cells, *Proc. Natl. Acad. Sci. USA* **87:**3410–3414.

Wagner, E., Cotten, M., Foisner, R., and Birnstiel, M. L., 1991a, Transferrin-polycation-DNA complexes: The effect of polycations on the structure of the complex and DNA delivery to cells, *Proc. Natl. Acad. Sci. USA* **88:**4255–4259.

Wagner, E., Cotten, M., Mechtler, K., Kirlappos, H., and Birnstiel, M. L., 1991b, DNA-binding transferrin conjugates as functional gene-delivery agents: Synthesis by linkage of polylysine or ethidium homodimer to the transferrin carbohydrate moiety, *Bioconjugate Chem.* **2:**226–231.

Wagner, E., Plank, C., Zatloukal, K., Cotten, M., and Birnstiel, M. L., 1992a, Influenza virus hemagglutinin HA-2 N-terminal fusogenic peptides augment gene transfer by transferrin-polylysine-DNA complexes: Toward a synthetic virus-like gene-transfer vehicle, *Proc. Natl. Acad. Sci. USA* **89:**7934–7938.

Wagner, E., Zatloukal, K., Cotten, M., Kirlappos, H., Mechtler, K., Curiel, D. T., and Birnstiel, M. L., 1992b, Coupling of adenovirus to transferrin-polylysine/DNA complexes greatly enhances receptor-mediated gene delivery and expression of transfected genes, *Proc. Natl. Acad. Sci. USA* **89:**6099–6103.

Wagner, E., Curiel, D., and Cotten, M., 1994, Delivery of drugs, proteins and genes into cells using transferrin as a ligand for receptor-mediated endocytosis, *Adv. Drug Delivery Rev.* **14:**113–135.

Walther, R., Leibiger, I., Kiessling, U., Sarrach, D., and Zuhlke, H., 1988, Transfer of a human preproinsulin gene containing plasmid into non-pancreatic mammalian cells, *Biomed. Biochim. Acta* **47:**343–348.

Wang, C. Y., and Huang, L., 1987a, pH-sensitive immunoliposomes mediate target-cell-specific delivery and controlled expression of a foreign gene in mouse, *Proc. Natl. Acad. Sci. USA* **84:**7851–7855.

Wang, C. Y., and Huang, L., 1987b, Plasmid DNA adsorbed to pH-sensitive liposomes efficiently transforms the target cells, *Biochem. Biophys. Res. Commun.* **147:**980–985.

Wang, C. Y., and Huang, L., 1989, Highly efficient DNA delivery mediated by pH-sensitive immunoliposomes, *Biochemistry* **28:**9508–9514.

Wang, B., Ugen, K. E., Srikantan, V., Agadjanyan, M. G., Dang, K., Refaeli, Y., Sato, A. I., Boyer, J., Williams, W. V., and Weiner, D. B., 1993, Gene inoculation generates immune responses against human immunodeficiency virus type 1, *Proc. Natl. Acad. Sci. USA* **90:**4156–4160.

Wang, C., Chao, L., and Chao, J., 1995, Direct gene delivery of human tissue kallikrein reduces blood pressure in spontaneously hypertensive rats, *J. Clin. Invest.* **95:**1710–1716.

Wattiaux, R., Jadot, M., Dubois, F., Misquith, S., and Wattiaux De Coninck, S., 1995, Uptake of exogenous DNA by rat liver: Effect of cationic lipids, *Biochem. Biophys. Res. Commun.* **213:**81–87.

Wells, D. J., and Goldspink, G., 1992, Age and sex influence expression of plasmid DNA directly injected into mouse skeletal muscle, *FEBS Lett.* **306:**203–205.

Westbrook, C. A., Chmura, S. J., Arenas, R. B., Kim, S. Y., and Otto, G., 1994, Human APC gene expression in rodent colonic epithelium *in vivo* using liposomal gene delivery, *Hum. Mol. Genet.* **3:**2005–2010.

Williams, R. S., Johnston, S. A., Riedy, M., DeVit, M. J., McElligott, S. G., and Sanford, J. C., 1991, Introduction of foreign genes into tissues of living mice by DNA-coated microprojectiles, *Proc. Natl. Acad. Sci. USA* **88:**2726–2730.

Wilson, J. M., Grossman, M., Wu, C. H., Chowdhury, N. R., Wu, G. Y., and Chowdhury, J. R., 1992, Hepatocyte-directed gene transfer *in vivo* leads to transient improvement of hypercholesterolemia in low density lipoprotein receptor-deficient rabbits, *J. Biol. Chem.* **267:**963–967.

Wolfert, M. A., and Seymour, I. W., 1996, Atomic force microscopic analysis of the influence of poly(L)lysine on the size of polylelectrolyte complexes formed with DNA, *Gene Ther.* **3:**269–273.

Wolff, J. A., Malone, R. W., Williams, P., Chong, W., Acsadi, G., Jani, A., and Felgner, P. L., 1990, Direct gene transfer into mouse muscle *in vivo*, *Science* **247:**1465–1468.

Wolff, J. A., Williams, P., Williams, P., Acsadi, G., Jiao, S., Jani, A., and Chong, W., 1991, Conditions affecting direct gene transfer into rodent muscle *in vivo*, *Biotechniques* **11:**474–485.

Wolff, J. A., Dowty, M. E., Jiao, S., Repetto, G., Berg, R. K., Ludtke, J. J., Williams, P., and Slautterback, D. B., 1992, Expression of naked plasmids by cultured myotubes and entry of plasmids into T tubules and caveolae of mammalian skeletal muscle, *J. Cell Sci.* **103:**1249–1259.

van der Woude, I., Visser, H. W., ter Beest, M. B., Wagenaar, A., Ruiters, M. H., Engberts, J. B., and Hoekstra, D., 1995, Parameters influencing the introduction of plasmid DNA into cells by the use of synthetic amphiphiles as a carrier system, *Biochim. Biophys. Acta* **1240:**34–40.

Wu, G. Y., and Wu, C. H., 1987, Receptor-mediated *in vitro* gene transformation by a soluble DNA carrier system, *J. Biol. Chem.* **262:**4429–4432.

Wu, G. Y., and Wu, C. H., 1988a, Evidence for targeted gene delivery to Hep G2 hepatoma cells *in vitro*, *Biochemistry* **27:**887–892.

Wu, G. Y., and Wu, C. H., 1988b, Receptor-mediated gene delivery and expression *in vivo*, *J. Biol. Chem.* **263:**14621–14624.

Wu, C. H., Wilson, J. M., and Wu, G. Y., 1989, Targeting genes: Delivery and persistent expression of a foreign gene driven by mammalian regulatory elements *in vivo*, *J. Biol. Chem.* **264:**16985–16987.

Wu, G. Y., Wilson, J. M., Shalaby, F., Grossman, M., Shafritz, D. A., and Wu, C. H., 1991, Receptor-mediated gene delivery *in vivo*. Partial correction of genetic analbuminemia in Nagase rats, *J. Biol. Chem.* **266:**14338–14342.

Wu, G. Y., Zhan, P., Sze, L. L., Rosenberg, A. R., and Wu, C. H., 1994, Incorporation of adenovirus into a ligand-based DNA carrier system results in retention of original receptor specificity and enhances targeted gene expression, *J. Biol. Chem.* **269:**11542–11546.

Wu, P., de Fiebre, C. M., Millard, W. J., Elmstrom, K., Gao, Y., and Meyer, E. M., 1995, Sendai virosomal infusion of an adeno-associated virus-derived construct containing neuropeptide Y into primary rat brain cultures, *Neurosci. Lett.* **190:**73–76.

Wu, P., de Fiebre, C. M., Millard, W. J., King, M. A., Wang, S., Bryant, S. O., Gao, Y. P., Martin, E. J., and Meyer, E. M., 1996, An AAV promoter-driven neuropeptide Y gene delivery system using Sendai virosomes for neurons and rat brain, *Gene Ther.* **3:**246–253.

Xiang, Z. Q., Spitalnik, S., Tran, M., Wunner, W. H., Cheng, J., and Ertl, H. C., 1994, Vaccination with a plasmid vector carrying the rabies virus glycoprotein gene induces protective immunity against rabies virus, *Virology* **199:**132–140.

Yang, N. S., Burkholder, J., Roberts, B., Martinell, B., and McCabe, D., 1990, *In vivo* and *in vitro* gene transfer to mammalian somatic cells by particle bombardment, *Proc. Natl. Acad. Sci. USA* **87:**9568–9572.

Yang, T. A., Heiser, W. C., and Sedivy, J. M., 1995, Efficient in situ electroporation of mammalian cells grown on microporous membranes, *Nucleic Acids Res.* **23:**2803–2810.

Yin, W., and Cheng, P. W., 1994, Lectin conjugate-directed gene transfer to airway epithelial cells, *Biochem. Biophys. Res. Commun.* **205:**826–833.

Yovandich, J., O'Malley, B. W. Jr., Sikes, M., and Ledley, F. D., 1995, Gene transfer to synovial cells by intra-articular administration of plasmid DNA, *Hum. Gene Ther.* **6:**603–610.

Zabner, J., Fasbender, A. J., Moninger, T., Poellinger, K. A., and Welsh, M. J., 1995, Cellular and molecular barriers to gene transfer by a cationic lipid, *J. Biol. Chem.* **270:**18997–19007.

Zarozinski, C. C., Fynan, E. F., Selin, L. K., Robinson, H. L., and Welsh, R. M., 1995, Protective CTL-dependent immunity and enhanced immunopathology in mice immunized by particle bombardment with DNA encoding an internal virion protein, *J. Immunol.* **154:**4010–4017.

Zauner, W., Blaas, D., Kuechler, E., and Wagner, E., 1995, Rhinovirus-mediated endosomal release of transfection complexes, *J. Virol.* **69:**1085–1092.

Zenke, M., Steinlein, P., Wagner, E., Cotten, M., Beug, H., and Birnstiel, M. L., 1990, Receptor-mediated endocytosis of transferrin-polycation conjugates: An efficient way to introduce DNA into hematopoietic cells, *Proc. Natl. Acad. Sci. USA* **87:**3655–3659.

Zhou, X. H., Klibanov, A. L., and Huang, L., 1991, Lipophilic polylysines mediate efficient DNA transfection in mammalian cells, *Biochim. Biophys. Acta* **1065:**8–14.

Zhou, X., and Huang, L., 1994, DNA transfection mediated by cationic liposomes containing lipopolylysine: Characterization and mechanism of action, *Biochim. Biophys. Acta* **1189:**195–203.

Zhou, H., Zeng, G., Zhu, X., Tang, J., Chen, G., Huang, Q., Peng, T., and Hu, B., 1995, Enhanced adeno-associated virus vector expression by adenovirus protein-cationic liposome complex. A novel and high efficient way to introduce foreign DNA into endothelial cells, *Chin. Med. J. Engl.* **108:**332–337.

Zhu, N., Liggitt, D., Liu, Y., and Debs, R., 1993, Systemic gene expression after intravenous DNA delivery into adult mice, *Science* **261:**209–211.

Zeigler, S. T., Kerby, J. D., Curiel, D. T., Diethelm, A. G., and Thompson, J. A., 1996, Molecular conjugate-mediated gene transfer into isolated human kidneys, *Transplantation* **61:**812–817.

Chapter 6

Prospects for Gene Therapy of Inherited Immunodeficiency

Colin Casimir

1. INTRODUCTION TO GENE THERAPY

Gene therapy has been described as "the treatment of human disease by gene transfer" (Miller, 1992a). We are currently still some way from achieving this goal but we are probably closer to its realization in the realm of the inherited immunodeficiencies than with any other group of disorders. Moreover, much of the ground-breaking development work on gene therapy (safety aspects, testing of vector systems etc.) has been in immunodeficiency, culminating with the first clinical trials of gene therapy in 1990.

1.1. Immunodeficiencies as Candidate Disorders for Gene Therapy

Of all the areas of human disease, the immunodeficiencies represent fertile ground for the development of gene therapy. They fulfill the basic criterion of being serious, often fatal disorders, and also the currently available therapies are usually extremely limited in scope. Moreover, most of the inherited immunodeficiencies have also stood the ultimate test for a gene therapy candidate disorder, correction through bone marrow transplantation in the rare instance where a matched sibling donor has been available. This, of course, also highlights the great advantage that the hematopoietic system has over other organ systems as a potential recipient of gene therapy approaches, the relative accessibility of the pluripotent stem cells. In addi-

---

Colin Casimir Department of Haematology, Imperial College School of Medicine at St. Mary's, Norfolk Place, London W2 1PG, United Kingdom.

Blood Cell Biochemistry, Volume 8: Hematopoiesis and Gene Therapy, edited by Fairbairn and Testa. Kluwer Academic/Plenum Publishers, New York, 1999.

tion, these remarkable cells can reconstitute all the lineages of mature blood cells to a transplant recipient and also can regenerate themselves, the process of self renewal. The accessibility of such cells in the bone marrow, or now, from the peripheral blood of cytokine-mobilized individuals, or even neo-natal cord blood, makes the hematopoietic system unique in its suitability for therapies dependent on gene transfer technology. This also brings with it some attendant disadvantages, most specifically, the necessity of affecting the phenotype of a terminally differentiated cell that may be removed from the gene transfer target by many cell generations.

As will become apparent in this chapter, the rapid progress during the last few years in identifying and isolating the genes underlying the various immunodeficiency syndromes has now made many of these disorders realistic and prime candidates for the development of gene therapy technologies.

1.2. Target Cell Populations

The optimal target cell for gene therapy of immunodeficiency is the pluripotent hematopoietic stem cell (PHSC). These cells are the source of all of the body's mature blood cells, and they produce progeny cells for the lifetime of the individual. Inherent in this ability to produce daughter cells that differentiate into one or more of the mature cell lineages is the property of self-renewal. This unique property of stem cells allows them to give rise to daughter cells identical to themselves that still possess all the developmental potential of the parent stem cell. Whether naturally occurring PHSCs truly subscribe to this somewhat idealized view of self-renewal is debatable, but their ability for something akin to this property is unchallenged. PHSCs can repopulate the complete blood system under the correct circumstances, so clearly they have phenomenal proliferative capacity, greatly in excess of the demands that would normally be placed on them in a single lifetime.

Until relatively recently, the only available source of PHSCs was the bone marrow. Now there are two alternative sources of long-term repopulating cells, the peripheral blood from individuals whose progenitors have been mobilized with recombinant cytokines (Chen *et al.*, 1995; Heimfeld *et al.*, 1992; Yan *et al.*, 1995) and the cord blood of neonates (Broxmeyer, 1995; Van Epps *et al.*, 1994; Wagner, 1995; Williams and Moritz, 1994). Both can be abundant sources of immature cells, though whether these populations contain cells functionally equivalent to bone marrow derived PHSCs remains to be evaluated through their continued clinical usage. It should be noted, however, that now at many centers performing bone marrow transplantation mobilized peripheral blood has almost completely replaced the use of marrow as a source of stem cells. Presently the most popular regimen for mobilizing cells typically involves the use of granulocyte colony-stimulating factor (G-CSF) often in conjunction with stem cell factor (SCF) (Donahue *et al.*, 1996; Drize *et al.*, 1995; Heimfeld *et al.*, 1992; Yan *et al.*, 1994, 1995) which, after approximately five days of daily administration, can produce circulating levels as high as 3–4%, of cells positive for the progenitor-cell-specific surface antigen CD34, about double that seen with marrow.

There has been considerable recent interest in using neonatal cord blood, particularly for its apparently lower incidence of graft-versus-host-disease (GVHD)

(Stephenson, 1995; Wagner, 1995). Banking of different cord blood serotypes has been going on for a number of years worldwide, but its application in transplantation has been restricted to pediatric use because there is rarely sufficient material in a single cord blood harvest for adult recipients. Time will show us whether it is acceptable to pool cord blood of identical HLA type for such usage. The results obtained clinically with cord blood have been impressive but the ability of cord blood PHSC to sustain long term hematopoiesis (greater than 5 yrs.) has not yet been established.

2. IMMUNODEFICIENCY DISORDERS

The history of immunodeficiency is in one sense the history of the mapping of the X-chromosome because a surprising number of these disorders are caused by defects in genes carried on the X-chromosome (Figure 1).

2.1. Severe Combined Immunodeficiency (SCID)

2.1.1. X-SCID

Although a fraction of SCIDs are of the "Swiss" type that lack both T and B cells, the classic, primary immunodeficiency disorder must be X-linked severe combined immunodeficiency (X-SCID), which accounts for over 50% of cases (Fischer, 1992; Leonard *et al.*, 1994b). Patients who have this disorder have severely compromised cellular and humoral immunity. T cells are absent or extremely low in number, and B cells, though sometimes present in larger numbers than normal, are nonfunctional. Thus, X-SCID patients are effectively without an immune system. The typical clinical pattern is one of early onset of infections, such as oral candidiasis or pneumonia and severe viral infections. Infants manifest the condition as a "failure to thrive" as early as three months of age (Fischer, 1992).

This disorder has captured the popular imagination because of its images of a sufferer encapsulated inside a sterile environment, the so-called "Bubble Boy" (Lawrence, 1985; Leonard *et al.*, 1994b). This picture emerges because current therapies are inadequate. The only treatment for X-SCID is allogeneic bone

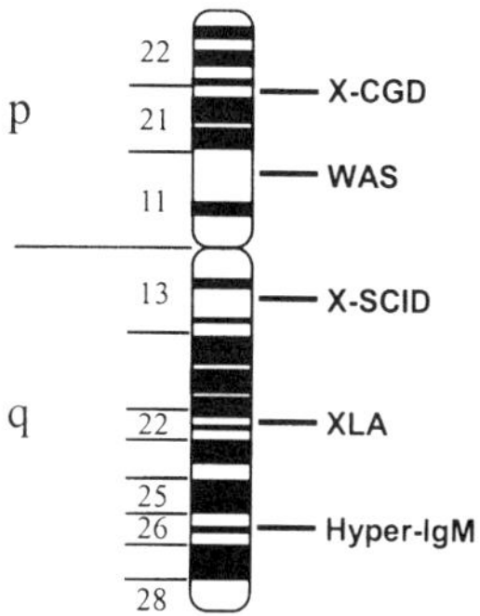

FIGURE 1. Schematic diagram of the human X-chromosome showing the positions of five immunodeficiency disorders that are candidates for gene therapy: X-CGD, X-linked chronic granulomatous disease; WAS, Wiskott–Aldrich syndrome; X-SCID, X-linked severe combined immunodeficency; XLA, X-linked agammaglobulinemia; Hyper IgM, X-linked immunodeficiency with raised IgM.

marrow transplantation. Even in this scenario the defective B cell function is often not properly restored, and such transplants have a high risk of graft-versus-host-disease (GVHD) when the recipient is immunocompromised. In the absence of a suitable donor the prognosis for the patients is very poor, and all succumb to a fatal opportunistic infection within the first years of life (Fischer, 1992) .

2.1.1a. The IL-2 Cytokine Receptor. The discovery of the molecular basis of X-SCID is an interesting one that brought together the efforts of researchers purposefully closing in on the SCID locus by gene mapping techniques and those investigating the function of lymphocyte cytokines.

The cytokine IL-2 has profound effects on the development of T cells and is key to a T-cell-based immune response. It is synthesized by T cells in response to antigen challenge and leads to specific clonal amplification (Leonard *et al.*, 1994b; Puck, 1994b).

From study of the structure and function of the IL-2 receptor a picture eventually emerged involving three different classes of receptors that have low, intermediate, and high affinity for IL-2. The low-affinity receptor is the IL-2R α-chain, and the intermediate-affinity receptor consists of a β-chain and a γ-chain heterodimer. The high-affinity receptor includes all three chains (Taniguchi and Minami, 1993). This is achieved in activated T cells by potent induction of the IL-2Rα, which is not found on resting cells. The α-chain alone is not capable of internalization and cytoplasmic signaling. These functions reside with the intermediate-affinity receptor structure. The α-chain, however, binds IL-2 very efficiently by virtue of a rapid on rate, and the stabilization of this interaction by the β/γ chain heterodimer produces the high-affinity receptor function (Leonard *et al.*, 1994b).

2.1.1b. Identification of IL-2 γ Chain Defects as the Origin of X-SCID. The IL-2Rγ was discovered more recently than the other two receptor chains and therefore was not cloned until 1992 (Takeshita *et al.*, 1992). The structure of the gene shows that the IL-2Rγ is homologous to the β-chain of the receptor and to the superfamily of cytokine receptors, and motifs in the cytoplasmic portion are consistent with a signal transduction function (Noguchi *et al.*, 1993a).

Mapping of the genetic locus for IL2Rγ by analyzing somatic cell hybrids indicated an X-chromosomal location (Noguchi *et al.*, 1993c). Mapping experiments in a number of laboratories had eventually narrowed the location of the X-SCID gene to Xq13 (Puck *et al.*, 1993a). Further mapping of the IL2Rγ gene, using known translocations and *in situ* hybridization, refined this position to Xq13.1 (Noguchi *et al.*, 1993c; Puck *et al.*, 1993c; Puck, 1994c). Given the concordance of map position and the role of IL-2 in T cell maturation and proliferation, this strongly suggested that the IL2Rγ is the gene affected in X-SCID. Linkage analysis in X-SCID pedigrees using probes from within the IL-2Rγ gene demonstrated very tight linkage between this gene and the X-SCID locus. The final demonstration that X-SCID is caused by defects in the IL-2Rγ gene came from direct sequencing of PCR products from the gene (Noguchi *et al.*, 1993c) and the transcript (Puck *et al.*, 1993b) in EBV-immortalized B cell lines derived from X-SCID patients.

2.1.1c. Mutations. Many mutations in the IL-2γ have now been identified and paint a similar picture to that seen with other genetic diseases. Examples of most of the common mechanisms for mutation have been observed, such as insertions, deletions, and point mutations. A number occur at RNA splice junctions (Leonard *et al.*, 1994; Pepper *et al.*, 1995; Puck, 1993, 1994a; Schmalstieg *et al.*, 1995). In addition, an unusually large number of single-base changes in the N-terminal region of the protein lead to the generation of stop codons. Indeed, all three of the original patient groups analyzed had mutations of this kind (Leonard *et al.*, 1994b). Two true mutational hot spots have been identified though, mapping at nucleotides 690 (amino acid R226) and 879 (Pepper *et al.*, 1995). Data of this kind along with other amino acid residues that are crucial for receptor activity provide information on γ-chain function.

2.1.1d. Cytokine Receptor Family. Despite the unequivocal assignment of IL-2Rγ as the gene affected in X-SCID, a number of factors indicated that this was not a complete story. First, it was not immediately apparent why IL-2Rγ mutations produce the defective B cell function observed in X-SCID (Fischer, 1992; Leonard *et al.*, 1994b). Moreover, IL-2 deficient individuals with normal T cell numbers were previously identified (Weinberg and Parkman, 1990), and IL-2 gene "knockouts" in mice produced a much milder phenotype than seen in X-SCID (Belmont, 1995; Kundig *et al.*, 1993). The implication was that the X-SCID mutations may affect other cytokine receptors in addition to IL-2R. This stimulated the investigation of the role of the IL-2Rγ in other such receptors, particularly those that play a role in B cell development, such as IL-4R and IL-7R. Coexpression of these receptors in Cos 7 cells revealed that both of these receptors interact with the IL-2Rγ to produce receptors that have higher affinity for their respective ligands (Leonard *et al.*, 1994a,b; Noguchi *et al.*, 1993b). For IL-7R the heterodimeric receptor that contains IL-2Rγ is strikingly higher in its affinity for IL-7, some 50-fold increase over that of the homodimeric form of IL-7R (Noguchi *et al.*, 1993b). The IL-4 receptor, however showed an increase in affinity of only a three- to fourfold following inclusion of IL-2Rγ, indicating that there could be two different classes of IL-4 receptors (Leonard *et al.*, 1994b; Matthews *et al.*, 1995). The crucial role demonstrated for IL-7 in B cell development and differentiation makes it very likely that the involvement of the "common gamma chain" (γ_c), as it has now been termed, in multiple cytokine pathways can explain the full spectrum of the X-SCID phenotype. Indeed a role for γ_c in the receptors for IL-13 and IL-15 has also been proposed, though the former has come somewhat into doubt (Matthews *et al.*, 1995). Interestingly, however, although it is thought that the γ_c functions primarily in signal transduction, there is not a common downstream pathway for all of the cytokines involved (unlike IL-3, IL-6 and GM-CSF that share the gp130 chain, for example) because the spectrum of activities and downstream phosphorylation targets differ for the different ligands.

2.2. Defects of Purine Metabolism

2.2.1. ADA-Deficient SCID

A second major cause of the SCID phenotype is a deficiency of the enzyme adenosine deaminase (ADA), which accounts for about one fifth of all SCID patients (Fischer, 1992; Hirschhorn, 1990). This defect is distinct from X-SCID because it is autosomally inherited. The gene has been mapped to chromosome 20

(Fischer, 1992; Hirschhorn, 1990). Phenotypically the disease is similar to X-SCID though there is often T and B cell lymphocytopenia. The first presentation occurs somewhat later than in X-SCID but there is a great deal of variability in clinical severity, and neurological disturbances occur in the worst cases. Allogeneic bone marrow transplantation from matched sibling donors has been quite successful for these patients. In the absence of a sibling donor the prognosis is poorer, and there is a much greater risk of severe GVHD (Fischer, 1992). A number of patients have also been quite successfully treated with recombinant bovine ADA coupled to polyethylene glycol (PEG-ADA) to stabilize it. The enzyme is administered by intramuscular injection and helps to reduce the levels of poisonous metabolites in the serum (Hershfield, 1995).

2.2.1a. Biochemistry of ADA Deficiency. ADA is a component of the purine nucleotide salvage pathway and converts adenosine to inosine. In its absence there is an intracellular accumulation of dATP (in T cells this can be 100 times the normal level) which is highly toxic to the enzyme ribonucleotide reductase and blocks DNA synthesis. Although ADA is expressed in all cells, the T cell population is particularly sensitive to the toxic effects of dATP, and T cells rely heavily on the purine nucleotide salvage pathway because they exhibit very low *de novo* purine biosynthesis. The thymus and thymic lymphocytes also have the highest levels of ADA activity.

2.2.1b. Identification and Cloning of the ADA Gene. As described previously, the gene was mapped to chromosome 20q13.4 (Fischer, 1992), though the precise localization proved more difficult to resolve. The gene spans some 32 kb, has 12 exons, and the transcript is approximately 1.5 kb in size. All cells express the gene, though as stated earlier, the level varies among tissues (Hirschhorn, 1993).

Much of the phenotypic variability can be accounted for by heterogeneity in the genetic lesions involved. The most severe cases arise from gene deletions, which may be mediated by "alu" repeat sequences within the gene, whereas milder forms that often exhibit residual ADA activity are caused by point mutations.

The ADA gene was the first of the immunodeficiency genes cloned (Valerio *et al.*, 1983; Wiginton *et al.*, 1983). Because of its small size and generally "housekeeping" nature, gene transfer experiments began soon after, and it has been the earliest target for clinical gene therapy trials.

2.2.2. Purine Nucleoside Phosphorylase Deficiency (PNP)

A less well recognized form of SCID derives from purine nucleoside phosphorylase (PNP) deficiency. This enzyme lies immediately downstream of ADA in the purine metabolic pathway, so the effects of PNP deficiency are very similar to those of ADA. PNP, however, is also involved in conversion of deoxyguanosine into guanine, and therefore PNP is associated with accumulation of dGTP. Like dATP, this nucleotide inhibits ribonucleotide reductase and DNA synthesis (Markert, 1991). The resulting loss of T cells may result from high levels of deoxyguanosine phosphorylating activity in the thymus and spleen, but B cells are spared giving rise to a T cells immunodeficiency characterized by unresponsive, hypersensitive skin reactions and recurrent infections (Fischer, 1992; Markert, 1991). The disorder is also associated with neurological damage but the reasons for this complication are unclear. The condition accounts for about 5% of autosomal SCIDs (there are about 33 reported cases), and the gene has been mapped to chromosome 14 (Cournoyer and Caskey, 1993; Markert, 1991).

2.3. B- and T-Cell Immunodeficiencies

2.3.1. Hyper IgM Syndrome

The Hyper IgM syndrome is an immunodeficiency disorder, most commonly found in an X-linked form (HIGM 1), but also seen as an autosomal recessive condition (HIGM 2) that is characterized by an inability to produce soluble antibodies of classes other than IgM or IgD (Kroczek *et al.*, 1994; Notarangelo *et al.*, 1992; Ramesh *et al.*, 1994). There are normal numbers of B cells, and these can be stimulated by pokeweed mitogen to secrete IgM but never IgG or IgA (Kroczek *et al.*, 1994; Notarangelo *et al.*, 1992). It was inferred from this pattern that the disease stems from a defect in the mechanism of antibody class switching. Analysis of the DNA of the immunoglobulin loci of HIGM lymphocytes showed that recombination between "switch" regions does not occur and that the constant regions are in their germ-line configuration (Notarangelo *et al.*, 1992). Therefore, the failure to produce IgG was confirmed as a failure of the switch recombination, though it was not apparent whether this was an intrinsic B cell defect or a problem of B and T cell cooperation. Both helper and suppressor T cell populations are essentially normal in HIGM patients, and coculture experiments using healthy allogeneic T cells were unable to stimulate class switching in HIGM B cells, implying that the defect is B cell specific (Notarangelo *et al.*, 1992). A number of features, however, also suggested that the T cells are not totally normal. For example, patients displayed an increased sensitivity to *Pneumocystis carinii* pneumonia and cryptosporidial diarrhea, both usually associated with T cell immunodeficiencies (Kroczek *et al.*, 1994; Notarangelo *et al.*, 1992), and coculture of HIGM B cells with a malignant T cell line enables the production of IgG IgA and IgE (Mayer *et al.*, 1986).

Mapping of the HIGM 1 locus on the X-chromosome located the disease gene to the region Xq26 and helped to distinguish it from X-linked agammaglobulinemia (for XLA, see Section 2.3.2), which is can resemble phenotypically (Padayachee *et al.*, 1993). This location is very similar to that assigned to a molecule, called CD40 ligand (CD40L), found on the surface of T cells (Kroczek *et al.*, 1994). CD40L interacts with B cells through a surface receptor CD40, which is also found on cells of the thymic epithelium and on monocytes. Ligation of B cell CD40 using antibodies directed against it induces LFA-1 dependent homotypic adhesion and, in combination with anti-IgM, stimulates B cell proliferation. The CD40L was, therefore, a strong candidate as the gene affected in HIGM 1. In 1993 no fewer than five different laboratories identified mutations in the CD40L gene in DNA from HIGM 1 patients (Allen *et al.*, 1993; Aruffo *et al.*, 1993; DiSanto *et al.*, 1993; Fuleihan *et al.*, 1993; Korthauer *et al.*, 1993). With one exception, all of these mutations mapped to the carboxy-terminal region of the protein that is homologous to tumor necrosis factor (TNF) (Callard *et al.*, 1993; Kroczek *et al.*, 1994). Further experience has not suggested a major hot spot for mutations in this gene, except for possibly Trp_{140} (Kroczek *et al.*, 1994), though the majority are point mutations and splice junction defects. The commonest cause of defective CD40L function is failures in folding of the protein's extracellular domain. Only one mutation in the proposed binding site for CD40 has been identified (Callard *et al.*, 1993).

2.3.2. X-Linked Agammaglobulinaemia

The archetypal immunodeficiency disorder is X-linked agammaglobulinaemia (XLA). XLA was first described by Bruton in 1952 and has often since been called Bruton's disease. The syndrome is characterized by a complete absence of all classes of immunoglobulin and of mature B cells. Consequently, patients display extreme susceptibility to infections, especially those of bacterial origin. Since the discovery that carriers of XLA show non-random X-inactivation patterns in their B cells but not granulocytes (Alterman *et al.*, 1993; Kinnon *et al.*, 1993; Rawlings and Witte, 1994; Smith *et al.*, 1994), XLA has been considered intrinsically a B cell disorder. Moreover, it became clear that, although mature B cell numbers are affected, the numbers of B cell progenitors (pre-B and pro B cells) are not (Rawlings and Witte, 1994), a strong indication that the XLA defect leads to the failure of differentiation and/or survival of B lineage cells.

The elucidation the gene responsible for XLA arrived simultaneously by two independent routes, one a "tour de force" of the use of positional cloning (Vetrie *et al.*, 1993) and the other a very astute use of a candidate gene approach (Tsukada *et al.*, 1993), which came out of an *in vitro* study of mouse B cell development (Faust *et al.*, 1993; Rawlings and Witte, 1994; Tsukada *et al.*, 1994).

Much of the positional cloning strategy became possible because a long range genomic map assembled from pulse field gel electrophoresis was generated (Kinnon *et al.*, 1995; Lovering *et al.*, 1993; O'Reilly *et al.*, 1992, 1993; Parkar *et al.*, 1994; Sweatman *et al.*, 1993). The knowledge obtained from the mapping allowed assigning the gene to the region Xq22. Yeast artificial chromosomes (YACs) incorporating DNA from this region were used to isolate B-cell-specific cDNA transcripts, which could be analyzed for mutations in XLA patients. In three out of eight XLA patients analyzed, mutations were found in one particular gene mapping to this region (Vetrie *et al.*, 1993). The sequencing of this gene revealed that it is a kinase related to the src family of nonreceptor tyrosine kinases. This kinase was also identified independently in murine pre-B cell lines (Tsukada *et al.*, 1993, 1994) using a reduced homology search strategy to look for such molecules by probing with the src kinase catalytic domain. Because differences in original nomenclature, this kinase has now been termed Btk, standing for Bruton's tyrosine kinase.

2.3.2a. Mutation Analysis in XLA. Extensive mutational analysis on *btk* has now been performed in over 250 XLA patients, revealing mutations spread right across the gene. Not surprisingly, many are located in the protein's kinase domain (see later), but there has been little evidence of mutational hot spots. Also, despite the existence of large and small deletions, insertions (Hagemann *et al.*, 1995), chain terminations and splicing defects, the predominant mutations are missense mutations, originating mainly at CpG dinucleotides (Bradley *et al.*, 1994; Conley and Rohrer, 1995; Jin *et al.*, 1995; Saffran *et al.*, 1994; Vihinen *et al.*, 1996; Vorechovsky *et al.*, 1995; Zhu *et al.*, 1994), which are particularly susceptible to sequence alterations (Jones *et al.*, 1992). *btk* remains the only gene where a mutation in a pleckstrin homology domain (see below) leads to a disease phenotype (Vihinen *et al.*, 1995; Yao *et al.*, 1994). One mutation in the unique region of *btk* an Arg_{28} is found in XLA, and an identical change is also the underlying defect in X-linked immunodeficiency in the mouse, the so-called *xid* mouse, though the phenotype of *xid* is significantly less severe than that of XLA (de Weers *et al.*, 1994b; Rawlings *et al.*, 1993; Thomas *et al.*, 1993).

2.3.2b. The Btk Protein. The protein encoded by the *btk* gene shares homology with a number of other cytoplasmic nonreceptor tyrosine kinases of which the prototype is the *src* proto-oncogene. The C-terminal region is the kinase domain, but the protein also shares peptide motifs with *src* regions known as SH2 and SH3 domains. These peptide motifs function in protein–protein binding interactions. The SH2 domain functions in binding to phospho-tyrosine residues, and the SH3 domain to a proline-rich binding motif (Feller *et al.*, 1994). In addition, now it has been shown that the N-terminal "unique region" contains a pleckstrin homology (PH) domain (Frech *et al.*, 1995; Shaw, 1996), another motif thought to play a role in protein–protein interactions, which also binds a proline-rich stretch similar to those bound by SH3 domains. In addition, there is an overall similarity to two other cytoplasmic tyrosine kinases Itk (interleukin 2 inducible kinase) (Siliciano *et al.*, 1992; Silvennoinen *et al.*, 1996) and Tec (Mano *et al.*, 1990; Silvennoinen *et al.*, 1996) which are expressed in T cells and in T cells and myeloid cells, respectively.

2.3.2c. Signal Transduction and Btk. Although this structure identifies Btk fairly positively as a molecule involved in signal transduction, the identity of its intracellular targets is still somewhat obscure. In intact B cells, it autophosphorylates in response to cross-linking of surface immunoglobulin (Aoki *et al.*, 1994; de Weers *et al.*, 1994a; Hinshelwood *et al.*, 1995). *In vitro*, Btk binds to cCbl (Cory *et al.*, 1995), a major docking protein involved in signal transduction which carries a number of proline-rich binding motifs, and, interestingly, to WASP (Cory *et al.*, 1996), the protein affected in the Wiskott–Aldrich syndrome (see Section 2.3.3), an immunodeficiency disorder that has some similarities to XLA. Neither of these interactions occurs *in vivo*, however.

Perhaps the most interesting associations are in the IL-5 pathway where both IL-5, a major regulator of B cell proliferation, and CD38, a surface receptor that augments the IL-5 response, show evidence of interaction with Btk. Although it was not observed initially (Silvennoinen *et al.*, 1996), now it is established that ligation of cd38 leads to tyrosine phosphorylation of Btk (Kikuchi *et al.*, 1995), as does IL-5 dependent growth factor stimulation (Sato *et al.*, 1994). Significantly, in the *xid* mouse the proliferative response to Cd38 ligation (Santos Argumedo *et al.*, 1995) and to IL-5 (Koike *et al.*, 1995) are significantly impaired, and the constitutively active form of Btk confers IL-5-independent growth on a cytokine-dependent cell line (Li *et al.*, 1995).

Other reports have suggested that Btk is activated by interaction with the IL-6 receptor (but not IL-3R) (Matsuda *et al.*, 1995) and that *in vivo* the plextrin homology (PH) domain is bound to protein kinase C (Yao *et al.*, 1994).

The identity of Btk as a nonreceptor tyrosine kinase has implicated it as a possible culprit in generating B cell leukemias. No such association emerged from a study of 20 patients with acute lymphoblastic leukemia (ALL) (Katz *et al.*, 1994), but a chronically activated variant that arises spontaneously *in vitro* exerts transforming activity on mouse fibroblasts (Li *et al.*, 1995), suggesting that this may not be an idle speculation.

2.3.3. Wiskott–Aldrich Syndrome

The Wiskott–Aldrich syndrome (WAS) has always been one of the most perplexing of the immunodeficiency disorders, both for the extreme variability observed in the disorder's severity and also for the involvement of both T cells and platelets which leads to a thrombocytopenia highly characteristic of WAS (Remold-O'Donnell *et al.*, 1996). Indeed, its relationship to a very similar disease, X-linked thrombocytopenia (XLT), which has no immunological consequences, proved elusive until recently, when the gene affected in WAS was identified and cloned (Derry *et al.*, 1994a,b).

WAS is an X-linked disorder usually presenting as a thrombocytopenia with small platelet size in the first years of life. The thrombocytopenia is caused by accelerated platelet destruction because megakaryocyte number and morphology are normal (Remold-O'Donnell *et al.*, 1996). With increasing age the immunological consequences become more apparent, with marked impairment of T cell function and lymphopenia. WAS patients also often exhibit eczema and fail to produce antipolysaccharide antibodies. There is also increased susceptibility to opportunistic and pyrogenic infection.

The treatment of WAS by BMT has been quite successful and has demonstrated the cell-specific nature of the disorder. In one case where there was only engraftment of T cells, all of the immune functions were restored (Parkman *et al.*, 1978), implying that B cells are normally unaffected. This is borne out by findings normal B cell numbers and levels of serum immunoglobulins in affected individuals. In older patients however, an increased frequency of non-Hodgkin's lymphoma has been noted. Although there is no apparent defect in the myeloid and B cell lineages in WAS patients, analysis of X inactivation patterns in obligate carriers has shown nonrandom X inactivation patterns in essentially all hematologic lineages (with the possible exception of the erythroid lineage), including early progenitors such as CD34+ cells. Therefore cells that inactivate the normal X-chromosome fail to survive, implying that *was* gene function is required in all blood cells (Remold-O'Donnell *et al.*, 1996).

2.3.3a. Identification and Cloning of the WAS Gene. The WAS defect was originally mapped to Xp11.22 by using a pair of highly polymorphic markers DXS255 and TIMP (Derry *et al.*, 1994a; Remold-O'Donnell *et al.*, 1996). A positional cloning approach was used to localise the affected gene which has been termed *WASP* (Derry *et al.*, 1994a,b). The gene was analyzed in three unrelated WAS patients and was affected by a frameshift mutation in one case and in the other two by substitution of the same Arg residue for a His or Leu, respectively.

Now a number of groups have analyzed mutations in *WASP* and mutations of essentially all types have been identified (Derry *et al.*, 1994a, 1995; Kolluri *et al.*, 1995; Kwan *et al.*, 1995, 1996; Villa *et al.*, 1995; Wengler *et al.*, 1995; Zhu *et al.*, 1995). These studies have shown unequivocally that WAS and XLT are allelic diseases caused by mutations in the same gene (Derry *et al.*, 1994a, 1995; Kolluri *et al.*, 1995; Kwan *et al.*, 1996; Villa *et al.*, 1995; Zhu *et al.*, 1995). In XLT, which can be considered a milder form, the changes tend towards missense mutations, clustered to some extent in the first two exons (Remold-O'Donnell *et al.*, 1996), whereas in WAS, the pattern tends toward the more complex, and has a preponderance of frameshift, chain-terminating mutations, insertions, deletions, and splicing defects, all of which have more serious consequences for the structure of the protein (Wengler *et al.*, 1995; Zhu *et al.*, 1995). Identical missense mutations, though, are the underlying cause of WAS in some patients and XLT in others, including a $Arg_{86} \rightarrow Cys$ change found in two cases of severe WAS. This suggests that the relationship between genotype and phenotype is not as strict as the mutational analysis might imply (Derry *et al.*, 1995; Kolluri *et al.*, 1995; Kwan *et al.*, 1996; Zhu *et al.*, 1995). The pattern of missense mutations has indicated a few mutational hot spots because the same mutations have appeared in a number of different families, and this has highlighted a number of residues critical for WASP function.

The function of WASP is still poorly understood, and the amino acid sequence in this case reveals little in terms of homology to other known proteins. WASP has some very proline-rich regions which could be targets for SH3 domains, and one such interaction has been found with Nck (Rivero Lezcano *et al.*, 1995) a non-receptor tyrosine kinase. But equally it may suggest an interaction with elements of the cytoskeleton (Musacchio *et al.*, 1992). The latter would be consistent with the extreme variability in the WAS phenotype, many of the observed cell surface changes, and the increased level of platelet destruction, which are similar to changes in other cytoskeletal disorders (Remold-O'Donnell *et al.*, 1996). A cytoskeletal role for WASP has been given further credence by the recent finding that it interacts *in vivo* with Cdc42 (Kolluri *et al.*, 1996; Symons *et al.*, 1996), a member of the rac/rho family of GTPases, which are involved in regulating cell architecture (Hall, 1992; Ridley *et al.*, 1992) and are also associated with increases in actin polymerization (Symons *et al.*, 1996).

2.4. Myeloid Cell-Specific Disorders

2.4.1. Chronic Granulomatous Disease

As long ago as 1957, an inherited immunodeficiency characterized by an unusual susceptibility to pyogenic infection was described. The disorder led to the formation of large granulomata filled with neutrophils and was termed "fatal granulomatosus of childhood" (Berendes *et al.*, 1957). Subsequently it has be come known as chronic granulomatous disease (CGD). Quite soon after, it was established that CGD abolishes the *respiratory burst* of neutrophils (and other phagocytes), a rapid uptake of oxygen associated with their microbicidal activity (Casimir and Teahan, 1994).

The disease was first described as an X-linked condition, but later became associated with forms which affected boys and girls equally, and thus had an autosomal recessive inheritance pattern (Segal and Jones, 1980). In total, CGD affects around 1 in 500,000 to 1 in 250,000 individuals (Casimir and Teahan, 1994; Roos, 1994). Four distinct genetic loci that can be affected in CGD are now known. Defects in any one produces the CGD phenotype (Casimir and Teahan, 1994; Curnutte, 1993; Dinauer, 1993; Roos, 1994; Thrasher *et al.*, 1994). All four of these genes encode components of an electron transport system called the NADPH oxidase (Roos, 1994; Segal, 1989; Segal, 1991; Smith and Curnutte, 1991), so-called because it generates superoxide by passing electrons from NADPH to molecular oxygen. The superoxide generates a number of highly reactive oxidative intermediates and effects a major upward shift in the pH of the phagocytic vacuole (Segal *et al.*, 1981). These mechanisms play crucial role in the oxidative killing of microorganisms (Dinauer and Orkin, 1992; Dinauer, 1993; Roos, 1994). Therefore, the classic granulomata of the disease are caused by accumulations of neutrophils that have engulfed pathogens but cannot kill them.

2.4.1a. NADPH Oxidase. The central component of NADPH oxidase is the (flavo) cytochrome b_{558} (Segal *et al.*, 1986). This is a multifunctional protein located in the plasma membrane (and in the membrane of cytoplasmic granules) that controls all of the redox functions of the Oxidase, using flavin adenine dinucleotide (FAD) and heme as cofactors (Rotrosen *et al.*, 1992; Segal *et al.*, 1992). The flavocytochrome has two subunits (Dinauer *et al.*, 1987; Parkos *et al.*, 1987; Segal, 1987; Teahan *et al.*, 1987), the larger of which is homologous to the ferredoxin reductase (FNR) family of reductases (Casimir and Teahan, 1994; Segal *et al.*, 1992) and to the yeast ferric reductase (Dancis *et al.*, 1992). It is not homologous to bacterial or mitochondrial cytochromes, though a tentative similarity between the small subunit of cytochrome b_{558} and the heme binding region of cytochrome c oxidase (Parkos *et al.*, 1988) has been described. The remaining two core components of NADPH oxidase are two cytosolic proteins of 47 kDa (p47*phox*) and 67 kDa (p67*phox*), respectively (Leto *et al.*, 1990; Lomax *et al.*, 1989; Nunoi *et al.*, 1988; Volpp *et al.*, 1988) (the four specific core components all take the suffix *phox*, for *ph*agocyte *ox*idase). On activation of the oxidase, these molecules translocate to the membrane where they bind to the cytochrome, to form an active oxidase complex (Dusi *et al.*, 1993; Dusi and Rossi, 1993; Heyworth *et al.*, 1989, 1991; Rotrosen and Leto, 1990). The interaction between the components of the oxidase are mediated by specific protein domains, known as SH3 domains, that bind to proline-rich motifs and function in a large number of protein–protein interactions (Feller *et al.*, 1994). The SH3 domains of p47*phox*, specifically, interact with proline-rich domains in gp91*phox* and p22*phox* (de Mendez *et al.*, 1994, 1996; Finan *et al.*, 1994; Leto *et al.*, 1994; Sumimoto *et al.*, 1994). Although the precise functions of the two cytosolic components are not established, their role as essential components of the oxidase has been unequivocally demonstrated by the *in vitro* reconstitution of oxidase activity in a cell-free system comprising wholly recombinant or purified components (Abo and Segal, 1995; Rotrosen *et al.*, 1993). In addition to the four *phox* components, a further essential element of NADPH oxidase is the small GTPase p21rac[1]or rac[2] (Abo *et al.*, 1991, 1994; Abo and Pick, 1991; Abo, 1995; Abo and Segal, 1995; Diekmann *et al.*, 1994; Dorseuil *et al.*, 1996; Heyworth *et al.*, 1994; Knaus *et al.*, 1991, 1992; Philips *et al.*, 1995; Rotrosen *et al.*, 1993). The bound nucleotide state (GTP or GDP) acts as a switch to regulate oxidase activity (Segal and Abo, 1993). The rac protein also translocates from the cytosol to membrane but is independent of p47 and p67*phox* (Abo *et al.*, 1994; Dusi *et al.*, 1996; Heyworth *et al.*, 1994). Though essential for oxidase activity, mutations in p21rac have not been associated with CGD, most likely because the rac protein is an essential component of many other enzyme systems and defects in this gene would prove lethal.

The last known component of the oxidase, termed p40*phox* (Dusi *et al.*, 1996; Fuchs *et al.*, 1995, 1996; Ito *et al.*, 1996; Tsunawaki *et al.*, 1994; Wientjes *et al.*, 1993, 1996), is complexed with p47*phox* and p67*phox* in resting cell cytosol, though its affinity for the latter is much greater. The function of this molecule is not understood at present, though it contains an SH3 domain and shares quite extensive sequence homology with p47*phox* (Wientjes *et al.*, 1993).

2.4.1b. Molecular Genetics. The genes for all four specific oxidase components have been cloned and sequenced. The large subunit of the cytochrome, gp91*phox*, is encoded by the gene carried on the X-chromosome and derived a certain celebrity by being the first gene to be isolated solely from knowledge of its map location (Royer Pokora *et al.*, 1986a,b) at Xp21 (Baehner *et al.*, 1986; de Saint Basile *et al.*, 1988). Defects in gp91*phox* account for about two-thirds of all CGD cases, and about one quarter arise from defects in the cytosolic component p47*phox*. The remaining 5–10% of CGD cases are accounted for by mutations in the other two autosomally inherited components, p67*phox* and the smaller subunit of the cytochrome, p22*phox* (Casimir *et al.*, 1992; Clark *et al.*, 1989).

A substantial number of mutations in gp91*phox* have been characterized, and these cover most of the usual causes of mutation, including large and small deletions (Bu Ghanim *et al.*, 1995; Casimir and Teahan, 1994; Curnutte, 1993; Roos, 1994), frameshifts (Bu Ghanim *et al.*, 1995; Curnutte, 1993; Rabbani *et al.*, 1993; Roos, 1994), chain terminators (Bolscher *et al.*, 1991; Curnutte, 1993; Newburger *et al.*, 1994a; Roos, 1994), missense mutations (Bolscher *et al.*, 1991; Curnutte, 1993; Dinauer *et al.*, 1989; Roos, 1994), and splice junction defects (Curnutte, 1993; de Boer *et al.*, 1992; Roos, 1994; Schapiro *et al.*, 1991). These last account for about a third of the total, so are perhaps unexpectedly prevalent. One very interesting missense mutation is the Pro-His 415 mutation, which results in the synthesis of normal amounts of a totally nonfunctional cytochrome b_{558} (Bolscher *et al.*, 1991; Dinauer *et al.*, 1989). The Pro 415 lies in a highly conserved region of the molecule that is strongly homologous to the NADPH binding site of other FNR reductases and fails to bind radiolabeled NADPH analogs (Segal *et al.*, 1992). Therefore, this residue plays a crucial role in substrate binding. An additional single amino acid substitution lying at residue 500 (Asp→Gly) destroys the binding of the p47*phox* cytosolic factor to the cytochrome (Leusen *et al.*, 1994a).

Another interesting group of mutants are the so-called “variant” patients who have reduced but detectable oxidase activity. In a recent study of three such patients

(Bu Ghanim *et al.*, 1995), a pair of brothers both carried a three nucleotide deletion that gives rise to the deletion of a single lysine residue. Despite the fact that they still retain approximately 25% of normal cytochrome protein and oxidase activity, their ability to kill bacteria was profoundly affected, such that they were indistinguishable from classical X-linked patients. This compares strikingly with carrier mothers who may have as few as 5% normal circulating cells, yet still are free of symptoms. These observations have important implications for gene therapy in this disease, because they suggest that it should be possible to correct the phenotype with only relatively small numbers of functioning cells, but that these cells must function as efficiently as normal cells.

Another patient in this study had a short deletion of the C-terminal six amino acids of the protein. This had a disproportionate effect on the activity of the cytochrome, implicating the C-terminus in activation of electron transfer. This pattern was highly consistent with a structural model of the cytoplasmic portion of gp91*phox* that places the C-terminus in close apposition to the NADPH binding site, where it lies close enough to play a crucial role in substrate binding (Taylor *et al.*, 1993).

Three other very unusual variant cases have been described, two that had single-base mutations in the CAAT and TATA box regions of the gene promoter, respectively (Newburger *et al.*, 1994b), causing a reduction in the level of transcription and another single kindred where a subpopulation of about 5–15% of the neutrophils had normal oxidase activity against a background of "classical" X-linked CGD cells with no oxidase activity (Woodman *et al.*, 1995). The molecular basis of this defect has yet to be unraveled.

The pattern of mutations in the p47*phox* component, which account for between 25 and 30% of all CGD cases, could not be more different. Unlike gp91*phox*, where the same mutation has appeared in only a few unrelated individuals, for p47*phox* a single mutation (Casimir *et al.*, 1991) affects over 90% of the defective alleles. The overwhelming majority of patients were homozygous for this defect, and most of the remainder were compound heterozygotes (Casimir *et al.*, 1991; Roos, 1994; Volpp and Lin, 1993), where the common mutation is carried on one chromosome and a sporadic change is inherited on the other.

The genetic basis of this mutation proved to be a deletion of a GT dinucleotide pair at a GTGT repeat sequence located at the border of the first intron and first exon (Casimir *et al.*, 1991). Sequencing of genomic DNA confirmed the mutation as a deletion, not a splicing defect. What accounts for the unusual prevalence of this mutation is not clear. It is probably carried in the population at a frequency of around 1 in 2000, and consequently mutations in p47*phox* are approximately 200 times more prevalent than those in gp91*phox*.

Originally, evidence suggested that there may be local sequence features that render this region susceptible to errors in copying by polymerases (Casimir *et al.*, 1991). More recently, however, a picture has been emerging that involves the presence of at least one closely linked p47*phox* pseudogene (carrying the GT deletion) (S. Chanock, personal communication) on a duplicated region of this chromosome. Then, the high mutation rate could be accounted for by gene conversion.

As may be expected, no overall pattern of mutations exists for the rare mutations in the remaining two oxidase components, but one particularly interesting example has been found for p22*phox*. Similar to a mutation seen in gp91*phox*, a point mutation affecting function but not the synthesis or stability of cytochrome b_{558} was found in p22*phox*. This was a Pro→Gln substitution at residue 156 (Dinauer *et al.*, 1991) that affects the interaction of cytochrome b_{558} with p47*phox* (Leto *et al.*, 1994; Leusen *et al.*, 1994b).

2.4.2. Leukocyte Adhesion Deficiency

Leukocyte adhesion deficiency (LAD) has two known forms, termed LAD type I and LAD type II. Both forms affect the ability of white blood cells to attach to the surface of endothelial cells that block infiltration into the tissues across a vessel wall, a major component of the inflammatory response. Type II disease, recognized only quite recently, involves the sialyl Lewis X antigen, which in LAD type II is not correctly expressed on the cell surface (Etzioni *et al.*, 1993, 1995). The sialyl Lewis X carbohydrate is the ligand for the E and P selectins on the surface of endothelial cells, and this attachment mediates the process of "rolling", a precursor to the firm attachment required for neutrophils and monocytes in particular to pass through into the tissues (Etzioni *et al.*, 1993; Price *et al.*, 1994).

LAD type I affects this infiltration process because of the failure to express type-two (or β) integrins. The three type-two integrins are heterodimers that consist of a type-specific chain CD11a,b, or c and a common chain CD18. Mutations in the common CD18 chain are the underlying cause of LAD (Fischer *et al.*, 1988; Mazzone and Ricevuti, 1995). These integrins have also been known individually as LFA-1 (CD11a/CD18), Mac-1 (CD11b/CD18), and p150,95 (CD11c/CD18). Although LFA-1, is normally expressed on the surface of all leukocytes and many precursors, including early erythroid cells (Mazzone and Ricevuti, 1995), the other type-two integrins are more restricted, particularly CD11b/CD18 which is very abundant on the surface of activated granulocytes and monocytes. The consequences of CD18 deficiency on the phagocytes are the dominant feature of LAD. Most other cells, T cells, for example, have integrin-independent infiltration mechanisms (Fischer *et al.*, 1988; Kavanaugh *et al.*, 1991), though their function is undoubtedly compromised (Kavanaugh *et al.*, 1991; Tohma *et al.*, 1991).

Therefore, the characteristic symptoms of LAD are, recurrent and often life-threatening infectious episodes that commonly originate on the skin and other exposed tissues in conjunction with a failure to produce pus. Staphylococcus and enteric bacteria are frequently involved, and omphalitis is associated with first presentation (Fischer *et al.*, 1988; Paller *et al.*, 1994). LAD divides into moderate and severe phenotypes, and this correlates well with the expression level of CD18 on the cell surface. Patients who express little or no CD18 display the severe phenotype, and those with residual expression have the more moderate form (Fischer *et al.*, 1988). Prognosis for the latter patients is much better, and their disease is often well controlled by antibiotics and granulocyte infusions. The severe form suffects from significantly greater mortality, and although some patients survive infancy, actuarial data compiled some ten years ago indicate 75% mortality by age three (Fischer *et al.*, 1988). Since then many patients have benefited from bone marrow transplantation because LAD is more tolerant of HLA mismatch than many other conditions, probably because LFA-1 expression on T cells is absent (Fischer *et al.*, 1994).

Correlation of genotype and phenotype in LAD has been reasonably successful. Frameshift, nonsense, and splicing defects are more often associated with severe disease (Back *et al.*, 1992; Corbi *et al.*, 1992; Lopez Rodriguez *et al.*, 1993; Matsuura *et al.*, 1992; Nelson *et al.*, 1992; Wright *et al.*, 1995), and missense alterations correlate with a milder form (Back *et al.*, 1993; Nelson *et al.*, 1992; Sligh *et al.*, 1992; Wright *et al.*, 1995). Point mutations associated with the severe phenotype also cluster to two regions of the protein that are highly conserved among the integrin family (Back *et al.*, 1992; Corbi *et al.*, 1992; Matsuura *et al.*, 1992).

3. VECTOR SYSTEMS AND THEIR SUITABILITY FOR GENE THERAPY OF IMMUNODEFICIENCY

There are currently a number of viral and nonviral gene transfer vectors suitable for gene therapy. The main criteria for applying them to immunodeficiency disorders are efficiency and heritability. A high level of efficiency is required because the natural target cells for gene therapy of immune disorders are the pluripotent hematopoietic stem cells (PHSC) and these by their very nature are rare in the population of bone marrow cells, though protocols for enriching such cells are under constant development (see section 4.6.2). Secondly, because the defects in immunodeficiency are expressed in mature cells of a given lineage, the transgene must be passed on to the progeny of any transduced PHSC. Currently these constraints limit immunodeficiency gene therapy to virally based vector systems because the efficiency obtainable now with physical transfer methods is insufficient for transfer to PHSC.

The usable viral vectors are based on retroviruses, adenoviruses, or adeno-associated viruses. Because the adenovirus vectors have very high titers and a wide host range, they have some applicability to immunodeficiency and can transduce terminally differentiated cells. Their inability to integrate into the host genome, however, precludes their use for transducing PHSC. This has left the retroviral and adeno-associated virus vectors as the current systems of choice for gene therapy in the immunodeficiencies.

Retroviral vectors are by far the most highly developed of the gene transfer systems. They offer stable packaging lines of reasonably high titer and hence good gene transfer efficiencies, very good safety (all the viral genes are removed from the vector) profile, and highly efficient integration into the host genome (Miller, 1992b; Miller *et al.*, 1993; Vile and Russell, 1995). They are limited by their maximum packaging size of about 5 kb of DNA that makes them generally applicable only to cDNA inserts and by an inability to integrate their genome in the absence of cell division (Miller *et al.*, 1990; Roe *et al.*, 1993). This latter property has become of paramount importance in recent years (see section 4.6.3).

The adeno-associated virus (AAV), a defective parvovirus, has become very popular as a vector system in the past few years and although plagued by low titers and a small ~4 kb packaging limit, has much to commend it. Its safety profile is probably the best of all. The vectors require just two 145 bp hairpin structures from the virus, and the wild-type AAV has the attractive property that it integrates preferentially into a region on chromosome 19 that does not contain any genes (Flotte and Carter, 1995). This is not currently a property of the vectors, however. It was not thought thus host-cell entry is receptor-mediated providing a very wide host range (Flotte and Carter, 1995; Kotin, 1994; Kremer and Perricaudet, 1995). Thus far, AAV has not lived up to its promise as a vector, however, because of problems with the toxicity of the rep gene product (Hermonat, 1994; Yang *et al.*, 1994, 1995) and frequency of integration much lower than originally reported (Alexander *et al.*, 1994; Ferrari *et al.*, 1996; Fisher *et al.*, 1996; Flotte *et al.*, 1994; Halbert *et al.*, 1995; Russell *et al.*, 1994, 1995; Thrasher *et al.*, 1995b). Crucially perhaps, it also enters CD34+ hematopoietic progenitor cells with very low efficiency (M. de Alwis and A. Thrasher, personal commununication).

4. GENE THERAPY FOR IMMUNODEFICIENCY DISORDERS

4.1. ADA-SCID

Any discussion of gene therapy for immunodeficiency disease must center on the experience gained with ADA-SCID, in which there have been the longest running clinical trials (see later) and the most encouraging results. The unique position of ADA-SCID derives from a number of factors. First, the gene was cloned relatively early and has essentially a "housekeeping" nature, which mean that low level and relatively unregulated expression should correct the disease phenotype. The disorder also has some unique characteristics, such as the lack of conditioning required for BMT recipients (Hirschhorn, 1990; Hoogerbrugge *et al.*, 1995) and the selective survival advantage ADA-expressing cells have over their nonexpressing counterparts. These suggest that small numbers of genetically corrected cells should be sufficient for a therapeutic effect. Taken together these factors have always made ADA-SCID a very attractive candidate disorder for gene therapy trials.

The ADA gene therapy story began as long ago as 1987 when a retroviral vector containing ADA cDNA was introduced into human ADA-deficient fibroblasts and expressed functional ADA enzyme (Palmer *et al.*, 1987). Concomitant with this, similar vectors were used successfully to transduce bone marrow progenitor cells of murine (Belmont *et al.*, 1986; van Beusechem *et al.*, 1990; Williams *et al.*, 1986) and later, human (Bordignon *et al.*, 1989, 1993; Cournoyer *et al.*, 1991) origin. Protocols capable of long-term reconstituting the bone marrow of lethally irradiated mice (Lim *et al.*, 1987; Osborne *et al.*, 1990; van Beusechem *et al.*, 1990) and nonhuman primates were evolved (Bodine *et al.*, 1993a; Kantoff *et al.*, 1987; van Beusechem *et al.*, 1992, 1994). Finally, T cells from ADA patients were used as recipients, and it was found that the retrovirally encoded ADA corrects the metabolic defect in these cells (Bordignon *et al.*, 1993; Braakman *et al.*, 1992; Ferrari *et al.*, 1992). These experiments paved the way for a first clinical of trial of human gene therapy (Anonymous, 1990). The long-lived nature of T cells made it feasible to use them as recipients of a retroviral vector. This strategy necessitated repeating the therapy at regular intervals because the transduced T cells cannot effect a permanent reversal of the disorder.

In 1990 two teams, one led by Blaese and Anderson at NIH and another in Milan, under Bordignon, undertook the first clinical trials of human gene therapy, using patients who had been treated with PEG-ADA (Hershfield, 1995), but whose condition was again worsening. The approach at NIH was to harvest T cells from the patients' peripheral blood and expand these *in vitro* using human recombinant IL-2. This strategy was made possible because the PEG-ADA therapy had resulted in developing small numbers of circulating T cells in these patients. Then, the cycling T cells were cocultivated with retroviral packaging cells that produce retroviral vector encoding human ADA. The vector was a simple MULV- based vector, and the inserted sequence was driven from the retroviral LTR. There was a neo-selectable marker (see Figure 2A). Following retroviral transduction, the T cells were harvested and reinfused into the patient. This protocol was repeated nine

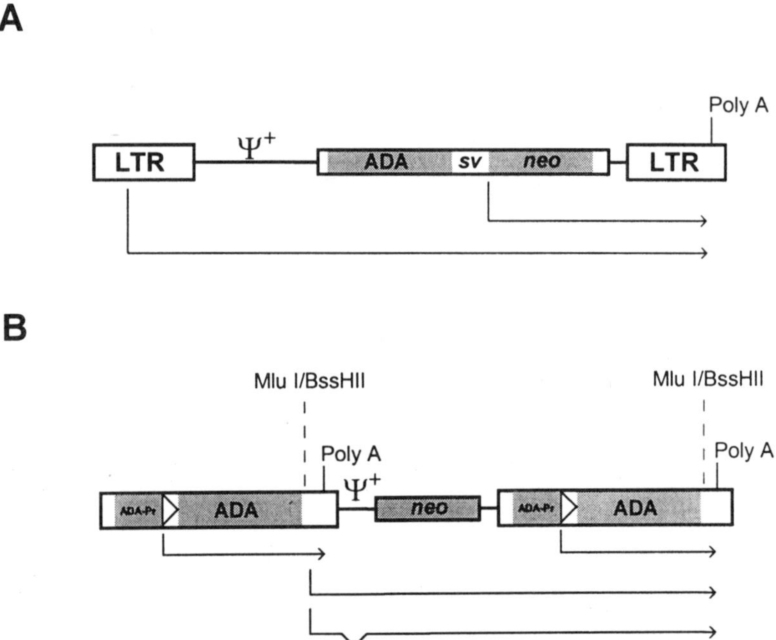

FIGURE 2. Schematic diagrams of vectors used in clinical trails of ADA gene therapy. (A) Vector used by NIH group. (B) Vector used by Italian group. ADA, adenosine deaminase cDNA; LTR, vector long terminal repeat; ADA-Pr, ADA promoter; PolyA, polyadenylation addition site; Ψ^+, packaging signal for vector genome. Lines with arrows indicate the transcripts from the vector. MluI/BssHII is the position of a single-base alteration creating different restriction sites made in the two vectors used to transduce peripheral blood or bone marrow, respectively. The origin of the reconstituting cells was identified by appropriate restriction enzyme digests.

times over the course of two years for one patient and eleven times in a year for the other.

The Italian trial was performed similarly, though in this case no *ex vivo* expansion of T cells was performed, but additionally, two almost identical retroviral constructs were employed, which because of a single-base change, could be distinguished by the presence or absence of a restriction enzyme site in the LTR. One vector was used, as before, to transduce peripheral blood T cells, and the other was used on harvested bone marrow cells. Then, the source of any reconstituting cells could be identified by restriction enzyme digestion. A type of vector slightly different from that used in the NIH trial was employed for this study. The vector conformed to the "double-copy" style (Figure 2B) where the transcription units are placed in the LTRs. The natural promoter of the ADA gene was used to drive transcription from the ADA cDNA, and the vector contained an internal *neo* gene conferring resistance to the drug G418. Further experience with vectors of this type has suggested that they are less stable than their simpler counterparts.

T cells were transduced by cocultivating the retroviral producers with the target cells. Bone marrow cells were transduced by using repeated additions of viral supernatants to bone marrow cells cultured on stromal layers in the absence of exogenous cytokines.

The results of both these trials have recently been published, some four years after the original starting date (Blaese *et al.*, 1995; Bordignon *et al.*, 1995). In both cases the patients remained on PEG-ADA therapy for the duration of the trial, though the dosage was left unaltered as the patients' body mass increased, effectively reducing the dose (PEG-ADA is now to be withdrawn from the patients in the Italian trial). Despite this proviso, the results of these trials are hugely encouraging for the future potential of gene therapy. Clinically, the patients have all shown major improvements in their conditions. They were free of major infections during the trial enabling them to return to some sort of normal life. More specifically, total lymphocyte counts were normalized and cellular and humoral antibody responses could be elicited. Analysis of specific immune responses, for example, to tetanus toxoid (Blaese *et al.*, 1995; Bordignon *et al.*, 1995) or influenza virus (Blaese *et al.*, 1995; Bordignon *et al.*, 1995) were greatly improved after gene therapy as was pokeweed mitogen-stimulated IgM production (Blaese *et al.*, 1995), which is T-cell-dependent.

The Italian study (Bordignon *et al.*, 1995) used restriction enzyme digestion to analyze the retroviral DNA in peripheral blood and bone marrow samples and establish the origin of the transduced cells. For the first year after gene therapy ceased, the lymphocytes were derived from T cell transductions. After this time bone marrow-derived gene marked lymphocytes and granulocytes started to appear in the circulation and by the end of the trial constituted the majority of cells. The conclusions from this gradual switch is that the hypothesized selective advantage of transduced over nontransduced cells is operating, and that retroviral vectors can transduce hematopoietic stem cells. The efficiency for accomplishing this, however, is some orders of magnitude lower than originally expected (see Section 4.4).

Two further clinical trials of gene therapy in ADA-SCID have been attempted that involve retroviral transduction of hematopoietic progenitors. These are discussed in Section 4.4.

4.2. Gene Therapy for Non-ADA Diseases

ADA-SCID has presented a unique opportunity for testing the clinical efficacy of gene therapy, though any T cell based therapy must be inherently limited by the need to repeat the therapy at regular intervals. To affect a permanent genetic correction, the aim is to target the pluripotent hematopoietic stem cells (PHSC). This aim has yet to be achieved in humans and other large animal models with a satisfactory degree of efficiency, though significant progress toward this goal has been made in the last few years. The picture is rather different in murine systems, and successful gene transfer protocols for PHSC have been evolved by a number of different groups. The fact that gene therapy is successful in the mouse makes it unlikely that the technical and biological problems of achieving this goal in human subjects cannot be overcome thereby making gene therapy a clinical reality for many patients suffering from inherited immunodeficiency disorders.

4.2.1. Chronic Granulomatous Disease

One of the problems for retroviral mediated gene transfer in CGD has been the fact that the cells displaying the phenotype (neutrophils) are terminally differentiated and have a very short life span, which makes them unsuitable as targets. Notwithstanding the fact that CGD monocytes were successfully transduced recently using adenoviral vectors (Thrasher *et al.*, 1995a), the existence of EBV-immortalized B cell lines with NADPH oxidase activity, albeit at significantly reduced levels compared to neutrophils (Chetty *et al.*, 1995; Morel *et al.*, 1993), has provided an advantageous model system for testing whether gene transfer can correct the CGD phenotype. B cell lines derived from CGD patients fail to express the oxidase component missing in their neutrophils and so, similarly, do not produce superoxide. A number of groups have shown that gene transfer into such cells restores their ability to produce superoxide. This was first achieved for a p47*phox*-deficient patient cell line by Thrasher *et al.* (1992, 1993), who were able to reconstitute approximately 30% of the normal level of oxidase activity by using a retroviral vector. Subsequently, a number of laboratories successfully reconstituted p47*phox*-deficient cell lines using EBV-based plasmids (Chanock *et al.*, 1992; Volpp and Lin, 1993) and with AAV vectors (Thrasher *et al.*, 1995b). Retroviral vectors were also successfully employed to correct gp91*phox*- (Porter *et al.*, 1993) and p22*phox*-deficient B cell lines (Maly *et al.*, 1993; Porter *et al.*, 1994), though the degree of correction was less than that observed for the p47*phox* deficiency. In addition, Dinauer and colleagues used similar technology to correct a myeloid cell line (PLB985) (Kume and Dinauer, 1994), in which they had inactivated gp91*phox via* homologous recombination (Zhen *et al.*, 1993). They made the interesting observation that a relatively low expression level of the cytochrome in these cells was sufficient to restore normal levels of oxidase activity completely (Kume and Dinauer, 1994), unlike the situation with the B cell lines.

Retrovirally mediated gene transfer was taken one step further by two groups who targeted CD34+ cells. Porter *et al.* (1996) reported efficient transfer of vectors to bone marrow-derived CD34+ cells and to some degree functionally corrected the

CGD defect in patient CD34+ cells differentiated *in vitro*. The group of Malech at the NIH also described similar results with CD34+ cells from the peripheral blood of cytokine-mobilized individuals (Li *et al.*, 1994; Sekhsaria *et al.*, 1993). Using a simple vector based on the MFG backbone and lacking a selectable marker, they demonstrated that superoxide generation is restored in hematopoietic colonies from autosomal recessive (Sekhsaria *et al.*, 1993) and X-linked CGD patients (Li *et al.*, 1994), by chemiluminescent detection of oxidase activity in pooled colonies and by classical nitroblue tetrazolium (NBT) staining of individual colonies *in situ* in semisolid media. The phenotypic correction achieved in these cases is considered high enough to extend this study to a clinical trial, though poor mobilization of CD34+ cells in CGD patients has been recently been described (Sekhsaria *et al.*, 1996).

4.2.2. Leukocyte Adhesion Deficiency (LAD)

B cell lines in LAD have been used similarly as recipients to test gene transfer. Two groups have successfully reconstituted cell-surface integrins by retrovirally mediated transfer of a vector encoding the CD18 cDNA (Back *et al.*, 1990; Hibbs *et al.*, 1990). This restores the ability of the B cells to bind to endothelial cells (Hibbs *et al.*, 1990). CD18 has also been successfully transferred to human bone marrow progenitors (Yorifuji *et al.*, 1993).

4.2.3. X-SCID

The identification of the γ_c chain of the IL2 interleukin receptor family as the underlying cause of X-SCID has led to a renewed interest in developing gene therapy for this serious disorder. A number of recent papers (Candotti *et al.*, 1996; Hacein Bey *et al.*, 1996; Taylor *et al.*, 1996) have shown that γ_c-deficient B cell lines from X-SCID individuals can be made to express the retrovirally encoded γ-chain and that this restores the ability of these cells to respond appropriately to growth factors.

4.3. Retrovirally Mediated Gene Transfer into Hematopoietic Stem Cells *in Vitro*

The aim of all gene therapy protocols directed at immunodeficiency disorders is to target genes at the pluripotent haematopoietic stem cells (PHSC). These cells are the source of all the mature blood elements and progenitor cell populations and have the unique property of self-renewal. For the gene therapist this means that a single therapeutic intervention could potentially produce a lifetime cure. Whether this aim can be realized, of course, remains to be established.

Introducing genes into PHSC, however, is not a straightforward task. PHSCs in bone marrow probably number approximately 1 in 10^5–10^4 mononuclear cells. There are no obvious morphological distinguishing features for these cells and, as yet, no adequate description of surface markers enabling their identification or isolation. Essentially, the definition of PHSC remains a functional one, namely the ability to repopulate the marrow of a lethally irradiated individual, either in hemopoietic cell transfers in animal models or in clinical bone marrow transplantation (Keller, 1992; Orlic and Bodine, 1994). Because of the difficulty in defining cells on this basis, particularly for human PHSC, other *in vitro* assays have sought to indicate the pluripotent potential of cell populations enriched for immature phenotypes. This has predominantly involved the use of colony assays in semisolid media and long-term bone marrow culture (LTC) techniques (Spooncer and Dexter, 1984). Cells that can initiate the latter type of culture (long-term culture initiating cells; LTC-IC), though probably more abundant than true PHSC, share many of their characteristics. They can proliferate extensively and can give rise to colony-forming cells of all myeloid and erythroid lineages in culture. For marrow transplantation there is good agreement on the numbers of LTC-IC in a population and its potential for engraftment (Hogge *et al.*, 1994; Sutherland *et al.*, 1993, 1995).

Targeting of PHSC for gene transfer has been particularly successful in murine systems. Retrovirally mediated transfer of the bacterial *neo* gene to murine stem cells was achieved as long ago as 1984 (Keller *et al.*, 1985; Williams *et al.*, 1984) and genes of eukaryotic origin followed soon after (Williams *et al.*, 1987). The role of the cytotoxic drug 5-fluorouracil (5FU) in achieving this should not be overlooked (see section 4.6.2c). Gene transfer to PHSC in large animals and humans has proven much more problematic. Successful gene transfer to committed progenitors was reported quite early (Bordignon *et al.*, 1989; Cournoyer *et al.*, 1991; Kantoff *et al.*, 1987) and since then the CD34 antigen (Krause *et al.*, 1996) has been used extensively to isolate target populations of the most immature progenitor cells in bone marrow, mobilized peripheral blood and umbilical cord blood. CD34 is an antigen found on the surface of approximately 1–2% of all bone marrow mononuclear cells, and this population is highly enriched for colony-forming cells (CFC) and LTC-IC. A large number of groups have successfully transduced CD34+ cells isolated from all the sources listed previously (Akatsuka *et al.*, 1994; Bagnis *et al.*, 1994; Bahnson *et al.*, 1994; Bertolini *et al.*, 1994; Bodine *et al.*, 1993a; Chen *et al.*, 1995; Conneally *et al.*, 1996; Crooks and Kohn, 1993; Humeau *et al.*, 1996; Li *et al.*, 1994; Lu *et al.*, 1993a, 1994, 1995; Mannion Henderson *et al.*, 1995; Medin *et al.*, 1996; Migita *et al.*, 1996; Nimgaonkar *et al.*, 1994; Nolta *et al.*, 1995b; O'Shaughnessy *et al.*, 1994; Porter *et al.*, 1996; Qazilbash *et al.*, 1995; Shi *et al.*, 1994; van Beusechem *et al.*, 1994, 1995; Walsh *et al.*, 1995; Ward *et al.*, 1994; Xu *et al.*, 1995). Typically, these results have rested on the transfer of a drug resistance marker gene, such as *neo*, or the multidrug resistance marker MDR (Bernad *et al.*, 1994; Bertolini *et al.*, 1994; Bordignon *et al.*, 1989; Hanania and Deisseroth, 1994; Licht *et al.*, 1995; Lu *et al.*, 1993; Nolta *et al.*, 1995; O'Shaughnessy *et al.*, 1994; Richardson and Bank, 1995; Schwarzenberger *et al.*, 1996; Sokolic *et al.*, 1996; Ward *et al.*, 1994) and, occasionally, the use of reporter genes, such as β-galactosidase (Bagnis *et al.*, 1994, 1995; Clapp *et al.*, 1995). In many instances the best results have been obtained by further incubation with cytokines during the infection process. The most popular combination is IL-3, IL-6, and SCF (Agrawal *et al.*, 1996; Bodine *et al.*, 1989; Cassel *et al.*, 1993; Conneally *et al.*, 1996; Crooks and Kohn, 1993; Flasshove *et al.*, 1995; Luskey *et al.*, 1992; Nolta *et al.*, 1992;

Shi *et al.*, 1994; Szilvassy and Cory, 1994). In other cases, optimum transfer has been achieved in the absence of exogenous cytokines but with stromal cell support under LTC conditions (Chertkov *et al.*, 1993; Moore *et al.*, 1992; Porter *et al.*, 1996b; Wells *et al.*, 1995; Xu *et al.*, 1995b). Despite the fact that cocultivation is the most efficient method for retroviral infection, the use of producer-cell supernatants for infection has proven sufficient where adequate retroviral titers have been obtained. Surprisingly, the impact of retroviral titer on transduction frequencies has not proven critical (van Beusechem *et al.*, 1993).

4.4. Clinical Gene Marking Trials

Two major investigations have reported on the general safety using retroviral vectors for gene therapy, the efficiency of gene transfer to PHSC, and the expression of the transduced gene in their mature descendants. One of these studies, performed at NIH by Dunbar and collaborators on 11 patients who had breast cancer or multiple myeloma, was designed to study whether peripheral blood mobilized stem cells might be better targets for gene therapy than bone marrow derived cells (Dunbar and Emmons, 1994; Dunbar *et al.*, 1995). Patients were given high-dose chemotherapy before cytokine mobilization. CD34+ cells were selected from marrow or peripheral blood harvests and then transduced with retroviral vectors after a 48 hr *ex vivo* stimulation with cytokines (IL-3, IL-6, and SCF). Initial transduction frequencies assayed by neo gene transfer in colony assay were reasonable encouraging (21%) and immediately after transplantation, all 10 evaluable patients showed evidence of successful transduction. Between 0.2% and 1% of peripheral blood cells were positive for the retroviral genome by PCR. This value rapidly declined, however, so that by one year after transplantation only three patients had a detectable peripheral blood PCR signal at a level indicating that approximately 0.01–0.1% of cells still harbored a retroviral genome. This study has shown, however, that retroviral gene transfer protocols are safe and that stable integration of retroviral genomes is still detectable more than one year posttransplant, especially in the patients receiving mobilized peripheral blood stem cells.

A second study involved juvenile patients receiving transplants for ALL (Brenner, 1995). These patients were given transplants following high-dose chemotherapy with cyclophosphamide, and the marrow graft was marked with retrovirus to investigate the source of relapse in the patients (Brenner *et al.*, 1993b). It also formed the basis of an effective gene marking trial for testing the potential of gene transfer to PHSC (Brenner *et al.*, 1993a; Brenner, 1995). Retroviral vectors were used to transduce whole marrow without use of exogenous cytokines. Unlike virtually all other studies, this trial indicated a reasonably high level of transfer to multipotent cells. As many as 5% of the peripheral blood cells were positive for the retroviral genome some six months posttransplantation (Brenner, 1995). In the time subsequent to that investigation, the level of representation of the retroviral genome in the blood and marrow of these patients has dwindled, so that at eighteen months posttransplantation levels similar to those obtained elsewhere were observed (Brenner, 1996; Brenner *et al.*, 1995). This study still probably represents the most successful transfer of new genetic material to human PHSC.

Two further attempts to use gene therapy clinically for ADA-SCID have been described. One was a collaboration between groups in Holland, France, and the United Kingdom (Fairbanks *et al.*, 1994), where bone marrow derived CD34+ cells were transduced by coculture with retroviral producers and some cytokine support before being returned to the three patients, who were not "conditioned." Despite good initial levels of gene transfer to colony-forming cells when assayed *in vitro* (around 14%), no evidence for gene transfer to PHSC was obtained, apart from a very weak PCR signal from a marrow aspirate in one of the patients at six months, which was not observed before or after this time.

The other study involved three ADA-SCID patients diagnosed by antenatal testing that opened up the possibility of using of cord blood cells as recipients for retrovirally mediated gene transfer (Kohn *et al.*, 1995). CD34+ cells were isolated from cord blood and transduced by supernatant infection in the presence of IL-3, IL-6, and SCF, using the same vector employed in the T cell gene therapy trial (Blaese *et al.*, 1995) (see above, section 4.1). Low levels of retrovirally mediated gene transfer have been detected some 18 months posttransplantation in the peripheral blood and marrow of these patients. Using PCR, the overall frequency of gene-marked cells was estimated as approximately 0.1% in bone marrow granulocytes and 0.001–0.03% in peripheral blood leukocytes. Interestingly, estimates for the numbers of transduced progenitors were considerably higher, at approximately 1%. These patients have also been receiving PEG-ADA, and it remains to be seen what may happen if the transduced cells are provided with a selective advantage by withdrawing the drug.

4.5. Strategies to Overcome the Low Level of Gene Transfer to Human PHSC

4.5.1. Increased Infectivity

A number of approaches have been adopted to improve gene transfer to PHSC. One strategy has been to perform gene transfer over an extended time period in LTC. There has been one recent report of improved levels of PHSC transduction, up to 5%, using this method in dogs, but further experience is necessary before this approach can be properly evaluated.

Other groups have sought to improve transduction frequencies by replacing the amphotropic retroviral envelope, whose receptor is thought to be poorly represented on the surface of human PHSC and progenitors, with one that is more abundant, such as that for the gibbon-ape leukemia virus (GALV). This has provided a marginal improvement in some cases (Bauer *et al.*, 1995; Eglitis *et al.*, 1995; von Kalle *et al.*, 1994). Alternatively, attempts have been made to increase infectivity by boosting retroviral titer by pseudotyping the virus with the envelope from vesicular stomatitis virus (VSV). This produces a viral particle that can withstand concentration by centrifugation and does not require a receptor to infect target cells (Burns *et al.*, 1993). Generally the improvement in titer achieved with these viruses has been offset by their greatly increased toxicity (Agrawal *et al.*, 1996; Akkina *et al.*, 1996; Eglitis *et al.*, 1995; Xu *et al.*, 1995a).

4.5.2. Enrichment of Stem Cell Populations

4.5.2a. Selection of Transduced Cells. Rather than attempt to improve the initial infection process, some groups have sought to enrich for the transduced cells by using a retrovirally encoded cell-surface marker or by selecting for drug resistance. The latter approach lends itself to the possibility of selection *in vivo*, mirroring the selective advantage that is conferred on ADA-competent cells in a SCID background.

Effective selection of transduced cells has been achieved with CD24 (also known as heat stable antigen in the mouse), a small membrane-anchored peptide that can be exploited to sort cells in the fluorescence activated cell sorter (FACS) (Conneally *et al.*, 1996; Migita *et al.*, 1996; Pawliuk *et al.*, 1994). Effectively a population of 100% transduced cells can be obtained in this way (Conneally *et al.*, 1996).

Drug selection of transduced cells using the multidrug resistance gene (MDR) has been exploited particularly by Bank and his collaborators (Bertolini *et al.*, 1994; Cournoyer *et al.*, 1991; Hanania and Deisseroth, 1994; Licht *et al.*, 1995; O'Shaughnessy *et al.*, 1994; Richardson and Bank, 1995; Schwarzenberger *et al.*, 1996; Sokolic *et al.*, 1996; Ward *et al.*, 1994). Development of hematopoietic colonies in the presence of taxol has demonstrated that efficient selection for transduced cells which express the MDR gene can be achieved *in vitro* (Bertolini *et al.*, 1994; Ward *et al.*, 1994). In mice, selection of cells positive for the expressing the MDR gene and sorting on the FACs before transplantation increased both the frequency and expression level in retrovirally transduced cells and led to greater sustained expression of MDR (Richardson and Bank, 1995). There is now a clinical trial using retroviral vectors that transduce MDR to genetically modify bone marrow grafts thus enabling the use of larger doses of taxol for therapy of cancer patients (Hesdorffer *et al.*, 1994).

4.5.2b. PHSC Enrichment Using Surface Phenotype. A number of laboratories have explored ways to enrich for PHSC and hope thereby to increase the effectiveness of vector-mediated gene transfer. The surface phenotype of the stem cell is not adequately defined to enable the purification of stem cell populations, though high levels of enrichment are attained. On the other hand, whether there is a surface phenotype uniquely defining stem cells is open to debate. In murine systems the Sca1 antigen (Dubois *et al.*, 1994; Fleming *et al.*, 1993; Ikuta and Weissman, 1992; Jacobsen *et al.*, 1995; Licht *et al.*, 1995; Morrison and Weissman, 1996; Okada *et al.*, 1992; Osawa *et al.*, 1996; Palacios *et al.*, 1996; Phillips *et al.*, 1992; Rebel *et al.*, 1994; Uchida *et al.*, 1996) has been very useful in enriching for stem cells, but there is no direct human homologue.

The commonest marker for enriching human progenitors for PHSC is the CD34 antigen described earlier. This population can be further enriched by combining CD34 positive selection with the rejection of cells expressing differentiation-specific markers and thus selecting the so-called "lin-"cells (Chen *et al.*, 1995; Cicuttini *et al.*, 1994; Conneally *et al.*, 1996; Lamkin *et al.*, 1994; Muench *et al.*, 1995; Murray *et al.*, 1994, 1995, 1996; Park *et al.*, 1995; Rowley *et al.*, 1993; Sutherland *et al.*,

1996; Young *et al.*, 1996). Cells that express the surface antigens CD33 and CD38 are also considered more mature cells. In fact, the CD34+/CD38– fraction is quite highly enriched for PHSCs (Agrawal *et al.*, 1996; Cicuttini *et al.*, 1994; Civin and Small, 1995; Conneally *et al.*, 1996; Graf and Torok Storb, 1995; Hao *et al.*, 1995; Olweus *et al.*, 1994; Petzer *et al.*, 1996; Rusten *et al.*, 1994a; Shah *et al.*, 1996; Sutherland *et al.*, 1996; Terstappen and Huang, 1994; Terstappen *et al.*, 1991). Other workers have used cytokine receptors to enrich for PHSC.

Bodine, in particular, has selected populations that express high levels of the receptor for the cytokine stem cell factor (also known as steel factor or kit-ligand) called the *kit-bright* population in this context. When coupled with selection for low levels of rhodamine staining and the "lin-" phenotype, highly enriched populations of murine PHSC have been obtained (Orlic *et al.*, 1993, 1995). Paradoxically, some evidence has emerged recently that murine PHSC may be CD34– (Goodell *et al.*, 1996) and/or CD38+ (Randall *et al.*, 1996) in strict contrast to their human counterparts.

4.5.2c. Enrichment by Functional Properties. Perhaps the one single property, apart from their long term repopulating ability that distinguishes PHSC from their progeny is another functional property, their quiescence. This has led Scadden and his colleagues to devise a highly original methodology for stem cell purification based on the cytotoxic effects of 5FU (Berardi *et al.*, 1995). This drug has been used extensively *in vivo*, particularly in mice where, by virtue of its toxic effects on progenitors, it plays a critical role in inducing cycling in murine PHSC. In large animals, its toxicity has limited its use, but a 5FU-dependent increase in gene transfer to PHSC in primates has been reported (Wieder *et al.*, 1991).

Berardi *et al.* (1995) exposed bone marrow cells *in vitro* in combination with a cocktail of growth factors predicted to stimulate all cells other than PHSC into division. Thereby, all progenitors are rendered susceptible to the effects of 5FU, but the PHSC, which remain quiescent, are spared. Bone marrow cells were incubated for one week in the presence of SCF, IL-3, and 5FU to select PHSC. The surviving cells numbered only 1 in 10^5 of the starting population and had properties suggesting they were PHSC. For example, they were very efficient LTC-IC but not clonogenic in semisolid media. It remains to be seen if they can function in two *in vivo* models of human PHSC, engratment of SCID mice (Dick, 1994; Larochelle *et al.*, 1995; Vormoor *et al.*, 1994) and fetal sheep (Sutherland *et al.*, 1996).

Analysis of single selected cells showed, as might be expected, that they were CD34+ and did not express receptors for IL-3 but did express the IL-1 receptor and the gp130 chain, common to the IL-6, IL11 and GM-CSF receptors. Intriguingly, however, they were also high level expressors of SCF receptor, something of a paradox considering the mode of selection used to obtain these cells. Unfortunately, these authors could not find a combination of growth factors able to stimulate this 5FU-selected population to divide.

4.5.3. Induction of Cycling in PHSC

As discussed earlier, the quiescence of stem cells is a major impediment to their transduction by retroviral vectors. Therefore, many research groups are actively researching combinations of cytokines that might be utilized to promote stem cell cycling. SCF, already mentioned, has effects on the more immature progenitors (Galli *et al.*, 1994; McNiece and Briddell, 1995) and on murine long-term repopulating cells (Bodine *et al.*, 1993b; Drize *et al.*, 1995, 1996; Yan *et al.*, 1994). Its synergistic properties in combination with other cytokines are also well documented (Cicuttini *et al.*, 1992; Firkin *et al.*, 1993; Heyworth *et al.*, 1992; Hoffman *et al.*, 1993; Lemoli *et al.*, 1994). There is good recent evidence from analysis of PHSC transplanted from the W/W^{41} mouse (Miller *et al.*, 1996), in which the SCF receptor function is impaired, that SCF has a central role in cycling of stem cells *in vivo*.

A great deal of interest currently surrounds the recently identified cytokine Flt-3 ligand (Brasel *et al.*, 1995; Broxmeyer *et al.*, 1995; Hannum *et al.*, 1994; Hudak *et al.*, 1995; Jacobsen *et al.*, 1995; Lyman *et al.*, 1993, 1994a,b; Lyman, 1995; Petzer *et al.*, 1996; Rusten *et al.*, 1996; Shah *et al.*, 1996; Small *et al.*, 1994; Zeigler *et al.*, 1994), a close relative of SCF that has a similar spectrum of activities, including strong synergistic properties. There has been one report that it is the crucial component in combinations of growth factors capable of stimulating the expansion of LTC-IC numbers *in vitro* in serum-free medium (Petzer *et al.*, 1996).

In addition, a number of laboratories have highlighted the role of negatively acting factors that may contribute to stem cell quiescence, such as TGF-β (Cardoso *et al.*, 1993; de Vos *et al.*, 1993; Dubois *et al.*, 1994; Eaves *et al.*, 1991; Elias *et al.*, 1994; Lardon *et al.*, 1994; Li *et al.*, 1994; Lu *et al.*, 1993; Mayani *et al.*, 1995), TNF-α (Maciejewski *et al.*, 1995; Mayani *et al.*, 1995; Oez *et al.*, 1993; Rusten *et al.*, 1994b), MIP-1α (Avalos *et al.*, 1994; Heyworth *et al.*, 1996; Lu *et al.*, 1993b; Mayani *et al.*, 1995; Verfaillie *et al.*, 1994; Wright and Pragnell, 1992), and IFN-γ (Selleri *et al.*, 1996; Shah *et al.*, 1983; Shiohara *et al.*, 1993; Snoeck *et al.*, 1994).

Whether a single factor exists to support the expansion of PHSC without pronoting their differentiation, much as the effect of leukemia inhibitory factor (LIF) on murine embryonal stem cells, still remains to be established.

In the past year there has been the exciting development of a vector system based on the HIV virus (Naldini *et al.*, 1996) which, in principle, can neatly sidestep the problem of stem cell cycling because this vector exploits the ability of lentiviruses to enter the nucleus of quiescent cells and integrate into the host genome. If this can be achieved with appropriate efficiency and necessary safety, it will represent a major step forward toward the goal of genetically transducing PHSC and evolving gene therapy protocols to permanently correct an inherited genetic defect.

5. CONCLUSION

Gene therapy has progressed remarkably in a very short time. This cutting edge technology has already proven itself clinically, showing that it can provide true therapeutic benefit. Inherited immunodeficiency disorders have been at the forefront of this research and will continue to be so for the foreseeable future. Major difficulties still exist with the current generation of vectors because of the need to obtain sustained high level and, in many cases, tissue-specific expression from the transferred genes and because of the rather intransigent nature of the pluripotent hematopoietic stem cell. There is little doubt, however, that gene therapy for inherited diseases will be a commonplace mode of treatment in the twenty-first century and that immunodeficiency will be one of its first major applications.

6. REFERENCES

Abo, A., Pick, E., Hall, A., Totty, N., Teahan, C. G., and Segal, A. W., 1991, Activation of the NADPH oxidase involves the small GTP-binding protein p21rac1, *Nature* **353:**668–670.

Abo, A., Webb, M. R., Grogan, A., and Segal, A. W., 1994, Activation of NADPH oxidase involves the dissociation of p21rac from its inhibitory GDP/GTP exchange protein (rhoGDI) followed by its translocation to the plasma membrane, *Biochem. J.* **298**(Pt 3):585–591.

Abo, A., 1995, Purification of Rac-GDP dissociation inhibitor complex from phagocyte cytosol, *Methods Enzymol.* **256:**33–41.

Abo, A., and Pick, E., 1991, Purification and characterization of a third cytosolic component of the superoxide-generating NADPH oxidase of macrophages, *J. Biol. Chem.* **266:**23577–23585.

Abo, A., and Segal, A. W., 1995, Reconstitution of cell-free NADPH oxidase activity by purified components, *Methods Enzymol.* **256:**268–278.

Agrawal, Y. P., Agrawal, R. S., Sinclair, A. M., Young, D., Maruyama, M., Levine, F., and Ho, A. D., 1996, Cell-cycle kinetics and VSV-G pseudotyped retrovirus-mediated gene transfer in blood-derived CD34+ cells, *Exp. Hematol.* **24:**738–747.

Akatsuka, Y., Emi, N., Kato, H., Abe, A., Tanimoto, M., Lupton, S. D., and Saito, H., 1994, Retrovirus-mediated transfer of a hygromycin phosphotransferase-thymidine kinase fusion gene into human CD34+ bone marrow cells, *Int. J. Hematol.* **60:**251–261.

Akkina, R. K., Walton, R. M., Chen, M. L., Li, Q. X., Planelles, V., and Chen, I. S., 1996, High-efficiency gene transfer into CD34+ cells with a human immunodeficiency virus type 1-based retroviral vector pseudotyped with vesicular stomatitis virus envelope glycoprotein G, *J. Virol.* **70:**2581–2585.

Alexander, I. E., Russell, D. W., and Miller, A. D., 1994, DNA-damaging agents greatly increase the transduction of nondividing cells by adeno-associated virus vectors, *J. Virol.* **68:**8282–8287.

Allen, R. C., Armitage, R. J., Conley, M. E., Rosenblatt, H., Jenkins, N. A., Copeland, N. G., Bedell, M. A., Edelhoff, S., Disteche, C. M., Simoneaux, D. K., *et al.*, 1993, CD40 ligand gene defects responsible for X-linked hyper-IgM syndrome, *Science* **259:**990–993.

Alterman, L. A., de Alwis, M., Genet, S., Lovering, R., Middleton Price, H., Morgan, G., Jones, A., Malcolm, S., Levinsky, R. J., and Kinnon, C., 1993, Carrier determination for X-linked agammaglobulinemia using X inactivation analysis of purified B cells, *J. Immunol. Methods* **166:**111–116.

Anonymous, 1990, The ADA human gene therapy clinical protocol. *Hum Gene Ther.* **1:**327–362.

Aoki, Y., Isselbacher, K. J., and Pillai, S., 1994, Bruton tyrosine kinase is tyrosine phosphorylated and activated in pre-B lymphocytes and receptor-ligated B cells, *Proc. Natl. Acad. Sci. USA* **91:**10606–10609.

Aruffo, A., Farrington, M., Hollenbaugh, D., Li, X., Milatovich, A., Nonoyama, S., Bajorath, J., Grosmaire, L. S., Stenkamp, R., Neubauer, M., *et al.*, 1993, The CD40 ligand, gp39, is defective in activated T cells from patients with X-linked hyper-IgM syndrome, *Cell* **72:**291–300.

Avalos, B. R., Bartynski, K. J., Elder, P. J., Kotur, M. S., Burton, W. G., and Wilkie, N. M., 1994, The active monomeric form of macrophage inflammatory protein-1 alpha interacts with high- and low-affinity classes of receptors on human hematopoietic cells, *Blood* **84:**1790–1801.

Back, A. L., Kwok, W. W., Adam, M., Collins, S. J., and Hickstein, D. D., 1990, Retroviral-mediated gene transfer of the leukocyte integrin CD18 subunit, *Biochem. Biophys. Res. Commun.* **171:**787–795.

Back, A. L., Kwok, W. W., and Hickstein, D. D., 1992, Identification of two molecular defects in a child with leukocyte adherence deficiency, *J. Biol. Chem.* **267:**5482–5487.

Back, A. L., Kerkering, M., Baker, D., Bauer, T. R., Embree, L. J., and Hickstein, D. D., 1993, A point mutation associated with leukocyte adhesion deficiency type 1 of moderate severity, *Biochem. Biophys. Res. Commun.* **193:**912–918.

Baehner, R. L., Kunkel, L. M., Monaco, A. P., Haines, J. L., Conneally, P. M., Palmer, C., Heerema, N., and Orkin, S. H., 1986, DNA linkage analysis of X chromosome-linked chronic granulomatous disease, *Proc. Natl. Acad. Sci. USA* **83:**3398–3401.

Bagnis, C., Gravis, G., Imbert, A. M., Herrera, D., Allario, T., Galindo, R., Lopez, M., Pavon, C., Sempere, C., and Mannoni, P., 1994, Retroviral transfer of the nlsLacZ gene into human CD34+ cell populations and into TF-1 cells: Future prospects in gene therapy, *Hum. Gene Ther.* **5:**1325–1333.

Bagnis, C., Imbert, A. M., Gravis, G., Herrera, D., Pavon, C., Galindo, R., Allario, T., Sempere, C., Imbert, J., Costello, R., *et al.*, 1995, Hematological reconstitution and gene therapy: Retroviral transfer of the bacterial beta-galactosidase activity into human hematopoietic CD34+ cell populations and into T lymphocytes derived from the peripheral blood, *Leukemia* **9**(Suppl 1)**:**S61–3.

Bahnson, A. B., Nimgaonkar, M., Fei, Y., Boggs, S. S., Robbins, P. D., Ohashi, T., Dunigan, J., Li, J., Ball, E. D., and Barranger, J. A., 1994, Transduction of CD34+ enriched cord blood and Gaucher bone marrow cells by a retroviral vector carrying the glucocerebrosidase gene, *Gene Ther.* **1:**176–184.

Bauer, T. R. J., Miller, D., and Hickstein, D. D., 1995, Improved transfer of the leukocyte integrin CD18 subunit into hematopoietic cell lines by using retroviral vectors having a gibbon ape leukemia virus envelope, *Blood* **86:**2379–2387.

Belmont, J. W., Henkel Tigges, J., Chang, S. M., Wager Smith, K., Kellems, R. E., Dick, J. E., Magli, M. C., Phillips, R. A., Bernstein, A., and Caskey, C. T., 1986, Expression of human adenosine deaminase in murine haematopoietic progenitor cells following retroviral transfer, *Nature* **322:**385–387.

Belmont, J. W., 1995, Insights into lymphocyte development from X-linked immune deficiencies, *Trends Genet.* **11:**112–116.

Berardi, A. C., Wang, A., Levine, J. D., Lopez, P., and Scadden, D. T., 1995, Functional isolation and characterization of human hematopoietic stem cells, *Science* **267:**104–108.

Berendes, H., and Bridges, R. A., Good, R. A., 1957, A fatal granulomatosus of childhood, *Minn. Med.* **40:**309.

Bernad, A., Varas, F., Gallego, J. M., Almendral, J. M., Bueren, J. A., 1994, Ex vivo expansion and selection of retrovirally transduced bone marrow: An efficient methodology for gene transfer to murine lympho-haemopoietic stem cells, *Br. J. Haematol.* **87:**6–17.

Bertolini, F., de Monte, L., Corsini, C., Lazzari, L., Lauri, E., Soligo, D., Ward, M., Bank, A., and Malavasi, F., 1994, Retrovirus-mediated transfer of the multidrug resistance gene into human haemopoietic progenitor cells, *Br. J. Haematol.* **88:**318–324.

Bienzle, D., Abrams, O. A., Krutn, S. A., Ackland, S. J., Carter, R. F., Dick, J. E., Jacobs, R. M., Kamel, R. S., and Dube, I. D., 1994, Gene transfer into hematopoietic stem cells: long-term maintenance of in vitro activated progenitors without marrow ablation, *Proc. Natl. Acad. Sci. USA* **91:**350–354.

Blaese, R. M., Culver, K. W., Miller, A. D., Carter, C. S., Fleisher, T., Clerici, M., Shearer, G., Chang, L., Chiang, Y., Tolstoshev, P., *et al.*, 1995, T lymphocyte-directed gene therapy for ADA- SCID: Initial trial results after 4 years, *Science* **270:**475–480.

Bodine, D. M., Karlsson, S., Nienhuis, A. W., 1989, Combination of interleukins 3 and 6 preserves stem cell function in culture and enhances retrovirus-mediated gene transfer into hematopoietic stem cells, *Proc. Natl. Acad. Sci. USA* **86:**8897–8901.

Bodine, D. M., Moritz, T., Donahue, R. E., Luskey, B. D., Kessler, S. W., Martin, D. I., Orkin, S. H., Nienhuis, A. W., and Williams, D. A., 1993a, Long-term in vivo expression of a murine adenosine deaminase gene in rhesus monkey hematopoietic cells of multiple lineages after retroviral mediated gene transfer into CD34+ bone marrow cells, *Blood* **82:**1975–1980.

Bodine, D. M., Seidel, N. E., Zsebo, K. M., and Orlic, D., 1993b, In vivo administration of stem cell factor to mice increases the absolute number of pluripotent hematopoietic stem cells, *Blood* **82:**445–455.

Bolscher, B. G., de Boer, M., de Klein, A., Weening, R. S., and Roos, D., 1991, Point mutations in the beta-subunit of cytochrome b558 leading to X-linked chronic granulomatous disease, *Blood* **77:**2482–2487.

Bordignon, C., Yu, S. F., Smith, C. A., Hantzopoulos, P., Ungers, G. E., Keever, C. A., O'Reilly, R. J., and Gilboa, E., 1989, Retroviral vector-mediated high-efficiency expression of adenosine deaminase

(ADA) in hematopoietic long-term cultures of ADA-deficient marrow cells, *Proc. Natl. Acad. Sci. USA* **86:**6748–6752.

Bordignon, C., Mavilio, F., Ferrari, G., Servida, P., Ugazio, A. G., Notarangelo, L. D., Gilboa, E., Rossini, S., O'Reilly, R. J., Smith, C. A., *et al.*, 1993, Transfer of the ADA gene into bone marrow cells and peripheral blood lymphocytes for the treatment of patients affected by ADA-deficient SCID, *Hum. Gene Ther.* **4:**513–520.

Bordignon, C., Notarangelo, L. D., Nobili, N., Ferrari, G., Casorati, G., Panina, P., Mazzolari, E., Maggioni, D., Rossi, C., Servida, P., *et al.*, 1995, Gene therapy in peripheral blood lymphocytes and bone marrow for ADA- immunodeficient patients, *Science* **270:**470–475.

Braakman, E., van Beusechem, V. W., Van Krimpen, B. A., Fischer, A., Bolhuis, R. L., and Valerio, D., 1992, Genetic correction of cultured T cells from an adenosine deaminase-deficient patient: Characteristics of non-transduced and transduced T cells, *Eur. J. Immunol.* **22:**63–69.

Bradley, L. A., Sweatman, A. K., Lovering, R. C., Jones, A. M., Morgan, G., Levinsky, R. J., and Kinnon, C., 1994, Mutation detection in the X-linked agammaglobulinemia gene, BTK, using single strand conformation polymorphism analysis, *Hum. Mol. Genet.* **3:**79–83.

Brasel, K., Escobar, S., Anderberg, R., de Vries, P., Gruss, H. J., and Lyman, S. D., 1995, Expression of the flt3 receptor and its ligand on hematopoietic cells, *Leukemia* **9:**1212–1218.

Brenner, M. K., Rill, D. R., Holladay, M. S., Heslop, H. E., Moen, R. C., Buschle, M., Krance, R. A., Santana, V. M., Anderson, W. F., and Ihle, J. N., 1993a, Gene marking to determine whether autologous marrow infusion restores long-term haemopoiesis in cancer patients, *Lancet* **342:**1134–1137.

Brenner, M. K., Rill, D. R., Moen, R. C., Krance, R. A., Mirro, J., Jr., Anderson, W. F., and Ihle, J. N., 1993b, Gene-marking to trace origin of relapse after autologous bone-marrow transplantation, *Lancet* **341:**85–86.

Brenner, M. K., 1995, Autologous bone-marrow transplantation in childhood acute lymphoblastic leukaemia, *Lancet* **346:**856–857.

Brenner, M. K., Cunningham, J. M., Sorrentino, B. P., and Heslop, H. E., 1995, Gene transfer into human hemopoietic progenitor cells, *Br. Med. Bull.* **51:**167–191.

Brenner, M. K., 1996, Gene transfer to hematopoietic cells, *N. Engl. J. Med.* **335:**337–339.

Broxmeyer, H. E., 1995, Growth factors and cord blood stem and progenitor cells, *Immunol. Invest.* **24:**391–402.

Broxmeyer, H. E., Lu, L., Cooper, S., Ruggieri, L., Li, Z. H., and Lyman, S. D., 1995, Flt3 ligand stimulates/costimulates the growth of myeloid stem/progenitor cells, *Exp. Hematol.* **23:**1121–1129.

Bu Ghanim, H. N., Segal, A. W., Keep, N. H., and Casimir, C. M., 1995, Molecular analysis in three cases of X91- variant chronic granulomatous disease, *Blood* **86:**3575–3582.

Burns, J. C., Friedmann, T., Driever, W., Burrascano, M., and Yee, J. K., 1993, Vesicular stomatitis virus G glycoprotein pseudotyped retroviral vectors: Concentration to very high titer and efficient gene transfer into mammalian and nonmammalian cells, *Proc. Natl. Acad. Sci. USA* **90:**8033–8037.

Callard, R. E., Armitage, R. J., Fanslow, W. C., and Spriggs, M. K., 1993, CD40 ligand and its role in X-linked hyper-IgM syndrome, *Immunol. Today* **14:**559–564.

Candotti, F., Johnston, J. A., Puck, J. M., Sugamura, K., O'Shea, J. J., and Blaese, R. M., 1996, Retroviral-mediated gene correction for X-linked severe combined immunodeficiency, *Blood* **87:**3097–3102.

Cardoso, A. A., Li, M. L., Batard, P., Hatzfeld, A., Brown, E. L., Levesque, J. P., Sookdeo, H., Panterne, B., Sansilvestri, P., Clark, S. C., *et al.*, 1993, Release from quiescence of CD34+ CD38– human umbilical cord blood cells reveals their potentiality to engraft adults, *Proc. Natl. Acad. Sci. USA* **90:**8707–8711.

Casimir, C., Chetty, M., Bohler, M. C., Garcia, R., Fischer, A., Griscelli, C., Johnson, B., and Segal, A. W., 1992, Identification of the defective NADPH-oxidase component in chronic granulomatous disease: A study of 57 European families, *Eur. J. Clin. Invest.* **22:**403–406.

Casimir, C. M., Bu Ghanim, H. N., Rodaway, A. R., Bentley, D. L., Rowe, P., and Segal, A. W., 1991, Autosomal recessive chronic granulomatous disease caused by deletion at a dinucleotide repeat, *Proc. Natl. Acad. Sci. USA* **88:**2753–2757.

Casimir, C. M., and Teahan, C, G., 1994, The respiratory burst of neutrophils and its deficiency, in *Immunopharmacology of Neutrophils*, (C. A. Chapman ed.), Academic Press, London, pp. 27–54.

Cassel, A., Cottler Fox, M., Doren, S., and Dunbar, C. E., 1993, Retroviral-mediated gene transfer into CD34-enriched human peripheral blood stem cells, *Exp. Hematol.* **21:**585–591.

Chanock, S. J., Faust, L. R., Barrett, D., Bizal, C., Maly, F. E., Newburger, P. E., Ruedi, J. M., Smith, R. M., and Babior, B. M., 1992, O_2 production by B lymphocytes lacking the respiratory burst oxidase subunit p47phox after transfection with an expression vector containing a p47phox cDNA, *Proc. Natl. Acad. Sci. USA* **89:**10174–10177.

Chen, B. P., Fraser, C., Reading, C., Murray, L., Uchida, N., Galy, A., Sasaki, D., Tricot, G., Jagannath, S., Barlogie, B., *et al.*, 1995, Cytokine-mobilized peripheral blood CD34+Thy-1+Lin- human hematopoietic stem cells as target cells for transplantation-based gene therapy, *Leukemia* **9**(Suppl. 1):S17–25.

Chertkov, J. L., Jiang, S., Lutton, J. D., Harrison, J., Levere, R. D., Tiefenthaler, M., and Abraham, N. G., 1993, The hematopoietic stromal microenvironment promotes retrovirus-mediated gene transfer into hematopoietic stem cells, *Stem Cells* **11:**218–227.

Chetty, M., Thrasher, A. J., Abo, A., and Casimir, C. M., 1995, Low NADPH oxidase activity in Epstein–Barr-virus-immortalized B-lymphocytes is due to a post-transcriptional block in expression of cytochrome b558, *Biochem. J.* **306:**141–145.

Cicuttini, F. M., Begley, C. G., and Boyd, A. W., 1992, The effect of recombinant stem cell factor (SCF) on purified CD34-positive human umbilical cord blood progenitor cells, *Growth Factors* **6:**31–39.

Cicuttini, F. M., Welch, K., and Boyd, A. W., 1994, Characterization of CD34+HLA-DR-CD38+ and CD34+HLA-DR-CD38-progenitor cells from human umbilical cord blood, *Growth Factors* **10:**127–134.

Civin, C. I., and Small, D., 1995, Purification and expansion of human hematopoietic stem/progenitor cells, *Ann. NY Acad. Sci.* **770:**91–98.

Clapp, D. W., Freie, B., Srour, E., Yoder, M. C., Fortney, K., and Gerson, S. L., 1995, Myeloproliferative sarcoma virus directed expression of beta-galactosidase following retroviral transduction of murine hematopoietic cells, *Exp. Hematol.* **23:**630–638.

Clark, R. A., Malech, H. L., Gallin, J. I., Nunoi, H., Volpp, B. D., Pearson, D. W., Nauseef, W. M., and Curnutte, J. T., 1989, Genetic variants of chronic granulomatous disease: Prevalence of deficiencies of two cytosolic components of the NADPH oxidase system, *N. Engl. J. Med.* **321:**647–652.

Conley, M. E., and Rohrer, J., 1995, The spectrum of mutations in Btk that cause X-linked agammaglobulinemia, *Clin. Immunol. Immunopathol.* **76:**S192–197.

Conneally, E., Bardy, P., Eaves, C. J., Thomas, T., Chappel, S., Shpall, E. J., and Humphries, R. K., 1996, Rapid and efficient selection of human hematopoietic cells expressing murine heat-stable antigen as an indicator of retroviral-mediated gene transfer, *Blood* **87:**456–464.

Corbi, A. L., Vara, A., Ursa, A., Garcia Rodriguez, M. C., Fontan, G., and Sanchez Madrid, F. 1992, Molecular basis for a severe case of leukocyte adhesion deficiency, *Eur. J. Immunol.* **22:**1877–1881.

Cory, G. O., Lovering, R. C., Hinshelwood, S., MacCarthy Morrogh, L., Levinsky, R. J., and Kinnon, C., 1995, The protein product of the c-cbl protooncogene is phosphorylated after B cell receptor stimulation and binds the SH3 domain of Bruton's tyrosine kinase, *J. Exp. Med.* **182:**611–615.

Cory, G. O. C., MacCarthy Morrogh, L., Banin, S., Gout, I., Brickell, P. M., Levinsky, R. J., Kinnon, C., and Lovering, R. C., 1996, Evidence that the Wiskott–Aldrich syndrome protein may be involved in lymphoid cell signalling pathways, *J. Immunol.* **157:**3791–3795.

Cournoyer, D., Scarpa, M., Mitani, K., Moore, K. A., Markowitz, D., Bank, A., Belmont, J. W., and Caskey, C. T., 1991, Gene transfer of adenosine deaminase into primitive human hematopoietic progenitor cells, *Hum. Gene Ther.* **2:**203–213.

Cournoyer, D., and Caskey, C. T., 1993, Gene therapy of the immune system, *Annu. Rev. Immunol.* **11:**297–329.

Crooks, G. M., and Kohn, D. B., 1993, Growth factors increase amphotropic retrovirus binding to human CD34+ bone marrow progenitor cells, *Blood* **82:**3290–3297.

Curnutte, J. T., 1993, Chronic granulomatous disease: The solving of a clinical riddle at the molecular level, *Clin. Immunol. Immunopathol.* **67:**S2–15.

Dancis, A., Roman, D. G., Anderson, G. J., Hinnebusch, A. G., and Klausner, R. D., 1992, Ferric reductase of *Saccharomyces cerevisiae*: Molecular characterization, role in iron uptake, and transcriptional control by iron, *Proc. Natl. Acad. Sci. USA* **89:**3869–3873.

de Boer, M., Bolscher, B. G., Dinauer, M. C., Orkin, S. H., Smith, C. I., Ahlin, A., Weening, R. S., and Roos, D., 1992, Splice site mutations are a common cause of X-linked chronic granulomatous disease, *Blood* **80:**1553–1558.

de Mendez, I., Garrett, M. C., Adams, A. G., and Leto, T. L., 1994, Role of p67-phox SH3 domains in assembly of the NADPH oxidase system, *J. Biol. Chem.* **269:**16326–16332.

de Mendez, I., Adams, A. G., Sokolic, R. A., Malech, H. L., and Leto, T. L., 1996, Multiple SH3 domain interactions regulate NADPH oxidase assembly in whole cells, *EMBO J.* **15:**1211–1220.

de Saint Basile, G., Bohler, M. C., Fischer, A., Cartron, J., Dufier, J. L., Griscelli, C., and Orkin, S. H., 1988, Xp21 DNA microdeletion in a patient with chronic granulomatous disease, retinitis pigmentosa, and McLeod phenotype, *Hum. Genet.* **80:**85–89.

de Vos, S., Brach, M. A., Asano, Y., Ludwig, W. D., Bettelheim, P., Gruss, H. J., and Herrmann, F., 1993, Transforming growth factor-beta 1 interferes with the proliferation-inducing activity of stem cell factor in myelogenous leukemia blasts through functional down-regulation of the c-kit proto-oncogene product, *Cancer Res.* **53:**3638–3642.

de Weers, M., Brouns, G. S., Hinshelwood, S., Kinnon, C., Schuurman, R. K., Hendriks, R. W., and Borst, J., 1994a, B-cell antigen receptor stimulation activates the human Bruton's tyrosine kinase, which is deficient in X-linked agammaglobulinemia, *J. Biol. Chem.* **269:**23857–23860.

de Weers, M., Mensink, R. G., Kraakman, M. E., Schuurman, R. K., and Hendriks, R. W., 1994b, Mutation analysis of the Bruton's tyrosine kinase gene in X-linked agammaglobulinemia: Identification of a mutation which affects the same codon as is altered in immunodeficient xid mice, *Hum. Mol. Genet.* **3:**161–166.

Derry, J. M., Ochs, H. D., and Francke, U., 1994a, Isolation of a novel gene mutated in Wiskott–Aldrich syndrome, *Cell* **78:**635–644.

Derry, J. M., Ochs, H. D., and Francke, U., 1994b, Isolation of a novel gene mutated in Wiskott–Aldrich syndrome, *Cell* **79:**923.

Derry, J. M., Kerns, J. A., Weinberg, K. I., Ochs, H. D., Volpini, V., Estivill, X., Walker, A. P., and Francke, U., 1995, WASP gene mutations in Wiskott–Aldrich syndrome and X-linked thrombocytopenia, *Hum. Mol. Genet.* **4:**1127–1135.

Dick, J. E., 1994, Future prospects for animal models created by transplanting human haematopoietic cells into immune-deficient mice, *Res. Immunol.* **145:**380–384.

Diekmann, D., Abo, A., Johnston, C., Segal, A. W., and Hall, A., 1994, Interaction of Rac with p67phox and regulation of phagocytic NADPH oxidase activity, *Science* **265:**531–533.

Dinauer, M. C., Orkin, S. H., Brown, R., Jesaitis, A. J., and Parkos, C. A., 1987, The glycoprotein encoded by the X-linked chronic granulomatous disease locus is a component of the neutrophil cytochrome b complex, *Nature* **327:**717–720.

Dinauer, M. C., Curnutte, J. T., Rosen, H., and Orkin, S. H., 1989, A missense mutation in the neutrophil cytochrome b heavy chain in cytochrome-positive X-linked chronic granulomatous disease, *J. Clin. Invest.* **84:**2012–2016.

Dinauer, M. C., Pierce, E. A., Erickson, R. W., Muhlebach, T. J., Messner, H., Orkin, S. H., Seger, R. A., and Curnutte, J. T., 1991, Point mutation in the cytoplasmic domain of the neutrophil p22-phox cytochrome b subunit is associated with a nonfunctional NADPH oxidase and chronic granulomatous disease, *Proc. Natl. Acad. Sci. USA.* **88:**11231–11235.

Dinauer, M. C., 1993, The respiratory burst oxidase and the molecular genetics of chronic granulomatous disease, *Crit. Rev. Clin. Lab. Sci.* **30:**329–369.

Dinauer, M. C., and Orkin, S. H., 1992, Chronic granulomatous disease, *Annu. Rev. Med.* **43:**117–124.

DiSanto, J. P., Bonnefoy, J. Y., Gauchat, J. F., Fischer, A., and de Saint Basile, G., 1993, CD40 ligand mutations in X-linked immunodeficiency with hyper-IgM, *Nature* **361:**541–543.

Donahue, R. E., Kirby, M. R. M., Metzger, M. E., Agricola, B. A., Sellers, S. E., and Cullis, H. M., 1996, Peripheral blood CD34+ cells differ from bone marrow CD34+ cells in Thy-1 expression and cell cycle status in nonhuman primates mobilized or not mobilized with granulocyte colony-stimulating factor and/or stem cell factor, *Blood* **87:**1644–1653.

Dorseuil, O., Reibel, L., Bokoch, G. M., Camonis, J., and Gacon, G., 1996, The Rac target NADPH oxidase p67phox interacts preferentially with Rac2 rather than Rac1, *J. Biol. Chem.* **271:**83–88.

Drize, N., Chertkov, J., and Zander, A., 1995, Hematopoietic progenitor cell mobilization into the peripheral blood of mice using a combination of recombinant rat stem cell factor (rrSCF) and recombinant human granulocyte colony-stimulating factor (rhG-CSF), *Exp. Hematol.* **23:**1180–1186.

Drize, N., Chertkov, J., Samoilina, N., and Zander, A., 1996, Effect of cytokine treatment (granulocyte colony-stimulating factor and stem cell factor) on hematopoiesis and the circulating pool of hematopoietic stem cells in mice, *Exp. Hematol.* **24:**816–822.

Dube First Symposium on Hematopoietic Stem Cell Gene Therapy. Rockville. M. Oct. 1995.

Dubois, C. M., Ruscetti, F. W., Stankova, J., and Keller, J. R., 1994, Transforming growth factor-beta regulates c-kit message stability and cell-surface protein expression in hematopoietic progenitors, *Blood* **83:**3138–3145.

Dunbar, C. E., Cottler Fox, M., O'Shaughnessy, J. A., Doren, S., Carter, C., Berenson, R., Brown, S., Moen, R. C., Greenblatt, J., Stewart, F. M., *et al.*, 1995, Retrovirally marked CD34-enriched peripheral blood and bone marrow cells contribute to long-term engraftment after autologous transplantation, *Blood* **85:**3048–3057.

Dunbar, C. E., and Emmons, R. V., 1994, Gene transfer into hematopoietic progenitor and stem cells: Progress and problems, *Stem Cells* **12:**563–576.

Dusi, S., Della Bianca, V., Grzeskowiak, M., and Rossi, F., 1993, Relationship between phosphorylation and translocation to the plasma membrane of p47phox and p67phox and activation of the NADPH oxidase in normal and Ca(2+)-depleted human neutrophils, *Biochem. J.* **290:**173–178.

Dusi, S., Donini, M., and Rossi, F., 1996, Mechanisms of NADPH oxidase activation: Translocation of p40phox, Rac1 and Rac2 from the cytosol to the membranes in human neutrophils lacking p47phox or p67phox, *Biochem. J.* **314:**409–412.

Dusi, S., and Rossi, F., 1993, Activation of NADPH oxidase of human neutrophils involves the phosphorylation and the translocation of cytosolic p67phox, *Biochem. J.* **296:**367–371.

Eaves, C. J., Cashman, J. D., Kay, R. J., Dougherty, G. J., Otsuka, T., Gaboury, L. A., Hogge, D. E., Lansdorp, P. M., Eaves, A. C., and Humphries, R. K., 1991, Mechanisms that regulate the cell cycle status of very primitive hematopoietic cells in long-term human marrow cultures. II. Analysis of positive and negative regulators produced by stromal cells within the adherent layer, *Blood* **78:**110–117.

Eglitis, M. A., Schneiderman, R. D., Rice, P. M., and Eiden, M. V., 1995, Evaluation of retroviral vectors based on the gibbon ape leukemia virus, *Gene Ther.* **2:**486–492.

Elias, J. A., Zheng, T., Whiting, N. L., Trow, T. K., Merrill, W. W., Zitnik, R., Ray, P., and Alderman, E. M., 1994, IL-1 and transforming growth factor-beta regulation of fibroblast-derived IL-11, *J. Immunol.* **152:**2421–2429.

Etzioni, A., Harlan, J. M., Pollack, S., Phillips, L. M., Gershoni Baruch, R., and Paulson, J. C., 1993, Leukocyte adhesion deficiency (LAD) II: A new adhesion defect due to absence of sialyl Lewis X, the ligand for selectins, *Immunodeficiency* **4:**307–308.

Etzioni, A., Phillips, L. M., Paulson, J. C., and Harlan, J. M., 1995, Leukocyte adhesion deficiency (LAD) II, *Ciba Found. Symp.* **189:**51–58.

Fairbanks, L. D., Simmonds, H. A., Hoogerbrugge, P. M., van Beusechem, V. W., Valerio, D., Moseley, A., Levinsky, R. J., Gaspar, H. B., and Morgan, G., 1994, Biochemical and immunological status following gene therapy and PEG-ADA therapy for adenosine deaminase (ADA) deficiency, *Adv. Exp. Med. Biol.* **370:**391–394.

Faust, E. A., Saffran, D. C., Toksoz, D., Williams, D. A., and Witte, O. N., 1993, Distinctive growth requirements and gene expression patterns distinguish progenitor B cells from pre-B cells, *J. Exp. Med.* **177:**915–923.

Feller, S. M., Ren, R., Hanafusa, H., and Baltimore, D., 1994, SH2 and SH3 domains as molecular adhesives: The interactions of Crk and Abl, *Trends Biochem. Sci.* **19:**453–458.

Ferrari, F. K., Samulski, T., Shenk, T., and Samulski, R. J., 1996, Second-strand synthesis is a rate-limiting step for efficient transduction by recombinant adeno-associated virus vectors, *J. Virol.* **70:**3227–3234.

Ferrari, G., Rossini, S., Nobili, N., Maggioni, D., Garofalo, A., Giavazzi, R., Mavilio, F., and Bordignon, C., 1992, Transfer of the ADA gene into human ADA-deficient T lymphocytes reconstitutes specific immune functions, *Blood* **80:**1120–1124.

Finan, P., Shimizu, Y., Gout, I., Hsuan, J., Truong, O., Butcher, C., Bennett, P., Waterfield, M. D., and Kellie, S., 1994, An SH3 domain and proline-rich sequence mediate an interaction between two components of the phagocyte NADPH oxidase complex, *J. Biol. Chem.* **269:**13752–13755.

Firkin, F., Dunlop, J., and Bertoncello, I., 1993, Expansion of hemopoietic activity in long-term culture of human bone marrow by c-kit ligand (stem cell factor), *Growth Factors* **8:**135–140.

Fischer, A., Lisowska Grospierre, B., Anderson, D. C., and Springer, T. A., 1988, Leukocyte adhesion deficiency: Molecular basis and functional consequences, *Immunodefic. Rev.* **1:**39–54.

Fischer, A., 1992, Severe combined immunodeficiencies. *Immunodeficiency Rev.* **3:**83–100.

Fischer, A., Landais, P., Friedrich, W., Gerritsen, B., Fasth, A., Porta, F., Vellodi, A., Benkerrou, M., Jais, J. P., Cavazzana Calvo, M., *et al.*, 1994, Bone marrow transplantation (BMT) in Europe for primary immunodeficiencies other than severe combined immunodeficiency: A report from the European Group for BMT and the European Group for Immunodeficiency, *Blood* **83:**1149–1154.

Fisher, K. J., Gao, G. P., Weitzman, M. D., DeMatteo, R., Burda, J. F., and Wilson, J. M., 1996, Transduction with recombinant adeno-associated virus for gene therapy is limited by leading-strand synthesis, *J. Virol.* **70:**520–532.

Flasshove, M., Banerjee, D., Mineishi, S., Li, M. X., Bertino, J. R., and Moore, M. A., 1995, Ex vivo expansion and selection of human CD34+ peripheral blood progenitor cells after introduction of a mutated dihydrofolate reductase cDNA via retroviral gene transfer, *Blood* **85:**566–574.

Fleming, W. H., Alpern, E. J., Uchida, N., Ikuta, K., and Weissman, I. L., 1993, Steel factor influences the distribution and activity of murine hematopoietic stem cells in vivo, *Proc. Natl. Acad. Sci. USA* **90:**3760–3764.

Flotte, T. R., Afione, S. A., and Zeitlin, P. L., 1994, Adeno-associated virus vector gene expression occurs in nondividing cells in the absence of vector DNA integration, *Am. J. Respir. Cell. Mol. Biol.* **11:**517–521.

Flotte, T. R., and Carter, B. J., 1995, Adeno-associated virus vectors for gene therapy, *Gene Ther.* **2:**357–362.

Frech, M., Ingley, E., Andjelkovic, M., and Hemmings, B. A., 1995, Pleckstrin homology domains, *Biochem. Soc. Trans.* **23:**616–618.

Fuchs, A., Dagher, M. C., and Vignais, P. V., 1995, Mapping the domains of interaction of p40phox with both p47phox and p67phox of the neutrophil oxidase complex using the two-hybrid system, *J. Biol. Chem.* **270:**5695–5697.

Fuchs, A., Dagher, M. C., Faure, J., and Vignais, P. V., 1996, Topological organization of the cytosolic activating complex of the superoxide-generating NADPH-oxidase. Pinpointing the sites of interaction between p47phoz, p67phox and p40phox using the two-hybrid system, *Biochim. Biophys. Acta.* 1**312:**39–47.

Fuleihan, R., Ramesh, N., Loh, R., Jabara, H., Rosen, R. S., Chatila, T., Fu, S. M., Stamenkovic, I., and Geha, R. S., 1993, Defective expression of the CD40 ligand in X chromosome-linked immunoglobulin deficiency with normal or elevated IgM, *Proc. Natl. Acad. Sci. USA* **90:**2170–2173.

Galli, S. J., Zsebo, K. M., and Geissler, E. N., 1994, The kit ligand, stem cell factor, *Adv. Immunol.* **55:**1995.

Goodell, M. A., Brose, K., Paradis, G., Conner, A. S., and Mulligan, R. C., 1996, Isolation and functional properties of murine hematopoietic stem cells that are replicating in vivo, *J. Exp. Med.* **183:**1797–1806.

Graf, L., and Torok Storb, B., 1995, Identification of a novel DNA sequence differentially expressed between normal human CD34+CD38hi and CD34+CD38lo marrow cells, *Blood* **86:**548–556.

Hacein Bey, H., Cavazzana Calvo, M., Le Deist, F., Dautry Varsat, A., Hivroz, C., Riviere, I., Danos, O., Heard, J. M., Sugamura, K., Fischer, A., *et al.*, 1996, gamma-c gene transfer into SCID X1 patients' B-cell lines restores normal high-affinity interleukin-2 receptor expression and function, *Blood* **87:**3108–3116.

Hagemann, T. L., Rosen, F. S., and Kwan, S. P., 1995, Characterization of germline mutations of the gene encoding Bruton's tyrosine kinase in families with X-linked agammaglobulinemia. *Hum. Mutation* **5:**296–302.

Halbert, C. L., Alexander, I. E., Wolgamot, G. M., and Miller, A. D., 1995, Adeno-associated virus vectors transduce primary cells much less efficiently than immortalized cells, *J. Virol.* **69:**1473–1479.

Hall, A., 1992, Ras-related GTPases and the cytoskeleton, *Mol. Biol. Cell* **3:**475–479.

Hanania, E. G., and Deisseroth, A. B., 1994, Serial transplantation shows that early hematopoietic precursor cells are transduced by MDR-1 retroviral vector in a mouse gene therapy model, *Cancer Gene Ther.* **1:**21–25.

Hannum, C., Culpepper, J., Campbell, D., McClanahan, T., Zurawski, S., Bazan, J. F., Kastelein, R., Hudak, S., Wagner, J., Mattson, J., *et al.*, 1994, Ligand for FLT3/FLK2 receptor tyrosine kinase regulates growth of haematopoietic stem cells and is encoded by variant RNAs, *Nature* **368:**643–648.

Hao, Q. L., Shah, A. J., Thiemann, F. T., Smogorzewska, E. M., and Crooks, G. M., 1995, A functional comparison of CD34 + CD38– cells in cord blood and bone marrow, *Blood* **86:**3745–3753.

Heimfeld, S., Fogarty, B., McGuire, K., Williams, S., and Berenson, R. J., 1992, Peripheral blood stem cell mobilization after stem cell factor or G-CSF treatment: Rapid enrichment for stem and progenitor cells using the CEPRATE immunoaffinity separation system, *Transplant. Proc.* **24:**2818.

Hermonat, P. L., 1994, Down-regulation of the human c-fos and c-myc proto-oncogene promoters by adeno-associated virus Rep78, *Cancer Lett.* **81:**129–136.

Hershfield, M. S., 1995, PEG-ADA replacement therapy for adenosine deaminase deficiency: An update after 8.5 years, *Clin. Immunol. Immunopathol.* **76:**S228–32.

Hesdorffer, C., Antman, K., Bank, A., Fetell, M., Mears, G., and Begg, M., 1994, Human MDR gene transfer in patients with advanced cancer, *Hum. Gene Ther.* **5:**1151–1160.

Heyworth, C. M., Whetton, A. D., Nicholls, S., Zsebo, K., and Dexter, T. M., 1992, Stem cell factor directly stimulates the development of enriched granulocyte-macrophage colony-forming cells and promotes the effects of other colony-stimulating factors, *Blood* **80:**2230–2236.

Heyworth, C. M., Pearson, M. A., Dexter, T. M., Wark, G., Owen Lynch, P. J., and Whetton, A. D., 1996, Macrophage inflammatory protein-1 alpha mediated growth inhibition in a haemopoietic stem cell line is associated with inositol 1,4,5-triphosphate generation, *Growth Factors* **12:**165–172.

Heyworth, P. G., Shrimpton, C. F., and Segal, A. W., 1989, Localization of the 47 kDa phosphoprotein involved in the respiratory-burst NADPH oxidase of phagocytic cells, *Biochem. J.* **260:**243–248.

Heyworth, P. G., Curnutte, J. T., Nauseef, W. M., Volpp, B. D., Pearson, D. W., Rosen, H., and Clark, R. A., 1991, Neutrophil nicotinamide adenine dinucleotide phosphate oxidase assembly. Translocation of p47-phox and p67-phox requires interaction between p47-phox and cytochrome b558, *J. Clin. Invest.* **87:**352–356.

Heyworth, P. G., Bohl, B. P., Bokoch, G. M., and Curnutte, J. T., 1994, Rac translocates independently of the neutrophil NADPH oxidase components p47phox and p67phox. Evidence for its interaction with flavocytochrome b558, *J. Biol. Chem.* **269:**30749–30752.

Hibbs, M. L., Wardlaw, A. J., Stacker, S. A., Anderson, D. C., Lee, A., Roberts, T. M., and Springer, T. A., 1990, Transfection of cells from patients with leukocyte adhesion deficiency with an integrin beta subunit (CD18) restores lymphocyte function-associated antigen-1 expression and function, *J. Clin. Invest.* **85:**674–681.

Hinshelwood, S., Lovering, R. C., Genevier, H. C., Levinsky, R. J., and Kinnon, C., 1995, The protein defective in X-linked agammaglobulinemia, Bruton's tyrosine kinase, shows increased autophosphorylation activity in vitro when isolated from cells in which the B cell receptor has been cross-linked, *Eur. J. Immunol.* **25:**1113–1116.

Hirschhorn, R., 1990, Adenosine deaminase deficiency, *Immunodeficiency Rev.* **2:**175–198.

Hirschhorn, R., 1993, Overview of biochemical abnormalities and molecular genetics of adenosine deaminase deficiency, *Pediatr Res.* **33:**S35–41.

Hoffman, R., Tong, J., Brandt, J., Traycoff, C., Bruno, E., McGuire, B. W., Gordon, M. S., McNiece, I., and Srour, E. F., 1993, The in vitro and in vivo effects of stem cell factor on human hematopoiesis, *Stem Cells* **11**(Suppl. 2)**:**76–82.

Hogge, D. E., Sutherland, H. J., Cashman, J. D., Lansdorp, P. M., Humphries, R. K., and Eaves, C. J., 1994, Cytokines acting early in human haematopoiesis, *Baillieres Clin. Haematol.* **7:**49–63.

Hoogerbrugge, P. M., von Beusechem, V. W., Kaptein, L. C., Einerhand, M. P., and Valerio, D., 1995, Gene therapy for adenosine deaminase deficiency, *Br. Med. Bull.* **51:**72–81.

Hudak, S., Hunte, B., Culpepper, J., Menon, S., Hannum, C., Thompson Snipes, L., and Rennick, D., 1995, FLT3/FLK2 ligand promotes the growth of murine stem cells and the expansion of colony-forming cells and spleen colony-forming units, *Blood* **85:**2747–2755.

Humeau, L., Bardin, F., Maroc, C., Alario, T., Galindo, R., Mannoni, P., and Chabannon, C., 1996, Phenotypic, molecular, and functional characterization of human peripheral blood CD34+/THY1+ cells, *Blood* **87:**949–955.

Ikuta, K., and Weissman, I. L., 1992, Evidence that hematopoietic stem cells express mouse c-kit but do not depend on steel factor for their generation, *Proc. Natl. Acad. Sci. USA* **89:**1502–1506.

Ito, T., Nakamura, R., Sumimoto, H., Takeshige, K., and Sakaki, Y., 1996, An SH3 domain-mediated interaction between the phagocyte NADPH oxidase factors p40phox and p47phox, *FEBS Lett.* **385:**229–232.

Jacobsen, S. E., Okkenhaug, C., Myklebust, J., Veiby, O. P., and Lyman, S. D., 1995, The FLT3 ligand potently and directly stimulates the growth and expansion of primitive murine bone marrow progenitor cells in vitro: Synergistic interactions with interleukin (IL) 11, IL-12, and other hematopoietic growth factors, *J. Exp. Med.* **181:**1357–1363.

Jin, H., Webster, A. D., Vihinen, M., Sideras, P., Vorechovsky, I., Hammarstrom, L., Bernatowska Matuszkiewicz, E., Smith, C. I., Bobrow, M., and Vetrie, D., 1995, Identification of Btk mutations in 20 unrelated patients with X-linked agammaglobulinaemia (XLA). *Hum. Mol. Genet.* **4:**693–700.

Jones, P. A., Rideout, W. M., Shen, J. C., Spruck, C. H., and Tsai, Y. C., 1992, Methylation, mutation and cancer, *Bioessays* **14:**33–36.

Kantoff, P. W., Gillio, A. P., McLachlin, J. R., Bordignon, C., Eglitis, M. A., Kernan, N. A., Moen, R. C., Kohn, D. B., Yu, S. F., Karson, E., *et al.*, 1987, Expression of human adenosine deaminase in nonhuman primates after retrovirus-mediated gene transfer, *J. Exp. Med.* **166:**219–234.

Katz, F. E., Lovering, R. C., Bradley, L. A., Rigley, K. P., Brown, D., Cotter, F., Chessells, J. M., Levinsky, R. J., and Kinnon, C., 1994, Expression of the X-linked agammaglobulinemia gene, btk in B-cell acute lymphoblastic leukemia, *Leukemia* **8:**574–577.

Kavanaugh, A. F., Lightfoot, E., Lipsky, P. E., and Oppenheimer Marks, N., 1991, Role of CD11/CD18 in adhesion and transendothelial migration of T cells. Analysis utilizing CD18-deficient T cell clones, *J. Immunol.* **146:**4149–4156.

Keller, G., Paige, C., Gilboa, E., and Wagner, E. F., 1985, Expression of a foreign gene in myeloid and lymphoid cells derived from multipotent haematopoietic precursors, *Nature* **318:**149–154.

Keller, G., 1992, Hematopoietic stem cells, *Curr. Opinion Immunol.* **4:**133–139.

Kikuchi, Y., Yasue, T., Miyake, K., Kimoto, M., and Takatsu, K., 1995, CD38 ligation induces tyrosine phosphorylation of Bruton tyrosine kinase and enhanced expression of interleukin 5-receptor alpha chain: Synergistic effects with interleukin 5, *Proc. Natl. Acad. Sci. USA* **92:**11814–11818.

Kinnon, C., Hinshelwood, S., Levinsky, R. J., and Lovering, R. C., 1993, X-linked agammaglobulinemia—gene cloning and future prospects, *Immunol. Today* **14:**554–558.

Kinnon, C., Lovering, R., O'Reilly, M. A., Sweatman, A., Bradley, L., Parkar, M., Alterman, L., and Levinsky, R., 1995, Physical and genetic approaches to the isolation of the gene for X-linked agammaglobulinemia, *Immunodeficiency* **5:**179–185.

Knaus, U. G., Heyworth, P. G., Evans, T., Curnutte, J. T., and Bokoch, G. M., 1991, Regulation of phagocyte oxygen radical production by the GTP-binding protein Rac 2, *Science* **254:**1512–1515.

Knaus, U. G., Heyworth, P. G., Kinsella, B. T., Curnutte, J. T., and Bokoch, G. M., 1992, Purification and characterization of Rac 2. A cytosolic GTP-binding protein that regulates human neutrophil NADPH oxidase, *J. Biol. Chem.* **267:**23575–23582.

Kohn, D. B., Weinberg, K. I., Nolta, J. A., Heiss, L. N., Lenarsky, C., Crooks, G. M., Hanley, M. E., Anette, G., Brooks, J. S., El Khoureiy, A., *et al.*, 1995, Engraftment of gene-modified umbilical cord blood cells in neonates with adenosine deaminase deficiency, *Nat. Med.* **1:**1017–1023.

Koike, M., Kikuchi, Y., Tominaga, A., Takaki, S., Akagi, K., Miyazaki, J., Yamamura, K., and Takatsu, K., 1995, Defective IL-5-receptor-mediated signaling in B cells of X-linked immunodeficient mice, *Int. Immunol.* **7:**21–30.

Kolluri, R., Shehabeldin, A., Peacocke, M., Lamhonwah, A. M., Teichert Kuliszewska, K., Weissman, S. M., and Siminovitch, K. A., 1995, Identification of WASP mutations in patients with Wiskott–Aldrich syndrome and isolated thrombocytopenia reveals allelic heterogeneity at the WAS locus, *Hum. Mol. Genet.* **4:**1119–1126.

Kolluri, R., Tolias, K. F., Carpenter, C. L., Rosen, F. S., and Kirchhausen, T., 1996, Direct interaction of the Wiskott–Aldrich syndrome protein with the GTPase Cdc42, *Proc. Natl. Acad. Sci. USA* **93:**5615–5618.

Korthauer, U., Graf, D., Mages, H. W., Briere, F., Padayachee, M., Malcolm, S., Ugazio, A. G., Notarangelo, L. D., Levinsky, R. J., and Kroczek, R. A., 1993, Defective expression of T-cell CD40 ligand causes X-linked immunodeficiency with hyper-IgM, *Nature* **361:**539–541.

Kotin, R. M., 1994, Prospects for the use of adeno-associated virus as a vector for human gene therapy, *Hum. Gene Ther.* **5:**793–801.

Krause, D. S., Fackler, M. J., Civin, C. I., and May, W. S., 1996, CD34: Structure, biology and clinical utility, *Blood* **87:**1–13.

Kremer, E. J., and Perricaudet, M., 1995, Adenovirus and adeno-associated virus mediated gene transfer, *Br. Med. Bull.* **51:**31–44.

Kroczek, R. A., Graf, D., Brugnoni, D., Giliani, S., Korthuer, U., Ugazio, A., Senger, G., Mages, H. W., Villa, A., and Notarangelo, L. D., 1994, Defective expression of CD40 ligand on T cells causes "X-linked immunodeficiency with hyper-IgM (HIGM1)," *Immunol. Rev.* **138:**39–59.

Kume, A., and Dinauer, M. C., 1994, Retrovirus-mediated reconstitution of respiratory burst activity in X-linked chronic granulomatous disease cells, *Blood* **84:**3311–3316.

Kundig, T. M., Schorle, H., Bachmann, M. F., Hengartner, H., Zinkernagel, R. M., and Horak, I., 1993, Immune responses in interleukin-2-deficient mice, *Science* **262:**1059–1061.

Kwan, S. P., Hagemann, T. L., Radtke, B. E., Blaese, R. M., and Rosen, F. S., 1995, Identification of mutations in the Wiskott–Aldrich syndrome gene and characterization of a polymorphic dinucleotide repeat at DXS6940, adjacent to the disease gene, *Proc. Natl. Acad. Sci. USA* **92:**4706–4710.

Kwan, S. P., Hagemann, T. L., Blaese, R. M., Knutsen, A., and Rosen, F. S., 1996, Scanning of the Wiskott–Aldrich syndrome (WAS) gene: Identification of 18 novel alterations including a possible mutation hotspot at Arg86 resulting in thrombocytopenia, a mild WAS phenotype, *Hum. Mol. Genet.* **4:**1995–1998.

Lamkin, T., Brooks, J., Annett, G., Roberts, W., Weinberg, K., 1994, Immunophenotypic differences between putative hematopoietic stem cells and childhood B-cell precursor acute lymphoblastic leukemia cells, *Leukemia* **8:**1871–1878.

Lardon, F., Snoeck, H. W., Nijs, G., Lenjou, M., Peetermans, M. E., Rodrigus, I., Berneman, Z. N., and Van Bockstaele, D. R., 1994, Transforming growth factor-beta regulates the cell cycle status of interleukin-3 (IL-3) plus IL-1, stem cell factor, or IL-6 stimulated CD34+ human hematopoietic progenitor cells through different cell kinetic mechanisms depending on the applied stimulus, *Exp. Hematol.* **22:**903–909.

Larochelle, A., Vormoor, J., Lapidot, T., Sher, G., Furukawa, T., Li, Q., Shultz, L. D., Olivieri, N. F., Stamatoyannopoulos, G., and Dick, J. E., 1995, Engraftment of immune-deficient mice with primitive hematopoietic cells from beta-thalassemia and sickle cell anemia patients: Implications for evaluating human gene therapy protocols, *Hum. Mol. Genet.* **4:**163–172.

Lawrence, R. J., 1985, David the "bubble boy" and the boundaries of the human, *JAMA* **253:**74–76.

Lemoli, R. M., Fortuna, A., Fogli, M., Motta, M. R., Rizzi, S., Benini, C., and Tura, S., 1994, Stem cell factor (c-kit ligand) enhances the interleukin-9-dependent proliferation of human CD34+ and CD34+CD33-DR- cells, *Exp. Hematol.* **22:**919–923.

Leonard, W. J., Noguchi, M., and Russell, S. M., 1994a, Sharing of a common gamma chain, gamma c, by the IL-2, IL-4, and IL-7 receptors: Implications for X-linked severe combined immunodeficiency (XSCID), *Adv. Exp. Med. Biol.* **365:**225–232.

Leonard, W. J., Noguchi, M., Russell, S. M., and McBride, O. W., 1994b, The molecular basis of X-linked severe combined immunodeficiency: The role of the interleukin-2 receptor gamma chain as a common gamma chain, gamma c, *Immunol. Rev.* **138:**61–86.

Leto, T. L., Lomax, K. J., Volpp, B. D., Nunoi, H., Sechler, J. M., Nauseef, W. M., Clark, R. A., Gallin, J. I., and Malech, H. L., 1990, Cloning of a 67-kD neutrophil oxidase factor with similarity to a noncatalytic region of p60c-src, *Science* **248:**727–730.

Leto, T. L., Adams, A. G., and de Mendez, I., 1994, Assembly of the phagocyte NADPH oxidase: Binding of Src homology 3 domains to proline-rich targets, *Proc. Natl. Acad. Sci. USA* **91:**10650–10654.

Leusen, J. H., de Boer, M., Bolscher, B. G., Hilarius, P. M., Weening, R. S., Ochs, H. D., Roos, D., and Verhoeven, A. J., 1994a, A point mutation in gp91-phox of cytochrome b558 of the human NADPH oxidase leading to defective translocation of the cytosolic proteins p47-phox and p67-phox, *J. Clin. Invest.* **93:**2120–2126.

Leusen, J. H., Bolscher, B. G., Hilarius, P. M., Weening, R. S., Kaulfersch, W., Seger, R. A., Roos, D., and Verhoeven, A. J., 1994b, 156Pro→Gln substitution in the light chain of cytochrome b558 of the human NADPH oxidase (p22-phox) leads to defective translocation of the cytosolic proteins p47-phox and p67-phox, *J. Exp. Med.* **180:**2329–2334.

Li, F., Linton, G. F., Sekhsaria, S., Whiting Theobald, N., Katkin, J. P., Gallin, J. I., and Malech, H. L., 1994, CD34+ peripheral blood progenitors as a target for genetic correction of the two flavocytochrome b558 defective forms of chronic granulomatous disease, *Blood* **84:**53–58.

Li, M. L., Cardoso, A. A., Sansilvestri, P., Hatzfeld, A., Brown, E. L., Sookdeo, H., Levesque, J. P., Clark,

S. C., and Hatzfeld, J., 1994, Additive effects of steel factor and antisense TGF-beta 1 oligodeoxynucleotide on CD34+ hematopoietic progenitor cells, *Leukemia* **8:**441–445.

Li, T., Tsukada, S., Satterthwaite, A., Havlik, M. H., Park, H., Takatsu, K., and Witte, O. N., 1995, Activation of Bruton's tyrosine kinase (BTK) by a point mutation in its pleckstrin homology (PH) domain, *Immunity* **2:**451–460.

Licht, T., Aksentijevich, I., Gottesman, M. M., Pastan, I., 1995, Efficient expression of functional human MDR1 gene in murine bone marrow after retroviral transduction of purified hematopoietic stem cells, *Blood* **86:**111–121.

Lim, B., Williams, D. A., and Orkin, S. H., 1987, Retrovirus-mediated gene transfer of human adenosine deaminase: Expression of functional enzyme in murine hematopoietic stem cells in vivo, *Mol. Cell. Biol.* **7:**3459–3465.

Lomax, K. J., Leto, T. L., Nunoi, H., Gallin, J. I., and Malech, H. L., 1989, Recombinant 47-kilodalton cytosol factor restores NADPH oxidase in chronic granulomatous disease, *Science* **245:**409–412.

Lopez Rodriguez, C., Nueda, A., Grospierre, B., Sanchez Madrid, F., Fischer, A., Springer, T. A., and Corbi, A. L., 1993, Characterization of two new CD18 alleles causing severe leukocyte adhesion deficiency, *Eur. J. Immunol.* **23:**2792–2798.

Lovering, R., Sweatman, A. K., O'Reilly, M. A., Genet, S. A., Middleton Price, H., Malcolm, S., Levinsky, R. J., and Kinnon, C., 1993, Physical mapping identifies DXS265 as a useful genetic marker for carrier detection and prenatal diagnosis of X-linked agammaglobulinemia, *Hum. Genet.* **91:**178–180.

Lu, L., Xiao, M., Clapp, D. W., Li, Z. H., and Broxmeyer, H. E., 1993a, High efficiency retroviral mediated gene transduction into single isolated immature and replatable CD34(3+) hematopoietic stem/progenitor cells from human umbilical cord blood, *J. Exp. Med.* **178:**2089–2096.

Lu, L., Xiao, M., Grigsby, S., Wang, W. X., Wu, B., Shen, R. N., and Broxmeyer, H. E., 1993b, Comparative effects of suppressive cytokines on isolated single CD34(3+) stem/progenitor cells from human bone marrow and umbilical cord blood plated with and without serum, *Exp. Hematol.* **21:**1442–1446.

Lu, L., Ge, Y., Li, Z. H., Freie, B., Clapp, D. W., and Broxmeyer, H. E., 1995, CD34 stem/progenitor cells purified from cryopreserved normal cord blood can be transduced with high efficiency by a retroviral vector and expanded ex vivo with stable integration and expression of Fanconi anemia complementation C gene, *Cell Transplant.* **4:**493–503.

Lu, M., Maruyama, M., Zhang, N., Levine, F., Friedmann, T., and Ho, A. D., 1994, High efficiency retroviral-mediated gene transduction into CD34+ cells purified from peripheral blood of breast cancer patients primed with chemotherapy and granulocyte-macrophage colony-stimulating factor, *Hum. Gene Ther.* **5:**203–208.

Luskey, B. D., Rosenblatt, M., Zsebo, K., and Williams, D. A., 1992, Stem cell factor, interleukin-3, and interleukin-6 promote retroviral-mediated gene transfer into murine hematopoietic stem cells, *Blood* **80:**396–402.

Lyman, S. D., James, L., Vanden Bos, T., de Vries, P., Brasel, K., Gliniak, B., Hollingsworth, L. T., Picha, K. S., McKenna, H. J., Splett, R. R., *et al.*, 1993, Molecular cloning of a ligand for the flt3/flk-2 tyrosine kinase receptor: A proliferative factor for primitive hematopoietic cells, *Cell* **75:**1157–1167.

Lyman, S. D., Brasel, K., Rousseau, A. M., and Williams, D. E., 1994a, The flt3 ligand: A hematopoietic stem cell factor whose activities are distinct from steel factor, *Stem Cells* **12**(Suppl 1)**:**99–107.

Lyman, S. D., James, L., Johnson, L., Brasel, K., de Vries, P., Escobar, S. S., Downey, H., Splett, R. R., Beckmann, M. P., and McKenna, H. J., 1994b, Cloning of the human homologue of the murine flt3 ligand: a growth factor for early hematopoietic progenitor cells, *Blood* **83:**2795–2801.

Lyman, S. D., 1995, Biology of flt3 ligand and receptor, *Int. J. Hematol.* **62:**63–73.

Maciejewski, J., Selleri, C., Anderson, S., and Young, N. S., 1995, Fas antigen expression on CD34+ human marrow cells is induced by interferon gamma and tumor necrosis factor alpha and potentiates cytokine-mediated hematopoietic suppression in vitro, *Blood* **85:**3183–3190.

Maly, F. E., Schuerer Maly, C. C., Quilliam, L., Cochrane, C. G., Newburger, P. E., Curnutte, J. T., Gifford, M., and Dinauer, M. C., 1993, Restitution of superoxide generation in autosomal cytochrome-negative chronic granulomatous disease (A22(0) CGD)-derived B lymphocyte cell lines by transfection with p22phox cDNA, *J. Exp. Med.* **178:**2047–2053.

Mannion Henderson, J., Kemp, A., Mohney, T., Nimgaonkar, M., Lancia, J., Beeler, M. T., Mierski, J.,

Bahnson, A. B., Ball, E. D., and Barranger, J. A., 1995, Efficient retroviral mediated transfer of the glucocerebrosidase gene in CD34+ enriched umbilical cord blood human hematopoietic progenitors, *Exp. Hematol.* **23:**1628–1632.

Mano, H., Ishikawa, F., Nishida, J., Hirai, H., and Takaku, F., 1990, A novel protein-tyrosine kinase, tec, is preferentially expressed in liver, *Oncogene* **5:**1781–1786.

Markert, M. L., 1991, Purine nucleoside phosphorylase deficiency, *Immunodeficiency Rev.* **3:**45–81.

Matsuda, T., Takahashi Tezuka, M., Fukada, T., Okuyama, Y., Fujitani, Y., Tsukada, S., Mano, H., Hirai, H., Witte, O. N., and Hirano, T., 1995, Association and activation of Btk and Tec tyrosine kinases by gp130, a signal transducer of the interleukin-6 family of cytokines, *Blood* **85:**627–633.

Matsuura, S., Kishi, F., Tsukahara, M., Nunoi, H., Matsuda, I., Kobayashi, K., and Kajii, T., 1992, Leukocyte adhesion deficiency: Identification of novel mutations in two Japanese patients with a severe form, *Biochem. Biophys. Res. Commun.* **184:**1460–1467.

Matthews, D. J., Clark, P. A., Herbert, J., Morgan, G., Armitage, R. J., Kinnon, C., Minty, A., Grabstein, K. H., Caput, D., Ferrara, P., *et al.*, 1995, Function of the interleukin-2 (IL-2) receptor gamma-chain in biologic responses of X-linked severe combined immunodeficient B cells to IL-2, IL-4, IL-13, and IL-15, *Blood* **85:**38–42.

Mayani, H., Little, M. T., Dragowska, W., Thornbury, G., and Lansdorp, P. M., 1995, Differential effects of the hematopoietic inhibitors MIP-1 alpha, TGF-beta, and TNF-alpha on cytokine-induced proliferation of subpopulations of CD34+ cells purified from cord blood and fetal liver, *Exp. Hematol.* **23:**422–427.

Mayer, L., Kwan, S. P., Thompson, C., Ko, H. S., Chiorazzi, N., Waldmann, T., and Rosen, F., 1986, Evidence for a defect in "switch" T cells in patients with immunodeficiency and hyperimmunoglobulinemia M, *N. Engl. J. Med.* **314:**409–413.

Mazzone, A., and Ricevuti, G., 1995, Leukocyte CD11/CD18 integrins: biological and clinical relevance. *Haematologica.* **80:**161–175.

McNiece, I. K., and Briddell, R. A., 1995, Stem cell factor, *J. Leukocyte Biol.* **58:**14–22.

Medin, J. A., Migita, M., Pawliuk, R., Jacobson, S., Amiri, M., Kluepfel Stahl, S., Brady, R. O., Humphries, R. K., and Karlsson, S., 1996, A bicistronic therapeutic retroviral vector enables sorting of transduced CD34+ cells and corrects the enzyme deficiency in cells from Gaucher patients, *Blood* **87:**1754–1762.

Migita, M., Medin, J. A., Pawliuk, R., Jacobson, S., Nagle, J. W., Anderson, S., Amiri, M., Humphries, R. K., and Karlsson, S., 1996, Selection of transduced CD34+ progenitors and enzymatic correction of cells from Gaucher patients, with bicistronic vectors, *Proc. Natl. Acad. Sci. USA* **92:**12075–12079.

Miller, A. D., 1992a, Human gene therapy comes of age, *Nature* **357:**455–460.

Miller, A. D., 1992b, Retroviral vectors *Curr. Top. Microbiol. Immunol.* **158:**1–24.

Miller, A. D., Miller, D. G., Garcia, J. V., and Lynch, C. M., 1993, Use of retroviral vectors for gene transfer and expression, *Methods Enzymol.* **217:**581–599.

Miller, C. L., Rebel, V. I., Lemieux, M. E., Helgason, C. D., Lansdorp, P. M., and Eaves, C. J., 1996, Studies of W mutant mice provide evidence for alternate mechanisms capable of activating hematopoietic stem cells, *Exp. Hematol.* **24:**185–194.

Miller, D. G., Adam, M. A., and Miller, A. D., 1990, Gene transfer by retrovirus vectors occurs only in cells that are actively replicating at the time of infection, *Mol. Cell. Biol.* **10:**4239–4242.

Moore, K. A., Deisseroth, A. B., Reading, C. L., Williams, D. E., and Belmont, J. W., 1992, Stromal support enhances cell-free retroviral vector transduction of human bone marrow long-term culture-initiating cells, *Blood* **79:**1393–1399.

Morel, F., Cohen Tanugi Cholley, L., Brandolin, G., Dianoux, A. C., Martel, C., Champelovier, P., Seigneurin, J. M., Francois, P., Bost, M., and Vignais, P. V., 1993, The O_2-generating oxidase of B lymphocytes: Epstein–Barr virus-immortalized B lymphocytes as a tool for the identification of defective components of the oxidase in chronic granulomatous disease, *Biochim. Biophys. Acta* **1182:**101–109.

Morrison, S. J., and Weissman, I. L., 1996, The long-term repopulating subset of hematopoietic stem cells is deterministic and isolatable by phenotype, *Immunity* **1:**661–673.

Muench, M. O., Roncarolo, M. G., Menon, S., Xu, Y., Kastelein, R., Zurawski, S., Hannum, C. H., Culpepper, J., Lee, F., and Namikawa, R., 1995, FLK-2/FLT-3 ligand regulates the growth of early myeloid progenitors isolated from human fetal liver, *Blood* **85:**963–972.

Murray, L., DiGiusto, D., Chen, B., Chen, S., Combs, J., Conti, A., Galy, A., Negrin, R., Tricot, G., and Tsukamoto, A., 1994, Analysis of human hematopoietic stem cell populations, *Blood Cells* **20:**364–369.

Murray, L., Chen, B., Galy, A., Chen, S., Tushinski, R., Uchida, N., Negrin, R., Tricot, G., Jagannath, S., Vesole, D., *et al.*, 1995, Enrichment of human hematopoietic stem cell activity in the CD34+Thy-1+Lin- subpopulation from mobilized peripheral blood, *Blood* **85:**368–378.

Murray, L. J., Mandich, D., Bruno, E., DiGiusto, R. K., Fu, W. C., Sutherland, D. R., Hoffman, R., and Tsukamoto, A., 1996, Fetal bone marrow CD34+CD41+ cells are enriched for multipotent hematopoietic progenitors, but not for pluripotent stem cells, *Exp. Hematol.* **24:**236–245.

Musacchio, A., Gibson, T., Lehto, V. P., and Saraste, M., 1992, SH3—an abundant protein domain in search of a function, *FEBS Lett.* **307:**55–61.

Naldini, L., Blomer, U., Gallay, P., Ory, D., Mulligan, R., Gage, F. H., Verma, I. M., and Trono, D., 1996, In vivo gene delivery and stable transduction of nondividing cells by a lentiviral vector, *Science* **272:**263–267.

Nelson, C., Rabb, H., and Arnaout, M. A., 1992, Genetic cause of leukocyte adhesion molecule deficiency. Abnormal splicing and a missense mutation in a conserved region of CD18 impair cell surface expression of beta 2 integrins, *J. Biol. Chem.* **267:**3351–3357.

Newburger, P. E., Malawista, S. E., Dinauer, M. C., Gelbart, T., Woodman, R. C., Chada, S., Shen, Q., van Blaricom, G., Quie, P. G., and Curnutte, J. T., 1994a, Chronic granulomatous disease and glutathione peroxidase deficiency, revisited, *Blood* **84:**3861–3869.

Newburger, P. E., Skalnik, D. G., Hopkins, P. J., Eklund, E. A., and Curnutte, J. T., 1994b, Mutations in the promoter region of the gene for gp91-phox in X-linked chronic granulomatous disease with decreased expression of cytochrome b558, *J. Clin. Invest.* **94:**1205–1211.

Nimgaonkar, M. T., Bahnson, A. B., Boggs, S. S., Ball, E. D., and Barranger, J. A., 1994, Transduction of mobilized peripheral blood CD34+ cells with the glucocerebrosidase cDNA, *Gene Ther.* **1:**201–207.

Noguchi, M., Adelstein, S., Cao, X., and Leonard, W. J., 1993a, Characterization of the human interleukin-2 receptor gamma chain gene, *J. Biol. Chem.* **268:**13601–13608.

Noguchi, M., Nakamura, Y., Russell, S. M., Ziegler, S. F., Tsang, M., Cao, X., and Leonard, W. J., 1993b, Interleukin-2 receptor gamma chain: A functional component of the interleukin-7 receptor, *Science* **262:**1877–1880.

Noguchi, M., Yi, H., Rosenblatt, H. M., Filipovich, A. H., Adelstein, S., Modi, W. S., McBride, O. W., and Leonard, W. J., 1993c, Interleukin-2 receptor gamma chain mutation results in X-linked severe combined immunodeficiency in humans, *Cell* **73:**147–157.

Nolta, J. A., Crooks, G. M., Overell, R. W., Williams, D. E., and Kohn, D. B., 1992, Retroviral vector-mediated gene transfer into primitive human hematopoietic progenitor cells: Effects of mast cell growth factor (MGF) combined with other cytokines, *Exp. Hematol.* **20:**1065–1071.

Nolta, J. A., Smogorzewska, E. M., and Kohn, D. B., 1995, Analysis of optimal conditions for retroviral-mediated transduction of primitive human hematopoietic cells, *Blood* **86:**101–110.

Notarangelo, L. D., Duse, M., and Ugazio, A. G., 1992, Immunodeficiency with hyper-IgM (HIM), *Immunodeficiency Rev.* **3:**101–121.

Nunoi, H., Rotrosen, D., Gallin, J. I., and Malech, H. L., 1988, Two forms of autosomal chronic granulomatous disease lack distinct neutrophil cytosol factors, *Science* **242:**1298–1301.

O'Reilly, M. A., Alterman, L. A., Malcolm, S., Levinsky, R. J., and Kinnon, C., 1992, Identification of CpG islands around the DXS178 locus in the region of the X-linked agammaglobulinaemia gene locus in Xq22, *Hum. Genet.* **90:**275–278.

O'Reilly, M. A., Sweatman, A. K., Bradley, L. D., Alterman, L. A., Lovering, R., Malcolm, S., Levinsky, R. J., and Kinnon, C., 1993, Isolation and mapping of discrete DXS101 loci in Xq22 near the X-linked agammaglobulinaemia gene locus, *Hum. Genet.* **91:**605–608.

O'Shaughnessy, J. A., Cowan, K. H., Nienhuis, A. W., McDonagh, K. T., Sorrentino, B. P., Dunbar, C. E., Chiang, Y., Wilson, W., Goldspiel, B., Kohler, D., *et al.*, 1994, Retroviral mediated transfer of the human multidrug resistance gene (MDR-1) into hematopoietic stem cells during autologous transplantation after intensive chemotherapy for metastatic breast cancer, *Hum. Gene Ther.* **5:**891–911.

Oez, S., Birkmann, J., Smetak, M., Corbacioglu, S., Hofmann Wackersreuther, G., Welte, K., and Gallmeier, W. M., 1993, Regulation of the density of the stem cell factor receptor (c-kit) by tumor necrosis factor alpha on a human myeloid cell line, *Eur. Cytokine Netw.* **4:**439–445.

Okada, S., Nakauchi, H., Nagayoshi, K., Nishikawa, S., Miura, Y., and Suda, T., 1992, In vivo and in vitro stem cell function of c-kit- and Sca-1-positive murine hematopoietic cells, *Blood* **80:**3044–3050.

Olweus, J., Lund Johansen, F., and Terstappen, L. W., 1994, Expression of cell surface markers during differentiation of CD34+, CD38-/lo fetal and adult bone marrow cells, *Immunomethods* **5:**179–188.

Orlic, D., Fischer, R., Nishikawa, S., Nienhuis, A. W., and Bodine, D. M., 1993, Purification and characterization of heterogeneous pluripotent hematopoietic stem cell populations expressing high levels of c-kit receptor, *Blood* **82:**762–770.

Orlic, D., Anderson, S., Biesecker, L. G., Sorrentino, B. P., and Bodine, D. M., 1995, Pluripotent hematopoietic stem cells contain high levels of mRNA for c-kit, GATA-2, p45 NF-E2, and c-myb and low levels or no mRNA for c-fms and the receptors for granulocyte colony-stimulating factor and interleukins 5 and 7, *Proc. Natl. Acad. Sci. USA* **92:**4601–4605.

Orlic, D., and Bodine, D. M., 1994, What defines a pluripotent hematopoietic stem cell (PHSC): Will the real PHSC please stand up! *Blood* **84:**3991–3994.

Osawa, M., Nakamura, K., Nishi, N., Takahasi, N., Tokuomoto, Y., Inoue, H., and Nakauchi, H., 1996, In vivo self-renewal of c-Kit+ Sca-1+ Lin(low/-) hemopoietic stem cells, *J. Immunol.* **156:**3207–3214.

Osborne, W. R., Hock, R. A., Kaleko, M., and Miller, A. D., 1990, Long-term expression of human adenosine deaminase in mice after transplantation of bone marrow infected with amphotropic retroviral vectors, *Hum. Gene Ther.* **1:**31–41.

Padayachee, M., Levinsky, R. J., Kinnon, C., Finn, A., McKeown, C., Feighery, C., Notarangelo, L. D., Hendriks, R. W., Read, A. P., and Malcolm, S., 1993, Mapping of the X linked form of hyper IgM syndrome (HIGM1), *J. Med. Genet.* **30:**202–205.

Palacios, R., Bucana, C., and Xie, X., 1996, Long-term culture of lymphohematopoietic stem cells, *Proc. Natl. Acad. Sci. USA* **93:**5247–5252.

Paller, A. S., Nanda, V., Spates, C., and O'Gorman, M., 1994, Leukocyte adhesion deficiency: Recurrent childhood skin infections, *J. Am. Acad. Dermatol.* **31:**316–319.

Palmer, T. D., Hock, R. A., Osborne, W. R., and Miller, A. D., 1987, Efficient retrovirus-mediated transfer and expression of a human adenosine deaminase gene in diploid skin fibroblasts from an adenosine deaminase-deficient human, *Proc. Natl. Acad. Sci. USA* **84:**1055–1059.

Park, J. R., Bernstein, I. D., and Hockenbery, D. M., 1995, Primitive human hematopoietic precursors express Bcl-x but not Bcl-2, *Blood* **86:**868–876.

Parkar, M., Lovering, R., Levinsky, R. J., and Kinnon, C., 1994, Genetic mapping of two loci, DXS454 and DXS458, with respect to the X-linked agammaglobulinemia gene locus, *Hum. Genet.* **93:**89–90.

Parkman, R., Rappeport, J., Geha, R., Belli, J., Cassady, R., Levey, R., Nathan, D. G., and Rosen, F. S., 1978, Complete Correction of the Wiskott–Aldrich syndrome by allogeneic bone-marrow transplantation, *N. Engl. J. Med.* **298:**921–927.

Parkos, C. A., Allen, R. A., Cochrane, C. G., and Jesaitis, A. J., 1987, Purified cytochrome b from human granulocyte plasma membrane is comprised of two polypeptides with relative molecular weights of 91,000 and 22,000, *J. Clin. Invest.* **80:**732–742.

Parkos, C. A., Dinauer, M. C., Walker, L. E., Allen, R. A., Jesaitis, A. J., and Orkin, S. H., 1988, Primary structure and unique expression of the 22-kilodalton light chain of human neutrophil cytochrome b, *Proc. Natl. Acad. Sci. USA* **85:**3319–3323.

Pawliuk, R., Kay, R., Lansdorp, P., and Humphries, R. K., 1994, Selection of retrovirally transduced hematopoietic cells using CD24 as a marker of gene transfer, *Blood* **84:**2868–2877.

Pepper, A. E., Buckley, R. H., Small, T. N., and Puck, J. M., 1995, Two mutational hotspots in the interleukin-2 receptor gamma chain gene causing human X-linked severe combined immunodeficiency, *Am. J. Hum. Genet.* **57:**564–571.

Petzer, A. L., Hogge, D. E., Landsdorp, P. M., Reid, D. S., and Eaves, C. J., 1996, Self-renewal of primitive human hematopoietic cells (long-term-culture-initiating cells) in vitro and their expansion in defined medium, *Proc. Natl. Acad. Sci. USA* **93:**1470–1474.

Philips, M. R., Feoktistov, A., Pillinger, M. H., and Abramson, S. B., 1995, Translocation of p21rac2 from cytosol to plasma membrane is neither necessary nor sufficient for neutrophil NADPH oxidase activity, *J. Biol. Chem.* **270:**11514–11521.

Phillips, R. L., Reinhart, A. J., and Van Zant, G., 1992, Genetic control of murine hematopoietic stem cell pool sizes and cycling kinetics, *Proc. Natl. Acad. Sci. USA* **89:**11607–11611.

Porter, C. D., Parkar, M. H., Levinsky, R. J., Collins, M. K., and Kinnon, C., 1993, X-linked chronic granulomatous disease: Correction of NADPH oxidase defect by retrovirus-mediated expression of gp91-phox, *Blood* **82:**2196–2202.

Porter, C. D., Parkar, M. H., Verhoeven, A. J., Levinsky, R. J., Collins, M. K., and Kinnon, C., 1994, p22-phox-deficient chronic granulomatous disease: Reconstitution by retrovirus-mediated expression and identification of a biosynthetic intermediate of gp91-phox, *Blood* **84:**2767–2775.

Porter, C. D., Parkar, M. H., Collins, M. K., Levinsky, R. J., and Kinnon, C., 1996, Efficient retroviral transduction of human bone marrow progenitor and long-term culture-initiating cells: Partial reconstitution of cells from patients with X-linked chronic granulomatous disease by gp91-phox expression, *Blood* **87:**3722–3730.

Price, T. H., Ochs, H. D., Gershoni Baruch, R., Harlan, J. M., and Etzioni, A., 1994, In vivo neutrophil and lymphocyte function studies in a patient with leukocyte adhesion deficiency type II, *Blood* **84:**1635–1639.

Puck, J. M., 1993, X-linked immunodeficiencies, *Adv. Hum. Genet.* **21:**107–144.

Puck, J. M., Conley, M. E., and Bailey, L. C., 1993a, Refinement of linkage of human severe combined immunodeficiency (SCIDX1) to polymorphic markers in Xq13, *Am. J. Hum. Genet.* **53:**176–184.

Puck, J. M., Deschenes, S. M., Porter, J. C., Dutra, A. S., Brown, C. J., Willard, H. F., and Henthorn, P. S., 1993b, The interleukin-2 receptor gamma chain maps to Xq13.1 and is mutated in X-linked severe combined immunodeficiency, SCIDX1, *Hum. Mol. Genet.* **2:**1099–1104.

Puck, J. M., 1994a, Molecular basis for three X-linked immune disorders, *Hum. Mol. Genet.* **3:**1457–1461.

Puck, J. M., 1994b, Molecular and genetic basis of X-linked immunodeficiency disorders, *J. Clin. Immunol.* **14:**81–89.

Qazilbash, M. H., Walsh, C. E., Russell, S. M., Noguchi, M., Mann, M. M., Leonard, W. J., and Liu, J. M., 1995, Retroviral vector for gene therapy of X-linked severe combined immunodeficiency syndrome, *J. Hematother.* **4:**91–98.

Rabbani, H., de Boer, M., Ahlin, A., Sundin, U., Elinder, G., Hammarstrom, L., Palmblad, J., Smith, C. I., and Roos, D., 1993, A 40-base-pair duplication in the gp91-phox gene leading to X-linked chronic granulomatous disease, *Eur. J. Haematol.* **51:**218–222.

Ramesh, N., Fuleihan, R., and Geha, R., 1994, Molecular pathology of X-linked immunoglobulin deficiency with normal or elevated IgM (HIGMX-1), *Immunol. Rev.* **138:**87–104.

Randall, T. D., Lund, F. E., Howard, M. C., and Weissman, I. L., 1996, Expression of murine CD38 defines a population of long-term reconstituting hematopoietic stem cells, *Blood* **87:**4057–4067.

Rawlings, D. J., Saffran, D. C., Tsukada, S., Largaespada, D. A., Grimaldi, J. C., Cohen, L., Mohr, R. N., Bazan, J. F., Howard, M., Copeland, N. G., *et al.*, 1993, Mutation of unique region of Bruton's tyrosine kinase in immunodeficient XID mice, *Science* **261:**358–361.

Rawlings, D. J., and Witte, O. N., 1994, Bruton's tyrosine kinase is a key regulator in B-cell development, *Immunol. Rev.* **138:**105–119.

Rebel, V. I., Dragowska, W., Eaves, C. J., Humphries, R. K., and Lansdorp, P. M., 1994, Amplification of Sca-1+ Lin- WGA+ cells in serum-free cultures containing steel factor, interleukin-6, and erythropoietin with maintenance of cells with long-term in vivo reconstituting potential, *Blood* **83:**128–136.

Remold-O'Donnell, E., Rosen, F. S., and Kenney, D. M., 1996, Defects in Wiskott–Aldrich syndrome blood cells, *Blood* **87:**2621–2631.

Richardson, C., and Bank, A., 1995, Preselection of transduced murine hematopoietic stem cell populations leads to increased long-term stability and expression of the human multiple drug resistance gene, *Blood* **86:**2579–2589.

Ridley, A. J., Paterson, H. F., Johnston, C. L., Diekmann, D., and Hall, A., 1992, The small GTP-binding protein rac regulates growth factor-induced membrane ruffling, *Cell* **70:**401–410.

Rivero Lezcano, O. M., Marcilla, A., Sameshima, J. H., and Robbins, K. C., 1995, Wiskott–Aldrich syndrome protein physically associates with Nck through Src homology 3 domains, *Mol. Cell. Biol.* **15:**5725–5731.

Roe, T., Reynolds, T. C., Yu, G., and Brown, P. O., 1993, Integration of murine leukemia virus DNA depends on mitosis, *EMBO J.* **12:**2099–2108.

Roos, D., 1994, The genetic basis of chronic granulomatous disease, *Immunol. Rev.* **138:**121–157.

Rotrosen, D., Yeung, C. L., Leto, T. L., Malech, H. L., and Kwong, C. H., 1992, Cytochrome b558: The flavin-binding component of the phagocyte NADPH oxidase, *Science* **256:**1459–1462.

Rotrosen, D., Yeung, C. L., and Katkin, J. P., 1993, Production of recombinant cytochrome b558 allows reconstitution of the phagocyte NADPH oxidase solely from recombinant proteins, *J. Biol. Chem.* **268:**14256–14260.

Rotrosen, D., and Leto, T. L., 1990, Phosphorylation of neutrophil 47-kDa cytosolic oxidase factor. Translocation to membrane is associated with distinct phosphorylation events, *J. Biol. Chem.* **265:**19910–19915.

Rowley, S. D., Brashem Stein, C., Andrews, R., and Bernstein, I. D., 1993, Hematopoietic precursors resistant to treatment with 4-hydroperoxycyclophosphamide: Requirement for an interaction with marrow stroma in addition to hematopoietic growth factors for maximal generation of colony-forming activity, *Blood* **82:**60–65.

Royer Pokora, B., Kunkel, L. M., Monaco, A. P., Goff, S. C., Newburger, P. E., Baehner, R. L., Cole, F. S., Curnutte, J. T., and Orkin, S. H., 1986a, Cloning the gene for the inherited disorder chronic granulomatous disease on the basis of its chromosomal location, *Cold Spring Harb or. Symp. Quant. Biol.* **51(**Pt 1**):**177–183.

Royer Pokora, B., Kunkel, L. M., Monaco, A. P., Goff, S. C., Newburger, P. E., Baehner, R. L., Cole, F. S., Curnutte, J. T., and Orkin, S. H., 1986b, Cloning the gene for an inherited human disorder—chronic granulomatous disease—on the basis of its chromosomal location, *Nature* **322:**32–38.

Russell, D. W., Miller, A. D., and Alexander, I. E., 1994, Adeno-associated virus vectors preferentially transduce cells in S phase, *Proc. Natl. Acad. Sci. USA* **91:**8915–8919.

Russell, D. W., Alexander, I. E., and Miller, A. D., 1995, DNA synthesis and topoisomerase inhibitors increase transduction by adeno-associated virus vectors, *Proc. Natl. Acad. Sci. USA* **92:**5719–5723.

Rusten, L. S., Jacobsen, S. E., Kaalhus, O., Veiby, O. P., Funderud, S., and Smeland, E. B., 1994a, Functional differences between CD38– and DR-subfractions of CD34+ bone marrow cells, *Blood* **84:**1473–1481.

Rusten, L. S., Smeland, E. B., Jacobsen, F. W., Lien, E., Lesslauer, W., Loetscher, H., Dubois, C. M., and Jacobsen, S. E., 1994b, Tumor necrosis factor-alpha inhibits stem cell factor-induced proliferation of human bone marrow progenitor cells in vitro. Role of p55 and p75 tumor necrosis factor receptors, *J. Clin. Invest.* **94:**165–172.

Rusten, L. S., Lyman, S. D., Veiby, O. P., and Jacobsen, S. E., 1996, The FLT3 ligand is a direct and potent stimulator of the growth of primitive and committed human CD34+ bone marrow progenitor cells in vitro, *Blood* **87:**1317–1325.

Saffran, D. C., Parolini, O., Fitch Hilgenberg, M. E., Rawlings, D. J., Afar, D. E., Witte, O. N., and Conley, M. E., 1994, Brief report: A point mutation in the SH2 domain of Bruton's tyrosine kinase in atypical X-linked agammaglobulinemia, *N. Engl. J. Med.* **330:**1488–1491.

Santos Argumedo, L., Lund, F. E., Heath, A. W., Solvason, N., Wu, W. W., Grimaldi, J. C., Parkhouse, R. M., and Howard, M., 1995, CD38 unresponsiveness of xid B cells implicates Bruton's tyrosine kinase (btk) as a regulator of CD38 induced signal transduction, *Int. Immunol.* **7:**163–170.

Sato, S., Katagiri, T., Takaki, S., Kikuchi, Y., Hitoshi, Y., Yonehara, S., Tsukada, S., Kitamura, D., Watanabe, T., Witte, O., *et al.*, 1994, IL-5 receptor-mediated tyrosine phosphorylation of SH2/SH3-containing proteins and activation of Bruton's tyrosine and Janus 2 kinases, *J. Exp. Med.* **180:**2101–2111.

Schapiro, B. L., Newburger, P. E., Klempner, M. S., and Dinauer, M. C., 1991, Chronic granulomatous disease presenting in a 69-year-old man, *N. Engl. J. Med.* **325:**1786–1790.

Schmalstieg, F. C., Leonard, W. J., Noguchi, M., Berg, M., Rudloff, H. E., Denney, R. M., Dave, S. K., Brooks, E. G., and Goldman, A. S., 1995, Missense mutation in exon 7 of the common gamma chain gene causes a moderate form of X-linked combined immunodeficiency, *J. Clin. Invest.* **95:**1169–1173.

Schuening, F., Miller, A. D., Torok Storb, B., Bensinger, W., Storb, R., Reynolds, T., Fisher, L., Buckner, C. D., and Appelbaum, F. R., 1994, Study on contribution of genetically marked peripheral blood repopulating cells to hematopoietic reconstitution after transplantation, *Hum. Gene Ther.* **5:**1523–1534.

Schwarzenberger, P., Spence, S., Lohrey, N., Kmiecik, T., Longo, D. L., Murphy, W. J., Ruscetti, F. W., and Keller, J. R., 1996, Gene transfer of multidrug resistance into a factor-dependent human hematopoietic progenitor cell line: In vivo model for genetically transferred chemoprotection, *Blood* **87:**2723–2731.

Segal, A. W., Geisow, M., Garcia, R., Harper, A., and Miller, R., 1981, The respiratory burst of phagocytic cells is associated with a rise in vacuolar pH, *Nature* **290:**406–409.

Segal, A. W., Harper, A. M., Cross, A. R., and Jones, O. T., 1986, Cytochrome b-245, *Methods Enzymol.* **132:**378–394.

Segal, A. W., 1987, Absence of both cytochrome b-245 subunits from neutrophils in X-linked chronic granulomatous disease, *Nature* **326:**88–91.

Segal, A. W., 1989, The electron transport chain of the microbicidal oxidase of phagocytic cells and its involvement in the molecular pathology of chronic granulomatous disease, *J. Clin. Invest.* **83:**1785–1793.

Segal, A. W., 1991, Components of the microbicidal oxidase of phagocytes, *Biochem. Soc. Trans.* **19:**49–50.

Segal, A. W., West, I., Wientjes, F., Nugent, J. H., Chavan, A. J., Haley, B., Garcia, R. C., Rosen, H., and Scrace, G., 1992, Cytochrome b-245 is a flavocytochrome containing FAD and the NADPH-binding site of the microbicidal oxidase of phagocytes, *Biochem. J.* **284:**781–788.

Segal, A. W., and Abo, A., 1993, The biochemical basis of the NADPH oxidase of phagocytes, *Trends Biochem. Sci.* **18:**43–47.

Segal, A. W., and Jones, O. T., 1980, Absence of cytochrome b reduction in stimulated neutrophils from both female and male patients with chronic granulomatous disease, *FEBS Lett.* **110:**111–114.

Sekhsaria, S., Gallin, J. I., Linton, G. F., Mallory, R. M., Mulligan, R. C., and Malech, H. L., 1993, Peripheral blood progenitors as a target for genetic correction of p47phox-deficient chronic granulomatous disease, *Proc. Natl. Acad. Sci. USA* **90:**7446–7450.

Sekhsaria, S., Fleisher, T. A., Vowells, S., Brown, M., Miller, J., Gordon, I., Blaese, R. M., Dunbar, C. E., Leitman, S., and Malech, H. L., 1996, Granulocyte colony-stimulating factor recruitment of CD34+ progenitors to peripheral blood: Impaired mobilization in chronic granulomatous disease and adenosine deaminase—deficient severe combined immunodeficiency disease patients, *Blood* **88:** 1104–1112.

Selleri, C., Maciejewski, J. P., Sato, T., and Young, N. S., 1996, Interferon-gamma constitutively expressed in the stromal microenvironment of human marrow cultures mediates potent hematopoietic inhibition, *Blood* **87:**4149–4157.

Shah, A. J., Smogorzewska, E. M., Hannum, C., and Crooks, G. M., 1996, Flt3 ligand induces proliferation of quiescent human bone marrow CD34+CD38– cells and maintains progenitor cells in vitro, *Blood* **87:**3563–3570.

Shah, G., Dexter, T. M., and Lanotte, M., 1983, Interferon production by human marrow stromal cells, *Br. J. Haematol.* **54:**365–372.

Shaw, G., 1996, The pleckstrin homology domain: An intriguing multifunctional protein module, *Bioessays* **18:**35–46.

Shi, Y. J., Shen, R. N., Lu, L., and Broxmeyer, H. E., 1994, Comparative analysis of retroviral-mediated gene transduction into CD34+ cord blood hematopoietic progenitors in the presence and absence of growth factors, *Blood Cells* **20:**517–524.

Shiohara, M., Koike, K., and Nakahata, T., 1993, Synergism of interferon-gamma and stem cell factor on the development of murine hematopoietic progenitors in serum-free culture, *Blood* **81:**1435–1441.

Siliciano, J. D., Morrow, T. A., and Desiderio, S. V., 1992, itk, a T-cell-specific tyrosine kinase gene inducible by interleukin 2, *Proc. Natl. Acad. Sci. USA* **89:**11194–11198.

Silvennoinen, O., Nishigaki, H., Kitanaka, A., Kumagai, M., Ito, C., Malavasi, F., Lin, Q., Conley, M. E., and Campana, D., 1996, CD38 signal transduction in human B cell precursors. Rapid induction of tyrosine phosphorylation, activation of syk tyrosine kinase, and phosphorylation of phospholipase C-gamma and phosphatidylinositol 3-kinase, *J. Immunol.* **156:**100–107.

Sligh, J. E., Jr., Hurwitz, M. Y., Zhu, C. M., Anderson, D. C., and Beaudet, A. L., 1992, An initiation codon mutation in CD18 in association with the moderate phenotype of leukocyte adhesion deficiency, *J. Biol. Chem.* **267:**714–718.

Small, D., Levenstein, M., Kim, E., Carow, C., Amin, S., Rockwell, P., Witte, L., Burrow, C., Ratajczak, M. Z., Gewirtz, A. M., *et al.*, 1994, STK-1, the human homolog of Flk-2/Flt-3, is selectively expressed in CD34+ human bone marrow cells and is involved in the proliferation of early progenitor/stem cells, *Proc. Natl. Acad. Sci. USA* **91:**459–463.

Smith, C. I., Islam, K. B., Vorechovsky, I., Olerup, O., Wallin, E., Rabbani, H., Baskin, B., and Hammarstrom, L., 1994, X-linked agammaglobulinemia and other immunoglobulin deficiencies, *Immunol. Rev.* **138:**159–183.

Smith, R. M., and Curnutte, J. T., 1991, Molecular basis of chronic granulomatous disease, *Blood* **77:**673–686.

Snoeck, H. W., Van Bockstaele, D. R., Nys, G., Lenjou, M., Lardon, F., Haenen, L., Rodrigus, I., Peetermans, M. E., and Berneman, Z. N., 1994, Interferon gamma selectively inhibits very primitive CD342+CD38– and not more mature CD34+CD38+ human hematopoietic progenitor cells, *J. Exp. Med.* **180:**1177–1182.

Sokolic, R. A., Sekhsaria, S., Sugimoto, Y., Whiting Theobald, N., Linton, G. F., Li, F., Gottesman, M. M., and Malech, H. L., 1996, A bicistronic retrovirus vector containing a picornavirus internal ribosome entry site allows for correction of X-linked CGD by selection for MDR1 expression, *Blood* **87:**42–50.

Spooncer, E., and Dexter, T. M., 1984, Long-term bone marrow cultures, *Bibl. Haematol.* **48:**366–383.

Stephenson, J., 1995, Terms of engraftment: Umbilical cord blood transplants arouse enthusiasm, *JAMA* **273:**1813–1815.

Sumimoto, H., Kage, Y., Nunoi, H., Sasaki, H., Nose, T., Fukumaki, Y., Ohno, M., Minakami, S., and Takeshige, K., 1994, Role of Src homology 3 domains in assembly and activation of the phagocyte NADPH oxidase, *Proc. Natl. Acad. Sci. USA* **91:**5345–5349.

Sutherland, D. R., Yeo, E. L., Stewart, A. K., Nayar, R., DiGiusto, R., Zanjani, E., Hoffman, R., and Murray, L. J., 1996, Identification of CD34+ subsets after glycoprotease selection: Engraftment of CD34+Thy-1+Lin- stem cells in fetal sheep, *Exp. Hematol.* **24:**795–806.

Sutherland, H. J., Hogge, D. E., and Eaves, C. J., 1993, Growth factor regulation of the maintenance and differentiation of human long-term culture-initiating cells (LTC-IC), *Leukemia* **7**(Suppl. 2)**:**S122–125.

Sutherland, H. J., Hogge, D. E., Lansdorp, P. M., Phillips, G. L., Eaves, A. C., and Eaves, C. J., 1995, Quantitation, mobilization, and clinical use of long-term culture-initiating cells in blood cell autografts, *J. Hematother.* **4:**3–10.

Sweatman, A., Lovering, R., Middleton Price, H., Jones, A., Morgan, G., Levinsky, R., and Kinnon, C., 1993, A new restriction fragment length polymorphism at the DXS101 locus allows carrier detection in a family with X linked agammaglobulinaemia, *J. Med. Genet.* **30:**512–514.

Symons, M., Derry, J. M., Karlak, B., Jiang, S., Lemahieu, V., McCormick, F., Francke, U., and Abo, A., 1996, Wiskott–Aldrich syndrome protein, a novel effector for the GTPase CDC42Hs, is implicated in actin polymerization, *Cell* **84:**723–734.

Szilvassy, S. J., and Cory, S., 1994, Efficient retroviral gene transfer to purified long-term repopulating hematopoietic stem cells, *Blood* **84:**74–83.

Takeshita, T., Asao, H., Ohtani, K., Ishii, N., Kumaki, S., Tanaka, N., Munakata, H., Nakamura, M., and Sugamura, K., 1992, Cloning of the gamma chain of the human IL-2 receptor, *Science* **257:**379–382.

Taniguchi, T., and Minami, Y., 1993, The IL-2/IL-2 receptor system: A current overview, *Cell* **73:**5–8.

Taylor, N., Uribe, L., Smith, S., Jahn, T., Kohn, D. B., and Weinberg, K., 1996, Correction of interleukin-2 receptor function in X-SCID lymphoblastoid cells by retrovirally mediated transfer of the gamma-c gene, *Blood* **87:**3103–3107.

Taylor, W. R., Jones, D. T., and Segal, A. W., 1993, A structural model for the nucleotide binding domains of the flavocytochrome b-245 beta-chain, *Protein Sci.* **2:**1675–1685.

Teahan, C., Rowe, P., Parker, P., Totty, N., and Segal, A. W., 1987, The X-linked chronic granulomatous disease gene codes for the beta-chain of cytochrome b-245, *Nature* **327:**720–721.

Terstappen, L. W., Huang, S., Safford, M., Lansdorp, P. M., and Loken, M. R., 1991, Sequential generations of hematopoietic colonies derived from single nonlineage-committed CD34+CD38– progenitor cells, *Blood* **77:**1218–1227.

Terstappen, L. W., and Huang, S., 1994, Analysis of bone marrow stem cell, *Blood Cells* **20:**45–61.

Thomas, J. D., Sideras, P., Smith, C. I., Vorechovsky, I., Chapman, V., and Paul, W. E., 1993, Colocalization of X-linked agammaglobulinemia and X-linked immunodeficiency genes, *Science* **261:**355–358.

Thrasher, A., Chetty, M., Casimir, C., and Segal, A. W., 1992, Restoration of superoxide generation to a chronic granulomatous disease-derived B-cell line by retrovirus mediated gene transfer, *Blood* **80:**1125–1129.

Thrasher, A., Segal, A., and Casimir, C., 1993, Chronic granulomatous disease: Toward gene therapy, *Immunodeficiency* **4:**327–333.

Thrasher, A. J., Keep, N. H., Wientjes, F., and Segal, A. W., 1994, Chronic granulomatous disease, *Biochim. Biophys. Acta* **1227:**1–24.

Thrasher, A. J., Casimir, C. M., Kinnon, C., Morgan, G., Segal, A. W., and Levinsky, R. J., 1995a, Gene transfer to primary chronic granulomatous disease monocytes, *Lancet* **346:**92–93.

Thrasher, A. J., de Alwis, M., Casimir, C. M., Kinnon, C., Page, K., Lebkowski, J., Segal, A. W., and Levinsky, R. J., 1995b, Functional reconstitution of the NADPH-oxidase by adeno-associated virus gene transfer, *Blood* **86:**761–765.

Tohma, S., Hirohata, S., and Lipsky, P. E., 1991, The role of CD11a/CD18-CD54 interactions in human T cell-dependent B cell activation, *J. Immunol.* **146:**492–499.

Tsukada, S., Saffran, D. C., Rawlings, D. J., Parolini, O., Allen, R. C., Klisak, I., Sparkes, R. S., Kubagawa, H., Mohandas, T., Quan, S., *et al.*, 1993, Deficient expression of a B cell cytoplasmic tyrosine kinase in human X-linked agammaglobulinemia, *Cell* **72:**279–290.

Tsukada, S., Rawlings, D. J., and Witte, O. N., 1994, Role of Bruton's tyrosine kinase in immunodeficiency, *Curr. Opinion Immunol.* **6:**623–630.

Tsunawaki, S., Mizunari, H., Nagata, M., Tatsuzawa, O., and Kuratsuji, T., 1994, A novel cytosolic component, p40phox, of respiratory burst oxidase associates with p67phox and is absent in patients with chronic granulomatous disease who lack p67phox, *Biochem. Biophys. Res. Commun.* **199:**1378–1387.

Uchida, N., Jerabek. L., and Weissman, I. L., 1996, Searching for hematopoietic stem cells. II. The heterogeneity of Thy-1.1(lo)Lin(-/lo)Sca-1+ mouse hematopoietic stem cells separated by counterflow centrifugal elutriation, *Exp. Hematol.* **24:**649–659.

Valerio, D., Duyvesteyn, M. G., Meera Khan, P., Geurts and van Kessel, A., de Waard, A., van der Eb, A. J., 1983, Isolation of cDNA clones for human adenosine deaminase, *Gene* **25:**231–240.

van Beusechem, V. W., Kukler, A., Einerhand, M. P., Bakx, T. A., van der Eb, A. J., van Bekkum, D. W., and Valerio, D., 1990, Expression of human adenosine deaminase in mice transplanted with hemopoietic stem cells infected with amphotropic retroviruses, *J. Exp. Med.* **172:**729–736.

van Beusechem, V. W., Kukler, A., Heidt, P. J., and Valerio, D., 1992, Long-term expression of human adenosine deaminase in rhesus monkeys transplanted with retrovirus-infected bone-marrow cells, *Proc. Natl. Acad. Sci. USA* **89:**7640–7644.

van Beusechem, V. W., Bakx, T. A., Kaptein, L. C., Bart Baumeister, J. A., Kukler, A., Braakman, E., and Valerio, D., 1993, Retrovirus-mediated gene transfer into rhesus monkey hematopoietic stem cells: The effect of viral titers on transduction efficiency, *Hum. Gene Ther.* **4:**239–247.

van Beusechem, V. W., Bart Baumeister, J. A., Bakx, T. A., Kaptein, L. C., Levinsky, R. J., and Valerio, D., 1994, Gene transfer into nonhuman primate CD34+CD11b- bone marrow progenitor cells capable of repopulating lymphoid and myeloid lineages, *Hum. Gene Ther.* **5:**295–305.

van Beusechem, V. W., Bart Baumeister, J. A., Hoogerbrugge, P. M., and Valerio, D., 1995, Influence of interleukin-3, interleukin-6, and stem cell factor on retroviral transduction of rhesus monkey CD34+ hematopoietic progenitor cells measured in vitro and in vivo, *Gene Ther.* **2:**245–255.

Van Epps, D. E., Bender, J., Lee, W., Schilling, M., Smith, A., Smith, S., Unverzagt, K., Law, P., and Burgess, J., 1994, Harvesting, characterization, and culture of CD34+ cells from human bone marrow, peripheral blood, and cord blood, *Blood Cells* **20:**411–423.

Verfaillie, C. M., Catanzarro, P. M., and Li, W. N., 1994, Macrophage inflammatory protein 1 alpha, interleukin 3 and diffusible marrow stromal factors maintain human hematopoietic stem cells for at least eight weeks in vitro, *J. Exp. Med.* **179:**643–649.

Vetrie, D., Vorechovsky, I., Sideras, P., Holland, J., Davies, A., Flinter, F., Hammarstrom, L., Kinnon, C., Levinsky, R., Bobrow, M., *et al.*, 1993, The gene involved in X-linked agammaglobulinaemia is a member of the src family of protein-tyrosine kinases, *Nature* **361:**226–233.

Vihinen, M., Zvelebil, M. J., Zhu, Q., Brooimans, R. A., Ochs, H. D., Zegers, B. J., Nilsson, L., Waterfield, M. D., and Smith, C. I., 1995, Structural basis for pleckstrin homology domain mutations in X-linked agammaglobulinemia, *Biochemistry* **34:**1475–1481.

Vihinen, M., Iwata, T., Kinnon, C., Kwan, S. P., Ochs, H. D., Vorechovsky, I., and Smith, C. I., 1996, BTKbase, mutation database for X-linked agammaglobulinemia (XLA), *Nucleic Acids Res.* **24:**160–165.

Vile, R. G., and Russell, S. J., 1995, Retroviruses as vectors, *Br. Med. Bull.* **51:**12–30.

Villa, A., Notarangelo, L., Macchi, P., Mantuano, E., Cavagni, G., Brugnoni, D., Strina, D., Patrosso, M. C., Ramenghi, U., Sacco, M. G., *et al.*, 1995, X-linked thrombocytopenia and Wiskott–Aldrich syndrome are allelic diseases with mutations in the WASP gene, *Nat. Genet.* **9:**414–417.

Volpp, B. D., Nauseef, W. M., and Clark, R. A., 1988, Two cytosolic neutrophil oxidase components absent in autosomal chronic granulomatous disease, *Science* **242:**1295–1297.

Volpp, B. D., and Lin, Y., 1993, In vitro molecular reconstitution of the respiratory burst in B lymphoblasts from p47-phox-deficient chronic granulomatous disease, *J. Clin. Invest.* **91:**201–207.

von Kalle, C., Kiem, H. P., Goehle, S., Darovsky, B., Heimfeld, S., Torok Storb, B., Storb, R., and Schuening, F. G., 1994, Increased gene transfer into human hematopoietic progenitor cells by extended in vitro exposure to a pseudotyped retroviral vector, *Blood* **84:**2890–2897.

Vorechovsky, I., Vihinen, M., de Saint Basile, G., Honsova, S., Hammarstrom, L., Muller, S., Nilsson, L., Fischer, A., and Smith, C. I., 1995, DNA-based mutation analysis of Bruton's tyrosine kinase gene in patients with X-linked agammaglobulinaemia, *Hum. Mol. Genet.* **4:**51–58.

Vormoor, J., Lapidot, T., Pflumio, F., Risdon, G., Patterson, B., Broxmeyer, H. E., and Dick, J. E., 1994, Immature human cord blood progenitors engraft and proliferate to high levels in severe combined immunodeficient mice, *Blood* **83:**2489–2497.

Wagner, J. E., 1995, Umbilical cord blood transplantation, *Transfusion* **35:**619–621.

Walsh, C. E., Mann, M. M., Emmons, R. V., Wang, S., and Liu, J. M., 1995, Transduction of CD34-enriched human peripheral and umbilical cord blood progenitors using a retroviral vector with the Fanconi anemia group C gene, *J. Invest. Med.* **43:**379–385.

Ward, M., Richardson, C., Pioli, P., Smith, L., Podda, S., Goff, S., Hesdorffer, C., and Bank, A., 1994, Transfer and expression of the human multiple drug resistance gene in human CD34+ cells, *Blood* **84:**1408–1414.

Weinberg, K., and Parkman, R., 1990, Severe combined immunodeficiency due to a specific defect in the production of interleukin-2, *N. Engl. J. Med.* **322:**1741–1743.

Wells, S., Malik, P., Pensiero, M., Kohn, D. B., and Nolta, J. A., 1995, The presence of an autologous marrow stromal cell layer increases glucocerebrosidase gene transduction of long-term culture initiating cells (LTCICs) from the bone marrow of a patient with Gaucher disease, *Gene Ther.* **2:**512–520.

Wengler, G. S., Notarangelo, L. D., Berardelli, S., Pollonni, G., Mella, P., Fasth, A., Ugazio, A. G., and Parolini, O., 1995, High prevalence of nonsense, frameshift, and splice-site mutations in 16 patients with full-blown Wiskott–Aldrich syndrome, *Blood* **86:**3648–3654.

Wieder, R., Cornetta, K., Kessler, S. W., and Anderson, W. F., 1991, Increased efficiency of retroviral-mediated gene transfer and expression in primate bone marrow progenitors after 5-fluorouracil-induced hematopoietic suppression and recovery, *Blood* **77:**448–455.

Wientjes, F. B., Hsuan, J. J., Totty, N. F., and Segal, A. W., 1993, p40phox, a third cytosolic component of the activation complex of the NADPH oxidase to contain src homology 3 domains, *Biochem. J.* **296:**557–561.

Wientjes, F. B., Panayotou, G., Reeves, E., and Segal, A. W., 1996, Interactions between cytosolic components of the NADPH oxidase: p40phox interacts with both p67phox and p47phox, *Biochem. J.* **317:**919–924.

Wiginton, D. A., Adrian, G. S., Friedman, R. L., Suttle, D. P., and Hutton, J. J., 1983, Cloning of cDNA sequences of human adenosine deaminase, *Proc. Natl. Acad. Sci. USA* **80:**7481–7485.

Williams, D. A., Lemischka, I. R., Nathan, D. G., and Mulligan, R. C., 1984, Introduction of new genetic material into pluripotent haematopoietic stem cells of the mouse, *Nature* **310:**476–480.

Williams, D. A., Orkin, S. H., and Mulligan, R. C., 1986, Retrovirus-mediated transfer of human adenosine deaminase gene sequences into cells in culture and into murine hematopoietic cells in vivo, *Proc. Natl. Acad. Sci. USA* **83:**2566–2570.

Williams, D. A., Lim, B., and Orkin, S. H., 1987, Transfer and expression of human ADA in murine hematopoietic stem cells, *Prog. Clin. Biol. Res.* **251:**567–580.

Williams, D. A., and Moritz, T., 1994, Umbilical cord blood stem cells as targets for genetic modification: New therapeutic approaches to somatic gene therapy, *Blood Cells* **20:**504–515.

Woodman, R. C., Newburger, P. E., Anklesaria, P., Erickson, R. W., Rae, J., Cohen, M. S., and Curnutte, J. T., 1995, A new X-linked variant of chronic granulomatous disease characterized by the existence of a normal clone of respiratory burst-competent phagocytic cells, *Blood* **85:**231–241.

Wright, A. H., Douglass, W. A., Taylor, G. M., Lau, Y. L., Higgins, D., Davies, K. A., and Law, S. K., 1995, Molecular characterization of leukocyte adhesion deficiency in six patients, *Eur. J. Immunol.* **25:**717–722.

Wright, E. G., and Pragnell, I. B., 1992, Stem cell proliferation inhibitors, *Baillieres Clin. Haematol.* **5:**723–739.

Xu, L. C., Karlsson, S., Byrne, E. R., Kluepfel Stahl, S., Kessler, S. W., Agricola, B. A., Sellers, S., Kirby, M., Dunbar, C. E., Brady, R. O., *et al.*, 1995a, Long-term in vivo expression of the human glucocerebrosidase gene in nonhuman primates after CD34+ hematopoietic cell transduction with cell-free retroviral vector preparations, *Proc. Natl. Acad. Sci. USA* **92:**4372–4376.

Xu, L. C., Kluepfel Stahl, S., Blanco, M., Schiffmann, R., Dunbar, C., and Karlsson, S., 1995b, Growth factors and stromal support generate very efficient retroviral transduction of peripheral blood CD34+ cells from Gaucher patients, *Blood* **86:**141–146.

Yan, X. Q., Briddell, R., Hartley, C., Stoney, G., Samal, B., and McNiece, I., 1994, Mobilization of long-term hematopoietic reconstituting cells in mice by the combination of stem cell factor plus granulocyte colony-stimulating factor, *Blood* **84:**795–799.

Yan, X. Q., Hartley, C., McElroy, P., Chang, A., McCrea, C., and McNiece, I., 1995, Peripheral blood progenitor cells mobilized by recombinant human granulocyte colony-stimulating factor plus recombinant rat stem cell factor contain long-term engrafting cells capable of cellular proliferation for more than two years as shown by serial transplantation in mice, *Blood* **98:**2303–2307.

Yang, Q., Chen, F., and Trempe, J. P., 1994, Characterization of cell lines that inducibly express the adeno-associated virus Rep proteins, *J. Virol.* **68:**4847–4856.

Yang, Q., Chen, F., Ross, J., and Trempe, J. P., 1995, Inhibition of cellular and SV40 DNA replication by the adeno-associated virus Rep proteins, *Virology* **207:**246–250.

Yao, L., Kawakami, Y., and Kawakami, T., 1994, The pleckstrin homology domain of Bruton tyrosine kinase interacts with protein kinase C, *Proc. Natl. Acad. Sci. USA* **91:**9175–9179.

Yorifuji, T., Wilson, R. W., and Beaudet, A. L., 1993, Retroviral mediated expression of CD18 in normal and deficient human bone marrow progenitor cells, *Hum. Mol. Genet.* **2:**1443–1448.

Young, J. C., Varma, A., DiGiusto, D., and Backer, M. P., 1996, Retention of quiescent hematopoietic cells with high proliferative potential during ex vivo stem cell culture, *Blood* **87:**545–556.

Zeigler, F. C., Bennett, B. D., Jordan, C. T., Spencer, S. D., Baumhueter, S., Carroll, K. J., Hooley, J., Bauer, K., and Matthews, W., 1994, Cellular and molecular characterization of the role of the flk-2/flt-3 receptor tyrosine kinase in hematopoietic stem cells, *Blood* **84:**2422–2430.

Zhen, L., King, A. A., Xiao, Y., Chanock, S. J., Orkin, S. H., and Dinauer, M. C., 1993, Gene targeting of X chromosome-linked chronic granulomatous disease locus in a human myeloid leukemia cell line and rescue by expression of recombinant gp91phox, *Proc. Natl. Acad. Sci. USA* **90:**9832–9836.

Zhu, Q., Zhang, M., Rawlings, D. J., Vihinen, M., Hagemann, T., Saffran, D. C., Kwan, S. P., Nilsson, L., Smith, C. I., Witte, O. N., *et al.*, 1994, Deletion within the Src homology domain 3 of Bruton's tyrosine kinase resulting in X-linked agammaglobulinemia (XLA), *J. Exp. Med.* **180:**461–470.

Zhu, Q., Zhang, M., Blaese, R. M., Derry, J. M., Junker, A., Francke, U., Chen, S. H., and Ochs, H. D., 1995, The Wiskott–Aldrich syndrome and X-linked congenital thrombocytopenia are caused by mutations of the same gene, *Blood* **86:**3797–3804.

Chapter 7

Gene Therapy for Lysosomal Disorders

L. J. Fairbairn and L. S. Lashford

The lysosomal storage disorders (LSDs) represent a wide group of clinically diverse types of disorders that include the mucopolysaccharidoses, sphingolipidoses, and defects in glycoprotein catabolism (Neufeld, 1991). All are characterized by the inability of cellular lysosomes to degrade complex substrates, which stems from a deficiency in one or more lysosomal enzymes. Accumulation of undegraded macromolecules in the lysosomes of cells leads to massive lysosomal distension, anatomical distortion of cells, and functional impairment of affected tissues.

1. DEFINING A POPULATION OF PATIENTS SUITABLE FOR TREATMENT

The tissues affected and the clinical symptoms shown in LSD depend on the particular disorder and also on the severity of that disorder. For example, individuals who have the severe mucopolysaccharidosis, MPSI(H) (Hurler syndrome), exhibit severe bone abnormalities and progressive neurological dysfunction with multiple soft tissue defects that lead to death in the first decade. On the other hand, patients who have the milder Scheie syndrome, MPSI(S), have reduced bone involvement, no neurological dysfunction, fewer soft tissue abnormalities, and a normal life span (Neufeld and Muenzer, 1989). The severity of the disorder is also often reflected in the age at which clinically detectable disease is seen. In general, early onset of clinical disease is associated with the more severe forms of LSD that progress rapidly and have poor prognosis. Thus, one important requirement in the treatment of LSDs is to identify patients at an age where the phenotypic effects of the disorder are still amenable to therapy.

L. J. Fairbairn and L. S. Lashford Paterson Institute for Cancer Research, Christie Hospital (NHS) Trust, Manchester M20 4BX, United Kingdom.

Blood Cell Biochemistry, Volume 8: Hematopoiesis and Gene Therapy, edited by Fairbairn and Testa. Kluwer Academic/Plenum Publishers, New York, 1999.

An important consideration when evaluating an experimental treatment, such as gene therapy, is that it is usual to do so in patients whose prognosis in the absence of effective treatment is poor. Furthermore, in such a clinically heterogeneous group of disorders, such as the LSDs, it is essential to ascertain correctly the likely clinical course of disease in a particular patient group to facilitate analysis of any potential therapeutic effect. All of these issues require defining the patient population accurately and swiftly in terms of severity of disease and likely outcome, and this is currently being addressed by attempting to correlate the genotype of individuals with their phenotype.

1.1. The Relationship between Genotype and Expected Clinical Outcome

Despite the variation of phenotype within individual LSDs and the wide range of mutations which give rise to each disorder, it is becoming clear that certain mutations are associated predominantly with poor prognosis of disease when present as homozygotes or as heterozygotes with other "severe" mutations. For example, in the most common mucopolysaccharidosis, α-L-iduronidase deficiency (MPSI), over 50 mutations have been described which give rise to one or other form of the disorder. However, individuals who are homozygous for the nonsense mutations W402X and Q70X have no detectable IDUA and progress early to severe disease with CNS, bony, and soft tissue defects [MPSI(H)]. Compound heterozygotes, where one of two alleles encodes a truncated protein and the other an enzyme with reduced activity show reduced, but detectable (1–5% of normal), activity and milder but varied phenotype, often with no CNS involvement and a better overall prognosis (Scott *et al.*, 1995).

Similarly, in metachromatic leukodystrophy (MLD, arylsulphatase deficiency), almost 40 mutations have been identified which give rise to the disorder. Homozygotes for deletions and splice site mutations which do not produce functional enzyme, again show early onset of disease which progresses quickly and severely. Heterozygotes, which combine a null mutation with one which produces an active but unstable enzyme (P426L), show 1–5% normal enzyme levels which, because of substantial overcapacity in the wild-type system, account for as much as 30% of normal degradative activity and leads to the less progressive, juvenile form of the disease. Homozygotes for P426L show the mildest form of the disease and have 50% of normal degradative activity and onset in the second decade (Gieselmann *et al.*, 1994).

Thus in these cases and in others, such as homozygosity for N307S in type I Gaucher disease and L44P in a subset of individuals with type III Gaucher disease, it is possible to predict the occurrence of a severe phenotype based on genotype. It should be stressed, however, that this area is still tremendously complex, and often unexpected genotype–phenotype relationships can be seen. However it is hoped that as understanding of the genetics of each disorder improves, the ability to reliably predict phenotype will increase.

1.2. The Availability of Alternative Treatments

A second important consideration when proposing experimental treatment of patients with any inherited or acquired disease or disorder, is the availability of alternative treatment strategies and their efficacy. For the lysosomal storage diseases, this varies from disorder to disorder, but the available treatments fall broadly into three types: supportive care and enzyme replacement by either the administration of exogenous, purified enzyme or by transplantation of cells that synthesize and secrete functional enzyme.

1.2.1. Supportive Care

Supportive care forms the baseline of treatment in all individuals and is used whether or not other treatments are also administered. This can involve surgical intervention to correct skeletal problems in some of the mucopolysaccharidoses or splenectomy in individuals who have Gauchers disease and suffer from massive macrophage infiltration in soft tissues, transfusions to reduce the clinical effects of profound anaemia in Gauchers, and good analgesic care. All of these help prolong and/or improve the quality of life.

1.2.2. Enzyme Therapy

The other alternatives, namely, enzyme and cellular therapy, use what is known about the biosynthesis and intracellular targeting of lysosomal enzymes (Hasilik, 1992; see Figure 1). In general, lysosomal proteins are synthesized and cotranslationally inserted into the rough endoplasmic reticulum where they become N-glycosylated. Then one or more mannose residues are phosphorylated, and the mannose-6-phosphate (M6P) residues act as signals for lysosomal targeting *via* the binding of the M6P receptor (M6P-R) in the Golgi. Then regions of membrane that contain the M6P-R form vesicles which transport the lysosomal enzymes to the lysosomes. Upon fusion of the transport vesicles with the lysosomes, the acidic pH of the lysosomes causes dissociation of the enzymes from the receptor, and proteolytic activation of the lysosomal precursors occurs. Significantly, a proportion of the newly synthesized, mannose-6-phosphorylated enzyme escapes this intracellular targeting mechanism and is secreted from the cells. This extracellular enzyme can be sequestered and retargeted at intracellular lysosomes *via* the binding of receptors at the cell surface (Bou Gharios *et al.*, 1993). Generally this is through the widely expressed M6P-R, although other receptors also contribute, for example, mannose and *N*-acetylglucosamine receptors in the monocyte/macrophage lineage; sialic acid receptors on glial cells; fucose receptors in fibroblasts; and asialogalactose-containing proteins on hepatocytes (Rodman *et al.*, 1990). The phenomenon of enzyme secretion and capture has been demonstrated in classical "cross-correction" studies for a number of disorders. In these studies, cocultivation of wild-type and enzyme-deficient fibroblasts resulted in sequestration of enzyme by the normally deficient cells and correction of lysosomal storage in the "cross-corrected" cells (Vladutiu and Rattazzi, 1979; Willcox and Rattray, 1979). Furthermore, incubation of enzyme-deficient cells in culture medium, previously conditioned by the growth of wild-type cells and containing secreted lysosomal enzymes, also leads to correcting the enzyme defect in those cells. These studies have since been extended to demonstrate cross-correction of other important target cells, including macrophages

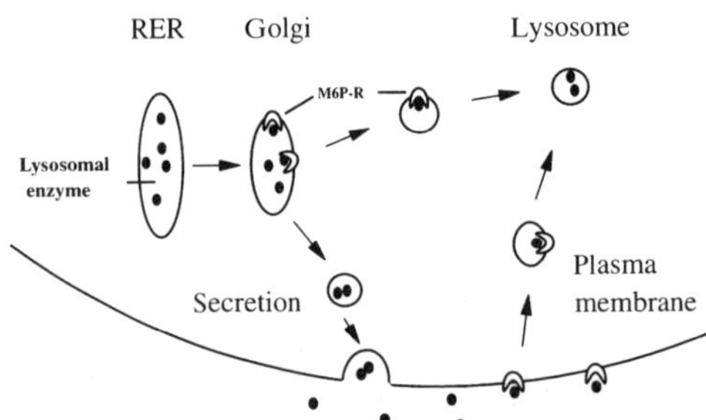

FIGURE 1. Trafficking of lysosomal proteins. Nascent protein, cotranslationally inserted into the rough endoplasmic reticulum (RER) is N-glycosylated. Then one or more mannose residues are phosphorylated, and the protein interacts with the mannose-6-phosphate receptor (M6P-R) in the Golgi. Then regions of membrane containing the M6P-R form vesicles that traffic to and fuse with the lysosomes. The acidic pH of the lysosomes causes dissociation of the enzymes from the receptor, and proteolytic activation of the lysosomal precursors occurs. Extracellular mannose-6-phosphorylated enzyme can be sequestered and targeted at intracellular lysosomes via the binding of receptors at the cell surface.

and cells of the central nervous system (Hill *et al.*, 1985; Stewart *et al.*, 1997). Thus, based on a rationale for correction provided by the synthetic pathway of lysosomal enzymes and experimental evidence of *in vitro* efficacy, both enzyme and cell therapy are being exploited to treat some lysosomal storage diseases.

Enzyme replacement therapy is currently proving useful in treating some forms of Gaucher disease (glucocerebrocidase deficiency). This deficiency stems from an inability to effectively degrade glucosylceramide and because the major source of this substrate is the membranes of haemopoietic cells, it is not surprising that one of the principally affected cell types are the tissue macrophages (Beutler, 1988). Although it conforms to the usual characteristics of lysosomal storage disorders in terms of diversity in time of onset of disease and severity of clinical symptoms, Gaucher's disease exists in at least one mild form (Type I nonneuropathic), which is also the most prevalent form of the disease. For this reason, considerable effort has been put into developing purified enzyme as a pharmacological treatment for Type I Gaucher disease. Early clinical trials of enzyme replacement used native enzyme, and although some clinical effects were seen, this was largely inconsistent and it became clear that hepatic sequestration of enzyme was resulting in an inefficient supply of enzyme to the tissue macrophages (Brady, 1984; Furbish *et al.*, 1978). This problem of inappropriate targeting of glucocerebrocidase has been overcome by modifying the native enzyme so that it contains exposed mannose residues which facilitate preferential entry into macrophages (Barton *et al.*, 1991; Brady *et al.*, 1994). This modified enzyme has been successful in achieving regression of clinical signs in patients with Type I Gaucher's and is becoming the treatment of choice in an important subset of these patients (Barton *et al.*, 1992; Brady and Barton, 1994; Frenkel, 1993; Grabowski *et al.*, 1995; Parker *et al.*, 1991).

As a result of this success, preclinical assessment of enzyme replacement using recombinant proteins is underway for a number of other LSDs, including aspartylglucosaminuria and some of the mucopolysaccharidoses (Anson *et al.*, 1992; Bielicki *et al.*, 1993; Crawley *et al.*, 1996; Fuller *et al.*, 1995; Sands *et al.*, 1994; Shull *et al.*, 1994; Unger *et al.*, 1994; Vogler *et al.*, 1996). However, there a number of reasons to believe that the efficacy of enzyme replacement in some of these disorders may be attenuated. Firstly, unlike in Gaucher's disease where residual enzyme activity can generally be detected in most if not all patients, many other LSDs stem from mutations that induce a null phenotype in terms of enzyme levels, protein production, or both. When administration of exogenous enzyme has been tried in animal models of some of these disorders, immune complications have arisen. Thus in MPS-I, administration of recombinant α-L-iduronidase in a null dog model led to an immunological reaction to the administered protein and deposition of immune complexes in the kidneys (Kakkis *et al.*, 1996; Shull *et al.*, 1994). In this model, enzyme therapy failed to correct the pathology in the CNS, cornea, heart valves, or articular cartilage. Similarly, immunological complications arose in a cat model of Maroteaux–Lamy syndrome (MPS-VI) (King *et al.*, 1996). Obviously, careful evaluation of immunological responses in patients will play an important role in assessing the clinical effectiveness of enzyme replacement therapy in these disorders.

A second consideration stems from the nature of the pathologies of different disorders. In Type I Gaucher's disease, there is one target system, namely, the macrophage lineage. For more complex disorders, a number of tissues need to be targeted. These include the CNS, where the blood brain barrier makes it unlikely that systemically administered enzyme is available to the brain cells.

For cellular therapy, in principle, any HLA matched tissue that secretes the missing enzyme may constitute a therapeutic graft, and clinical trials of fibroblast (Gibbs *et al.*, 1983), amniotic membrane (Scaggiante *et al.*, 1987; Yeager *et al.*, 1985) and kidney (Berty *et al.*, 1990; Moser, 1992) transplantation have taken place. However, the treatment which has most successful in lysosomal storage diseases is bone marrow transplantation. This has a number of potential advantages over administering purified enzyme. These include lifelong production of enzyme after a single treatment, which obviates the need for repeated administration of a costly pharmaceutical product; replacement of the immune system with that of the donor, thus preventing an immunological response to the enzyme; and transport of enzyme around the body by the cells of the hematopoietic system, which avoids sequestration by any single tissue. This latter is particularly important in multisystem disorders, especially those that involve the CNS, where bone marrow-derived microglial cells can act as carriers of enzyme across the blood–brain barrier (Krall *et al.*, 1994; Krivit *et al.*, 1995b). A number of issues relating to bone marrow transplantation including the risks of profound immunosuppression after conditioning, the effects of conditioning regimens on other tissues (such as the CNS), and the risks of chronic graft versus host disease. All of these considerations mean that transplantation is not generally indicated for patients with mild disease, such as those with type I Gaucher disease. Conversely, however, as discussed earlier, the severe disorders are often early onset diseases and treatment must be given before irreversible changes occur. Thus patients need to be transplanted early in life, and this raises a number of problems associated with the toxicity of a myeloablative conditioning regimen in young individuals.

Notwithstanding all of this, bone marrow transplantation (using grafts from matched related donors) has been used in a number of disorders (see Chapter 2) and depending on the disease has met with some success in at least slowing disease progression. For example, matched related transplantation in patients with MPS-IH leads to a reduction in lysosomal storage in a number of soft tissues and provided transplantation is performed early enough, some slowing of neurological deterioration although the overall neurological prognosis of these patients remains guarded (Hoogerbrugge *et al.*, 1995; Hopwood *et al.*, 1993). Similar results are seen for adrenoleukodystrophy and globoid cell leukodystrophy (Aubourg *et al.*, 1990; Krivit *et al.*, 1995a; Moser *et al.*, 1984; Shapiro *et al.*, 1995; Yeager *et al.*, 1986). In severe MPS-II and metachromatic leukodystrophy, little or no benefit for the most severe neurological effects of these disorders and current opinion does not recommend BMT as a treatment for severely affected individuals (Shapiro *et al.*, 1995).

Even in those disorders where a clear clinical benefit can be seen after BMT, the availability of this treatment has been diminished because few children have HLA identical siblings at an age when transplantation is considered useful. In those for whom no matched related donor has been found, matched unrelated donor (MUD) transplantation has and continues to be tried. In the most extensive report thus far of MUD transplantation for a LSD, morbidity and mortality were high. Fifty percent of patients died within 24 months of transplantation, and a high incidence of graft versus host disease was reported (Peters *et al.*, 1996).

In summary, therefore, genetic analysis permits selecting patients who may be candidates for treatment before the onset of progressive disease. For these, enzyme replacement therapy or bone marrow transplantation may be indicated, but there is clearly a group of patients for whom current therapeutic options are not available. For these patients new treatment strategies are required, one of which may be gene therapy.

2. GENE THERAPY

One of the cornerstones of successful gene therapy in any disorder is the ability to target expression or delivery of a therapeutic gene product at the tissue(s) where it is required. As discussed previously, the phenomenon of cross-correction may be useful for treating lysosomal storage disorders. This means that direct gene targeting of affected tissues may not be necessary and thus one can concentrate on appropriate gene delivery and expression in tissues which may be easier to manipulate than some of those (e.g., CNS, skeleton, heart) most heavily affected by the disorder. Thus far, three gene therapy approaches have been taken in the LSDs, utilizing three different cell delivery systems. Two of these are of hematopoietic (T-lymphocytes and hematopoietic stem cells) origin, and one (the neo-organ approach) utilizes cells from outside the hematopoietic system.

2.1. Autologous Hematopoietic Stem Cells

Because of the relative success of bone marrow transplantation in treating some LSDs, the use of autologous haemopoietic stem cells and their progeny as enzyme carriers after gene transfer is of considerable interest. The genetic therapy approach to bone marrow transplantation has the advantage of extending the availability of therapy to patients who do not have an allogeneic donor or whose donor is heterozygous for a disorder and consequently produces lower levels of enzyme. As discussed earlier, matched unrelated transplantation suffers from a number of disadvantages, none the least of which is the high morbidity and mortality of the conditioning regimes. This is especially the case with young children who, because of the progressive nature of many disorders and the subsequent need for early intervention, are often preferred for transplant therapy. Autologous stem cells engraft in the absence of conditioning or with only mild conditioning (Barquinero *et al.*, 1995; Wu and Keating, 1993). If this is so, then transplantation of genetically manipulated autologous stem cells should prove a less toxic therapeutic option than matched unrelated donor transplantation, particularly because complications of graft versus host disease will also have been avoided. Thus, gene therapy should extend corrective transplantation to children in the first few months after birth and to patients who have milder but chronically debilitating disease and for whom the risks of allogeneic transplantation are not justified.

Preclinical assessment of gene transfer into primitive hematopoietic cells has focused primarily on cells obtained from bone marrow or from peripheral blood following cytokine mobilization. As in most gene therapy studies in the hematopoietic system, retroviral vectors are the main means of gene transfer. Two models of hematopoiesis have been utilized to define the extent of transduction and expression in primitive hematopoietic cells. The first has been the use of potentially lethally conditioned animals as recipients of transduced hematopoietic cells. This can be considered the most rigorous test of the long-term reconstitutive potential of transduced cells and is particularly useful when an appropriate animal model of the disease is available. In assessing transduction of primitive human hematopoietic cells, no suitable *in vivo* model outside the clinical trial has thus far been available (although the recently described Nod/SCID mouse, that allows generating human hematopoiesis in an otherwise immunocompromised murine host may eventually prove to be such a model) (Larochelle *et al.*, 1996; Pflumio *et al.*, 1996). The best *in vitro* measure of long-term human hematopoiesis stems from a modification of the Dexter culture system, where human hematopoiesis is maintained in *in vitro* culture in the presence of a (autologous or allogeneic) bone marrow stromal layer for up to six months and can be used to study gene transfer into primitive hematopoietic cells from bone marrow, peripheral blood, or umbilical cord blood. In such a system, the less primitive cells rapidly commit to differentiation and clonal extinction. After five to six weeks, most if not all hematopoiesis in the cultures stems from the more primitive hematopoietic cells, the so called long-term culture initiating cells (LTCIC; Sutherland *et al.*, 1989). This cell population likely includes the hematopoietic stem cells, although it should be remembered that the LTCIC represent a wide range of cells in various stages of commitment to differentiation and that transduction of LTCIC is not a measure of stem cell transduction.

Notwithstanding this, a number of groups have used such *in vitro* systems to provide supporting evidence before moving on to clinical trials. For example, transfer and expression of the glucocerebrocidase gene has been demonstrated in LTCIC assays at five weeks post transduction of cord blood, peripheral blood, and bone marrow progenitors. In these studies, the standard cocktail of cytokines (IL-3, IL-6, SCF) combined with stromal support gave the highest levels of transduction and expression at five weeks (Xu *et al.*, 1995). In a similar study, bone marrow cells from patients with Hurler syndrome (MPS I) were successfully transduced with a retroviral vector carrying an α-L-iduronidase cDNA. In this case, transduction was performed during the genesis of the LTBMC and around 50% of LTCIC-derived GM-CFC at week nine of culture were transduced with the vector. Moreover, expression of α-L-iduronidase persisted for the life of the cultures (up to six months), and functional correction (in terms of cell morphology and reduced storage of sulfated glycosaminoglycans) of the disorder was demonstrated (Fairbairn *et al.*, 1996). Interestingly, this study found no advantage in transduction frequency or expression levels in using growth factors or intensive schedules of retroviral exposure. Although the reasons for this remain obscure, the advantage of the transduction protocol may be that minimal manipulation of the hematopoietic cells may prevent loss of stem cell function and hence reduce or prevent clonal extinction of transduced cells in the patient. A clinical trial of bone marrow gene therapy in Hurler syndrome has begun, and the results will be of great interest.

In Gaucher's disease, murine models have been used to demonstrate persistence of the transgene in hematopoietic cells after reconstitution of mice (Correll *et al.*, 1992; Ohashi *et al.*, 1992). Thus, after transduction of murine bone marrow with retroviral vectors encoding human GC, the human enzyme was expressed well in tissue macrophages for as long as seven months posttransplantation. In one study, macrophages derived from the transduced graft progressively accumulated in peripheral tissues, such that at six months posttransplantation up to 70% of liver macrophages and 20% of CNS microglial cells were donor derived. This bodes well for the concept of tissue macrophages as mobile producers of enzyme for uptake in distal target tissues (Krall *et al.*, 1994). Similar studies have been performed in a mouse model of MPS-VII (Sly syndrome, β-glucuronidase deficiency) where, despite low levels of gene transfer in bone marrow, enzyme was detected in a number of tissues, including brain, and lysosomal storage was alleviated in tissues, such as liver and spleen (Wolfe *et al.*, 1992b).

2.2. Lymphocyte Gene Transfer

T- and B-lymphocytes are suggested as targets for gene therapy in the LSD by early experiments where fibroblasts from patients with MPSII, and MPS VII were "cross-corrected" by direct contact with lymphocytes from unaffected individuals (Abraham *et al.*, 1985; Olsen *et al.*, 1986, 1988). Further to this, one group has shown transfer and expression of iduronate-2-sulfatase in T-lymphocytes from patients with Hunter syndrome (MPSII), using a retroviral vector (Braun *et al.*, 1996). The transduced cells corrected the enzyme deficiency in patient fibroblasts *in vitro* and based on this a clinical trial of lymphocyte gene therapy in mild MPSII has opened (Whitley *et al.*, 1996). The use of lymphocytes, particularly in patients with mild disease, offers a number of advantages, none the least of which is that collection of target cells for transduction is achieved by a relatively noninvasive procedure. Furthermore, the ease of collecting target cells will facilitate the use of multiple treatments of patients with gene therapy, and additionally it is anticipated that the current range of (Moloney murine leukemia virally based) retroviral vectors will express better in lymphoid cells compared with myeloid cells and their precursors.

It is worth noting, however, that lymphocytes do not repopulate the CNS to any real extent and therefore the utility of this approach is restricted to those disorders/patients where there is no significant CNS involvement.

2.3. Neo-Organs

A further approach which may be amenable for therapy in patients with milder disease is the *neo*-organ approach. In this, fibroblasts are transduced with a retrovirus vector that expresses a protein of interest, and the cells are grown in a polytetrafluoroethylene fibre/collagen mesh that is supplemented with basic fibroblast growth factor and epidermal growth factor. As the cells grow, the lattices contract to form small organ-like structures, which can be implanted into the peritoneum. There they become vascularized and act as "factories" of secreted enzyme. This approach has been used to investigate the potential for *neo*-organ gene therapy of MPSI and MPSVII. In MPSVII mice, implantation of *neo*-organs led to low but significant (around 0.5–6% normal levels) of β-glucuronidase that were detected as long as five months in the liver, spleen, and lungs of animals, and lower levels were detected in the brain, kidney, heart, and bone marrow (Moullier *et al.*, 1993a,b). The presence of enzyme was not associated with transferring retroviral DNA to distal tissues, indicating that neither the vector nor the fibroblasts in the *neo*-organ were directly responsible for the levels of β-glucuronidase in the distal sites. Furthermore, surgical removal of the *neo*-organ resulted in loss of enzyme in the peripheral tissues. Histochemically, enzyme was demonstrated only in the macrophage populations of the various tissues. However, storage lesions were cleared in liver and (to some extent) spleen, even in cell types where no histologically demonstrable enzyme was seen. The low levels of activity in the brain were present in a few scattered cells, and these are also presumed to be tissue macrophages because secreted enzyme would be unlikely to cross the blood–brain barrier. Similar results were obtained by using (larger) *neo*-organs implanted in the peritoneum of dogs (Moullier *et al.*, 1995), and these studies were extended to include the use of *neo*-organs that secrete α-L-iduronidase (Salvetti *et al.*, 1995). The latter studies led to a clinical trial of *neo*-organ gene therapy in MPS I, and the results of this study should be interesting.

3. TARGETING THE BRAIN

3.1. Bone Marrow Macrophages

As discussed earlier, one of the proposed benefits of bone marrow transplantation/HSC gene therapy is that tissue macrophages which express the missing enzyme may act as carriers of enzyme across the blood–brain barrier. There is certainly good evidence that such cells can provide this function under transplant conditions. For example, in mice reconstituted with bone marrow cells that express retrovirally encoded glucocerebrocidase, the CNS is repopulated by donor macrophages and reaches 20% of cells by six months (Krall *et al.*, 1994). Similarly, in transplantation experiments in the α-mannosidase-deficient cat model, transplantation of bone marrow from phenotypically normal littermates restored CNS enzyme to 9–40% of normal levels (Walkley *et al.*, 1994). Furthermore neurons and glia accumulate lysosomal proteins from an extracellular source. Given these observations, one important question is, why are the clinical effects of bone marrow transplantation on brain function in severe disorders so variable?

There are a number of different factors that affect the efficacy of bone marrow therapy for disorders which have a neurological component. Not the least of these will be the extent of preexisting damage and the rate at which neurodegeneration is occurring. This latter point means that treatment becomes a race against time for the clinician and in the case of bone marrow transplantation, because repopulation is a gradual process that occurs over several months, then even early transplantation may not prevent critical levels of damage in the early years. A further point worth considering here is that those animal studies which investigated the utility of BMT to correct abnormalities in other tissues have mostly used myeloablative conditioning *via* irradiation. Some studies have shown a clear relationship between the dose of radiation in conditioning and subsequent enzyme levels in distal tissues (Birkenmeier *et al.*, 1991; Sands *et al.*, 1993). Although it is likely that some of this is results from improved engraftment, there is also some suggestion that higher irradiation doses may lead to a transient breakdown in the blood–brain barrier and improved macrophage migration into the CNS. Because one advantage of autologous reconstitution might be a reduced need for myeloablative conditioning, the effects of reduced conditioning on CNS engraftment require careful examination.

3.2. Neurotropic Vectors

If it is proved that BMT-mediated enzyme transfer to the CNS is insufficient to halt neurodegeneration significantly, then it may of some benefit to consider directly targeting the brain. Obviously, because retroviral vectors successfully transduce only cycling cells, such vectors are unlikely to be of any great utility within the (largely quiescent) CNS. Two alternative viruses are currently under investigation as potential vectors for gene transfer to tissues, such as the CNS. These are the adenoviruses and Herpes simplex virus (HSV). HSV is a recognizably neurotropic virus which can cause life-threatening encephalitis (Olson *et al.*, 1967; Spear and Roizman, 1980). It can also exist in a latent state, and this latent state, in which the virus exists as an episome within the nucleus of infected cells (Latchman, 1990), is exploited in the HSV vectors under development. Unlike the retroviral vectors, the genome of HSV is quite complex and has a number of genes necessary for infecting or maintaining the episome. Consequently, thus far it has proved difficult to develop an optimized HSV vector for gene transfer into neuronal cells. Approaches thus far taken include deleting the viral thymidine kinase gene to disable the replicative function of the virus in neurones and deleting (with provision *in trans*) the immediate early genes of the virus (Dobson *et al.*, 1990; Palella *et al.*, 1989). Unfortunately both approaches generate vectors that are less than optimal for clinical use, have severe toxic effects in animals and produce replication competent virus that create major complications. Strategies are being formulated, however, to produce a packaging system analogous to that used with the retroviral vectors, where *cis* acting packaging signals are separated from *trans* acting packaging functions. It is expected that these will eventually bear fruit. Added to this major challenge will be the identification of promoter/enhancer sequences which can direct transcription from the (normally transcriptionally silent) latent-phase HSV genome. One obvious choice is the viral LAT promoter, which remains transcriptionally active during latent infection. Expression of β-glucuronidase has been demonstrated in the brains of MPSVII mice after infection with an HSV-LAT-β-glucuronidase virus (Wolfe *et al.*, 1992a).

The second viral system, which is receiving much attention, is the adenoviral vector system. Like HSV, adenovirus vectors transduce cells of the CNS (Akli *et al.*, 1993; Le Gal La Salle *et al.*, 1993), infect postmitotic cells, and establish themselves as episomes. Removing one or more immediate early genes from the rather complex genome of the adenovirus leads to a loss of replicative function and the creation of space for inserting therapeutic sequences. Adenoviral vectors have been successfully used to achieve expression of the ARA gene, which is defective in MLD, in fibroblasts and oligodendrocytes *in vitro* (Ohashi *et al.*, 1995) and of iduronate-2-sulfatase in primary fibroblasts from MPSII patients. However, there is still some way to go before sustainable levels of transgene expression will be demonstrable *in vivo* in the brain. Furthermore, the first generation adenoviral vectors were severely toxic, mainly because of inflammatory responses to viral proteins (Byrnes *et al.*, 1996; Kaplan *et al.*, 1996; Yang *et al.*, 1996). Clearly alternative vectors are required and, as with the HSV vectors, the production of high titer empty (or "gutless") vectors is a priority.

Regardless of the vector used and the efficacy of transduction/expression, a further complication is likely to arise from the mechanism of viral delivery to the brain. The blood–brain barrier is likely to prevent significant viral ingress into the CNS after systemic administration. Although disruption of the blood–brain barrier with osmotic agents leads to a small amount of viral gene transfer into brain (Nilaver *et al.*, 1995), it is likely that most of the systemically administered virus would be sequestered by liver and epithelial tissues. Faced with this, the prospects for direct viral installation into the brain have been investigated. However, with current vectors, viral spread around the injection site is limited to only a few millimeters. Clearly this is unsatisfactory and awaits development of a neurotropic vector for widespread, safe, and effective gene delivery in the CNS.

3.3. Neural Progenitor Cells

One alternative to *in vivo* installation of virus is the *ex vivo* expansion and transduction of neural progenitors. The prospects for this approach are encouraging because of the early studies of fetal neuronal grafts in patients with Parkinson's disease, where persistence of grafts was seen for more than a year and clinical signs improved (Kordower *et al.*, 1995). However, again the effects were localized to the region of cell installation, and this effect is also anticipated with autologous neuronal progenitors. In animal studies, using immortalized neuronal cells as therapeutic agents has been investigated, and here the prospects for disseminated transfer of functions is brighter. For example, cells from the cerebellum, immortalized *via* expression of the c-*myc* oncogene, stably engraft and disseminate throughout the brain after intraventricular injection (Snyder *et al.*, 1992). In MPSVII mice, such engraftment resulted in increased β-glucuronidase levels throughout the brain and a lack of neurodegenerative symptoms (Snyder *et al.*, 1995). Similarly, gene transfer of β-hexosaminidase into immortalized neuronal progenitors and engraftment into mice resulted in disseminated expression of the enzyme throughout the brain (Lacorazza *et al.*, 1996). Obviously, there are concerns regarding the use of immortalized cells in humans, but notwithstanding these, the prospects for using such cells in human transplants should and will be intensively investigated.

4. CONCLUSIONS

There are a large number of difficulties in formulating any gene therapy for multisystem disorders, such as the lysosomal storage diseases. Intervention *via* bone marrow transplantation or hematopoietic cell gene therapy offer the prospect of gene product delivery to a large number of organs. Where major CNS pathology is involved, however, the bone marrow approach may not prove sufficient, and other strategies, such as the use of neurotropic vectors or genetically manipulated neuronal progenitors, may be required.

5. REFERENCES

Abraham, D., Muir, H., Olsen, I., and Winchester, B., 1985, Direct enzyme transfer from lymphocytes corrects a lysosomal storage disease, *Biochem. Biophys. Res. Commun.* **129**(2)**:**417–425.

Akli, S., Caillaud, C., Vigne, E., Stratford Perricaudet, L. D., Poenaru, L., Perricaudet, M., Kahn, A., and Peschanski, M. R., 1993, Transfer of a foreign gene into the brain using adenovirus vectors [see comments], *Nat. Genet.* **3**(3)**:**224–228.

Anson, D. S., Taylor, J. A., Bielicki, J., Harper, G. S., Peters, C., Gibson, G. J., and Hopwood, J. J., 1992, Correction of human mucopolysaccharidosis type-VI fibroblasts with recombinant N-acetylgalactosamine-4-sulphatase, *Biochem. J.* **284**(Pt 3)**:**789–794.

Aubourg, P., Blanche, S., Jambaque, I., Rocchiccioli, F., Kalifa, G., Naud Saudreau, C., Rolland, M. O., Debre, M., Chaussain, J. L., Griscelli, C., *et al.*, 1990, Reversal of early neurologic and neuroradiologic manifestations of X-linked adrenoleukodystrophy by bone marrow transplantation, *N. Engl. J. Med.* **322**(26)**:**1860–1866.

Barquinero, J., Kiem, H. P., von Kalle, C., Darovsky, B., Goehle, S., Graham, T., Seidel, K., Storb, R., and Schuening, F. G., 1995, Myelosuppressive conditioning improves autologous engraftment of genetically marked hematopoietic repopulating cells in dogs, *Blood* **85**(5)**:**1195–1201.

Barton, N. W., Brady, R. O., Dambrosia, J. M., Di Bisceglie, A. M., Doppelt, S. H., Hill, S. C., Mankin, H. J., Murray, G. J., Parker, R. I., Argoff, C. E., *et al.*, 1991, Replacement therapy for inherited enzyme deficiency—macrophage-targeted glucocerebrosidase for Gaucher's disease [see comments], *N. Engl. J. Med.* **324**(21)**:**1464–1470.

Barton, N. W., Brady, R. O., Dambrosia, J. M., Doppelt, S. H., Hill, S. C., Holder, C. A., Mankin, H. J., Murray, G. J., Zirzow, G. C., and Parker, R. I., 1992, Dose-dependent responses to macrophage-targeted glucocerebrosidase in a child with Gaucher disease, *J. Pediatr.* **120**(2 Pt 1)**:**277–280.

Berty, R. M., Adler, S., Basu, A., and Glew, R. H., 1990, Effect of acid-base changes on urinary hydrolases in Fabry's disease after renal transplantation, *J. Lab. Clin. Med.* **115**(6)**:**696–703.

Beutler, E., 1988, Gaucher disease, *Blood Rev.* **2**(1)**:**59–70.

Bielicki, J., Hopwood, J. J., Wilson, P. J., and Anson, D. S., 1993, Recombinant human iduronate-2-

sulphatase: Correction of mucopolysaccharidosis-type II fibroblasts and characterization of the purified enzyme, *Biochem. J.* **289**(Pt 1):241–246.

Birkenmeier, E. H., Barker, J. E., Vogler, C. A., Kyle, J. W., Sly, W. S., Gwynn, B., Levy, B., and Pegors, C., 1991, Increased life span and correction of metabolic defects in murine mucopolysaccharidosis type VII after syngeneic bone marrow transplantation, *Blood* **78**(11):3081–3092.

Bou Gharios, G., Abraham, D., and Olsen, I., 1993, Lysosomal storage diseases: Mechanisms of enzyme replacement therapy, *Histochem. J.* **25**(9):593–605.

Brady, R. O., 1984, Enzyme replacement in the sphigolipidoses, in *The Molecular Basis of Lysosomal Storage Disorders* (J. A. Barranger, and R. O. Brady, eds.), Academic Press, Orlando Florida, pp. 461–478.

Brady, R. O., and Barton, N. W., 1994, Enzyme replacement therapy for Gaucher disease: critical investigations beyond demonstration of clinical efficacy, *Biochem. Med. Metab. Biol.* **52**(1):1–9.

Brady, R. O., Murray, G. J., and Barton, N. W., 1994, Modifying exogenous glucocerebrosidase for effective replacement therapy in Gaucher disease, *J. Inherited Metab. Dis.* **17**(4):510–519.

Braun, S. E., Pan, D., Aronovich, E. L., Jonsson, J. J., McIvor, R. S., and Whitley, C. B., 1996, Preclinical studies of lymphocyte gene therapy for mild Hunter syndrome (mucopolysaccharidosis type II), *Hum. Gene Ther.* **7**(3):283–290.

Byrnes, A. P., MacLaren, R. E., and Charlton, H. M., 1996, Immunological instability of persistent adenovirus vectors in the brain: Peripheral exposure to vector leads to renewed inflammation, reduced gene expression, and demyelination, *J. Neurosci.* **16**(9):3045–3055.

Correll, P. H., Colilla, S., Dave, H. P., and Karlsson, S., 1992, High levels of human glucocerebrosidase activity in macrophages of long-term reconstituted mice after retroviral infection of hematopoietic stem cells, *Blood* **80**(2):331–336.

Crawley, A. C., Brooks, D. A., Muller, V. J., Petersen, B. A., Isaac, E. L., Bielicki, J., King, B. M., Boulter, C. D., Moore, A. J., Fazzalari, N. L., Anson, D. S., Byers, S., and Hopwood, J. J., 1996, Enzyme replacement therapy in a feline model of Maroteaux–Lamy syndrome, *J. Clin. Invest.* **97**(8):1864–1873.

Dobson, A. T., Margolis, T. P., Sedarati, F., Stevens, J. G., and Feldman, L. T., 1990, A latent, nonpathogenic HSV-1-derived vector stably expresses beta-galactosidase in mouse neurons, *Neuron* **5**(3):353–360.

Fairbairn, L. J., Lashford, L. S., Spooncer, E., McDermott, R. H., Lebens, G., Arrand, J. E., Arrand, J. R., Bellantuono, I., Holt, R., Hatton, C. E., Cooper, A., Besley, G. T., Wraith, J. E., Anson, D. S., Hopwood, J. J., and Dexter, T. M., 1996, Long-term in vitro correction of alpha-L-iduronidase deficiency (Hurler syndrome) in human bone marrow, *Proc. Natl. Acad. Sci. USA* **93**(5):2025–2030.

Frenkel, E. P., 1993, Gaucher disease: A heterogeneous clinical complex for which effective enzyme replacement has come of age, *Am. J. Med. Sci.* **305**(5):331–344.

Fuller, M., Van der Ploeg, A., Reuser, A. J., Anson, D. S., and Hopwood, J. J., 1995, Isolation and characterisation of a recombinant, precursor form of lysosomal acid alpha-glucosidase, *Eur. J. Biochem.* **234**(3):903–909.

Furbish, F. S., Steer, C. J., Barranger, J. A., Jones, E. A., and Brady, R. O., 1978, Uptake and distribution of placental glucocerebrosidase in rat hepatic cells and effects of sequential deglycosylation, *Biochim. Biophys. Acta* **673**:425–434.

Gibbs, D. A., Spellacy, E., Tompkins, R., Watts, R. W., and Mowbray, J. F., 1983, A clinical trial of fibroblast transplantation for the treatment of mucopolysaccharidoses, *J. Inherited Metab. Dis.* **6**(2):62–81.

Gieselmann, V., Zlotogora, J., Harris, A., Wenger, D. A., and Morris, C. P., 1994, Molecular genetics of metachromatic leukodystrophy, *Hum. Mutation* **4**(4):233–242.

Grabowski, G. A., Barton, N. W., Pastores, G., Dambrosia, J. M., Banerjee, T. K., McKee, M. A., Parker, C., Schiffmann, R., Hill, S. C., and Brady, R. O., 1995, Enzyme therapy in type 1 Gaucher disease: Comparative efficacy of mannose-terminated glucocerebrosidase from natural and recombinant sources, *Ann. Intern. Med.* **122**(1):33–39.

Hasilik, A., 1992, The early and late processing of lysosomal enzymes: Proteolysis and compartmentation, *Experientia* **48**(2):130–151.

Hill, D. F., Bullock, P. N., Chiappelli, F., and Rome, L. H., 1985, Binding and internalization of lysosomal enzymes by primary cultures of rat glia, *J. Neurosci. Res.* **14**(1):35–47.

Hoogerbrugge, P. M., Brouwer, O. F., Bordigoni, P., Ringden, O., Kapaun, P., Ortega, J. J., O'Meara, A., Cornu, G., Souillet, G., Frappaz, D., *et al.*, 1995, Allogeneic bone marrow transplantation for lysosomal storage diseases. The European Group for Bone Marrow Transplantation [see comments], *Lancet* **345**(8962)**:**1398–1402.

Hopwood, J. J., Vellodi, A., Scott, H. S., Morris, C. P., Litjens, T., Clements, P. R., Brooks, D. A., Cooper, A., and Wraith, J. E., 1993, Long-term clinical progress in bone marrow transplanted mucopolysaccharidosis type I patients with a defined genotype, *J. Inherited Metab. Dis.* **16**(6)**:**1024–1033.

Kakkis, E. D., McEntee, M. F., Schmidtchen, A., Neufeld, E. F., Ward, D. A., Gompf, R. E., Kania, S., Bedolla, C., Chien, S. L., and Shull, R. M., 1996, Long-term and high-dose trials of enzyme replacement therapy in the canine model of mucopolysaccharidosis I, *Biochem. Mol. Med.* **58**(2)**:**156–167.

Kaplan, J. M., St. George, J. A., Pennington, S. E., Keyes, L. D., Johnson, R. P., Wadsworth, S. C., and Smith, A. E., 1996, Humoral and cellular immune responses of nonhuman primates to long-term repeated lung exposure to Ad2/CFTR-2, *Gene Ther.* **3**(2)**:**117–127.

King, B. M., Crawley, A. C., and Byers, S., 1996, Immune response to enzyme replacement therapy in MPS VI cats, *Proceedings 4th International Symposium on Mucopolysaccharide and Related Diseases*, Wollogon, NSW, Australia.

Kordower, J. H., Freeman, T. B., Snow, B. J., Vingerhoets, F. J., Mufson, E. J., Sanberg, P. R., Hauser, R. A., Smith, D. A., Nauert, G. M., Perl, D. P., *et al.*, 1995, Neuropathological evidence of graft survival and striatal reinnervation after the transplantation of fetal mesencephalic tissue in a patient with Parkinson's disease [see comments], *N. Engl. J. Med.* **332**(17)**:**1118–1124.

Krall, W. J., Challita, P. M., Perlmutter, L. S., Skelton, D. C., and Kohn, D. B., 1994, Cells expressing human glucocerebrosidase from a retroviral vector repopulate macrophages and central nervous system microglia after murine bone marrow transplantation, *Blood* **83**(9)**:**2737–2748.

Krivit, W., Lockman, L. A., Watkins, P. A., Hirsch, J., and Shapiro, E. G., 1995a, The future for treatment by bone marrow transplantation for adrenoleukodystrophy, metachromatic leukodystrophy, globoid cell leukodystrophy, and Hurler syndrome, *J. Inherited Metab. Dis.* **18**(4)**:**398–412.

Krivit, W., Sung, J. H., Shapiro, E. G., and Lockman, L. A., 1995b, Microglia: The effector cell for reconstitution of the central nervous system following bone marrow transplantation for lysosomal and peroxisomal storage diseases, *Cell Transplant.* **4**(4)**:**385–392.

Lacorazza, H. D., Flax, J. D., Snyder, E. Y., and Jendoubi, M., 1996, Expression of human beta-hexosaminidase alpha-subunit gene (the gene defect of Tay–Sachs disease) in mouse brains upon engraftment of transduced progenitor cells, *Nat. Med.* **2**(4)**:**424–429.

Larochelle, A., Vormoor, J., Hanenberg, H., Wang, J. C., Bhatia, M., Lapidot, T., Moritz, T., Murdoch, B., Xiao, X. L., Kato, I., Williams, D. A., and Dick, J. E., 1996, Identification of primitive human hematopoietic cells capable of repopulating NOD/SCID mouse bone marrow: Implications for gene therapy, *Nat. Med.* **2**(12)**:**1329–1337.

Latchman, D. S., 1990, Current status review: Molecular biology of herpes simplex virus latency, *J. Exp. Pathol. Oxford* **71**(1)**:**133–141.

Le Gal La Salle, G., Robert, J. J., Berrard, S., Ridoux, V., Stratford Perricaudet, L. D., Perricaudet, M., and Mallet, J., 1993, An adenovirus vector for gene transfer into neurons and glia in the brain, *Science* **259**(5097)**:**988–990.

Moser, H. W., 1992, New concepts in the diagnosis and treatment of lysosomal and peroxisomal disorders, *Curr. Opinion Neurol. Neurosurg.* **5**(3)**:**355–358.

Moser, H. W., Tutschka, P. J., Brown, F. R. D., Moser, A. E., Yeager, A. M., Singh, I., Mark, S. A., Kumar, A. A., McDonnell, J. M., White, C. L. D., *et al.*, 1984, Bone marrow transplant in adrenoleukodystrophy, *Neurology* **34**(11)**:**1410–1417.

Moullier, P., Bohl, D., Cardoso, J., Heard, J. M., and Danos, O., 1995, Long-term delivery of a lysosomal enzyme by genetically modified fibroblasts in dogs, *Nat. Med.* **1**(4)**:**353–357.

Moullier, P., Bohl, D., Heard, J. M., and Danos, O., 1993a, Correction of lysosomal storage in the liver and spleen of MPS VII mice by implantation of genetically modified skin fibroblasts [see comments], *Nat. Genet.* **4**(2)**:**154–159.

Moullier, P., Marechal, V., Danos, O., and Heard, J. M., 1993b, Continuous systemic secretion of a lysosomal enzyme by genetically modified mouse skin fibroblasts, *Transplantation* **56**(2)**:**427–432.

Neufeld, E. F., 1991, Lysosomal storage diseases, *Annu. Rev. Biochem.* **60:**257–280.

Neufeld, E. F., and Muenzer, J., 1989, The mucopolysaccharidoses, in *The Molecular Basis of Inherited Disease*, (C. J. Scriver, W. S. Beaudet, W. S. Sly, and D. Valle, eds.), McGraw-Hill, New York, pp. 1565–1587.

Nilaver, G., Muldoon, L. L., Kroll, R. A., Pagel, M. A., Breakefield, X. O., Davidson, B. L., and Neuwelt, E. A., 1995, Delivery of herpesvirus and adenovirus to nude rat intracerebral tumors after osmotic blood-brain barrier disruption, *Proc. Natl. Acad. Sci. USA* **92**(21)**:**9829–9833.

Ohashi, T., Boggs, S., Robbins, P., Bahnson, A., Patrene, K., Wei, F. S., Wei, J. F., Li, J., Lucht, L., Fei, Y., *et al.*, 1992, Efficient transfer and sustained high expression of the human glucocerebrosidase gene in mice and their functional macrophages following transplantation of bone marrow transduced by a retroviral vector, *Proc. Natl. Acad. Sci. USA* **89**(23)**:**11332–11336.

Ohashi, T., Watabe, K., Sato, Y., Saito, I., Barranger, J. A., and Eto, Y., 1995, Successful transduction of oligodendrocytes and restoration of arylsulfatase A deficiency in metachromatic leukodystrophy fibroblasts using an adenovirus vector, *Gene Ther.* **2**(7)**:**443–449.

Olsen, I., Abraham, D., Shelton, I., Bou Gharios, G., Muir, H., and Winchester, B., 1988, Cell contact induces the synthesis of a lysosomal enzyme precursor in lymphocytes and its direct transfer to fibroblasts, *Biochim. Biophys. Acta* **968**(3)**:**312–322.

Olsen, I., Oliver, T., Muir, H., Smith, R., and Partridge, T., 1986, Role of cell adhesion in contact-dependent transfer of a lysosomal enzyme from lymphocytes to fibroblasts, *J. Cell Sci.* **85:**231–244.

Olson, L. C., Bueschler, E. L., Artenstein, M. S., and Parkman, P. D., 1967, Herpes simplex virus infections of the human central nervous system, *N. Engl. J. Med.* **277:**1271–1277.

Palella, T. D., Hidaka, Y., Silverman, L. J., Levine, M., Glorioso, J., and Kelley, W. N., 1989, Expression of human HPRT mRNA in brains of mice infected with a recombinant herpes simplex virus-1 vector, *Gene* **80**(1)**:**137–144.

Parker, R. I., Barton, N. W., Read, E. J., and Brady, R. O., 1991, Hematologic improvement in a patient with Gaucher disease on long-term enzyme replacement therapy: Evidence for decreased splenic sequestration and improved red blood cell survival, *Am. J. Hematol.* **38**(2)**:**130–137.

Peters, C., Balthazor, M., Shapiro, E. G., King, R. J., Kollman, C., Hegland, J. D., Henslee Downey, J., Trigg, M. E., Cowan, M. J., Sanders, J., Bunin, N., Weinstein, H., Lenarsky, C., Falk, P., Harris, R., Bowen, T., Williams, T. E., Grayson, G. H., Warkentin, P., Sender, L., Cool, V. A., Crittenden, M., Packman, S., Kaplan, P., Lockman, L. A., *et al.*, 1996, Outcome of unrelated donor bone marrow transplantation in 40 children with Hurler syndrome, *Blood* **87**(11)**:**4894–4902.

Pflumio, F., Izac, B., Katz, A., Shultz, L. D., Vainchenker, W., and Coulombel, L., 1996, Phenotype and function of human hematopoietic cells engrafting immune-deficient CB17-severe combined immunodeficiency mice and nonobese diabetic-severe combined immunodeficiency mice after transplantation of human cord blood mononuclear cells, *Blood* **88**(10)**:**3731–3740.

Rodman, J. S., Mercer, R. W., and Stahl, P. D., 1990, Endocytosis and transcytosis, *Curr. Opinion Cell Biol.* **2**(4)**:**664–672.

Salvetti, A., Moullier, P., Cornet, V., Brooks, D., Hopwood, J. J., Danos, O., and Heard, J. M., 1995, In vivo delivery of human alpha-L-iduronidase in mice implanted with neo-organs, *Hum. Gene Ther.* **6**(9)**:**1153–1159.

Sands, M. S., Barker, J. E., Vogler, C., Levy, B., Gwynn, B., Galvin, N., Sly, W. S., and Birkenmeier, E., 1993, Treatment of murine mucopolysaccharidosis type VII by syngeneic bone marrow transplantation in neonates, *Lab. Invest.* **68**(6)**:**676–686.

Sands, M. S., Vogler, C., Kyle, J. W., Grubb, J. H., Levy, B., Galvin, N., Sly, W. S., and Birkenmeier, E. H., 1994, Enzyme replacement therapy for murine mucopolysaccharidosis type VII, *J. Clin. Invest.* **93**(6)**:**2324–2331.

Scaggiante, B., Pineschi, A., Sustersich, M., Andolina, M., Agosti, E., and Romeo, D., 1987, Successful therapy of Niemann-Pick disease by implantation of human amniotic membrane, *Transplantation* **44**(1)**:**59–61.

Scott, H. S., Bunge, S., Gal, A., Clarke, L. A., Morris, C. P., and Hopwood, J. J., 1995, Molecular genetics of mucopolysaccharidosis type I: Diagnostic, clinical, and biological implications, *Hum. Mutation* **6**(4)**:**288–302.

Shapiro, E. G., Lockman, L. A., Balthazor, M., and Krivit, W., 1995, Neuropsychological outcomes of several storage diseases with and without bone marrow transplantation, *J. Inherited Metab. Dis.* **18**(4)**:**413–429.

Shull, R. M., Kakkis, E. D., McEntee, M. F., Kania, S. A., Jonas, A. J., and Neufeld, E. F., 1994, Enzyme replacement in a canine model of Hurler syndrome, *Proc. Natl. Acad. Sci. USA* **91**(26)**:**12937–12941.

Snyder, E. Y., Deitcher, D. L., Walsh, C., Arnold Aldea, S., Hartwieg, E. A., and Cepko, C. L., 1992, Multipotent neural cell lines can engraft and participate in development of mouse cerebellum, *Cell* **68**(1)**:**33–51.

Snyder, E. Y., Taylor, R. M., and Wolfe, J. H., 1995, Neural progenitor cell engraftment corrects lysosomal storage throughout the MPS VII mouse brain, *Nature* **374**(6520)**:**367–370.

Spear, P. G., and Roizman, B., 1980, Herpes simplex viruses, in *DNA Tumour Viruses*, (J. Touze, ed.), Cold Spring Harbor Laboratory, Cold Spring Harbor, New York, pp. 615–746.

Stewart, K., Brown, O. A., Morelli, A. E., Fairbairn, L. J., Lashford, L. S., Cooper, A., Hatton, C. E., Dexter, T. M., Castro, M. G., and Lowenstein, P. R., 1997, Uptake of alpha-(L)-iduronidase produced by retrovirally transduced fibroblasts into neuronal and glial cells in vitro, *Gene Ther.* **4**(1)**:**63–75.

Sutherland, H. J., Eaves, C. J., Eaves, A. C., Dragowska, W., and Lansdorp, P. M., 1989, Characterization and partial purification of human marrow cells capable of initiating long-term hematopoiesis in vitro, *Blood* **74**(5)**:**1563–1570.

Unger, E. G., Durrant, J., Anson, D. S., and Hopwood, J. J., 1994, Recombinant alpha-L-iduronidase: Characterization of the purified enzyme and correction of mucopolysaccharidosis type I fibroblasts, *Biochem. J.* **304**(Pt 1)**:**43–49.

Vladutiu, G. D., and Rattazzi, M. C., 1979, Excretion-reuptake route of β-hexosaminidase in normal and I-cell disease cultured fibroblasts, *J. Clin. Invest.* **63:**595–601.

Vogler, C., Sands, M. S., Levy, B., Galvin, N., Birkenmeier, E. H., and Sly, W. S., 1996, Enzyme replacement with recombinant beta-glucuronidase in murine mucopolysaccharidosis type VII: Impact of therapy during the first six weeks of life on subsequent lysosomal storage, growth, and survival, *Pediatr. Res.* **39**(6)**:**1050–1054.

Walkley, S. U., Thrall, M. A., Dobrenis, K., Huang, M., March, P. A., Siegel, D. A., and Wurzelmann, S., 1994, Bone marrow transplantation corrects the enzyme defect in neurons of the central nervous system in a lysosomal storage disease, *Proc. Natl. Acad. Sci. USA* **91**(8)**:**2970–2974.

Whitley, C. B., McIvor, R. S., Aronovich, E. L., Berry, S. A., Blazar, B. R., Burger, S. R., Kersey, J
H., King, R. A., Faras, A. J., Latchaw, R. E., McCullough, J., Pan, D., Ramsay, N. K., and Stroncek, D. F., 1996, Retroviral-mediated transfer of the iduronate-2-sulfatase gene into lymphocytes for treatment of mild Hunter syndrome (mucopolysaccharidosis type II), *Hum. Gene Ther.* **7**(4)**:**537–549.

Willcox, P., and Rattray, S., 1979, Secretion and reuptake of β-N-acetylglucosaminidase by fibroblasts. Effect of chloroquine and mannose-6-phosphate, *Biochim. Biophys. Acta* **586:**442–452.

Wolfe, J. H., Deshmane, S. L., and Fraser, N. W., 1992a, Herpesvirus vector gene transfer and expression of beta-glucuronidase in the central nervous system of MPS VII mice, *Nat. Genet.* **1**(5)**:**379–384.

Wolfe, J. H., Sands, M. S., Barker, J. E., Gwynn, B., Rowe, L. B., Vogler, C. A., and Birkenmeier, E. H., 1992b, Reversal of pathology in murine mucopolysaccharidosis type VII by somatic cell gene transfer, *Nature* **360**(6406)**:**749–753.

Wu, D. D., and Keating, A., 1993, Hematopoietic stem cells engraft in untreated transplant recipients, *Exp. Hematol.* **21**(2)**:**251–256.

Xu, L. C., Kluepfel Stahl, S., Blanco, M., Schiffmann, R., Dunbar, C., and Karlsson, S., 1995, Growth factors and stromal support generate very efficient retroviral transduction of peripheral blood CD34+ cells from Gaucher patients, *Blood* **86**(1)**:**141–146.

Yang, Y., Jooss, K. U., Su, Q., Ertl, H. C., and Wilson, J. M., 1996, Immune responses to viral antigens versus transgene product in the elimination of recombinant adenovirus-infected hepatocytes in vivo, *Gene Ther.* **3**(2)**:**137–144.

Yeager, A. M., Moser, H. W., Tutschka, P. J., Saral, R., Moser, A. E., Kumar, A. A., and Santos, G. W., 1986, Allogeneic bone marrow transplantation in adrenoleukodystrophy: Clinical, pathologic, and biochemical studies, *Birth Defects* **22**(1)**:**79–100.

Yeager, A. M., Singer, H. S., Buck, J. R., Matalon, R., Brennan, S., O'Toole, S. O., and Moser, H. W., 1985, A therapeutic trial of amniotic epithelial cell implantation in patients with lysosomal storage diseases, *Am. J. Med. Genet.* **22**(2)**:**347–355.

Chapter 8

Genetic Approaches to Therapy for the Hemoglobinopathies

Michael Antoniou and Frank Grosveld

1. INTRODUCTION

Hemoglobinopathies constitute the most common, heterogenous group of genetically inherited disorders. They are caused by an imbalance in the α to β polypeptide ratio (thalassaemia) of hemoglobin (Hb) or abnormalities in the function of the β-globin chain (sickle cell disease) (see Stamatoyannopoulos *et al.*, 1987; Weatherall and Clegg, 1981). It is estimated that approximately 250 million people carry hemoglobinopathies worldwide. This gives rise to more than 300,000 births each year that are homozygous for either thalassaemia or sickle cell disease.

β-Thalassaemia is caused by the absence (or decrease) of β-globin chains which results in the precipitation of untetramerized α-chains and consequent damage to the red blood cells. More than one hundred different mutations that affect β-globin gene expression have been identified (Kazazian *et al.*, 1990). Most are point mutations that affect transcription, splicing, or translation of β-globin mRNA which results in a lack or decrease in β-globin synthesis and early destruction of red blood cells.

The most common cause of sickle cell anemia results from a single amino acid change in the β-globin protein caused by a base change (G<u>A</u>T > G<u>T</u>T) in codon 6 of exon 1 and a consequent glutamic acid to valine substitution (β^6Val). The resulting β^s hemoglobin (HbS) undergoes aggregation in conditions of low oxygen tension and subsequently distorts red blood cell morphology to a characteristic rigid crescent ("sickle") shape (Huisman, 1993). Two other but much rarer mutations increase the

---

Michael Antoniou Department of Experimental Pathology, GKT Medical and Dental School, King's College, London, Guy's Hospital, London SE1 9RT, United Kingdom. **Frank Grosveld** Department of Cell Biology, Erasmus University-Rotterdam, 3000DR Rotterdam, The Netherlands.

Blood Cell Biochemistry, Volume 8: Hematopoiesis and Gene Therapy, edited by Fairbairn and Testa. Kluwer Academic/Plenum Publishers, New York, 1999.

tendency for Hb polymerization and red-cell sickling. The $\beta^{Antilles}$ allele is a double mutant that has an isoleucine residue at position 23 *in cis* with β^s (β^6Val β^{23}Ile). In contrast to individuals carrying a single β^s mutation, patients who are heterozygous for $\beta^{Antilles}$ have a very severe sickle cell phenotype (Monplaisir *et al.*, 1986). Similarly, compound heterozygotes of HbS and HbD Punjab (β^{121}Gln), also result in a marked sickle cell syndrome (Milner *et al.*, 1970; Padlan and Love, 1985). The mild to severe anemia (6–10 g Hb per 100 ml) associated with this disease is normally well tolerated. The main clinical manifestations arise from vaso-occlusion by the sickle cells within the microvasculature. This results in crises of extreme pain in the limbs, back, chest and abdomen and also in damage to organs, such as heart, lungs, spleen, and kidneys. Accumulated damage from repeated microinfarcts ultimately gives rise to organ failure and possibly death (see Noguchi *et al.*, 1993).

The aim of this review is to critically assess the current state and future prospects for developing genetic approaches to therapy for hemoglobinopathies, the pharmaceutical activation of the fetal γ-globin genes and gene therapy targeted at the hematopoietic stem cells. We begin with an assessment of the current therapies employed for hemoglobinopathies which highlights why there is a great deal of scope for improvement in this area. This is followed by a brief overview of the molecular mechanisms controlling gene expression from the human β-globin locus, an understanding of which lays the foundation for the genetic approaches to therapy that hold such promise for the future.

2. CURRENT THERAPIES FOR β-THALASSAEMIA

2.1. Blood Transfusions and Iron Chelation

Maintenance therapy for β-thalassaemia consists of transfusions of packed red blood cells every 2–3 weeks. This in turn results in iron overload which gives rise to internal organ damage if untreated. The only iron chelator currently approved is desferrioxamine (Desferal, Ciba Geigy) which has to be administered by slow subcutaneous infusion *via* a pump for 12 h per day, 6 days per week. Overall this treatment is time-consuming expensive, and is also very painful and stressful for the patient. Compliance with chelation therapy in particular is a major problem. Orally administered iron chelators are under development (see al-Refaie and Hoffbrand, 1994; Kontoghiorghes, 1995; Olivieri *et al.*, 1995) and would be a great asset when available. Generally, chelation retards rather than completely prevents organ damage from iron overload, even with well chelated patients who succumb in their 30's.

2.2. Allogeneic Hematopoietic Stem Cell Transplantation

Allogeneic hematopoietic stem cell (HSC) transplantation is a therapy that offers the potential for a long-term cure of β-thalassaemia and sickle cell disease. There are three main sources of HSC, bone marrow, umbilical cord blood (UCB), and cytokine-mobilized peripheral blood stem cells.

Bone marrow transplantation (BMT) from an HLA-identical donor (preferably a sibling) has been performed in cases of β-thalassaemia for several years now (see Apperley, 1993; Evans, 1992; Giardini *et al.*, 1995). A long-term success rate greater than 90% that has an 85% probability of disease-free survival for more than 10 years has been reported for patients less than 17 years of age who have been well chelated and show no signs of organ damage (Lucarelli *et al.*, 1990, 1993). Results from other centers show an overall survival rate of only 70% post-BMT (Vellodi *et al.*, 1994). Generally, success rates are lower for older patients or those who have reduced overall health status caused by inadequate chelation (Giardini *et al.*, 1993a; Lucarelli *et al.*, 1992, 1996). These observations indicate that careful regard of a patient's history and pathological condition is important when considering their suitability for treatment by BMT.

Human umbilical cord blood (UCB), which can be collected at birth and cryopreserved, offers an alternative source of HSC for transplantation (see Almici *et al.*, 1995). The advantages of UCB-derived stem cells compared with those obtained from bone marrow are a higher proliferative capacity and a lower immunologic reactivity which reduces the risks of graft-versus-host disease (GVHD). UCB is readily available and because of the establishment of cord blood banks (see Gluckman, 1994; McCullough *et al.*, 1994; Rubinstein *et al.*, 1994), the probability of finding an unrelated, HLA-matched donor for transplant are increased significantly. The results of only four UCB transplants in thalassaemia patients have been published (Issaragrisih, 1994; Issaragrisih *et al.*, 1995) or reported to the International Cord Blood Transplant Registry to date. All have been carried out with cord blood from a matched sibling. Three have been completely successful. The fourth was performed with far too few stem cells (10% of the required number) and was unsuccessful.

Autologous cytokine-mobilized peripheral blood stem cell transplantation has been used extensively to provide HSC in patients who are receiving intensive chemotherapy (Anderson, 1995). Now there are indications that heterologous grafts create a far lower risk of acute GVHD than originally envisaged which also makes them potentially suitable sources of HSC for transplantation in cases of inherited blood disorders, such as the hemoglobinopathies (Tanaka *et al.*, 1995). However, further trials are needed to assess the possibilities of chronic GVHD before this application is considered more seriously.

A recent further development with potential application in the hemoglobinopathies is *in utero* hematopoietic transplantation (see Cowan and Golbus, 1994; Flake and Zanjani, 1993; Touraine, 1992). Before 14–15 weeks of gestation, the immunocompetency of the fetus is extremely low. Therefore, introducing allogeneic HSC derived from early (<10–12 week) fetal liver or adult bone marrow (purged of T-cells), can result in successful engraftment. However, fetal manipulation of this type, especially with donor cells derived from aborted fetal tissue, clearly creates a major new set of ethical problems. Thus it may be that this procedure will only be indicated if no viable alternatives exist.

The main limitations of transplantation procedures include the availability of a suitably matched donor and relapse from GVHD at any stage after transplant. The selection of an unrelated donor whose "extended" HLA haplotype is identical to the patient's, may improve the chances of success and increasing the number of potential donors (Contu *et al.*, 1994).

3. CURRENT THERAPIES FOR SICKLE CELL DISEASE

The frequency of vaso-occlusive crises and the severity of the resulting clinical manifestations of sickle cell disease are highly variable and unpredictable (Noguchi *et al.*, 1993). Therefore, the general use of blood transfusion/chelation therapy and allogeneic HSC transplantation used for thalassaemia is not justified and must be assessed on a case by case basis. Transfusions are normally administered during and after crises. The indications for BMT for patients with sickle cell disease are a major debating point (Davies, 1993; Roberts and Davies, 1993). However, it is clearly a viable option for patients who have a propensity for frequent vaso-occlusive crises from a young age (Ferster *et al.*, 1992; Giardini *et al.*, 1993b; Vermylen and Cornu, 1993).

3.1. Antisickling Agents

Currently available antisickling agents which directly inhibit HbS polymerization (e.g., urea, peptide competitors) or increase erythrocyte cell volume to reduce Hb concentration (e.g., desmopressin acetate), are not sufficiently effective or safe to be administered prophylactically.

A main obstacle to developing more effictive antisickling agents has been the lack of a suitable small animal model system of the disease in which new pharmaceuticals could be easily tested. Now, however, a number of transgenic mouse models have been described (Greaves *et al.*, 1990; Rubin *et al.*, 1991; Ryan *et al.*, 1990; Trudel *et al.*, 1991) and are currently being assessed for similarity to the human condition (Fabry *et al.*, 1992, 1995; Lutty *et al.*, 1994; Trudel *et al.*, 1994). Unfortunately, some of these transgenic animals have the HbS-Antilles mutation, and therefore it is not clear how representative they are of the common HbS-codon 6 phenotype (Rubin *et al.*, 1991; Trudel *et al.*, 1991). The construction of more suitable models are under way in several laboratories (T. Townes, personal communication; G. Stamatoyannopoulos, personal communication).

The treatment options for thalassaemia and sickle cell disease are clearly far from satisfactory. Furthermore, blood transfusions and HSC transplantation require sophisticated and expensive medical services which are unavailable in many parts of the world where the hemoglobinopathies are most prevalent. Genetic therapeutic approaches offer the hope of overcoming these problems by establishing easily administered procedures that require less hospital support.

4. REGULATION OF GENE EXPRESSION FROM THE HUMAN β-GLOBIN LOCUS

The design of genetic therapeutic strategies for hemoglobinopathies requires a clear understanding of the molecular mechanisms of gene expression from the β-globin locus. This has a direct bearing on the structure of transcription units for gene therapy (see section 6) and the search for pharmaceuticals to reactivate adult fetal γ-globin genes (see section 5). Fortunately, great advances have been made in recent years in this area, and these are briefly summarized following.

The β-like globin genes are present as a multigene cluster on the short arm of chromosome 11 (Figure 1, upper panel). The cluster consists of five active genes arranged in the order in which they are expressed during development (Figure 1, lower panel). The embryonic ε-globin gene is located at the 5′ end of the cluster and is expressed in erythroid cells derived from yolk sac cells during the first few weeks of gestation. The γ-globin genes are expressed in yolk-sac and fetal-liver-derived erythrocytes until birth. The adult δ- and β-globin genes at the 3′ end of the locus are first activated in the fetal liver and increase in expression after birth when the site of haematopoiesis shifts to adult bone marrow. The expression of the δ-globin gene is very low and only a few percent of that of the β-globin gene.

Although erythroid-specific promoter and enhancer elements have been mapped for each of the active genes (Antoniou *et al.*, 1988; Behringer *et al.*, 1987; Bodine and Ley, 1987; Catala *et al.*, 1989; deBoer *et al.*, 1988; Gong *et al.*, 1991; Kollias *et al.*, 1987; McDonagh *et al.*, 1991; Peters *et al.*, 1993; Trepicchio *et al.*, 1994; Trudel *et al.*, 1987; Wall *et al.*, 1988; Wu *et al.*, 1990; Yu *et al.*, 1991), expression is under the primary control of the locus control region (LCR). The human β-globin LCR consists of five, developmentally stable, erythroid-specific DNaseI hypersensitive (HS) sites distributed over 16kb of DNA located 5′ of the

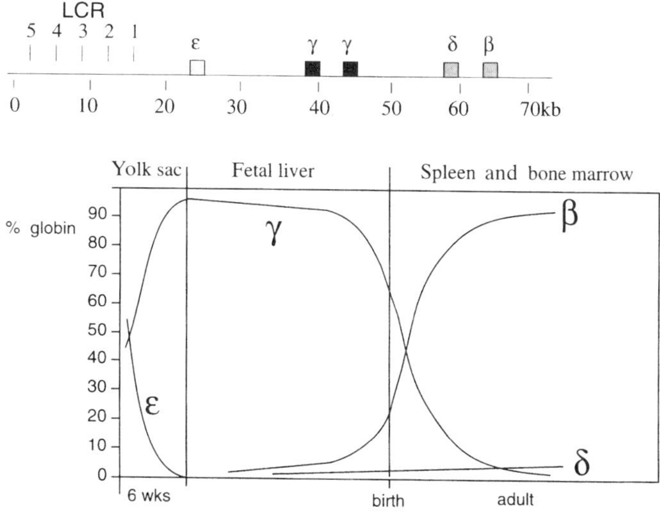

FIGURE 1. Structure and developmental pattern of gene expression of the human β-globin locus. Upper panel: The human β-globin locus that spans approximately 70kb on the short arm of chromosome 11. The embryonic ε-globin, two fetal γ-globin, adult δ- and β-globin genes are arranged in a 5′ to 3′ orientation and in the order in which they are expressed during development. The positions of the five DNaseI hypersensitive sites that constitute the locus control region (LCR) are also indicated. Lower panel: The site and pattern of expression of the genes from the β-globin locus during development.

entire β-globin gene cluster (Figure 1, upper panel). The βLCR was defined because it confers on a gene linked *in cis*, site-of-integration independent, physiological levels of erythroid-specific gene expression that are directly proportional to gene copy number in both transgenic mice (Grosveld *et al.*, 1987) and stably transfected tissue culture cells (Blom van Assendelft *et al.*, 1989). Each HS site of the βLCR maps to a 200–300 bp core region that consists of a high density of binding sites for both erythroid-specific and ubiquitous transcription factors (Philipsen *et al.*, 1990; Pruzina *et al.*, 1991; Talbot *et al.*, 1990; Zafaranga *et al.*, 1995). Testing these βLCR elements individually has shown that each HS site retains the essential properties of the LCR and possesses a degree of developmental specificity, albeit at a lower level of expression per gene (Fraser *et al.*, 1990 and 1993). These results imply that LCRs play a major role in developmental regulation and influence the expression level of a given gene.

The ability of the βLCR to override positional effects and confer transgenic copy-number-dependent expression suggests that it can open silent chromatin and establish and maintain a transcriptionally competent domain within an erythroid environment (Dillon and Grosveld, 1994; Felsenfeld, 1992; Grosveld *et al.*, 1987). The ability to open chromatin resides within HS3 because this is the only element that functions as a single copy in transgenic mice. HS sites 1, 2, and 4 function as LCRs only when present as multiple copies (Ellis *et al.*, 1996). These data suggest that the βLCR consists of two types of elements. First, the "core" of the LCR which has the capacity to generate an open chromatin domain, resides within HS3. Secondly, the other HS sites (numbers 1, 2, and 4) are powerful enhancer elements to boost the transcriptional potency of HS3 and hence give full dominant, transcriptional activaton at the physiologically required level. Therefore, the LCR acts as a master regulator because its activation which results in establishing an open chromatin structure, is a prerequisite for gene expression. Then transcription at the physiologically required level is achieved by an interaction between the LCR and the local promoter and enhancer elements of a gene.

Transgenic mouse experiments have also been conducted with the embryonic ε-globin (Raich *et al.*, 1990) and fetal γ-globin (Dillon and Grosveld, 1991) genes individually linked to the LCR. These studies show that the LCR confers full physiological levels of expression on these genes and that they are autonomously regulated during development. The ε-globin gene is expressed only in the embryonic yolk sack and not in fetal-liver or adult-bone-marrow-derived erythroid cells. The γ-globin gene is expressed at both embryonic and fetal stages of development but not in adult mice. The developmental pattern of expression observed with these transgenes mimics the situation in humans (Figure 1, lower panel) and is mediated primarily by the binding of developmental stage specific repressor proteins to the promoter regions of the ε-globin (Raich *et al.*, 1995) and γ-globin (see section 5) genes. These data suggest that a shift in the transcription factor complement during development results in changes in the relative strengths of the promoters of the β-like globin genes. This in turn dictates the capability of a given promoter to interact with the LCR and be transcribed. The binding of repressor protein(s) would weaken the interaction between the promoter and the LCR.

These experiments show that the first and most important level of developmental regulation of globin gene expression is activation of all of the genes by the LCR at all stages of development and repression of the early (ε and γ) genes by an, as yet unknown, number of factors (see section 5) that act on the sequences immediately flanking these genes. A second level of control that keeps the adult genes silenced early in development is superimposed on this repression mechanism. This does not occur through direct suppression acting on sequences immediately surrounding the gene, but *via* a mechanism in which the early (ε and γ) genes suppress the late (δ and β) genes by competing for the interaction with the LCR (Hanscombe *et al.*, 1991). The competitive ability of the genes is determined by their surrounding sequences and their ability to bind transcription factors and also by the position of the genes relative to the LCR. The shorter the relative distance to the LCR, the higher its competitive ability. Although this extra level of gene control is quantitatively less important than the direct repression mechanism in determining the relative levels of expression of the genes, it has significant implications and has provided an excellent assay system for probing transcriptional regulation at the single-cell level (see later).

The important implication of competitive gene interactions is that the βLCR complexes directly with each of the genes and that such interactions would be exclusive, that is, the LCR would be able to interact with only a single gene at a given time. *In situ* hybridization technology has allowed us to show that this is indeed the case when the γ- and β-glogin genes are expressed in the same cell during the period of switching from fetal to adult hemoglobin production (Wijgerde *et al.*, 1995). The results suggest that multiple genes are alternately, rather than cotranscribed, and the βLCR, stably complexes one gene at a time and switches back and forth between genes to generate multiple mRNAs in one cell. These data also imply that the βLCR is complexed with one of the genes almost all of the time. In a separate set of experiments we have shown that this is no longer the case when the βLCR is incomplete due to the deletion of any one of LCR HS sites. Such LCRs no longer provide the usual position-independent, transgenic copy-number-dependent expression when integrated into heterochromatic regions of the mouse genome (Milot *et al.*, 1996). Moreover, these studies confirmed that the level of transcription of the genes is determined by the frequency and duration of interactions with the LCR rather than by changes in the rate of transcription. Two disruption mechanisms of partial LCR activation were distinguished. One is a classical position effect variegation (PEV; see Hendrich and Willard, 1995; Karpen, 1994), that results in continuous transcription in some of the cells. The other is a novel mechanism that results in intermittent gene transcription and silencing in all red cells.

We have recently completed two independent sets of experiments that add further support to this dynamic, promoter-strength and distance-dependent transcriptional activation model of the βLCR. First, we have studied the regulation of the globin genes in both the absence of or at half the normal amount of the transcription factor EKLF by inactivating its gene in the mouse (Nuez *et al.*, 1995). This zinc-finger protein binds to promoter sequences of the β-globin gene but not to those of the ε- or γ-globin genes. A lack of EKLF leads to an absence of β-globin gene expression and a fatal anaemia just past midgestation in transgenic mice that carry the β-globin locus (Wijgerde *et al.*, 1996). Most interesting are the mice that express half the normal level of EKLF. They show a shift in expression from β- to γ-globin during HbF to HbA switching. The elevation in γ-globin expression is entirely accounted for by an increase in both the frequency and periods of transcription of the γ-globin genes. Secondly, we have analyzed the competition between two β-globin genes by placing an extra gene at different positions in the β-globin locus (Dillon *et al.*, 1997). This analysis confirms that competition depends on the relative distance to the LCR because the extra gene competes with the resident β-globin gene more effectively, the closer it is to the LCR. In addition, *in situ* hybridization analysis shows that the differences in transcription levels observed for different positions of the extra gene are entirely accounted for by a difference in the frequency of transcription of the extra gene versus the resident β-globin gene.

These observations that involve a dynamic, distance-dependent interaction between the βLCR and a given gene can be explained by looping of the chromatin between the LCR and individual genes, although a linear process (i.e., a process moving along the DNA) could also explain these data (Martin *et al.*, 1996).

In summary, the study of the β-globin genes has pointed us in directions that are directly relevant to the transcriptional regulation of this locus and possibly to the development of novel treatments for patients. However, most interestingly it has allowed us to start formulating the basics of a dynamic and general mechanism of gene transcription/regulation *in vivo*. This mechanism takes into account a new level of complexity in which space and time play important roles.

5. PHARMACEUTICAL ACTIVATION OF FETAL γ-GLOBIN GENE EXPRESSION IN THE ADULT

A number of mutations have been characterized that result in persistent fetal γ-globin gene expression in the adult (hereditary persistence of fetal hemoglobin, HPFH; see Wood, 1993). HPFH is a clinically benign condition characterized by levels of HbF as high as 30% of total hemoglobin in some cases. These elevated levels of γ-globin gene expression compensate for the deficiency or abnormality in β-globin within individuals who are compound heterozygotes for HPFH and thalassaemia or sickle cell disease. Such individuals are asymptomatic and transfusion-independent. The molecular mechanisms resulting in HPFH is an area of intense research in the hope that it will give rise to a pharmacological approach to activating the γ-globin genes in adults afflicted with a hemoglobinopathy, with resulting therapeutic benefit.

The HPFH phenotype results either from deletions that juxtapose an erythroid-specific enhancer downstream of the $^{A}\gamma$-globin gene (Anagnou *et al.*, 1995; Elder *et al.*, 1990; Feingold and Forget, 1989) or from point mutations in the promoters of the γ-globin genes (see Gilman, 1988). The promoter point mutations are generally of two types. First, several are located in the upstream part of the promoter (–158 to –202) and enhance the binding of the transcription factors Sp1 (Fischer and Nowock, 1990; Ronchi *et al.*, 1989; Sykes and Kaufman, 1990) or

GATA-1 (Gumucio *et al.*, 1990; Martin *et al.*, 1989; Nicolis *et al.*, 1989). In addition, point mutations mapping to the distal CCAAT box at –117 ("Greek HPFH"; Collins *et al.*, 1985; Gelinas *et al.*, 1985) and –114 (Japanese/Georgian C–T, Fucharoen *et al.*, 1990; Oner *et al.*, 1991; Australian C–G, Motum *et al.*, 1994) and a 13 bp deletion that spans this region (American black; Gilman *et al.*, 1988) have been described and may interfere with the binding of a transcriptional repressor protein complex. Perturbations in the complement of protein factors binding to the distal CCAAT box caused by these mutations have been documented (Mantovani *et al.*, 1988; Superti-Furga *et al.*, 1988). In particular, the –117 Greek HPFH mutation, which of the three CCAAT box mutations results in the highest levels of γ-globin (20%), markedly reduces the binding of GATA-1 (Berry *et al.*, 1992) and NF-E3 (Mantovani *et al.*, 1989). This suggests that GATA-1, NF-E3, or both are involved in supressing fetal globin gene expression after birth. However, analysis of transgenic mice carrying γ-globin genes harboring point mutations in the CCAAT box region, which specifically abolishes the binding of either GATA-1 or NF-E3, does not indicate a clear HPFH phenotype (Ronchi *et al.*, 1996). This suggests that neither of these two factors independently constitutes the repressor function but may be part of a large protein complex, in which the CCAAT box is a crucial although not necessarily exclusive DNA contact point.

The first pharmacological agents used to increase γ-globin gene expression in adults who have hemoglobinopathies were 5-azacytidine (5-azaC; Charache *et al.*, 1983; Ley *et al.*, 1983) and hydroxyurea (Platt *et al.*, 1984). These moderately increased HbF levels in a number of patients tested. The potential mutagenic nature of 5-azaC prevented its further implementation. However, hydroxyurea is continuing to be assessed on a long term basis (Charache, 1994; Charache *et al.*, 1995; Voskaridou *et al.*, 1995). More recently, butyric acid derivatives, such as sodium phenylbutyrate (Collins *et al.*, 1995; Dover *et al.*, 1994) and arginine butyrate (Sher *et al.*, 1995), have also entered clinical trials. In general, patient response in terms of HbF expression has proved very variable for all of these substances and clinically useful levels have been seen in only a few cases. Nevertheless, very encouraging results have been observed in sickle cell patients treated with hydroxyurea, alone (Charache *et al.*, 1995; Voskaridou *et al.*, 1995) or in combination with erythropoietin (el-Hazmi *et al.*, 1995; Rodgers *et al.*, 1993). These patients experience significantly fewer crises, an increase in the time between sickling episodes, and an overall reduction in painful discomfort. These trials showed that it may take several months for benefits to be felt and that each patient requires careful monitoring to avoid toxicity as the dose of agent is gradually increased during this period. The results obtained from a Multicentre Trial (Charache *et al.*, 1995) prompted the National Heart Lung and Blood Institute (USA) to issue a Clinical Alert on January 30th 1995 announcing the effectiveness of hydroxyurea for treating sickle cell disease (see Platt, 1995).

The mechanism of action of hydroxyurea is currently debatable. Given the variable levels of HbF production induced in patients, its overall efficacy may lie more in its anti-sickling properties rather than increases in γ-globin gene expression. In addition, cytostatic effects could suppress the anemia-induced, excessive bone marrow activity which normally causes severe pain.

A number of problems accompany the use of hydroxyurea in sickle cell disease. First, patient response is variable, and many patients are refractory to the action of this drug. Secondly, the long term effects of administering such a powerful metabolic toxin are still far from clear especially because complications have already been reported (Vichinsky and Lubin, 1994). Lastly, none of the drugs, including hydroxyurea, used to increase γ-globin gene expression, have been successful in treating transfusion-dependent, β-thalassaemia patients.

Therefore pharmaceuticals that have a more specific mode of action on the repressor(s) of the γ-globin genes in adults are still needed. Two possible approaches can be used to achieve this end. The first relies on thorough knowledge of the repressors and their mode of action. Ideally this should include three-dimensional structural data which reveal the connection between the various components and the regions of contact with the promoter DNA. Then, pharmaceuticals could be designed to interfere with one or more of these interactions. This approach would be quite feasible if a single or at most two proteins were involved. However, as described earlier in this section, on the basis of currently available data the mechanism of γ-globin gene repression involves a multicomponent complex which makes dissecting its mechanism and deriving structural information extremely difficult. Therefore technical constraints severely limit the practicality of this approach now.

An alternative strategy without the same restrictions is based on a random screening of compounds without prior detailed knowledge of the repressor complex. Drug discovery based on the activation or repression of transcription by the robotized, random screening of compounds is a new initiative within the pharmaceutical industry but one which in all likelihood will increase in importance. Nevertheless, this approach still relies on understanding the DNA regulatory elements responsible for conferring the observed pattern of expression on the target gene. This approach involves constructing a stable, transfected, test cell line harboring an easily assayable reporter gene (e.g., luciferase) driven by the desired genetic control elements into whose action one is seeking to intervene. Then the test cell line is subjected to treatment with substances to assess their ability to activate or repress the expression of the reporter gene. This whole automated process allows screening several thousand compounds per month. In the search for activators of the γ-globin genes, a murine erythroleukaemia cell line containing a γ-globin mini-locus (see Dillon and Grosveld, 1991) or preferably the entire human β-globin locus (see Strouboulis *et al.*, 1992) is required. The nature of the adult stage of these cells ensures that the γ-globin genes are normally silent. We have recently initiated a project to generate transgenic mice harboring such constructs from which the production of cell lines will be possible (Grosveld *et al.*, 1996).

6. GENE THERAPY

Three main components must be considered for any given gene therapy strategy. These are the target tissue and biology of the disease, the gene delivery system, and the regulation of expression of the therapeutic transcription unit. These are interdependent components, and each imposes restrictions on the other two. In hemoglobinopathies the cells that must be targeted for a long-term therapeutic effect are the HSC which are a major gene therapy target for a number of other inherited metabolic disorders (e.g., mucopolysaccharidoses) and acquired diseases (e.g., leukemia, AIDS). A number of excellent reviews that address gene transfer into HSC in general and within the context of the hemoglobinopathies have been published in recent years (Brenner *et al.*, 1995; Clapp, 1993; Dunbar and Emmons, 1994; Einerhand and Valerio, 1992; Kiem *et al.*, 1995; Kohn, 1995; Nienhuis, 1994; Smith, 1992; Walsh *et al.*, 1993). The aim of this review is to assess the status of the field primarily from the viewpoint of the latest findings regarding the mechanism of gene expression from the β-globin locus. This will highlight the improvements that need to be made, especially in designing the therapeutic transcription unit for an effictive gene therapy protocol.

It has been estimated from cases of thalassaemia intermedia that 25% of the normal level of β-globin chains would be sufficient to render a patient transfusion-independent. The quantity required for a therapeutic effect in patients who have sickle cell disease is unknown but is likely to be of the same order. This amount of β-globin could be achieved from a single copy of the gene introduced into the HSC of a patient and could function reproducibly at 50% of wild-type levels. However, in practice a much higher level of gene expression may be required because it may not be possible to modify all of the patient's HSC genetically. Another major limitation posed by the biology of HSCs is that they are very rare ($1{:}10^4$–10^5 of total bone marrow cells) and are normally quiescent. As discussed later, in the absence of an efficient *in vivo* targeted delivery system, gene therapy of HSC presently can be contemplated only by an *ex vivo* procedure where cells are first isolated, genetically modified in tissue culture, and then returned to the patient. However, autologous grafts of this type have clear advantages over allogeneic transplants (see section 2) because there is no risk of rejection or GVHD. As discussed previously (section 2), HSC can be obtained from bone marrow or from the periphery after cytokine mobilization. UCB stem cells are also a potential target for gene therapy. The cord blood of a prenatally diagnosed affected fetus can be collected at birth, and the stem cells can be purified and genetically modified before returning them to the infant (Bahnson *et al.*, 1994; Kohn *et al.*, 1995; Williams and Moritz, 1994).

There are two possible means by which stable retention of the therapeutic gene construct introduced within HSC can be achieved, namely the use of self-replicating episomal vectors or integration into the host cell genome. Self-replicating episomal vectors which utilise viral origins of replication, such as those from EBV (Yates *et al.*, 1985), human papovavirus BK (Cooper and Miron, 1993; De Benedetti and Rhoads, 1991), and BPV-1, (Piirsoo *et al.*, 1996) have been developed. In addition, combinations of human genomic and viral origins have been used (Krysan *et al.*, 1989; Wohlgemuth *et al.*, 1996). Many problems make these vectors currently impractical or unsafe to use. First, these vectors are generally large and can be introduced into cells only by using nonviral delivery systems which are presently inefficient. In addition, the viral protein components required for self-replication and maintenance of episomes (e.g., EBNA-1 of EBV-based vectors) are toxic when present in excessive amounts and are potentially oncogenic. This is a particular concern because there is no method of controlling episome copy number and therefore transgenic expression levels per cell. Now, therefore, stable integration of the therapeutic gene construct into the HSC genome remains the preferred option for obtaining long-term expression.

Presently, stable integration of foreign DNA within the host cell genome, can be achieved efficiently only by using retroviral (Miller, 1992; Miller, A. D. *et al.*, 1993) and adeno-associated viral (AAV; Flotte and Carter, 1995; Muzyczka, 1992) vectors. However, these vectors possess major limitations which greatly influences the design of the transcription unit which they can accommodate. First, both have limited capacity for genetic material, approximately 8kb for retroviruses and 4.4kb in the case of AAV. Additionally, retroviruses infect and integrate only into dividing cells. AAV transduces nondividing cells (Podsakoff *et al.*, 1994) but at a much lower efficiency than those in S-phase (Russell *et al.*, 1994). This is a major obstacle because at any given time most HSC are quiescent. However, vectors based on HIV, which in principle can infect nondividing cells, may overcome this difficulty (Naldini *et al.*, 1996). A second, but by nomeans insurmountable problem is that, obtaining sufficiently high viral titers can be difficult with these vectors, particularly when complex transcription units are incorporated into them.

The potential of retroviral vectors for delivering a human β-globin gene to HSC was demonstrated in animal (murine) model systems several years ago (Bender *et al.*, 1989; Dzierzak *et al.*, 1988; Karlsson *et al.*, 1988). These vectors contain a complete genomic β-globin gene that has all of the known local erythroid specific promoter and enhancer elements (Antoniou *et al.*, 1988; Behringer *et al.*, 1987; deBoer *et al.*, 1988; Kollias *et al.*, 1987; Trudel *et al.*, 1987; Wall *et al.*, 1988). However, the level of expression observed in these studies was very low and variable (0.1–5% of normal) and therefore well below a therapeutically useful value. The discovery of the βLCR (see section 4) made gene therapy for hemoglobinopathies a practical possibility. Included as part of the transcription unit the βLCR should overcome the chromatin positional effects that condemned these early experiments to failure and should provide a predictable, sustained physiological level of gene expression required for clinical benefit.

The four transcriptionally active DNaseI hypersensitive sites that constitute the βLCR (numbers 1–4), are normally distributed over 16kb (see Figure 1, upper panel). This is clearly too large to be accommodated within a retroviral or AAV vector. However, great efforts have been made to minimize the size and combination of elements required to produce LCR activity (Antoniou and Grosveld, 1990; Collis *et al.*, 1990; Fraser *et al.*, 1990; Philipsen *et al.*, 1990; Pruzina *et al.*, 1991; Raguz and Grosveld, unpublished; Talbot *et al.*, 1989, 1990). In addition, the β-globin gene must have both of its introns to accumulate stable cytoplasmic mRNA efficiently (Collis *et al.*, 1990). The second intervening sequence, which is needed for efficient polyadenylation and subsequent transport of mature mRNA to the cytoplasm, is absolutely required (Antoniou *et al.*, 1998). This has resulted in testing a number of βLCR/β-globin minigene transcription units within a retrovirus and more recently, in AAV.

Much attention has been paid to βLCR HS2 which possesses potent classical enhancer activity localized to an NF-E2/AP-1 dimer binding site within its core region (Ney *et al.*, 1990a,b; Tuan *et al.*, 1989). Retroviral vectors that incorporate this element, which drives a human β-globin gene, have been used to infect murine erythroleukaemic (MEL) cells in tissue culture (Chang *et al.*, 1992; Leboulch *et al.*, 1994; Takekoshi *et al.*, 1995). The data show clearly enhanced expression over that seen with the gene alone but levels are still too variable and low to be of therapeutic value. Furthermore, retroviral sequences are inhibitory to expression from an HS 2/β-globin gene combination (McCune and Townes, 1994). Similar results have been obtained with βLCR HS 2/γ-globin constructs in AAV vectors which were used to transduce human erythroleukaemic, K562 cells (Miller, J. L. *et al.*, 1993; Walsh *et al.*, 1992).

Recent results from transgenic mice (Ellis *et al.*, 1993, 1996; see section 4), have shown that the use of βLCR HS 2 alone will not be sufficient for stable, high level, lineage-specific gene expression. These studies demonstrate that this element functions only as an LCR at multiple copy number. In contrast, HS 3 gives significant but variable (20%–40%) levels of expression even as a single copy. Because retroviral and AAV vectors normally result in independent integration within the transduced cell, the βLCR transcription unit must function reproducibly at single copy, a condition which is met only if HS 3 is included. However, because the use of HS 3 alone still results in variable levels of expression which are below a therapeutic value (Ellis *et al.*, 1996), a combination of βLCR elements is clearly required. Because the deletion of individual LCR elements from within the whole locus results in the loss of full LCR activity (Milot *et al.*, 1996; see section 4), this strongly indicates that all HS sites must be included as part of the transcription unit to guarantee therapeutic levels of expression.

Retroviral (Leboulch *et al.*, 1994; Novak *et al.*, 1990; Plavec *et al.*, 1993; Sadelain *et al.*, 1995) and AAV (Einerhand *et al.*, 1995; Miller *et al.*, 1994) vectors containing multiple βLCR HS sites have been tested but, on the whole, with similarly disappointing results. In retrospect, two of the studies, which attempted to combine all four βLCR HS sites within a retroviral backbone (Novak *et al.*, 1990; Plavec *et al.*, 1993), resulted in the inadvertent omission of HS 4 (see Pruzina *et al.*, 1991) and the 5′ half of HS 3 (see Philipsen *et al.*, 1993). Therefore, the results obtained really reflect only the effect of the combination of HS 1 and 2. More recently, retroviral (Leboulch *et al.*, 1994; Sadelain *et al.*, 1995) and AAV (Einerhand *et al.*, 1995; Miller *et al.*, 1994) vectors that combine the core (200–300 bp) regions of the three most transcriptionally active sites (HS 2, 3, and 4), have been constructed and tested. These vectors, which contain such a highly simplified LCR of just over 900 bp long, allow much higher retroviral titers (Sadelain *et al.*, 1995). However the expression levels obtained with both retroviral (Sadelain *et al.*, 1995) and AAV (Miller *et al.*, 1994) based constructs, were still too variable (4%–146%) to indicate these vectors for therapeutic use. Therefore much larger fragments that encompass the βLCR HS sites are needed to preserve full activity and position-independent expression.

Including a neomycin resistance gene driven off the retroviral LTR (Chang *et al.*, 1992; Leboulch *et al.*, 1994; Novak *et al.*, 1990; Takekoshi *et al.*, 1995) or an internal promoter in AAV (Einerhand *et al.*, 1995; Walsh *et al.*, 1992) in many of the vectors tested gives further reason to interpret many of the published results cautiously. This allowed selecting stably transduced cells with G418 which automatically selects for transgenic integration into open, actively transcribed chromatin. This has the effect of skewing the observed gene expression to much higher levels and with less variability than in cases where no selection is applied (Leboulch *et al.*, 1994; Miller *et al.*, 1994; Sadelain *et al.*, 1995). Because transduction in gene therapy will, in all likelihood, have to be performed in the absence of selection, the testing of gene constructs should involve procedures that avoid this process.

Generally, studies with retroviral and AAV vectors have demonstrated the feasibility, in principle, of using these delivery vehicles for gene therapy of hemoglobinopathies. However, the constructs tested so far give expression levels of β- or γ-globin that are either too low or too variable to be of therapeutic value. However, a fully functional βLCR-driven transcription unit has not yet been assessed in either system. This indicates that further refinements in designing the vectors are needed before a guaranteed therapeutic effect can be achieved.

Recent insight into the mechanism of βLCR-mediated transcription from experiments in transgenic mice has provided a clearer insight into what further modifications need to be made (see section 4). The need to include all four HS sites to obtain maximum gene expression suggests that the LCR forms a "holo-complex" of elements (Ellis *et al.*, 1996) which then can activate transcription from a single gene within the locus at any given time by direct contact with the promoter *via* a chromatin looping mechanism (Wijgerde *et al.*, 1995). The analysis of 70 kb constructs that encompass an entire β-globin locus, from which a single LCR HS site has been deleted, has shown that position-independent expression is lost when any of these elements, including the transcriptionally weak HS 1, is missing (Milot *et al.*, 1996). Finally, the inability of small βLCR constructs that consist of the HS cores ligated together to produce site-of-integration independent expression in both tissue culture cells (Einerhand *et al.*, 1995; Sadelain *et al.*, 1995) and transgenic mice (Antoniou *et al.*, unpublished) implies the need for larger constructs. Because a 6.5 kb microlocus βLCR functions reproducibly as a single copy transgene (Ellis *et al.*, 1996), indications are that the spacing between HS sites may be crucial (Jackson *et al.*, 1996). Again this observation is consistent with the model that the LCR functions as a holo-complex which requires a sufficient distance between HS sites to allow efficient interactions between elements.

These data taken together suggest that all four βLCR HS sites with a minimal spacing between these elements must be incorporated in future transcriptional units to provide full position-independent expression at a sufficiently high level to be of therapeutic value. Current data indicate that the distance between sites must be of the order of 1–2 kb. Although not thoroughly tested, presumably a minimal distance from the center of the βLCR to the promoter also has to included. In addition, because the βLCR activates the nearest open promoter (Hanscombe *et al.*, 1991), a region of neutral, "spacer" DNA sequences may also be required upstream of the LCR to maintain a clear advantage for the linked gene of choice.

7. SUMMARY AND FUTURE PROSPECTS

Hemoglobinopathies were the first genetically inherited diseases whose molecular basis was clearly understood, and it was thought that they would be among the first to be treated by gene therapy. However, the development of genetic approaches to therapy for hemoglobinopathies is a good example how what appears straightforward in theory turns out to be far more difficult to achieve in practice. Nevertheless, our understanding of the molecular mechanisms underlying the regulation of expression from the human β-globin locus surpasses that for most other gene families and puts researchers in an almost unique position in designing genetic therapeutic strategies. As technological advances have been made and progressively more has been learned about the molecular mechanisms of gene expression from the β-globin locus, certain options have become feasible, and others have had to be discarded. The random screening of compounds for activating the γ-globin genes in adult patients would have been impossible more than six years ago. The evolution of this field in general illustrates that significant advances can be made only on the basis of insight gained through basic research into the genetics and biology of the disease and the gene delivery systems. In addition, it must also be kept in mind that the vast majority of individuals who have hemoglobinopathies are born in the less developed parts of the world which lack sophisticated, modern medical services. Therefore, any genetic therapy must be inexpensive and easy to administer if it is to benefit all those in need.

Now it is increasingly unlikely that retroviral or AAV vectors are going to be suitable because all four DNaseI hypersensitive sites must be included with minimal spacing between each element to obtain full reproducible βLCR activity and therefore guarantee therapeutic levels of gene expression. Given their limited capacity, it is doubtful whether all of the required genetic components can be acommodated within these vectors. However, from a practical standpoint this may not be such a great loss because these viral vectors are difficult and expensive to produce and can be administered only as part of an *ex vivo* protocol which severely limits their usefulness. Furthermore, although these vectors can infect HSC in animal model systems, they have proved very ineffective thus far in transducing human HSC.

Therefore, it is necessary to explore nonviral gene delivery which is not hampered by the potentially large size of the desired transcription unit and which can more efficiently deliver DNA to human HSC. Furthermore, because these vectors would be composed of synthetic chemical components that can be produced cheaply on a large scale and are easily stored with a long shelf life, they should have a far greater practical utility. In this regard, the system that holds the greatest promise is based on receptor-mediated endocytosis (RME; see Guy *et al.*, 1995). By coupling DNA to a ligand or antibody specific for an HSC cell-surface antigen, in principle, the therapeutic transcription unit can be targeted systemically. A number of technical problems must be overcome before this method is of practical value. The efficiency of delivery must be significantly improved, and, in particular, nuclear uptake in nondividing cells deserves careful study. Inactivation by serum complement must also be circumvented to achieve effective systemic delivery. In an ideal scenario, gene constructs would be included as part of self-replicating episomal vectors to avoid problems of insertional mutagenesis. However, if self-replicating episomal vectors prove difficult to control, then an efficient system of stable integration must be developed based on, for example, retroviral integrases or bacterial recombinases. Integration should preferably be targeted at noncoding, heterochromatic regions of the genome (e.g., centromeres) to prevent insertional mutagenesis. Including a fully functional LCR ensures that, even incorporating the therapeutic transcriptional unit into silent heterochromatin, physiological levels of gene expression will still result (Festenstein *et al.*, 1996; Milot *et al.*, 1996). Finally, RME can also be used to deliver short RNA-DNA hybrid oligonucleotides that correct the genetic defect in cells derived from patients who have sickle cell disease by site-directed gene conversion (Cole-Strauss *et al.*, 1996). Similar results have been obtained with a cDNA that spans a mutation which causes cystic fibrosis in lung epithelial cells (Kunzelmann *et al.*, 1996). If this type of gene repair by homologous recombination can be optimized, it may offer the best possible approach for gene therapy in many instances.

In this review we have emphasized that gene therapy is only one treatment option that may become possible from understanding the basic cell and molecular biology of a given tissue and disease. The pharmacological activation of latent gene functions or the supression of expressed genes offers a clear viable alternative. Although it may take 10–15 years to develop a new drug starting from a random screen of compounds, the ease of administration of this type of therapy makes it very attractive. Gene therapy and pharmacological manipulation of gene expression are complementary rather than mutually exclusive procedures. Drugs can be used to control a disease until an efficient and safe gene therapy protocol is established to provide a long-term cure. Clearly, these two approaches should be developed in parallel, whenever possible. In either case, a genetic therapy for hemoglobinopathies unfortunately lies many years in the future.

ACKNOWLEDGEMENTS. The authors would like to express their appreciation to the many organizations that have supported and continue to support their work in this field, namely, the Medical Research Council, U.K., Zeneca (formerly I.C.I.) Pharmaceuticals, Therexsys, U.K., Oncogene Science (USA), the NWO (Netherlands), the Howard Hughes Foundation, and the European Union Biomed and Biotech programs. The secretarial assistance of Brenda Williams is also gratefully acknowledged.

8. REFERENCES

al-Refaie, F. N., and Hoffbrand, A. V., 1994, Oral iron chelation therapy: The L1 experience, *Baillieres Clin. Haematol.* **7:**941–963.

Almici, C., Carlo-Stella, C., Wagner, J. E., and Rizzoli, V., 1995, Umbilical cord blood as a source of hematopoietic stem cells: From research to clinical application *Haematologica* **80:**473–479.

Anagnou, N. P., Perez-Stable, C., Gelinas, R., Costantini, F., Liapaki, K., Constantopoulou, M., Kosteas, T., Moschonas, N. K., and Stamatoyannopoulos, G., 1995, Sequences located 3′ to the breakpoint of the hereditary persistence of fetal hemoglobin-3 deletion exhibit enhancer activity and can modify the development of the human $^{A}\gamma$-globin gene in transgenic mice, *J. Biol. Chem.* **270:**10256–10263.

Anderson, K. C., 1995, Autologous peripheral blood progenitor cell transplantation, *J. Clin. Apheres.* **10:**131–138.

Antoniou M., deBoer, E., Habets, G., and Grosveld, F., 1988, The human β-globin gene contains multiple regulatory regions: Identification of one promoter and two downstream enhancers, *EMBO J.* **7:**377–384.

Antoniou, M., Geraghty, F., Hurst, J., and Grosveld, F., 1998, Efficient 3′-end formation of human β-globin mRNA *in vivo* requires sequences within the last intron but occurs indipendently of the splicing reaction, *Nucl. Acids. Res.* **26:**721–729.

Antoniou, M., and Grosveld, F., 1990, The β-globin gene dominant control region interacts differently with distal and proximal promoter elements, *Genes Dev.* **4:**1007–1012.

Apperley, J. F., 1993, Bone marrow transplant for the haemoglobinopathies, *Baillieres Clin. Haematol.* **6:**299–325.

Bahnson, A. B., Nimgaonkar, M., Fei, Y., Boggs, S. S., Robbins, P. D., Ohashi, T., Dunigan, J., Li, J., Ball, E. D., and Barranger, J. A., 1994, Transduction of CD34+ enriched cord blood and Gaucher bone marrow cells by a retroviral vector carrying the glucocerebrosidase gene, *Gene Ther.* **1:**176–184.

Behringer, R. R., Hammer, R. E., Brinster, R. L., Palmiter, R. D., and Townes, T. M., 1987, Two 3′ sequences direct adult erythroid specific expression of human -globin genes in transgenic mice, *Proc. Natl. Acad. Sci. USA* **84:**7056–7060.

Bender, M. A., Gelinas, R. E., and Miller, A. D., 1989, A majority of mice show long-term expression of a human β-globin gene after retrovirus transfer into hematopoietic stem cells, *Mol. Cell. Biol.* **9:**1426–1434.

Berry, M., Dillon, N., and Grosveld, F., 1992, A single point mutation is the cause of the Greek form of hereditary persistence of fetal hemoglobin, *Nature* **358:**499–452.

Blom van Assendelft, G., Hanscombe, O., Grosveld, F., and Greaves, D. R., 1989, The β globin dominant control region activates homologous and heterologous promoters in a tissue-specific manner, *Cell* **56:**969–977.

Bodine, D. M., and Ley, T. J., 1987, An enhancer element lies 3′ to the $^{A}\gamma$ globin gene, *EMBO J.* **6:**2997–3004.

Brenner, M. K., Cunningham, J. M., Sorrentino, B. P., and Heslop, H. E., 1995, Gene transfer into human hematopoietic progenitor cells, *Brit. Med. Bull.* **51:**167–191.

Catala, F., deBoer E., Habets, G., and Grosveld, F., 1989, Nuclear protein factors and erythroid transcription of the human $^{A}\gamma$-globin gene, *Nucleic Acids Res.* **17:**3811–3827.

Chang, J. C., Liu, D., and Kan, Y. W., 1992, A 36-base-pair core sequence of the locus control region enhances retrovirally transferred human β-globin gene expression, *Proc. Natl. Acad. Sci. USA* **89:**3107–3110.

Charache, S., 1994, Experimental therapy of sickle cell disease. Use of hydroxyurea, *Am. J. Pediat. Hematol.-Oncol.* **16:**62–66.

Charache, S., Dover, G., Smith, K., Talbot, C.C. Jr., Moyer, M., and Boyer, S., 1983, Treatment of sickle cell anemia with 5-azacytidine results in increased fetal hemoglobin production and is associated with nonrandom hypomethylation of DNA around the γ-δ-β-globin gene complex, *Proc. Natl. Acad. Sci. USA* **80:**4842–4846.

Charache, S., Terrin, M. L., Moore, R. D., Dover, G. J., Barton, F. B., Eckert, S. V., McMahon, R. P., and Bonds, D. R., 1995, Effect of hydroxyurea on the frequency of painful crises in sickle cell anemia. Investigators of the Multicentre Study Of Hydroxyurea in Sickle Cell Anemia, *N. Engl. J. Med.* **332:**1317–1322.

Clapp, D. W., 1993, Somatic gene therapy into hematopoietic cells. Current status and future implications, *Clin. Perinatol.* **20:**155–168.

Cole-Strauss, A., Yoon, K., Xiang, Y., Byrne, B. C., Rice, M. C., Gryn, J., Holloman, W. K., and Kmiec, E. B., 1996, Correction of the mutation responsible for sickle cell anemia by an RNA-DNA oligonucleotide, *Science* **273:**1386–1388.

Collins, A. F., Pearson, H. A., Giardina, P., McDonagh, K. T., Brusilow, S. W., and Dover, G. J., 1995, Oral sodium phenylbutyrate therapy in homozygous beta-thalassemia: A clinical trial, *Blood* **85:**43–49.

Collins, F., Metherall, J., Yamakawa, M., Pan, J., Weismann, S. M., and Forget, B., 1985, A point mutation in the A gamma-globin gene promoter in Greek hereditary persistence of fetal hemoglobin, *Nature* **313:**325–326.

Collis, P., Antoniou, M., and Grosveld, F., 1990, Definition of the minimal requirements within the human β-globin gene and the dominant control region for high level expression. *EMBO J.* **9:**233–240

Contu, L., La Nasa, G., Arras, M., Ledda, A., Pizzati, A., Vacca, A., Carcassi, C., Floris, L., Porcella, R., and Oru, S., 1994, Successful unrelated bone marrow transplantation in β-thalassaemia, *Bone Marrow Transplant.* **13:**329–331.

Cooper, M. J., and Miron, S., 1993, Efficient episomal expression vector for human transitional carcinoma cells, *Hum. Gene Ther.* **4:**557–566.

Cowan, M. J., and Golbus, M., 1994, In utero hematopoietic stem cell transplants for inherited diseases, *Am. J. Pediat. Hematol.-Oncol.* **16:**35–42.

Davies, S. C., 1993, Bone marrow transplant for sickle cell disease—the dilemma, *Blood Rev.* **7:**4–9.

De Benedetti, A., and Rhoads, R. E., 1991, A novel BK virus-based episomal vector for expression of foreign genes in mammalian cells, *Nucleic Acids Res.* **19:**1925–1931.

deBoer, E., Antoniou, M., Mignotte, V., Wall, L., and Grosveld, F., 1988, The human β-globin promoter; nuclear protein factors and erythroid specific induction of transcription, *EMBO J.* **7:**4203–4212

Dillon, N., and Grosveld, F., 1991, Human γ-globin genes silenced independently of other genes in the β-globin locus, *Nature* **350:**252–254.

Dillon, N., and Grosveld, F., 1994, Chromatin domains as potential units of eukaryotic gene function, *Curr. Opinion Genet. Dev.* **4:**260–264.

Dillon, N., Trimborn, T., Strouboulis, J., Fraser, P., and Grosveld, F., 1997, The effects of distance on long-range chromatin interactions, *Mol. Cell* **1:**131–139.

Dover, G. J., Brusilow, S. W., and Charache, S., 1994, Induction of fetal hemoglobin production in subjects with sickle cell anemia by oral sodium phenylbutyrate, *Blood* **84:**339–343.

Dunbar, C. E., and Emmons, R. V., 1994, Gene transfer into hematopoietic progenitor and stem cells: Progress and problems, *Stem Cells* **12:**563–576.

Dzierzak, E. A., Papayannopoulou, T., and Mulligan, R. C., 1988, Lineage-specific expression of a human β-globin gene in murine bone marrow transplant recipients reconstituted with retrovirus-transduced stem cells, *Nature* **331:**35–41

Einerhand, M. P., and Valerio, D., 1992, Gene transfer into hematopoietic stem cells: Prospects for human gene therapy, *Curr. Top. Microbiol. Immunol.* **177:**217–235.

Einerhand, M. P. W., Antoniou, M., Zolothukin, S., Muzyczka, N., Berns, K. I., Grosveld, F., and Valerio, D., 1995, Regulated high level human β-globin gene expression in erythroid cells following recombinant adeno-associated virus mediated gene transfer, *Gene Ther.* **2:**336–343.

Elder, J. T., Forrester, W. C., Thompson, C., Mager, D., Henthorn, P., Peretz, M., Papayannopoulou, T., and Groudine, M., 1990, Translocation of an erythroid-specific hypersensitive site in deletion-type hereditary persistence of fetal hemoglobin, *Mol. Cell. Biol.* **10:**1382–1389.

el-Hazmi, M. A., al-Momen, A., Kandaswamy, S., Huraib, S., Harakati, M., al-Mohareb, F., and Warsy, A. S., 1995, On the use of hydroxyurea/erythropoietin combination therapy for sickle cell disease, *Acta Haematol.* **94:**128–134.

Ellis, J., Tan-Un, K. C., Harper, A., Michalovich, D., Yannoutsos, N., Philipsen, J., and Grosveld, F., 1996, A dominant chromatin-opening activity in 5′ hypersensitive site 3 of the human β-globin locus control region, *EMBO J.* **15:**562–568.

Ellis J., Talbot, D., Dillon, N., and Grosveld, F., 1993, Synthetic human β-globin 5′HS2 constructs function as locus control regions only in multicopy transgene concatamers, *EMBO J.* **12:**127–134.

Evans, D. I., 1992, Bone marrow transplantation for thalassaemia major, *J. Clin. Pathol.* **45:**553–555.

Fabry, M. E., Sengupta, A., Suzuka, S. M., Costantini, F., Rubin, E. M., Hofrichter, J., Christoph, G., Manci, E., Culberson, D., Factor, S. M., 1995, A second generation transgenic mouse model expressing both hemoglobin S (HbS) and HbS-Antilles results in increased phenotypic severity, *Blood* **86:**2419–2428.

Fabry, M. E., Costantini, F., Pachnis, A., Suzuka, S. M., Bank, N., Aynedjian, H. S., Factor, S. M., and Nagel, R. L., 1992, High expression of human βS- and α-globins in transgenic mice: Erythrocyte abnormalities, organ damage and the effect of hypoxia, *Proc. Natl. Acad. Sci. USA* **89:**12155–12159.

Feingold, E. A., and Forget, B. G., 1989, The breakpoint of a large deletion causing hereditary persistence of fetal hemoglobin occurs within an erythroid DNA domain remote from the β-globin gene cluster, *Blood* **74:**2178–2186.

Felsenfeld, G., 1992, Chromatin as an essential part of the transcriptional mechanism, *Nature* **355:**219–224.

Ferster, A., De Valck, C., Azzi, N., Fondu, P., Toppet, M., and Sariban, E., 1992, Bone marrow transplantation for sickle cell anaemia, *Brit. J. Haematol.* **80:**102–105.

Festenstein, R., Tolaini, M., Corbella, P., Mamalaki, C., Parrington, J., Fox, M., Miliou, A., Jones, M., and Kioussis, D., 1996, Locus control region function and heterochromatin-induced position effect variegation, *Science* **271:**1123–1125.

Fischer, K. D., and Nowock, J., 1990, The T–C substitution at -198 of the $^{A}\gamma$-globin gene associated with the British form of HPFH generates overlapping recognition sites for two DNA-binding proteins, *Nucleic Acids Res.* **18:**5685–5693.

Flake, A. W., and Zanjani, E. D., 1993, In utero transplantation of hematopoietic stem cells, *Crit. Rev. Oncol.-Hematol.* **15:**35–48.

Flotte, T. R., and Carter, B. J., 1995, Adeno-associated virus vectors for gene therapy, *Gene Ther.* **2:**357–362.

Fraser, P., Hurst, J., Collis, P., and Grosveld, F., 1990, DNaseI hypersensitive sites 1, 2 and 3 of the human β-globin dominant control region directs position-independent expression, *Nucleic Acids Res.* **18:**3503–3508.

Fraser, P., Pruzina, S., Antoniou, M., and Grosveld, F., 1993, Each hypersensitive site of the human β-globin locus control region confers a different developmental pattern of expression to the globin genes, *Genes Dev.* **7:**106–113.

Fucharoen, S., Shimizu, K., and Fukumaki, Y., 1990, A novel C–T transition within the distal CCAAT motif of the G gamma globin gene in the Japanese HPFH: implication of factor binding in the elevated fetal globin expression, *Nucleic Acids Res.* **18:**5245–5253.

Gelinas, R., Endlich, B., Pfeiffer, C., Yagi, M., and Stamatoyannopoulos, G., 1985, G to A substitution in the distal CCAAT box of the A gamma-globin gene in Greek hereditary persistence of fetal hemoglobin, *Nature* **313:**323–325.

Giardini, C., Galimberti, M., and Lucarelli, G., 1995, Bone marrow transplantation in thalassaemia, *Ann. Rev. Med.* **46:**319–330.

Giardini, C., Galimberti, M., Lucarelli, G., Polchi, P., Baronciani, D., and Angelucci, E., 1993a, Bone marrow transplantation in Class 2 thalassaemia patients, *Bone Marrow Transplant.* **12**(Suppl. 1)**:**59–62.

Giardini, C., Galimberti, M., Lucarelli, G., Polchi, P., Angelucci, E., Baronciani, D., Agostinelli, F., Giorgi, C., and Muretto, P., 1993b, Bone marrow transplantation in sickle cell anemia in Pesaro, *Bone Marrow Transplant.* **12**(Suppl. 1)**:**122–123.

Gilman, J. G., 1988, Expression of Gγ and Aγ globin genes in human adults, *Hemoglobin* **12:**707–716.

Gilman, J. G., Mishima, N., Wen, X. J., Stoming, T. A., Lobel, J., and Huisman, T. H., 1988, Distal CCAAT box deletion in the A gamma globin gene of two black adolescents with elevated fetal A gamma globin, *Nucleic Acids Res.* **16:**10635–10642.

Gluckman, E., 1994, European organisation for cord blood banking, *Blood Cells* **20:**601–608.

Gong, Q. H., Stern, J., and Dean, A., 1991, Transcriptional role of a conserved GATA-1 site in the human epsilon-globin gene promoter, *Mol. Cell. Biol.* **11:**2558–2566.

Greaves, D. R., Fraser, P., Vidal, M. A., Hedges, M. J., Ropers, D., Luzzatto, L., and Grosveld, F., 1990, A transgenic mouse model of sickle cell disorder, *Nature* **343:**183–185.

Grosveld, F., Antoniou, M., Berry, M., Dillon, N., Drabek, D., Ellis, J., Fraser, P., Haley, J., Philipsen, S., Pruzina, S., Raguz-Bolognesi, S., Trimborn, T., and Wijgerde, M., 1996, Drug discovery and the transcriptional control of the human beta globin gene locus, *Genomes, Molecular Biology and Drug Discovery, SmithKlyne Beecham Symposium Proceedings*, Academic Press, New York, pp. 117–127.

Grosveld, F., Blom van Assendelft, G. B., Greaves, D. R., and Kollias, G., 1987, Position-independent high level expression of the human β-globin gene in transgenic mice, *Cell* **51:**975–985.

Gumucio, D. L., Lockwood, W. K., Weber, J. L., Saulino, A. M., Delgrosso, K., Surrey, S., Schwartz, E., Goodman, M., and Collins, F. S., 1990, The −175 T–C mutation increases promoter strength in erythroid cells: Correlation with evolutionary conservation of binding sites for two trans-acting factors, *Blood* **75:**756–761.

Guy, J., Drabek, D., and Antoniou, M., 1995, Delivery of DNA into mammalian cells by receptor mediated endocytosis and gene therapy, *Mol. Biotech.* **3:**237–248.

Hanscombe, O., Whyatt, D., Fraser, P., Yannoutsos, N., Greaves, D., Dillon, N., and Grosveld, F., 1991, Importance of globin gene order for correct developmental expression, *Genes Dev.* **5:**1387–1394.

Hendrich, B. D., and Willard, H. F., 1995, Epigenetic regulation of gene expression: The effect of altered chromatin structure from yeast to mammals, *Hum. Mol. Genet.* **4**(Spec No.)**:**1765–1777.

Huisman, T. H., 1993, The structure and function of normal and abnormal hemoglobins, *Baillieres Clin. Haematol.* **6:**1–30.

Issaragrisil, S., 1994, Cord blood transplantation in thalassaemia, *Blood Cells* **20:**259–262.

Issaragrisil, S., Visuthisakchai, S., Suvatte, V., Tanphaichitr, V. S., Chandanayingyong, D., Schreiner, T., Kanokpongsakdi, S., Siritanaratkul, N., and Piankijagum, A., 1995, Brief report: Transplantation of cord-blood stem cells into a patient with severe thalassaemia, *N. Engl. J. Med.* **332:**367–369.

Jackson J. D., Petrykowska, H., Philipsen, S., Miller, W., and Hardison, R., 1996, Role of DNA sequences outside the cores of DNase hypersensitive sites (HSs) in the functions of the β-globin locus control region, *J. Biol. Chem.* **271:**11871–11878.

Karlsson, S., Bodine, D. M., Perry, L., Papayannopoulou, T., and Nienhuis, A. W., 1988, Expression of the human β-globin gene following retroviral-mediated transfer into multipotential hematopoietic progenitors of mice, *Proc. Natl. Acad. Sci. USA* **85:**6062–6066.

Karpen, G. H., 1994, Position-effect variegation and the new biology of heterochromatin, *Curr. Opinion Genet. Dev.* **4:**281–291.

Kazazian, H. H., Jr., Dowling, C. E., Boehm, C. D., Warren, T. C., Economou, E. P., Katz, J., and Antonarakis, S. E., 1990, Gene defects in β-thalassemia and their prenatal diagnosis, *6th Cooley's Anemia Symposium,* Ann. NY Acad. Sci. Vol. 612 (A. Bank ed.), The New York Academy of Sciences, New York, pp. 1–14.

Kiem, H. P., von Kalle, C., Schuening, F., and Storb, R., 1995, Gene therapy and bone marrow transplantation, *Curr. Opinion Oncol.* **7:**107–114.

Kohn, D. B., 1995, The current status of gene therapy using hematopoietic stem cells, *Curr. Opinion Pediatr.* **7:**56–63.

Kohn, D. B., Weinberg, K. I., Nolta, J. A., Heiss, L. N., Lenarsky, C., Crooks, G. M., Hanley, M. E., Annet, G., Brooks, J. S., el-Khoureiy, A., Lawrence, K., Wells, S., Moen, R. C., Bastian, J., Williams-Herman, D. E., Elder, M., Wara, D., Bowen, T., Hershfield, M. S., Mullen, C. A., Blaese, R. M., and Parkman, R., 1995, Engraftment of gene-modified umbilical cord blood cells in neonates with adenosine deaminase deficiency, *Nat. Med.* **1:**1017–1023.

Kollias, G., Hurst, J., deBoer, E., and Grosveld, F., 1987, The human β-globin gene contains a downstream developmental specific enhancer, *Nucleic Acids Res.* **15:**5739–5745.

Kontoghiorghes, G. J., 1995, New concepts of iron and aluminium chelation therapy with oral L1 (deferiprone) and other chelators. A review, *Analyst* **120:**845–851.

Krysan, P. J., Haase, S. B., and Calos, M. P., 1989, Isolation of human sequences that replicate autonomously in human cells, *Mol. Cell. Biol.* **9:**1026–1033.

Kunzelmann, K., Legendre, J-Y., Knoell, D. L., Escobar, L. C., Xu, Z., and Gruenert, D. C., 1996, Gene targeting of CFTR DNA in CF epithelial cells, *Gene Ther.* **3:**859–867.

Leboulch, P., Huang, G. M. S., Humphries, R. K., Oh, Y. H., Eaves, C. J., Tuan, D. Y. H., and London, Y. M., 1994, Mutagenesis of retroviral vectors transducing human β-globin gene and β-globin locus control region derivatives results in stable transmission of an active transcriptional structure, *EMBO J.* **13:**3065–3076.

Ley, T. J., DeSimone, J., Noguchi, C. T., Turner, P. H., Schechter, A. N., Heller, P., and Nienhuis, A. W., 1983, 5-Azacytidine increases gamma-globin synthesis and reduces the proportion of dense cells in patients with sickle cell anemia, *Blood* **62:**370–380.

Lucarelli, G., Clift, R. A., Galimberti, M., Polchi, P., Angelucci, E., Baronciani, D., Giardini, C., Andreani, M., Manna, M., Nesci, S., Agostinelli, F., Rapa, S., Ripalti, M., and Albertini, F., 1996, Marrow transplantation for patients with thalassaemia: Results in Class 3 patients, *Blood* **87:**2082–2088.

Lucarelli, G., Galimberti, M., Polchi, P., Angelucci, E., Baronciani, D., Giardini, C., Politi, P., Durazzi, S. M. T., Muretto, P., and Albertini, F., 1990, Bone marrow transplantation in patients with thalassaemia, *N. Engl. J. Med.* **322:**417–421.

Lucarelli, G., Galimberti, M., Polchi, P., Angelucci, E., Baronciani, D., Giardini, C., Politi, P., Andreani, M., Agostinelli, F., Albertini, F., and Clift, R. A., 1993, Marrow transplantation in patients with thalassaemia major responsive to iron chelation therapy, *N. Engl. J. Med.* **329:**840–844.

Lucarelli, G., Galimberti, M., Polchi, P., Angelucci, E., Baronciani, D., Durazzi, D., Giardini, C., Albertini, F., and Clift, R. A., 1992, Bone marrow transplantation in adult thalassaemia, *Blood* **80:**1603–1607.

Lutty, G. A., McLeod, D. S., Pachnis, A., Costantini, F., Fabry, M. E., and Nagel, R. L., 1994, Retinal and choroidal neovascularization in a transgenic mouse model of sickle cell disease, *Am. J. Pathol.* **145:**490–497.

Mantovani, R., Malgaretti, N., Nicolis, S., Ronchi, A., Giglioni, B., and Ottolenghi, S., 1988, The effects of HPFH mutations in the γ-globin promoter on binding of ubiquitous and erythroid specific nuclear factors, *Nucleic Acids Res.* **16:**7783–7797.

Mantovani, R., Superti-Furga, G., Gilman, G., and Ottolenghi, S., 1989, The deletion of the distal CCAAT box region of the $^{A}\gamma$-globin gene in black HPFH abolishes the binding of the erythroid specific protein NF-E3 and of the CCAAT displacement protein, *Nucleic Acids Res.* **17:**6681–6691.

Martin, D., Fiering, S., and Groudine, M., 1996, Regulation of β-globin gene expression: Straightening out the locus, *Curr. Opinion Genet. Dev.* **8:**488–495.

Martin, D. I., Tsai, S. F., and Orkin, S. H., 1989, Increased γ-globin expression in a nondeletion HPFH mediated by an erythroid-specific DNA-binding factor, *Nature* **338:**435–438.

McCullough, J., Clay, M. E., Fautsch, S., Noreen, H., Segall, M., Perry, E., and Stroncek, D., 1994, Proposed policies and procedures for the establishment of a cord blood bank, *Blood Cells* **20:**609–626.

McCune, S. L., and Townes, T. M., 1994, Retroviral vector sequences inhibit human β-globin gene expression in transgenic mice, *Nucleic Acids Res.* **22:**4477–4481.

McDonagh, K. T., Lin, H. J., Lowrey, C. H., Bodine, D. M., and Nienhuis, A. W., 1991, The upstream region of the human gamma-globin gene promoter. Identification and functional analysis of nuclear protein binding sites, *J. Biol. Chem.* **266:**11965–11974.

Miller, A. D., 1992, Retroviral vectors, *Curr. Top. Microbiol. Immunol.* **158:**1–24.

Miller, A. D., Miller, D. G., Garcia, J. V., and Lynch, C. M., 1993, Use of retroviral vectors for gene transfer and expression, *Methods Enzymol.* **217:**581–599.

Miller, J. L., Walsh, C. E., Ney, P. A., Samulski, R. J., and Nienhuis, A. W., 1993, Single-copy transduction and expression of human γ-globin in K562 erythroleukemia cells using recombinant adeno-associated virus vectors: The effect of mutations in NF-E2 and GATA-1 binding motifs within the hypersensitive site 2 enhancer, *Blood* **82:**1900–1906.

Miller, J. L., Donahue, R. E., Sellers, S. E., Samulski, R. J., Young, N. S., and Nienhuis, A. W., 1994, Recombinant adeno-associated virus (rAAV)-mediated expression of a human γ-globin gene in human progenitor-derived erythroid cells, *Proc. Natl. Acad. Sci. USA* **91:**10183–10187.

Milner, P., Miller, L., Grey, L., Seakins, M., Dejong, W., and Went, L., 1970, Hemoglobin O arab in four negro families and its interaction with hemoglobin S and C, *N. Engl. J. Med.* **283:**1417–1425.

Milot, E., Strouboulis, J., Trimborn, T., Wijgerde, M., de Boer, E., Langeveld, A., Tan-Un, K., Vergeer, W., Yannoutsos, N., Grosveld, F., and Fraser, P., 1996, Heterochromatin effects on the frequency and duration of LCR-mediated gene transcription, *Cell* **87:**105–114.

Monplaisir, N., Merault, G., Poyart, C., Rhoda, M. D., Craescu, C. T., Vidaud, M., Galacteros, F., Blouquit, Y., and Rosa, J., 1986, Hemoglobin S Antilles: A variant with lower solubility than hemoglobin S and producing sickle cell disease in heterozygotes, *Proc. Natl. Acad. Sci. USA* **83:**9363–9367.

Motum, P. I., Deng, Z. M., Huong, L., and Trent, R. J., 1994, The Australian type of nondeletion G gamma-HPFH has a C–G substitution at nucleotide –114 of the G gamma gene, *Brit. J. Haematol.* **86:**219–221.

Muzyczka, N., 1992, Use of adeno-associated virus as a general transduction vector for mammalian cells, *Curr. Top. Microbiol. Immunol.* **158:**97–129.

Naldini, L., Blömer, U., Galley, P., Ory, D., Mulligan, R., Gage, F. H., Verma, I. M., and Trono, D., 1996, In vivo gene delivery and stable transduction of nondividing cells by a lentiviral vector, *Science* **272:**263–267.

Ney, P. A., Sorrentino, B. P., McDonagh, K. T., and Nienhuis, A. W., 1990a, Tandem AP-1-binding sites within the human beta-globin dominant control region function as an inducible enhancer in erythroid cells, *Genes Dev.* **4:**993–1006.

Ney, P. A., Sorrentino, B. P., Lowrey, C. H., and Nienhuis, A. W., 1990b, Inducibility of the HS II enhancer depends on binding of an erythroid specific nuclear protein, *Nucleic Acids Res.* **18:**6011–6017.

Nicolis, S., Ronchi, A., Malgaretti, N., Mantovani, R., Giglioni, B., and Ottolenghi, S., 1989, Increased erythroid-specific expression of a mutated HPFH γ-globin promoter requires the erythroid factor NF-E1, *Nucleic Acids Res.* **17:**5509–5516.

Nienhuis, A. W., 1994, Gene transfer into hematopoietic stem cells, *Blood Cells* **20:**141–148.

Noguchi, C. T., Schechter, A. N., and Rodgers, G. P., 1993, Sickle cell disease pathophysiology, *Baillieres Clin. Haematol.* **6:**57–91.

Novak, U., Harris, E. A., Forrester, W., Groudine, M., and Gelinas, R., 1990, High-level β-globin expression after retroviral transfer of locus activating region-containing human β-globin gene derivatives into murine erythroleukemia cells, *Proc. Natl. Acad. Sci. USA* **87:**3386–3390.

Nuez, B., Michalovich, D., Bygrave, A., Ploemacher, R., and Grosveld, F., 1995, Defective haematopoiesis in fetal liver resulting from inactivation of the EKLF gene, *Nature* **375:**316–318.

Olivieri, N. F., Brittenham, G. M., Matsui, D., Berkovitch, M., Blendis, L. M., Cameron R. G., McClelland, R. A., Liu, P. P., Templeton, D. M., and Koren, G., 1995, Iron-chelation therapy with oral deferipronein in patients with thalassaemia major, *N. Engl. J. Med.* **332:**918–922.

Oner, R., Kutlar, F., Gu, L. H., and Huisman, T. H. J., 1991, The Georgia type of nondeletional hereditary persistence of fetal hemoglobin has a C–T mutation at nucleotide –114 of the A gamma-globin gene, *Blood* **77:**1124–1128.

Padlan, E., and Love, W., 1985, Refined crystal structure of deoxyhemoglobin S. II. Molecular interactions in the crystal, *J. Biol. Chem.* **260:**8280–8291.

Peters, B., Merezhinskaya, N., Diffley, J. F., and Noguchi, C. T., 1993, Protein-DNA interactions in the epsilon-globin gene silencer, *J. Biol. Chem.* **268:**3430–3437.

Philipsen, S., Talbot, D., Fraser, P., and Grosveld, F., 1990, The β-globin dominant control region: Hypersensitive site 2, *EMBO J.* **9:**2159–2167.

Philipsen, S., Pruzina, S., and Grosveld, F., 1993, The minimal requirements for activity in transgenic mice of hypersensitive site 3 of the β-globin locus control region, *EMBO J.* **12:**1077–1085.

Piirsoo, M., Ustav, E., Mandel, T., Stenlund, A., and Ustav, M., 1996, *Cis* and *trans* requirements for stable episomal maintenance of the BPV-1 replicator, *EMBO J.* **15:**1–11.

Platt, O. S., 1995, Sickle cell paths converge on hydroxyurea, *Nat. Med.* **1:**307–308

Platt, O. S., Orkin, S. H., Dover, G. J., Beardsley, G. P., Miller, B., and Nathan, D. G., 1984, Hydroxyurea enhances fetal hemoglobin production in sickle cell anemia, *J. Clin. Invest.* **74:**652–656.

Plavec, I., Papayannopoulou, T., Maury, C., and Meyer, F., 1993, A human β-globin gene fused to the human β-globin locus control region is expressed at high levels in erythroid cells of mice engrafted with retrovirus-transduced hematopoietic stem cells, *Blood* **81:**1384–1392.

Podsakoff, G., Wong, K.K. Jr., and Chatterjee, S., 1994, Efficient gene transfer into nondividing cells by adeno-associated virus-based vectors, *J. Virol.* **68:**5656–5666.

Pruzina, S., Hanscombe, O., Whyatt, D., Grosveld, F., and Philipsen, S., 1991, Hypersensitive site 4 of the human β-globin locus control region, *Nucleic Acids Res.* **19:**1413–1419.

Raich, N., Enver, T., Nakamoto, B., Josephson, B., Papayannopoulou, T., and Stamatoyannopoulos G., 1990, Autonomous developmental control of human embryonic globin gene switching in transgenic mice, *Science* **250:**1147–1149.

Raich, N., Clegg, C. H., Grofti, J., Romeo, P. H., and Stamatoyannopoulos, G., 1995, GATA1 and YY1 are developmental repressors of the human epsilon-globin gene, *EMBO J.* **4:**801–809.

Roberts, I. A., and Davies, S. C., 1993, Sickle cell disease: The transplant issue, *Bone Marrow Transplant.* **11:**253–254.

Rodgers, G. P., Dover, G. J., Uyesaka, N., Noguchi, C. T., Schechter, A. N., and Nienhuis, A. W., 1993, Augmentation by erythropoietin of the fetal-hemoglobin response to hydroxyurea in sickle cell disease, *N. Engl. J. Med.* **328:**73–80.

Ronchi, A., Berry, M., Raguz, S., Imam, A., Yannoutsos, N., Ottolenghi, S., Grosveld, F., and Dillon, N., 1996, Role of the duplicated CCAAT box region in γ-globin gene regulation and hereditary persistence of fetal hemoglobin, *EMBO J.* **15:**143–149.

Ronchi, A., Nicolis, S., Santoro, C., and Ottolenghi, S., 1989, Increased Sp1 binding mediates erythroid-specific overexpression of a mutated (HPFH) γ-globulin promoter, *Nucleic Acids Res.* **17:**10231–10241.

Rubin, E. M., Witkowska, H. E., Spangler, E., Curtin, P., Lubin, B. H., Mohandas, N., and Clift, S. M., 1991, Hypoxia-induced in vivo sickling of transgenic mouse red cells, *J. Clin. Invest.* **87:**639–647.

Rubinstein P., Taylor P. E., Scaradavou, A., Adamson, J. W., Migliaccio, G., Emanuel, D., Berkowitz, R. L., Alvarez, E., and Stevens, C. E., 1994, Unrelated placental blood for bone marrow reconstitution: Organization of the placental blood program, *Blood Cells* **20:**504–515.

Russell, D. W., Miller, A. D., and Alexander, I. E., 1994, Adeno-associated virus vectors preferentially transduce cells in S phase, *Proc. Natl. Acad. Sci. USA* **91:**8915–8919.

Ryan, T. M., Townes, T. M., Reilly, M. P., Asakura, T., Palmiter, R. D., Brinster, R. L., and Behringer, R. R., 1990, Human sickle hemoglobin in transgenic mice, *Science* **247:**566–568.

Sadelain, M., Jason Wang, C. H., Antoniou, M., Grosveld, F., and Mulligan, R., 1995, Generation of a high-titer retroviral vector capable of expressing high levels of the human β-globin gene, *Proc. Natl. Acad. Sci. USA* **92:**6728–6732.

Sher, G. D., Ginder, G.D, Little, J., Yang, S., Dover, G. J., and Olivieri, N. F., 1995, Extended therapy with intravenous arginine butyrate in patients with beta-hemoglobinopathies, *N. Engl. J. Med.* **332:**1606–1610.

Smith, C., 1992, Retroviral vector-mediated gene transfer into hematopoietic cells: Prospects and issues, *J. Hematother.* **1:**155–166.

Stamatoyannopoulos, G., Nienhuis, A. W., Leder, P., and Majerus, P.W. (eds.), 1987, *The Molecular Basis of Blood Diseases,* Saunders, Philadelphia.

Strouboulis, J., Dillon, N., and Grosveld, F., 1992, Developmental regulation of a complete 70 kb human β-globin locus in transgenic mice, *Genes Dev.* **6:**1857–1864.

Superti-Furga, G., Barberis, A., Schaffner, G., and Busslinger, M., 1988, The -117 mutation in Greek HPFH affects the binding of three nuclear factors to the CCAAT region of the γ-globin gene, *EMBO J.* **7:**3099–3107.

Sykes, K., and Kaufman, R., 1990, A naturally occurring gamma globin gene mutation enhances Sp1 binding activity, *Mol. Cell. Biol.* **10:**95–102.

Takekoshi, K. J., Oh, Y. H., Westerman, K. W., London, I. M., and Leboulch, P., 1995, Retroviral transfer of a human beta-globin/delta-globin hybrid gene linked to a beta locus control region hypersensitive site 2 aimed at the gene therapy of sickle cell disease, *Proc. Natl. Acad. Sci. USA* **92:**3014–3018.

Talbot, D., Philipsen, S., Fraser, P., and Grosveld, F., 1990, Detailed analysis of the site 3 region of the human β-globin dominant control region, *EMBO J.* **9:**2169–2178.

Talbot, D., Collis, P., Antoniou, M., Vidal, M., Grosveld, F., and Greaves, D. R., 1989, A dominant control region from the human β-globin locus conferring integration site-independent gene expression, *Nature* **338:**352–355.

Tanaka, J., Kasai, M., Imamura, M., and Asaka, M., 1995, Clinical application of allogeneic peripheral blood stem cells transplantation, *Ann. Hematol.* **71:**265–269.

Touraine J. L., 1992, In utero transplantation of fetal liver stem cells into human fetuses, *Hum. Reprod.* **7:**44–48.

Trepicchio, W. L., Dyer, M. A., and Baron, M. H., 1994, A novel developmental regulatory motif required for stage-specific activation of the epsilon-globin gene and nuclear factor binding in embryonic erythroid cells, *Mol. Cell. Biol.* **14:**3763–3771.

Trudel, M., De Paepe M. E., Chretien, N., Saadane, N., Jacmain, J., Sorette, M., Hoang, T., and Beuzard, Y., 1994, Sickle cell disease of transgenic SAD mice, *Blood* **84:**3189–3197.

Trudel, M., Magram, J., Bruckner, L., and Constantini, F., 1987, Upstream $^{G}\gamma$-globin and downstream β-globin sequences required for stage-specific expression in transgenic mice, *Mol. Cell. Biol.* **7:**4024–4029.

Trudel, M., Saadane, N., Garel, M. C., Bardakdjian-Michau, J., Blouquit, Y., Guerquin-Kern, J. L., Rouyer-Fessard, P., Vidaud, D., Pachnis, A., Romeo, P.-H., Beuzard, Y., and Constantini, F., 1991, Towards a transgenic mouse model of sickle cell disease: Hemoglobin SAD, *EMBO J.* **10:**3157–3165.

Tuan, D. Y., Solomon, W. B., London, I. M., and Lee, D. P., 1989, An erythroid-specific, developmental-stage-independent enhancer far upstream of the human "beta-like globin" genes, *Proc. Natl. Acad. Sci. USA* **86:**2554–2558.

Vellodi, A., Picton, S., Downie, C. J., Eltumi, M., Stevens, R., and Evans, D. I., 1994, Bone marrow transplantation for thalassaemia: Experience of two English centres, *Bone Marrow Transplant.* **13:**559–562.

Vermylen, C., and Cornu, G., 1993, Bone marrow transplantation in sickle cell anaemia, *Blood Rev.* **7:**1–3.

Vichinsky, E. P., and Lubin, B. H., 1994, A cautionary note regarding hydroxyurea in sickle cell disease, *Blood* **83:**1124–1128.

Voskaridou, E., Kalotychou, V., and Loukopoulos, D., 1995, Clinical and laboratory effects of long-term administration of hydroxyurea to patients with sickle-cell/beta-thalassaemia, *Brit. J. Haematol.* **89:**479–484.

Wall, L., de Boer, E., and Grosveld, F. 1988. The human β-globin gene 3′ enhancer contains multiple binding sites for an erythroid-specific protein , *Genes Dev.* **2:**1089–1100.

Walsh, C. E., Liu, J. M., Xiao, X., Young, N. S., Nienhuis, A. W., and Samulski, R. J., 1992, Regulated high level expression of a human gamma-globin gene introduced into erythroid cells by an adeno-associated virus vector, *Proc. Natl. Acad. Sci. USA* **89:**7257–7261.

Walsh, C. E., Liu, J. M., Miller, J. L., Nienhuis, A. W., and Samulski, R. J., 1993, Gene therapy for human hemoglobinopathies, *Proc. Soc. Exp. Biol. Med.* **204:**289–300.

Weatherall, D. J., and Clegg, J. B., 1981, *The Thalassaemia Syndromes*, 3rd ed. Blackwell Scientific, Oxford, U.K.

Wijgerde, M., Grosveld, F., and Fraser, P., 1995, Transcription complex stability and chromatin dynamics *in vivo*, *Nature* **377:**209–213.

Wijgerde, M., Gribnau, J., Trimborn, T., Nuez, B., Philipsen, S., Grosveld, F., and Fraser, P., 1996, The role of EKLF in human β-globin gene competition, *Genes Dev.* **10:**2894–2902.

Williams, D. A., and Moritz, T., 1994, Umbilical cord blood stem cells as targets for genetic modification: New therapeutic approaches to somatic gene therapy, *Blood Cells* **20:**504–515.

Wohlgemuth, J. G., Kang, S. H., Bulboaca, G. H., Nawotka, K. A., and Calos, M. P., 1996, Long-term expression from autonomously replicating vectors in mammalian cells, *Gene Ther.* **3:**503–512.

Wood, W. G., 1993, Increased HbF in adult life, *Baillieres Clin. Haematol.* **6:**177–213.

Wu, J., Grindlay, G. J., Johnson, C., and Allan, M., 1990, Interaction of epsilon-globin cis-acting control elements with erythroid-specific regulatory macromolecules, *Proc. Natl. Acad. Sci. USA* **87:**8115–8119.

Yates, J. L., Warren, N., and Sugden, B., 1985, Stable replication of plasmids derived from Epstein–Barr virus in various mammalian cells, *Nature* **313:**812–815.

Yu, C. Y., Motamed, K., Chen, J., Bailey, A. D., and Shen, C. K., 1991, The CACC box upstream of human embryonic epsilon globin gene binds Sp1 and is a functional promoter element in vitro and in vivo, *J. Biol. Chem.* **266:**8907–8915.

Zafaranga, G., Raguz, S., Pruzina, S., Grosveld, F., and Meijer, D., 1995, The regulation of human β-globin gene expression: The analysis of hypersensitive site 5 (HS5) in the LCR. In, *Proceedings of the Ninth Conference on Hemoglobin Switching*, Cras Island, Washington, U.S.A., June 10–14, 1994, (Stamatoyannopoulos, G. ed.), Vol. 1 Intercept Ltd., Andover, Hampshire, UK, pp 39–44.

Chapter 9

Gene Marking and the Biology of Hematopoietic Cell Transfer in Human Clinical Trials

A. K. Stewart, I. D. Dubé, and R. G. Hawley

1. INTRODUCTION

Clinical investigation of gene transfer in humans began with the seminal trials of Rosenberg, Anderson and Blaese in 1989 and 1990 (Anderson, 1992; Blaese *et al.*, 1995; Cai *et al.*, 1995; Miller, 1992a; Mulligan, 1993; Morgan and Anderson, 1993; Rosenberg *et al.*, 1990). By 1996, gene marking or gene therapy protocols were underway worldwide (Anderson, 1994). Unexpectedly, a high percentage of early protocols were designed for cancer patients rather than, as had originally been anticipated, inherited single gene defects (Gutierrez *et al.*, 1992; Karlsson, 1991; Lotze, 1991). This shift in emphasis reflects early uncertainties regarding the safety and efficacy of gene transfer protocols and the resulting necessity to investigate these issues in groups of patients willing to undergo investigational treatment with minimal, or in some instances no, direct benefit to themselves. Indeed, many of the early developmental milestones in human gene transfer arose from trials in which no therapeutic benefit was intended. These so-called "gene-marking" studies have been singled out for praise by recent review committees which have generally criticized the early introduction of gene therapy clinical trials (Crystal, 1995; Friedmann, 1996). The biological outcomes of such marking studies have been

A. K. Stewart, I. D. Dubé, and R. G. Hawley Departments of Medicine, Medical Biophysics, Pediatrics, and Pathology, The University of Toronto, and The Toronto Hospital Oncology Gene Therapy Program, Toronto, Ontario M5G 2C4, Canada.

Blood Cell Biochemistry, Volume 8: Hematopoiesis and Gene Therapy, edited by Fairbairn and Testa. Kluwer Academic/Plenum Publishers, New York, 1999.

surprisingly rewarding, albeit at times disappointing. The purpose of this chapter is to reiterate the inherent promise and the remaining obstacles posed by the application of gene transfer, using hematopoietic cells.

2. GENE MARKING AND CANCER BIOLOGY

Gene marking of cells is a powerful approach for addressing biological questions in clinical trials of experimental cancer treatment (Crystal, 1995; Merrouche *et al.*, 1995; Miller *et al.*, 1993; Miller and Rosman, 1989; Van Zant *et al.*, 1991). Such cell marking facilitates studies of the long-term distribution and survival of transplanted cells *in vivo*. In most applications, the cells to be tagged are incubated *ex vivo* with a replication-defective retrovirus that bears a reporter gene (Miller, 1990a, 1992b; Miller and Rosman, 1989; Miller *et al.*, 1993). The reporter gene used exclusively in these studies to date is the bacterial neomycin phosphotransferase (*neo*) gene which, when expressed, confers resistance on the neomycin analog G418 (Bayever *et al.*, 1988; Eglitis, 1991; Marty *et al.*, 1990). The stable and unique integration pattern of proviral DNA in the genome of marked cells provides a permanent marker for individual hematopoietic or malignant cells and their clonal descendants (Hawley *et al.*, 1989; Miller *et al.*, 1992). The fates of marked hematopoietic stem cells or indeed contaminating malignant cells infused into autologous recipients is thus readily determined by using sensitive genetic detection systems (e.g., PCR) or by clonogenic assays for progenitors resistant to toxic concentrations of G418 (Bayever *et al.*, 1988; Bodine *et al.*, 1990; Dick *et al.*, 1991; Eglitis, 1991; O'Shaughnessy *et al.*, 1994; Williams, 1990). Clinical applications in which gene marking has provided new and important information include the infusion of retrovirally marked, autologous, tumor-infiltrating lymphocytes (TIL) into patients who have advanced melanoma (Economou *et al.*, 1996; Merrouche *et al.*, 1995; Rosenberg *et al.*, 1990), and the infusion of retrovirally marked bone marrow or peripheral blood into patients who have leukemia (Brenner *et al.*, 1993b, 1994; Cornetta *et al.*, 1992; Diesseroth *et al.*, 1994b), breast cancer (Dunbar *et al.*, 1995), myeloma (Dunbar *et al.*, 1995; Stewart *et al.*, 1995), and neuroblastoma (Rill *et al.*, 1992).

3. RETROVIRAL MARKING OF TUMOR-INFILTRATING LYMPHOCYTES

One approach to addressing the biology of hematopoietic cell engraftment involves using genetically modified human lymphocytes. The rational for such experiments has been to target the tumor-infiltrating lymphocytes (TILS), originally described as relatively tumor-specific (Morecki *et al.*, 1991; Rosenberg, 1991), and more recently to protect lymphoid cell populations from viral infection in HIV (Riddell *et al.*, 1996). Results from three groups studying TILs are published (Economou *et al.*, 1996; Merrouche *et al.*, 1995; Rosenberg *et al.*, 1990). In these studies TILs are isolated and expanded *in vitro*. Expanded cells are genetically marked and then infused intravenously. One group also included control peripheral blood lymphocytes marked by a second, distinguishable, *neo*-containing vector

(Merrouche *et al.*, 1995). These pioneering studies confirmed the safety of retrovirally mediated gene transfer and the successful engraftment of gene modified cells, in this case lymphocytes. Genetically marked lymphocytes are detectable by PCR in most patients during the first month after infusion and persist in some patients for many months postinfusion (Rosenberg *et al.*, 1990). Furthermore genetically marked lymphocytes can be retrieved from tumor biopsies and skin biopsies (Merrouche *et al.*, 1995). Using a control population of peripheral blood lymphocytes, no particular tumor-homing specificity of lymphocytes could be demonstrated (Merrouche *et al.*, 1995).

4. CLINICAL TRIALS OF STEM CELL GENE MARKING

Patients who have consented to undergo the rigors of high-dose chemo radiotherapy with autologous bone marrow transplantation (ABMT) or peripheral blood stem cell transplantation have frequently been identified as candidates in which to study the safety and efficacy of gene transfer. This approach requires that patients have hematopoietic cells collected and cryopreserved before myeloablative chemoradiotherapy. Immediately after high-dose chemoradiotherapy, the cryopreserved autograft is thawed and infused back into the patients to rescue them from permanent bone marrow aplasia. Using this approach, higher doses of chemotherapy are delivered to the patients and, consequently, survival rates have increased in many hematologic malignancies. Although often considered to confer a survival advantage, the results obtained using ABMT or autologous blood cell transplantation are far from satisfactory. In particular, cancer relapse rates after ABMT or blood cell rescue remain consistently higher than those observed after a sibling (allogeneic) transplant. Because autologous marrow is contaminated with malignant cells in many of the diseases cited, albeit at levels below that of microscopic detection, it has been postulated for many years that malignant cells that contaminate the autograft contribute to disease relapse. Nevertheless this assumption has been extraordinarily difficult to prove in traditional, controlled, randomized trials. Rill *et al.*, summarized this problem by noting that to demonstrate a 5% survival difference attributable to removing malignant neuroblastoma cells from the autograft would require the study of every patient in the United States undergoing autologous transplantation for neuroblastoma during the next 20 years (Rill *et al.*, 1992, 1994).

The selection of patients undergoing autologous hematopoietic stem cell transplantation for gene-marking trials reflects the willingness of such patients to undergo experimental therapy and also the promise of hematopoietic stem cells as vehicles for gene therapy (Correll *et al.*, 1994; Karlsson, 1991; Nienhuis *et al.*, 1991). Such cells are distinguishable by their accessibility, longevity, high proliferative potential and the wide systemic distribution of their progeny (Abkowitz *et al.*, 1990; Bodine *et al.*, 1991b, 1993; Bowtell *et al.*, 1987; Dunbar *et al.*, 1994; Harrison *et al.*, 1998; Harrison *et al.*, 1983; Jordan and Lemischka, 1990; Jordon *et al.*, 1990; Mauch *et al.*, 1989; Mintz *et al.*, 1984; Nienhuis *et al.*, 1991; Nolta and Kohn, 1990; Reincke *et al.*, 1982; Smith *et al.*, 1991; Snodgrass and Keller, 1987; Weider *et al.*, 1991).

Therefore, successfully demonstrating long-term engraftment of genetically marked hematopoietic stem cells is an important landmark in developing clinically relevant therapeutic gene replacement. Thus, the study of cancer patients who receive genetically altered hematopoietic stem cells offers three important lines of investigation: (1) Is retrovirally mediated gene transfer safe? (2) Do genetically altered bone marrow or blood stem cells contribute to long-term hematopoiesis? (3) Do malignant cells or their precursors contribute to the high relapse rates observed after myeloablative therapy and autologous hematopoietic stem cell transplantation? The purpose of this review is to describe the early results obtained in a number of pioneering studies of gene transfer into hematopoietic stem cells with particular reference to the contribution of contaminating malignant cells to disease relapse.

5. CLINICAL TRIAL DESIGN

Gene-marking studies in ABMT patients were pioneered by investigators at St. Jude Children's Research Hospital, the M.D. Anderson Cancer Center and at the U.S. National Institutes of Health (N.I.H.) (Brenner *et al.*, 1993b, 1994; Diesseroth *et al.*, 1994a; Dunbar *et al.*, 1993; Rill *et al.*, 1992). Their approach has subsequently been adopted in at least five other centers worldwide: Indiana, Seattle (Schuening *et al.*, 1994), University of Southern California (Anderson, 1994), Toronto (Stewart *et al.*, 1995), and the Karolinska Institute in Sweden (Bjorkstrand *et al.*, 1994b). Indeed, 19 of the first 83 (23%) ethically approved and published gene transfer or gene therapy trials describe variations on this methodology (Anderson, 1994). In this approach to gene transfer, bone marrow or peripheral blood is harvested from patients during a clinical remission of their disease. The product is split, and a proportion of the hematopoietic cells to be returned to the patient are genetically marked *ex vivo* with a replication-defective retrovirus that contains the bacterial *neo* gene. The retroviral vectors G1Na and LNL6 have most frequently been employed and were provided by Genetic Therapy Inc. (Rockville, Maryland) for many of the trials described later. Following myeloablative therapy, the genetically-marked hematopoietic cells are thawed and returned to the patient together with unmanipulated cells. Then, the fate of cells that bear the marker gene is tracked by clonogenic assays or molecular studies.

Despite the apparent similarities of many of the 19 trials, enough variations exist to make each study distinct. The most apparent variables are the diseases studied and, although initially overlooked as of potential interest, the age of the patient populations. More important are the wide variations in transduction protocols (Table I) employed and the sources of cells targeted. The transduction protocols at St. Jude's and M.D. Anderson utilized a six-hour *in vitro* culture and a single exposure to retrovirus without the addition of exogenous cytokines (Brenner *et al.*, 1993b, 1994; Diesseroth, 1994; Diesseroth *et al.*, 1994a; Dunbar *et al.*, 1995; Rill *et al.*, 1992). At the Karolinska Institute, a 24-hour, three-exposure culture in the presence of cytokines is utilized (Bjorkstrand *et al.*, 1994b), whereas at the N.I.H. a three-day, three-exposure culture, also in the presence cytokines, has been adopted (Dunbar *et al.*, 1993, 1995; Dunbar and Emmons, 1994). In Seattle, a five-day, five-exposure culture (Barquinero *et al.*, 1995; Schuening *et al.*, 1989, 1991b, 1994; von Kalle *et al.*, 1994) and in Toronto our own three-week, three-exposure, long-term bone marrow

Table I
Representative Examples of Transduction Protocols from Different Centers[a]

Transduction—variation	Time	Cytokines	Number of Exposures
St. Jude	6 hr	No	1
Karolinska	24 hr	Yes	3
N.I.H.	3 days	Yes	3
Seattle	5 days	Yes	5
Toronto	21 days	No	3

[a] The time of culture, presence, or absence of exogenous cytokines, and the number of exposures to retroviral supernatant are indicated.

Table II
The Hematopoietic Cells Targeted for Transduction in These Gene Marking Trials Are Varied

Cells targeted—variation	Marrow	Blood	CD34
St. Jude	+	—	—
Karolinska	+	+	+
N.I.H.	+	+	+
Seattle	—	+	+
Toronto	+	—	—

culture (Bienzle *et al.*, 1994; Carter *et al.*, 1992; Stewart *et al.*, 1995) strive for maximal transduction efficiency, albeit at the cost of convenience. In preclinical studies, these culture conditions have widely varying efficiencies: a 5–10% transduction of colony-forming units-granulocyte macrophage (CFU-GM) occurred after the six-hour culture (Brenner *et al.*, 1994), 21% efficiency was obtained with the three-day culture (Dunbar *et al.*, 1993), and 53% transduction efficiency followed long-term bone marrow culture (Dubé *et al.*, 1996). These latter figures may be misleading, however, because only 10% of starting CFU-GM are recovered from the long-term bone marrow culture. Furthermore, the mature progenitor cell readout of the CFU-GM assay does not reflect the "stem" cell content of the graft, and thus using marked CFU-GM as an indicator of gene transfer efficacy is inappropriate. Unfortunately, an assay for hematopoietic stem cells continues to elude investigators and only long-term follow-up of patients in clinical gene-marking studies can truly address the optimal *in vitro* transduction protocol.

The cells targeted for marking in clinical trials also differed (Table II). Although a number of studies continue to examine gene marking of whole bone marrow, the majority have targeted peripheral blood stem cells or bone marrow cells selected on the basis of CD34 antigen expression (Baum *et al.*, 1992; Berenson *et al.*, 1991; Cassel *et al.*, 1993; Schiller *et al.*, 1995; Sutherland and Keating, 1992) as discussed later. Because CD34 cell selection reduces contaminating tumor cells (Freedman and Nadler, 1993; Gazitt *et al.*, 1995; Vescio *et al.*, 1994), the likelihood of detecting gene marked tumor cells at relapse is lower in certain trials incorporating this step (Dunbar *et al.*, 1995).

The considerable heterogeneity of experimental design suggests that each trial will individually contribute to knowledge of therapeutic gene transfer using hematopoietic cells.

6. RETROVIRAL MARKING OF MALIGNANT CELLS

Variation in the efficiency of marking tumor cells is also expected to be important particularly because of the proliferation of trials that purport to study disease relapse as an end point. Nevertheless data regarding the efficiency of retroviral transduction of malignant cells is limited. Brenner and colleagues describe 0–16.5% gene transfer efficiency into clonogenic neuroblastoma cells (median 3.5%) (Rill *et al.*, 1992), and approximately 10% of leukemic myeloblasts are transduced after a six-hour culture (Brenner *et al.*, 1993b, 1994). Others have reported that the transduction efficiency of fresh unselected solid tumor explants is 20–82% (median 40%). For example, 28% of breast cancer cells were transduced after a four-hour retroviral exposure (Jaffee *et al.*, 1996). Bjorkstrand *et al.*, reported 5–50% transduction efficiency into myeloma cells (Bjorkstrand *et al.*, 1994a). In our own studies in multiple myeloma, we exposed tumor-contaminated bone marrow to retroviral vectors in a 21-day, long-term bone marrow culture. In all samples studied after 21 days of culture, evidence for persistence of the myeloma clone was obtained by morphology, flow cytometry, and molecular analysis. Definitive evidence for marking of the malignant clone was obtained by the simultaneous localization of the bacterial β-galactosidase (*lacZ*) marker gene and tumor-specific cytogenetic changes in single clonogenic myeloma colonies isolated from methylcellulose (Stewart *et al.*, 1995). Thus, myeloma cells are susceptible to retrovirally mediated gene transfer, and it is evident that at least a proportion of genetically marked cells returned to patients in our own trial may be informative. Nevertheless, in this as in all of the gene marking trials described here, only a positive result, the detection of genetically marked cells at relapse, will be informative.

It is unclear whether or not tumor cells are more likely to be marked than hematopoietic progenitors. However, because of the relative cycling frequencies of such cells, it is probable that tumor cells are marked at higher efficiency. Indeed, this is supported by the high frequency with which tumor cells contribute to disease relapse in the studies described later. Furthermore, it is entirely probable that the cells susceptible to retroviral marking within a heterogeneous tumor population may exhibit an entirely different biological profile than unmarked cells. It might be argued, for example, that the rapidly cycling tumor cells, which are most susceptible to gene marking, are also the cells most likely to contribute to disease recurrence. If true, this phenomenon may explain the high frequency of genetically marked cells at relapse in spite of the relatively low frequency of successful transduction of malignant cells *in vitro*. Whatever the explanation, the results of clinical trials already completed have proved remarkably rewarding in this regard.

7. CLINICAL TRIAL RESULTS

Four groups have reported the consequences of infusing genetically marked bone marrow cells into humans and the contribution of contaminating tumor cells in the graft to disease recurrence (Brenner *et al.*, 1993a,b; Diesseroth *et al.*, 1994a; Dunbar *et al.*, 1995; Rill *et al.*, 1994). The first important observation is that retrovirally mediated gene transfer is safe as currently practiced (Anderson *et al.*, 1993; Boris-Lawrie and Temin, 1994; Brenner *et al.*, 1993a, 1994; Cornetta *et al.*, 1990; Cornetta *et al.*, 1991; Cornetta, 1992; Diesseroth *et al.*, 1994a; Dunbar *et al.*, 1995; Greenberger *et al.*, 1983; Gribben *et al.*, 1991; Miller, 1990a; Miller *et al.*, 1992; Moolten and Cupples, 1992; Rill *et al.*, 1992). No deterimental effects on the autograft or in patients have been reported. Replication-competent virus has not been detected. The second important observation is that the marked hematopoietic stem cells contribute to long-term hematopoiesis albeit at relatively low levels (Brenner *et al.*, 1993a; Dunbar *et al.*, 1995). Interestingly, hematopoietic engraftment of genetically marked cells occurs at higher efficiency in the trials involving children. This finding has been variously interpreted as reflecting the timing of harvest after chemotherapy, the youth of the patients, or the short *in vitro* culture conditions used in these studies (Brenner *et al.*, 1994).

8. HEMATOPOIESIS AND GENE MARKING

Optimism for human hematopoietic stem cell gene transfer is based on early success with selectable marker genes in human and murine hematopoietic progenitors (Gruber *et al.*, 1985; Hock and Miller, 1986; Hogge and Humphries, 1987; Laneuville *et al.*, 1988) and prolonged expression of nonselectable genes from retroviral vectors in mice (Belmon *et al.*, 1988; Bodine *et al.*, 1990; Correll *et al.*, 1989, 1992, 1994; Cournoyer *et al.*, 1991; Demarquoy *et al.*, 1992; Dick *et al.*, 1991; Hawley *et al.*, 1989; Hock *et al.*, 1989; Hughes *et al.*, 1989, 1992; Kaleko *et al.*, 1990; Mitani *et al.*, 1993; Moore *et al.*, 1991; Morganstern and Land, 1990; Nolta *et al.*, 1990; Ohashi *et al.*, 1992; Osborne *et al.*, 1990; Szilvassy *et al.*, 1989; Weinthal *et al.*, 1991; Williams, 1990). Thus far the data accumulated from studies in large animal models (Bienzle *et al.*, 1994; Carter *et al.*, 1992; Cornetta *et al.*, 1989; Kantoff *et al.*, 1989; Lothrop *et al.*, 1991; Schuening *et al.*, 1989, 1991b; Stead *et al.*, 1988; van Beusechem *et al.*, 1993; Wieder, 1991) and the first human clinical trials have generally been disappointing although notable exceptions exist. Reported frequencies of retroviral transduction of hematopoietic long-term repopulating cells in large animal models have been in the range of 0.01 to 15% (Bienzle *et al.*, 1994; Carter *et al.*, 1992). Comparable frequencies of human hematopoietic cell gene marking have been achieved in the St. Jude studies in children, where 2–15% of clonogenic hematopoietic progenitor cells were marked after ABMT (Brenner *et al.*, 1993a). The marker gene was detectable as long as four years after transplant and was found in granulocytes, B cells, and T cells, at least by PCR (Brenner *et al.*, 1994). In the adult gene-marking studies reported to date, however, retroviral transduction of marrow or peripheral blood stem cells has resulted in detectable vector integration in only 0.01 to 0.5% of peripheral blood cells (Dunbar *et al.*, 1995). Although the marker gene persisted as long as two years, *neo* positive cells could be detected only intermittently with a sensitive PCR reaction and no detectable expression was obtained by *in vitro* colony assays (Dunbar *et al.*, 1995). Dunbar *et al.*, infused eleven patients who had breast cancer or myeloma with CD34 antigen positive (CD34+) bone marrow or peripheral blood hematopoietic progenitor cells marked in a three-day culture in the presence of stem cell factor (SCF), interleukin (IL)-3 and IL-6, for breast cancer. Distinguishable genetic markers were used to mark bone marrow or blood cells. Interestingly, the blood stem cells contributed to hematopoiesis earlier and for a longer period than genetically marked cells from bone marrow (Dunbar *et al.*, 1995). The biological explanation for this unexpected finding is still unclear.

A second generation of gene-marking trials is now underway addressing how levels of gene transfer may be consistently improved in adults (Stewart *et al.*, 1995), whether purging of tumor-contaminated bone marrow is efficacious (Brenner, 1996), and how different transduction protocols affect gene transfer efficiency. Recent work by a number of groups including our own suggest that modifying the transduction protocols will indeed result in a significant improvement in engrafting genetically modified stem cells.

9. GENETICALLY MARKED RELAPSE

In total, data on 34 patients enrolled on gene-marking studies during bone marrow transplantation have been presented. Fourteen of these patients have relapsed (Table III). Of the 14 relapsed patients genetically marked tumor cells have been detected in nine and if patients with breast cancer are excluded, a remarkable nine out of 11 patients had gene-marked relapse (Brenner *et al.*, 1994; Diesseroth *et al.*, 1994a; Dunbar *et al.*, 1995).

At St. Jude, two cohorts of children were studied between 1991 and 1993, 12 patients who had acute myeloid leukemia (AML) and nine patients who had neuroblastoma (Brenner *et al.*, 1994). Bone marrow without morphologically detectable

Table III
Summary of Clinical Data from Published Reports

	Number of Patients	Relapse	Marked
AML	12	4	2
Neuroblastoma	9	5	4
CML	2	2	2
Myeloma	6	0	0
Breast cancer	5	3	0

tumor cell contamination was split, and one third of the marrow was retrovirally marked before return to the patient. Four of the 12 AML patients have relapsed and genetically marked cells contributed to relapse in two of these patients (Brenner *et al.*, 1993b, 1994). Importantly, this was the first unequivocal report of relapse arising from the autograft. In one patient the simultaneous detection of a cytogenetic marker along with the *neo* gene confirmed that genetically marked cells contributed to relapse. At relapse 2.1% of the leukemic blast cells were resistant to G418 indicating expression of the *neo* gene (Brenner *et al.*, 1994).

In the neuroblastoma trial, five of nine patients have relapsed and in at least three cases the relapse tumor contained genetically marked cells. In this same patient group, a second critical observation was made when Rill *et al.*, reported that a multiplicity of cells in the graft contributed to relapse (Rill *et al.*, 1994). Only 33% of the bone marrow graft was exposed to retroviral vector, the tumor contamination was less than 1% of the graft, and the transduction efficiency was assumed to be approximately 3%. Thus it can be estimated that approximately 0.0099% of the cells returned to the patient were genetically marked tumor cells. At least two distinct clones were detected in 1×10^6 isolated neuroblastoma cells from each of two patients at relapse, as determined by Southern blot analysis of proviral integration sites. Thus the authors concluded that, given a frequency of marking of at least 1%, a minimum of 200 clonogenic tumor cells were present in the graft at infusion. The high frequency of genetically marked relapse, in the face of the very low frequency of transfused malignant cells, strongly suggests that a large percentage of tumor cells in the graft contributes to relapse or, alternatively, that tumor cells susceptible to retroviral gene marking are uniquely capable of engraftment and clonal expansion.

Diesseroth and colleagues at M.D. Anderson have examined tumor relapse in the hematopoietic stem cell malignancy, chronic myeloid leukemia (CML) in adults (Diesseroth, 1994). This group marked bone marrow which had been processed using the CellPro column system (CellPro Inc. Bothell, Washington) to enrich the CD34+ cell fraction (Berenson *et al.*, 1988, 1991; Schiller *et al.*, 1995). Marrow was harvested from patients who had advanced disease after induction chemotherapy, and one-third of the marrow was transduced with retrovirus in the six-hour culture described previously. Again, by demonstrating that clonogenic cells at relapse contained both the *neo* marker gene and the tumor-specific *bcr-abl* oncogene rearrangement, this group demonstrated that infused, genetically marked, tumor cells contribute to relapse (Diesseroth *et al.*, 1994b). This result may be particularly relevant for treating CML because of the substantially higher relapse rate in patients who receive autologous compared to allogeneic bone marrow transplantion. Besides lacking the contribution of a graft-versus-leukemia effect provided by allogeneic transplant, the consequences of infusing malignant cells are evident. Unfortunately for patients with CML, distinguishing leukemic stem cells from normal hematopoietic cells for purging is a formidable task, and demonstrating genetically marked disease relapse is indeed discouraging for advocates of ABMT in CML.

The final published report of genetically marking hematopoietic cells in cancer patients is from Dunbar and colleagues at the N.I.H. (Dunbar *et al.*, 1995). In eleven patients who had breast cancer or myeloma, CD34+ cells were isolated from bone marrow or peripheral blood and retrovirally marked. The positive selection of CD34+ hematopoietic stem cells is an attractive alternative to purging tumor cells in ABMT for cancer patients (Freedman and Nadler, 1993; Vescio *et al.*, 1994). Purification of CD34+ cells from the marrow or peripheral blood may be particularly valuable in breast cancer or myeloma in which tumor cells do not, on the whole, express CD34. Indeed it has been demonstrated that CD34 selection depletes tumor cells by 2–4 logs in myeloma and breast cancer (Vescio *et al.*, 1994). This may explain in part the failure by Dunbar and colleagues to detect genetically marked malignant cells in patients who had breast cancer and myeloma (Dunbar *et al.*, 1995). None of the six myeloma patients have yet relapsed nor have CD38 bright (plasma cells) in the marrow of two patients contained the marker gene as determined by PCR at one year post transplant. Similarly, no evidence for the *neo* gene has been found in tumor biopsies from three breast cancer patients who have relapsed. These results are not surprising. The CD34 selection and three-day culture may both deplete the graft of tumor cells, and consequently the frequency of breast cancer or myeloma cells available for transduction may be exceedingly low. An additional factor unconfirmed by laboratory studies is that the fraction of myeloma cells and breast cancer cells in cycle and susceptible to retroviral marking may be low. Furthermore, the relative resistance of breast cancer and myeloma cells to chemotherapy makes recurrence of chemotherapeutically resistant disease a more likely source of relapse than resurgence of disease as a result of infusing cancer cells.

10. RETROVIRAL GENE MARKING AND PURGING EFFICACY

The compelling evidence presented confirms that tumor cells in the autograft contribute to relapse and consequently removing such cells before ABMT assumes a higher priority. Previous attempts to remove tumor cells have focused on tumor depletion by cytotoxic agents, predominantly mafosfamide and 4-hydroperoxycyclophosphamide (4HC), but cytokines, such as IL-2, monoclonal antibodies to B cells, neuroblastoma cells (with or without complement lysis), and more recently photodynamic purging, have all been explored (Freedman and Nadler, 1993). Although such approaches certainly deplete tumor cells without significantly affecting the hematopoietic content of the graft, it is unlikely that this depletion is absolute (Gribben *et al.*, 1991). Nevertheless, the high frequency with which tumor cells in the autograft are present at relapse (Brenner *et al.*, 1994; Rill *et al.*, 1994) suggests that purging may be more efficacious in preventing relapse than previously supposed, and consequently important studies of tumor purging are now underway at St. Jude (Brenner, 1996). In these trials the graft from neuroblastoma or AML patients is genetically marked and then divided equally. In AML, one-half is purged with IL-2, and the other with 4HC. In neuroblastoma half the marrow is purged using monoclonal antibodies (Brenner, 1996). Distinguishable genetic markers are employed for each half of the grafts. These studies should quickly answer important questions about the value and relative merits of purging without the necessity of resorting to large, expensive, and time-consuming, randomized, controlled, clinical trials.

11. IMPLICATIONS OF GENE MARKING RESULTS IN CLINICAL PRACTICE

Together with retrospective molecular studies in the mature B cell malignancy, low grade lymphoma (Gribben *et al.*, 1991), the trials described have convinced investigators at many transplant centers that an uncontaminated or successfully purged bone marrow should be used for reinfusion (Freedman and Nadler, 1993; Gazitt *et al.*, 1995; Vescio *et al.*, 1994). Despite this, there is also evidence in some malignancies that purging is unlikely to be efficacious until superior treatment regimens are adopted. In this regard it is important to remember that tumor cells in the autograft contribute to but do not cause relapse (Brenner *et al.*, 1994). Indeed one school of thought is that purging autografts will have little impact on clinical practice because the predominant bulk of disease resides in the patient and not the autograft and thus relapse is more likely to result from ineffective chemoradiotherapy induction regimens than from the infusion of tumor cells in an unpurged graft. Indeed in multiple myeloma, the percentage of plasma cells in the antograft (below or above 30%) does not correlate with either remission rate or median survival after transplantation (Barlogie and Garthon, 1991). This suggests that even if reinfused malignant cells do contribute to relapse it is more likely that myeloma patients who relapse after ABMT do so because the pretransplantation conditioning regimen fails to eradicate all clonogenic tumor cells.

Furthermore, the observation of Rill *et al.*, that gene-marked relapse is oligoclonal, even when tumor cells in the graft are present at very low frequency (Rill *et al.*, 1994), suggests that purging modalities need to be extremely efficient to affect survival after transplantation.

12. *IN VITRO* STRATEGIES TO IMPROVE HEMATOPOIETIC STEM CELL TARGETING

Because gene-marking studies in humans have clearly demonstrated the failings of current approaches to gene transfer into primitive hematopoietic cells, many laboratories are investigating ways to improve stem cell transduction *in vitro* (summarized in Table IV). A number of the problems to be overcome and the potential solutions under investigation are discussed here.

12.1. *In Vitro* Cycling

One serious impediment to hematopoietic stem cell gene transfer relates to the inability of retroviruses to infect quiescent cells (Hajihosseini *et al.*, 1993; Miller *et al.*, 1990; Roe *et al.*, 1993). Because most cells that exhibit the phenotype of hematopoietic stem cells are quiescent or slowly cycling, they need to be induced into cell cycle during *in vitro* culture to allow successful retroviral integration. One means of inducing cycling is introducing exogenous cytokine growth factors. Different combinations of hematopoietic growth factors, including recombinant IL-1, IL-3, IL-6, and SCF have been used to induce cycling of murine hematopoietic repopulating

Table IV
Strategies for Optimizing Gene Transfer into Hematopoietic Stem Cells[a]

1.	Cytokine stimulation
2.	Collect cells in a proliferative phase after chemotherapy
3.	Culture on stromal layers or fibronectin
4.	Target immunoisolated stem cells
5.	Increase virus and cell contact by centrifugation or continuous flow culture
6.	Change retrovirus pseudotype
7.	Modified retroviral vectors
8.	Targeting via chimeric retroviral envelope
9.	Alternative vector systems

[a] See text for description.

cells (Bodine *et al.*, 1991a, 1992; Luskey *et al.*, 1992; Muench *et al.*, 1993). Unfortunately no human growth factor that of induces cycling of human hematopoietic stem cells without committing cells to differentiate has yet been identified. Consequently using cytokines improves gene transfer into committed progenitor cells but fails to target the cells of interest (Crooks and Kohn, 1993; Knaan-Shanzer *et al.*, 1996; Xu *et al.*, 1995). Indeed, one potential problem identified with such an approach is a reported engraftment defect in cytokine-stimulated cells (Peters *et al.*, 1995). However, patience in such sytems may be a virtue because delayed responsiveness to cytokine stimulation in culture is characteristic of immature human progenitor cells. For example, in one study, *in vitro* cycling of primitive human precursor cells was not observed until day two after adding IL-1, IL-3, IL-6, SCF, granulocyte-colony stimulating factor (G-CSF), GM-CSF, and erythropoietin. The maximum proliferative response was not detected until day three, and 28% of cells were in the S/G_2M phase of the cell cycle at this time (Reems and Torok-Storb, 1995). Therefore, if cell viability can be maintained without extensive differentiation, presumably the proportion of transduced candidate hematopoietic stem cells can be increased by extending the time of *in vitro* culturing. Recently, use of FL + 3L, thrombopoietin, and SCF in combination has improved gene transfer *in vivo* in large animal models.

12.2. *In Vivo* Cycling

The results of Brenner and colleagues suggest that long term gene transfer into bone marrow cells is best acheived in children (Brenner *et al.*, 1993b, 1994). Because it is hard to believe that the six-hour transduction protocol explains the excellent results obtained, the only feasible explanations for these excellent results are (1) that youth equates with a robust and easily transduced population of bone marrow stem cells or (2) that collecting marrow during the recovery period from cytoablation allows gene transfer into stem cells mobilized to cycle *in vivo*. This latter hypothesis is supported by the increased numbers of hematopoietic stem cells observed in S/G_2M during marrow regeneration (Knaan-Shanzer *et al.*, 1996) and deserves to be tested in further clinical studies.

12.3. Stromal Layers or Fibronectin

An alternative approach to using exogenous cytokines for hematopoietic stem cell activation and maintenance *in vitro* involves culturing the cells on a (preestablished) autologous stromal cell feeder layer. Such stromal cell-supported cultures sustain the viability of the most primitive human hematopoietic progenitors yet detectable *in vitro* (Holland *et al.*, 1989; Hughes *et al.*, 1989; Sutherland *et al.*, 1990). When maintained for extended periods, as in the long-term (Dexter-type) marrow culture (Dexter *et al.*, 1980), progenitor cells, called long-term, culture-initiating cells (LTC-IC) are present for at least five weeks and give rise to myeloid and, in some instances, erythroid clonogenic cell progeny. In the murine system, at least some LTC-ICs share phenotypic characteristics of transplantable, *in vivo* repopulating cells (Lemieux *et al.*, 1995). These findings are highly relevant because studies of retrovirally mediated gene transfer into hematopoietic repopulating cells of large animals and, recently, humans indicate that higher frequencies of transduction are obtained with stromal cell support (Bienzle *et al.*, 1994; Carter *et al.*, 1992; Moore *et al.*, 1992; Nolta *et al.*, 1995; Schuening *et al.*, 1991a; Xu *et al.*, 1995). These preliminary observations have led at least two centers involved in human clinical trials to adopt stromal support (Kelso, 1995; Xu *et al.*, 1995).

Also germane to these studies is the finding that more efficient retrovirally mediated transfer of an adenosine deaminase gene into rhesus monkey hematopoietic stem cells is achieved by coculturing CD34-enriched cells on a murine stromal cell line engineered to produce the membrane-bound form of human SCF that supports human hematopoiesis *in vitro* (Bodine *et al.*, 1993; Toksoz *et al.*, 1992). Because the use of stromal layers is technically challenging and not readily clinically applicable on a wide scale, other investigators have attempted to mimic the "anchoring" of stem cells to stroma by using fibronectin. A series of experiments by Williams and colleagues at Indiana University indicate that fibronectin binding increases retroviral transduction efficiency (Moritz *et al.*, 1994). Recently, use of fibronectin fragments to enhance gene transfer efficiency has been widely adopted.

12.4. Stem Cell Isolation

Although the activation of hematopoietic stem cells by cytokines, cytoablation, or stroma all increase the efficiency of retrovirally mediated gene transfer, other complementary approaches to the problem are being pursued. One approach is to isolate the target population, thus increasing the viral to target cell ratio. This is most frequently accomplished by selecting hematopoietic cells that express the CD34 antigen. The CD34 antigen represents the only cell-surface antigen yet identified by monoclonal antibodies whose expression within the hematopoietic system is restricted to primitive progenitor cells of all lineages (Berenson *et al.*, 1988; Krause *et al.*, 1996; Sutherland and Keating, 1992). The 1–3% of normal bone marrow cells that express CD34 include virtually all unipotent and multipotent progenitors that are responsible for initial rapid engraftment and sustained reconstitution (Berenson *et al.*, 1988; Dunbar *et al.*, 1995; Schiller *et al.*, 1995; Sutherland and Keating, 1992). Consequently, CD34 represents a suitable "target" structure for the affinity purification of candidate hematopoietic stem cells. Thus, it is thought that the lineage-uncommitted fraction, characterized by high level expression of CD34, minimal expression of CD38, CD71 (transferrin receptor), and HLA-DR antigens, plus expression of the Thy-1/CDw90 and 8A3/CDw109 antigens, contains *bona fide* hematopoietic stem cells (Baum *et al.*, 1992; Berardi *et al.*, 1995; Craig *et al.*, 1993; DiGusto *et al.*, 1994; Huang and Terstappen, 1994; Lansdorp and Dragowska, 1992; Murray *et al.*, 1994, 1995; Sutherland *et al.*, 1988, 1991).

The immediate benefit to be gained by using CD34-enriched marrow for clinical gene transfer (Cassel *et al.*, 1993; Conneally *et al.*, 1996; Hughes *et al.*, 1992; Lu *et al.*, 1993; Medin *et al.*, 1996; Nolta *et al.*, 1995; Sirard *et al.*, 1996; Ward *et al.*, 1994; Xu *et al.*, 1995) is that a higher multiplicity of infection, that is, viral particle to stem cell ratio, is achieved. Enrichment for CD34+ cells may also obviate potential growth inhibitory effects mediated by cytokines that are produced by differentiated hematopoietic cells during *in vitro* culture. There are other obvious practical advantages afforded by this approach. These include a reduction in the volume of cells that needs to be cryopreserved and smaller volumes of retroviral supernatant, culture media, and supplements that are required for all subsequent manipulations, resulting in important cost savings.

12.5. Cell to Retrovirus Contact

An extension to purifying target cells to increase the retrovirus-to-cell contact ratio comes from the appreciation that potential cell-retrovirus interactions occur suboptimally in static systems. Accordingly, a number of groups are exploring the possibility of raising the local concentration of retroviral particles by centrifugation onto target cells (Kotani *et al.*, 1994) or by using flow-through systems in which the target cells are grown on filters or engineered stromal lines (Bertolini *et al.*, 1996; Eipers *et al.*, 1995). Early reports suggest that these physical methods of increasing the frequency of cell retrovirus contact result in significantly higher transduction efficiencies.

12.6. Pseudotyped Recombinant Retroviruses

Because the problem of retroviral entry into the cell is paramount, investigators are trying to overcome this limitation by modifying the retrovirus virion rather than the target cell (DeLouis *et al.*, 1990). Retroviruses are classified according to their host range, which is largely determined by binding of the retroviral envelope protein to a cellular receptor (Weiss and Tailor, 1995). Retroviral vectors produced as replication-defective amphotropic pseudotypes of Moloney murine leukemia virus (MoMuLV) are the most extensively used for gene delivery to human cells and the only ones to date in clinical trials (Miller, 1990b, 1992b). Amphotropic retroviruses utilize Ram-1, an inorganic phosphate transporter, as their cellular receptor. It is now generally assumed that low level expression of Ram-1 on candidate hematopoietic stem cells may be a major factor limiting highly efficient retroviral transduction by amphotropic retroviral vectors.

The gibbon ape leukemia virus (GALV) uses a different inorganic phosphate transporter, GLVR1, as its internalization receptor (Kavanaugh *et al.*, 1994).

Replication-defective retroviral vectors produced from the PG13 packaging cell line as GALV-pseudotyped retroviruses efficiently infect human cells (Miller *et al.*, 1991). Transduction of CD34-enriched hematopoietic cells—clonogenic myeloid progenitors and LTC-IC—his increased with GALV-pseudotyped retroviral vectors prepared using the PG13 packaging cell line, compared with conventional amphotropic retroviral preparations (von Kalle *et al.*, 1994). These results suggest that transduction of candidate hematopoietic stem cells might also be more efficient with PG13-packaged retroviral vectors. Other pseudotyped retroviral vectors, using the vesicular stomatitis viral envelope glycoprotein G, also increase transduction of hematopoietic cells (Akkina *et al.*, 1996; Burns *et al.*, 1993).

12.7. MSCV Retroviral Vector System

Although gene transfer into murine hematopoietic stem cells has been routinely accomplished with conventional retroviral vectors based on MoMuLV and the related myeloproliferative sarcoma virus (MPSV), many investigators, including ourselves, have reported low levels of expression and frequent transcriptional extinction with these constructs (Bowtell *et al.*, 1988; Challita and Kohn, 1994; Hawley *et al.*, 1994b; Szilvassy and Cory, 1994). Thus, even if retroviral transduction is achieved at high frequency, expression of the gene product may be low. Hypothesizing that mechanisms similar to those responsible for restricting expression of MoMuLV-based vectors in undifferentiated murine embryonal carcinoma and embryonic stem cells might be operative in human hematopoietic stem cells, we constructed a retroviral vector, MSCV (for murine stem cell virus), that contains multiple modifications which cooperatively enable expression of MoMuLV-based vectors in undifferentiated embryonic cells. Subsequently, we demonstrated that MSCV-based vectors yield high-titer recombinant retroviruses which function efficiently in immature murine hematopoietic cells, including myeloid progenitors(de Lanux *et al.*, 1995; Hawley *et al.*, 1994a), B- and T-lymphoid precursors (Hawley *et al.*, 1995) and, most importantly, in hematopoietic stem cells (Conneally *et al.*, 1996; Hawley *et al.*, 1996; Yan *et al.*, 1995). Recognizing the potential utility of this vector for delivering therapeutic genes clinically, we created safety-modified versions of the basic MSCV backbone for use in human gene therapy (Hawley, 1994; Hawley *et al.*, 1994b). An initial report of successful transduction of CD34+ hematopoietic progenitors with functional MSCV-based retroviruses (Conneally *et al.*, 1996) validates the assertion that the MSCV backbone will be a useful platform for evaluating the parameters governing optimal, retrovirally mediated gene expression in human hematopoietic stem cells.

12.8. Targeting with Engineered Retroviral Envelope Proteins

The envelope proteins of retroviruses consist of oligomers of a transmembrane (TM) protein linked to a surface (SU) glycoprotein. The SU glycoprotein mediates binding to the specific cellular receptor (i.e., to Ram-1 or GLVR1 in the case of amphotropic retroviruses and GaLV, respectively), whereas fusion with the cell depends on both SU and TM. Several groups have recently demonstrated the feasibility of altering the viral host range by generating chimeric envelope proteins that incorporate a single-chain variable region fragment of an antibody (scFv) or ligands that recognize different cell-surface molecules (Cosset *et al.*, 1995; Kasahara *et al.*, 1994; Russell *et al.*, 1993; Schnierle *et al.*, 1996; Somia *et al.*, 1995). Results from these studies have shown that coexpression of wild-type envelope protein (TM + SU) with the chimeric envelope protein is essential for infection to occur, presumably because functional interaction between SU and TM is necessary to induce conformational changes required for virion–cell membrane fusion.

Initial attempts with chimeric envelopes that retain the complete SU domain have generally resulted in recombinant pseudotyped retroviral particles that have low effective titers, most likely because of the chimeric proteins cannot optimally transduce a signal to trigger fusion after binding. However, increased retroviral infectivity by pseudotyped retroviruses that express chimeric envelope receptors in the absence of wild-type receptors has recently been obtained by including a spacer between the targeting domain and the SU domain (Valsesia-Wittmann *et al.*, 1996). Therefore, it is possible, and it is a subject of intense investigation to engineer the retroviral envelope so that it recognizes target cells, including hematopoietic stem cells. Together with improvements in isolating the target population, cycling of the target cell, improved viral uptake and expression, targeting of retroviral vectors at specific cell types will ultimately greatly improve current approaches to clinical gene transfer.

12.9. Alternative Vector Systems

Because retroviral vectors are inherently flawed as agents for hematopoietic stem cell gene transfer, a number of alternative approaches to gene transfer are being investigated. For example, one recent paper describes gene transfer into CD34+ hematopoietic cells using E1-deleted adenoviral vectors (Neering *et al.*, 1996). Although adenoviral vectors offer the advantage of gene delivery to noncycling cells, the long term utility of such an approach is constrained by their inability to integrate into chromosomal DNA. In contrast, the recent demonstration of transducing CD34+ hematopoietic progenitors by lentiviral vectors shows great potential because the latter vectors are not constrained by cell cycle and yet integrate (Kotani *et al.*, 1994; Naldini *et al.*, 1996; Shimada *et al.*, 1991). Such vectors promise to expand the scope and breadth of gene therapy using hematopoietic stem cells.

13. FUTURE DIRECTIONS

The exciting observations made in the early gene-marking studies described previously raise as many questions as they answer. Most importantly, the long term engraftment of genetically altered hematopoietic cells must still be optimized, and the functional expression of therapeutic genes at clinically relevant levels must be demonstrated. Nevertheless, these studies set the stage for investigating a multiplicity of maneuvers for increasing gene transfer efficiency and long-term gene transfer using hematopoietic stem cells. Further investigation of traditional and novel purging mechanisms to prevent genetically marked relapse are underway, and clinical trials have begun. Examples of the latter include using drug resistance genes in cancer patients (Sorrentino *et al.*, 1992; Ward *et al.*, 1994), treating inherited Gauchers disease (Xu *et al.*, 1995), adenosine deaminase deficiency (Bordignon *et al.*, 1995; Hoogerbrugge *et al.*, 1996), chronic granulomatous disease, and Fanconis anemia and using genetically modified lymphocytes to treat viral infection from HIV (Riddell *et al.*, 1996) or EBV(Rooney *et al.*, 1995).

14. SUMMARY

A surprising number of early gene-marking studies have targeted autologous hematopoietic stem cell recipients. Trials completed or underway are heterogeneous in the patient population studied, the transduction methodology employed, and the cells targeted. Thus, each trial is likely to contribute uniquely to understanding the utility and deficiencies of hematopoietic stem cells as vehicles for gene therapy and the contribution of genetically marked cells in the autograft to disease relapse. Trials already reported confirm the apparent safety of retroviral gene marking, demonstrate that reinfused genetically marked, hematopoietic cells contribute to long-term hematopoieis, and illustrate that tumor cells which contaminate the bone marrow infusion can engraft and contribute to relapse in acute and chronic myeloid leukemia and in neuroblastoma. Future trials will attempt to optimize hematopoietic engraftment while providing maximal tumor depletion.

It is important to conclude by observing that only three years ago issues of safety dominated thinking about retroviral gene transfer. Therefore, it is encouraging and a testament to early investigators that a few short years later we may now address the impact of pioneering studies on daily clinical practice and look forward to continued rapid progress in understanding cancer biology and the role of hematopoietic cells in gene therapy.

15. REFERENCES

Abkowitz, J. L., Linenberger, M. L., Newton, M. A., Shelton, G. H., Ott, R. L., and Guttrop, P., 1990, Evidence for the maintenance of hematopoiesis in a large animal by the sequential activation of stem-cell clones, *Proc. Natl. Acad. Sci. USA* **87:**9060–9062.

Akkina, R. K., Walton, R. M., Chen, M. L., Li, Q.-X., Planelles, V., and Chen, I. S. Y., 1996, High-efficiency gene transfer into CD34+ cells with a human immunodeficiency virus type 1-based retroviral vector pseudotyped with vesicular stomatitis virus envelope glycoprotein G, *J. Virol.* **70:**2581–2585.

Anderson, F. W., 1994, Recombinant DNA advisory committee data management report, *Hum. Gene Ther.* **5:**1290–1295.

Anderson, W. F., 1992, Human gene therapy, *Science* **256:**808–813.

Anderson, W. F., McGarrity, G. J., and Moen, R. C., 1993, Report to the NIH Recombinant DNA Advisory Committee on murine replication-competent retrovirus (RCR) assays, *Hum. Gene Ther.* **4:**310–311.

Barlogie, B., and Garthon, G., 1991, Bone marrow transplantation in multiple myeloma, *Bone Marrow Transpl.* **7**:70–71.

Barquinero, J., Kiem, H. P., von Kalle, C., Darovsky, B., Goehle, S., Graham, T., Seidel, K., Storb, R., and Schuening, F. G., 1995, Myelosuppressive conditioning improves autologous engraftment of genetically marked hematopoietic repopulating cells in dogs, *Blood* **85:**1195–1201.

Baum, C. M., Weissman, I. L., Tsukamoto, A. S., Buckle, A.-M., and Peault, B., 1992, Isolation of a candidate human hematopoietic stem cell population, *Proc. Natl. Acad. Sci. USA* **89:**2804–2808.

Bayever, E., Haines, K., Duprey, S., Rappaport, E., Douglas, S. D., and Surrey, S., 1988, Protection of uninfected human bone marrow cells in long-term culture from G418 toxicity after retroviral-mediated transfer of the neoR gene, *Exp. Cell. Res.* **179:**160–168.

Belmon, J. W., MacGregor, G. R., Wager-Smith, K., Fletcher, F. A., Moore, K. A., Hawkins, D., Villalon, D., Chang, S. M. W., and Caskey, C. T., 1988, Expression of human adenosine deaminase in murine hematopoietic cells, *Mol. Cell. Biol.* **8:**5110–5116.

Berardi, A. C., Wang, A., Levine, J. D., Lopez, P., and Scadden, D. T., 1995, Functional isolation and characterization of human hematopoietic stem cells, *Science* **267:**104–108.

Berenson, R. J., Andrews, R. G., Bensinger, W. I., Kalamasz, D., Knitter, G., Buckner, C. D., and Bernstein, I. D., 1988, Antigen CD34+ marrow cells engraft lethally irradiated baboons, *J. Clin. Invest.* **81:**951–955.

Berenson, R. J., Bensinger, W. I., Hill, R. S., Andrews, R. G., Garcia-Lopez, J., Kalamaz, D. F., Still, B. J., Spitzer, G., Buckner, D., Bernstein, I. D., and Thomas, E. D., 1991, Engraftment after infusion of CD34+ marrow cells in patients with breast cancer or neuroblastoma, *Blood* **77:**1717–1722.

Bertolini, F., Battaglia, M., Corsini, C., Lazzari, L., Soligo, D., Zibera, C., and Thalmeier, K., 1996, Engineered stromal layers and continous flow culture enhance multidrug resistance gene transfer in hematopoietic progenitors, *Cancer Res.* **56:**2566–2572.

Bienzle, D., Abrams-Ogg, A. C., Kruth, S. A., Ackland-Snow, J., Carter, R. F., Dick, J. E., Jacobs, R. M., Kamel-Reid, S., and Dube, I. D., 1994, Gene transfer into hematopoietic stem cells: Long-term maintenance of in vitro activated progenitors without marrow ablation, *Proc. Natl. Acad. Sci. USA* **91:**350–354.

Bjorkstrand, B., Dilber, M. S., Smith, C. I. E., Gahrton, G., and Xanthopoulos, K. G., 1994a, Retroviral-mediated gene transfer into human myeloma cells, *Br. J. Haematol.* **88:**325–331.

Bjorkstrand, B., Gahrton, G., Dilber, M. S,, Ljungman, P., Smith, C. I. E., and Xanthopoulos, K. G., 1994b, Retroviral mediated gene transfer of CD34 enriched bone marrow and peripheral blood cells during autologous stem cell transplantation for multiple myeloma, *Hum. Gene. Ther.* **5:**1279–1286.

Blaese, R. M., Culver, K. W., Miller, A. D., Carter, C. S., Fleisher, T., Clerici, M., Shearer, G., Chang, L., Chiang, Y., Tolstoshev, P., Greenblatt, J. J., Rosenberg, S. A., Klein, H., Berger, M., Mullen, C. A., Ramsey, W. J., Muul, L., Morgan, R. A., and Anderson, W. F., 1995, T lymphocyte directed gene therapy for ADA-SCID: Initial trial results after 4 years, *Science* **270:**475–480.

Bodine, D. M., McDonagh, K. T., Brandt, S. J., Ney, P. A., Agricola, B., Byrne, R., and Nienhuis, A. W., 1990, Development of a high-titer retrovirus producer cell line capable of gene transfer into rhesus monkey hematopoietic stem cells, *Proc. Natl. Acad. Sci. USA* **87:**3738–3742.

Bodine, D. M., Crosier, P. S., and Clark, S. C., 1991a, Effects of hematopoietic growth factors on the survival of primitive stem cells in liquid suspension culture, *Blood* **78:**914–919.

Bodine, D. M., McDonagh, K. T., Seidel, N. E., and Nienhuis, A. W., 1991b, Survival and retrovirus infection of murine hematopoietic stem cells in vitro: Effects of 5-FU and method of infection, *Exp. Hematol.* **19:**206–212.

Bodine, D. M., Orlic, D., Birkett, N. C., Seidel, N. E., and Zsebo, K. M., 1992, Stem cell factor increases colony-forming unit-spleen number in vitro in synergy with interleukin-6, and in vivo in Sl/Sl^d mice as a single factor, *Blood* **79:**913–919.

Bodine, D. M., Moritz, T., Donahue, R. E., Luskey, B. D., Kessler, S. W., Martin, D. I. K., Orkin, S. H., Nienhuis, A. W., and Williams, D. A., 1993, Long-term in vivo expression of a murine adenosine deaminase gene in rhesus monkey hematopoietic cells of multiple lineages after retroviral mediated gene transfer into CD34+ bone marrow cells, *Blood* **82:**1975–1980.

Bordignon, C., Notarangelo, L. D., Nobili, N., Ferrari, G., Casorati, G., Panina, P., Mazzolari, E., Maggioni, D., Rossi, C., Servida, P., Ugazio, A. G., and Mavilio, F., 1995, Gene therapy in peripheral blood lymphocytes and bone marrow for ADA(−) immunodeficient patients, *Science* **270:**470–475.

Boris-Lawrie, K., and Temin, H. M., 1994, The retroviral vector. Replication cycle and safety considerations for retrovirus mediated gene therapy, *Ann. N.Y. Acad. Sci.* **716:**59–64.

Bowtell, D. D. L., Johnson, G. R., Kelso, A., and Cory, S., 1987, Expression of genes transferred to haemopoietic stem cells by recombinant retroviruses, *Mol. Biol. Med.* **4:**229–250.

Bowtell, D. D. L., Cory, S., Johnson, G. R., and Gonda, T. J., 1988, Comparison of expression in hemopoietic cells by retroviral vectors carrying two genes, *J. Virol.* **62:**2464–2473.

Brenner, M., Rill, D. R., Moen, R. C., Krance, R. A., Heslop, H., Mirro, J., Anderson, W. F., and Ihle, J. N., 1994, Gene marking and autologous bone marrow transplant, *Ann. N.Y. Acad. Sci.* **716:**204–215.

Brenner, M., 1996, Use of marker genes to investigate the mechanism of relapse and the effect of bone marrow purging in autologous transplantation for stage D neuroblastoma, *Hum. Gene Ther.* **4:**809–820.

Brenner, M. K., Rill, D. R., Holladay, M. S., Heslop, H. E., Moen, R. C., Buschle, M., Krance, R. A., Santana, V. M., Anderson, W. F., and Ihle, J. N., 1993a, Gene marking to determine whether autologous marrow infusion restores long term haemopoiesis in cancer patients, *Lancet* **342:**1134–1137.

Brenner, M. K., Rill, D. R., and Moen, R. C., 1993b, Gene marking to trace origin of relapse after autologous bone-marrow transplantation for acute myeloid leukemia, *Lancet* **341:**80–85.

Burns, J. C., Friedmann, T., Driever, W., Burrascano, M., and Yee, J.-K., 1993, Vesicular stomatitis virus G glycoprotein pseudotyped retroviral vectors: Concentration to very high titer and efficient gene transfer into mammalian and nonmammalian cells, *Proc. Natl. Acad. Sci. USA* **90:**8033–8037.

Cai, Q., Rubin, J. T., and Lotze, M. T., 1995, Genetically marked human cells—Results of the first clinical gene transfer studies, *Cancer Gene Ther.* **2:**125–136.

Carter, R. F., Abrams-Ogg, A. C., Dick, J. E., Kruth, S. A., Valli, V. E., Kamel-Reid, S., and Dube, I. D., 1992, Autologous transplantation of canine long-term marrow culture cells genetically marked by retroviral vectors, *Blood* **79:**356–364.

Cassel, A., Cottler-Fox, M., Doren, S., and Dunbar, C. E., 1993, Retroviral-mediated gene transfer into CD34-enriched human peripheral blood stem cells, *Exp. Hematol.* **21:**585–591.

Challita, P. M., and Kohn, D. B., 1994, Lack of expression from a retroviral vector after transduction of murine hematopoietic stem cells is associated with methylation *in vivo*, *Proc. Natl. Acad. Sci. USA* **91:**2567–2571.

Conneally, E., Bardy, P., Eaves, C. J., Thomas, T., Chappel, S., Shpall, E. J., and Humphries, R. K., 1996, Rapid and efficient selection of human hematopoietic cells expressing murine heat-stable antigen as an indicator of retroviral-mediated gene transfer, *Blood* **87:**456–464.

Cornetta, K., Wieder, R., and Anderson, W. F., 1989, Gene transfer into primates and prospects for gene therapy in humans, *Prog. Nucleic Acids Res. Mol. Biol.* **36:**310–311.

Cornetta, K., Moen, R. C., and Culver, K., 1990, Amphotropic murine leukemia retrovirus is not an acute pathogen for primates, *Hum. Gene Ther.* **1:**10–15.

Cornetta, K., Morgan, R. A., and Anderson, W. F., 1991, Safety issues related to retroviral-mediated gene transfer in humans, *Hum. Gene Ther.* **2:**5–14.

Cornetta, K., 1992, Safety aspects of gene therapy, *Br. J. Haematol.* **80:**420–421.

Cornetta, K., Tricot, G., Broun, E. R., Hromas, R., Srour, E., Hoffman, R., Anderson, W. F., Moen, R. C., and Morgan, R. A., 1992, Retroviral-mediated gene transfer of bone marrow cells during autologous bone marrow transplantation for acute leukemia, *Hum. Gene Ther.* **3:**300–305.

Correll, O. H., Colilla, S., Dave, H. P. G., and Karlsson, S., 1992, High levels of human glucocerebrosidase activity in macrophages of long-term reconstituted mice after retroviral infection of hematopoietic stem cells, *Blood* **80:**330–331.

Correll, P. H., Fink, J. D., Brady, R. O., Perry, L. K., and Karlsson, S., 1989, Production of human glucocerebrosidase in mice after retroviral gene transfer into multipotential hematopoietic progenitor cells, *Proc. Natl. Acad. Sci. USA* **86:**8910–8912.

Correll, P. H., Colilla, S., and Karlsson, S., 1994, Retroviral vector design for long-term expression in murine hematopoietic cells in vivo, *Blood* **84:**1812–1822.

Cosset, F.-L., Morling, F. J., Takeuchi, Y., Weiss, R. A., Collins, M. K. L., and Russell, S. J., 1995, Retroviral retargeting by envelopes expressing an N-terminal binding domain, *J. Virol.* **69:**6314–6322.

Cournoyer, D., Scarpa, M., Mitani, K., Moore, K. A., Markowitz, D., Bank, A., Belmont, J. W., and Caskey, T., 1991, Gene transfer of adenosine deaminase into primitive human hematopoietic progenitor cells, *Hum. Gene Ther.* **2:**200–203.

Craig, W., Kay, R., Cutler, R. L., and Lansdorp, P. M., 1993, Expression of Thy-1 on human hematopoietic progenitor cells, *J. Exp. Med.* **177:**1331–1342.

Crooks, G. M., and Kohn, D. B., 1993, Growth factors increase amphotropic retrovirus binding to human CD34+ bone marrow progenitor cells, *Blood* **82:**3290–3297.

Crystal, R. G., 1995, Transfer of genes to humans: Early lessons and obstacles to success, *Science* **270:**404–410.

de Lanux, V. M., Reis, M. D., and Hawley, R. G., 1995, Establishment of myeloid progenitor lines from primary cultures of murine bone marrow cells expressing a v-Myb oncoprotein, *Int. J. Oncol.* **7:**555–563.

DeLouis, C., Milan, D., L'Haridon, R., Gianquinto, L., Bonnerot, C., and Nicolas, J.-F., 1990, Xenotropic and amphotropic pseudotyped recombinant retrovirus to transfer genes into cells from various species, *Biochem. Biophys. Res. Commun.* **169:**8–14.

Demarquoy, J., Herman, G. E., Lorenzo, I., Trentin, J., Beaudet, A. L., and O'Brien, W. E., 1992, Long-term expression of human argininosuccinate synthetase in mice following bone marrow transplantation with retrovirus-transduced hematopoietic stem cells, *Hum. Gene Ther.* **3:**3–10.

Dexter, T. M., Garland, J., Scott, D., Scolnick, E., and Metcalf, D., 1980, Growth of factor-dependent hemopoietic precursor cell lines, *J. Exp. Med.* **152:**1036–1047.

Dick, J. E., Samel-Reid, S., Murdoch, B., and Doedens, M., 1991, Gene transfer into normal human hematopoietic cells using in vitro and in vivo assays, *Blood* **78:**620–624.

Diesseroth, A. B., 1994, Use of retroviral vectors to evaluate the efficacy of purging and to discriminate between relapse which arises from systemic disease remaining after preparative therapy versus relapse due to residual neoplastic cells in autologous marrow following purging in indolent B cell neoplasms, *Hum. Gene Ther.* **2:**359–364.

Diesseroth, A. B., Zu, S., and Claxton, D., 1994a, Genetic marking shows that Ph+ cells present in autologous transplants of chronic myelogenous leukemia (CML) contribute to relapse after autologous bone marrow in CML, *Blood* **83:**3068–3076.

DiGusto, D., Chen, S., Combs, J., Webb, S., Namikawa, R., Tsukamoto, A., Chen, B. P., and Galy, A. H. M., 1994, Human fetal bone marrow early progenitors for T, B, and myeloid cells are found exclusively in the population expressing high levels of CD34, *Blood* **84:**421–432.

Dube, I. D., Kruth, S., Abrams-Ogg, A., Kamel-Reid, S., Lutzko, C., Nanji, S., Ruedy, C., Singaraja, R., Wild, A., Krygsman, P., Chu, P., Messner, H., Reddy, V., McGarrity, G., and Stewart, A. K., 1996, Pre-clinical assessment of human hematopoietic progenitor cell gene transduction in long term marrow cultures, *Hum. Gene Ther.*, in press.

Dunbar, C. E., Nienhuis, A. W., Stewart, F. M., Quesenberry, P., O'Shaunessy, J., Cowan, K., Cottler, F. M., Leitman, S., Goodman, S., and Sorrentino, B. P., 1993, Amendment to clinical research projects. Genetic marking with retroviral vectors to study the feasibility of stem cell gene transfer and the biology of hematopoietic reconstitution after autologous transplantation in multiple myeloma, chronic myelogenous leukemia, or metastatic breast cancer, *Hum. Gene Ther.* **4:**200–205.

Dunbar, C. E., Bodine, D. M., Sorrentino, B., Donahue, D. M., McDonagh, K., Cottler-Fox, M., O'Shaughnessy, J., Cowan, K., Carter, C., Doren, S., Cassel, A., and Nienhuis, A. W., 1994, Gene transfer into hematopoietic cells—implications for cancer therapy, *Ann. N.Y. Acad. Sci.* **716:**216–224.

Dunbar, C. E., and Emmons, R. V. B., 1994, Gene transfer into hematopoietic progenitor and stem cells: Progress and problems, *Stem Cells* **12:**563–576.

Dunbar, C. E., Cottler-Fox, M., O'Shaughnessy, J. A., Doren, S., Carter, C., Berenson, R., Brown, S., Moen, R. C., Greenblatt, J., Stewart, F. M., Leitman, S. F., Wilson, W. H., Cowan, K., Young, N. S., and Nienhuis, A. W., 1995, Retrovirally marked CD34-enriched peripheral blood and bone marrow cells contribute to long-term engraftment after autologous transplantation, *Blood* **85:**3048–3057.

Economou, J. S., Belldegrun, A. S., Glaspy, J., Toloza, E. M., Figlin, R., Hobbs, J., Meldon, N., Kaboo, R., Tso, C., Miller, A., Lau, R., McBride, W., and Moen, R. C., 1996, In vivo trafficking of adoptively transferred interleukin 2 expanded tumor infiltrating lymphocytes and peripheral blood lymphocytes. Results of a double gene marking trial, *J. Clin. Invest.* **97:**515–521.

Eglitis, M. A., 1991, Positive selectable markers for use with mammalian cells in culture, *Hum. Gene Ther.* **2:**195–201.

Eipers, P. G., Krauss, J. C., Palsson, B. O., Emerson, S. G., Todd, R. F., and Clarke, M. F., 1995, Retroviral mediated gene transfer in human bone marrow cells grown in continous perfusion culture vessels, *Blood* **10:**3754–3762.

Freedman, A. S., and Nadler, L., 1993, Developments in purging in autotransplantation, *Hematol./Oncol. Clin. Nor. Am.* **7:**687–680.

Friedmann, T., 1996, Human gene therapy—an immature genie but certainly out of the bottle, *Nat. Med.* **2:**144–147.

Gazitt, Y., Reading, C. C., Hoffman, R., Wickrema, A., Vesole, D. H., Jagannath, S., Condino, J., Lee, B., Barlogie, B., and Tricot, G., 1995, Purified $CD34^+$ Lin^- Thy^+ stem cells do not contain clonal myeloma cells, *Blood* **86:**381–389.

Greenberger, J. S., Sakakeeny, M. A., Humphries, R. K., Eaves, C. J., and Eckner, R. J., 1983, Demonstration of permanent factor-dependent multipotential (erythroid/neutrophil/basophil) hematopoietic progenitor cell lines, *Proc. Natl. Acad. Sci. USA* **80:**2931–2935.

Gribben, J. G., Freedman, A. S., and Neuberg, D., 1991, Immunologic purging of marrow assessed by PCR before autologous bone marrow transplantation for B cell lymphoma, *N. Engl. J. Med.* **22:**1520–1525.

Gruber, H. E., Finley, K. D., Hershberg, R. M., Katzman, S. S., Laikind, P. K., Seegmiller, J. E., Friedmann, T., Yee, J.-K., and Jolly, D. J., 1985, Retroviral vector-mediated gene transfer into human hematopoietic progenitor cells, *Science* **230:**1057–1061.

Gutierrez, A. A., Lemoine, N. R., and Sikora, K., 1992, Gene therapy for cancer, *Lancet* **339:**710–715.

Hajihosseini, M., Iavachev, L., and Price, J., 1993, Evidence that retroviruses integrate into post-replication host DNA, *EMBO J.* **12:**4969–4974.

Harrison, D. E., Astle, C. M., and Lerner, C., 1988, Number and continuous proliferative pattern of transplanted primitve immunohematopoietic stem cells, *Proc. Natl. Acad. Sci. USA* **85:**820–822.

Harrison, D. E., Jordan, C. T., Zhong, R. K., and Astle, C. M., 1993, Primitive hemopoietic stem cells: Direct assay of most productive populations by competitive repopulation with simple binomial, correlation and covariance calculations, *Exp. Hematol.* **21:**206–219.

Hawley, R., Covarrubias, L., Hawley, T., and Mintz, B., 1989, Clonal contributions of small numbers of retrovirally marked hematopoietic stem cells engrafted in unirradiated neonatal W W mice, *Proc. Natl. Acad. Sci. USA* **86:**4550–4554.

Hawley, R. G., 1994, High titer retroviral vectors for efficient transduction of functional genes into murine hematopoietic stem cells, *Ann. N.Y. Acad. Sci.* **716:**327–330.

Hawley, R. G., Fong, A. Z. C., Lu, M., and Hawley, T. S., 1994a, The HOX11 homeobox-containing gene of human leukemia immortalizes murine hematopoietic precursors, *Oncogene* **9:**1–12.

Hawley, R. G., Lieu, F. H. L., Fong, A. Z. C., and Hawley, T. S., 1994b, Versatile retroviral vectors for potential use in gene therapy, *Gene Ther.* **1:**136–138.

Hawley, R. G., Fong, A. Z. C., Ngan, B.-Y., and Hawley, T. S., 1995, Hematopoietic transforming potential of activated *ras* in chimeric mice, *Oncogene* **11:**1113–1123.

Hawley, R. G., Hawley, T. S., Fong, A. Z. C., Quinto, C., Collins, M., Leonard, J. P., and Goldman, S. J., 1996, Thrombopoietic potential and serial repopulating ability of murine hematopoietic stem cells constitutively expressing interleukin-11, *Proc. Natl. Acad. Sci. USA*, in press.

Hock, R. A., and Miller, A. D., 1986, Retrovirus-mediated transfer and expression of drug resistance genes in human haematopoietic progenitor cells, *Nature* **320:**275–277.

Hock, R. A., Miller, A. D., and Osborne, W. R. A., 1989, Expression of human adenosine deaminase from various strong promoters after gene transfer into human hematopoietic cell lines, *Blood* **74**(2)**:**870–876.

Hogge, D. E., and Humphries, R. K., 1987, Gene transfer to primary normal and malignant human hemopoietic progenitors using recombinant retroviruses, *Blood* **69:**611–617.

Holland, C. A., Rothstein, L., Sakakeeny, M. A., Anklesaria, P., Griffin, J. D., Harigaya, K., Newburer, P. E., and Greenberger, J. S., 1989, Infection of hematopoietic and stromal cells in human continuous bone marrow cultures by a retroviral vector containing the neomycin resistance gene, *Acta Haematol.* **82:**130–136.

Hoogerbrugge, P. M., van Beusechem, V. W., Fischer, A., Debree, M., le Deist, F., Perignon, J. L., Morgan, G., Gaspar, B., Fairbanks, L. D., Skeoch, C. H., Moseley, A., Harvey, M., Levinsky, R. J., and Valerio, D., 1996, Bone marrow gene transfer in three patients with adenosine deaminase deficiency, *Gene Ther.* **3:**179–183.

Huang, S., and Terstappen, L. W. M. M., 1994, Lymphoid and myeloid differentiation of single human CD34+, HLA-DR+, CD38- hematopoietic stem cells, *Blood* **83:**1515–1526.

Hughes, P. F. D., Eaves, C. J., Hogge, D. E., and Humphries, R. K., 1989, High-efficiency gene transfer to human hematopoietic cells maintained in long-term marrow culture, *Blood* **74:**1910–1915.

Hughes, P. F. D., Thacker, J. D., Hogge, D., Sutherland, H. J., Thomas, T. E., Lansdorp, P. M., Eaves, C. J., and Humphries, R. K., 1992, Retroviral gene transfer to primitive normal and leukemic hematopoietic cells using clinically applicable procedures, *J. Clin. Invest.* **89:**1817–1824.

Jaffee, E. M., Dranoff, G., Cohen, L. K., Hauda, K. M., Clift, S., Marshall, F. F., Mulligan, R. C., and Pardoll, D. M., 1996, High efficiency gene transfer into primary human tumor explants without cell selection, *Cancer Res.* **53:**2221–2226.

Jordan, C. T., and Lemischka, I. R., 1990, Clonal and systemic analysis of long-term hematopoiesis in the mouse, *Genes Dev.* **4:**220–232.

Jordon, C. T., McKearn, J. P., and Lemischka, I. R., 1990, Cellular and developmental properties of fetal hematopoietic stem cells, *Cell* **61:**950–953.

Kaleko, M., Garcia, J. V., Osborne, W. A., and Miller, A. D., 1990, Expression of human adenosine deaminase in mice after transplantation of genetically modified bone marrow, *Blood* **75**(8)**:**1730–1733.

Kantoff, P. W., Flake, A. W., Eglitis, M. A., Scahrf, S., Bond, S., Gilboa, E., Erlich, H., Harrison, M. R., Zanjani, E. D., and Anderson, W. F., 1989, In utero gene transfer and expression: A sheep transplantation model, *Blood* **73:**1060–1066.

Karlsson, S., 1991, Treatment of genetic defects in hematopoietic cell function by gene transfer, *Blood* **78:**2481–2492.

Kasahara, N., Dozy, A. M., and Kan, Y. W., 1994, Tissue-specific targeting of retroviral vectors through ligand-receptor interactions, *Science* **266:**1373–1376.

Kavanaugh, M. P., Miller, D. G., Zhang, W., Law, W., Kozak, S. L., Kabat, D., and Miller, A. D., 1994, Cell-surface receptors for gibbon ape leukemia virus and amphotropic murine retrovirus are inducible sodium-dependent phosphate symporters, *Proc. Natl. Acad. Sci. USA* **91:**7071–7075.

Kelso, A., 1995, Th1 and Th2 subsets: Paradigms lost? *Immunol. Today* **16:**374–379.

Knaan-Shanzer, S., Valerio, D., and van Beuschem, V. W., 1996, Cell cycle state, response to hemopoietic growth factors and retroviral vector mediated transduction of human hemopoietic stem cells, *Gene Ther.* **3:**323–333.

Kotani, H., Newton, P. B. III, Zhang, S., Chiang, Y. L., Otto, E., Weaver, L., Blaese, R. M., Anderson, W. F., and McGarrity, G. J., 1994, Improved methods of retroviral vector transduction and production for gene therapy, *Hum. Gene Ther.* **5:**19–28.

Krause, D. S., Fackler, M. J., Civin, C. I., and May, W. S., 1996, CD34: Structure, biology, and clinical utility, *Blood* **87:**1–13.

Laneuville, P., Chang, W., Kamel-Reid, S., Fauser, A. A., and Dick, J. E., 1988, High-efficiency gene transfer and expression in normal human hematopoietic cells with retrovirus vectors, *Blood* **71:**811–814.

Lansdorp, P. M., and Dragowska, W., 1992, Long term erythropoiesis from constant numbers of CD34+ cells in serum-free cultures initiated with highly purified progenitor cells from human bone marrow, *J. Exp. Med.* **175:**1501–1509.

Lemieux, M. E., Rebel, V. I., Lansdorp, P. M., and Eaves, C. J., 1995, Characterization and purification of a primitive hematopoietic cell type in adult mouse marrow capable of lymphomyeloid differentiation in long-term marrow "switch" cultures, *Blood* **86:**1339–1347.

Lothrop, C. D., Jr., al-Lebban, Z. S., Niemeyer, G. P., Jones, J. B., Peterson, M. G., Smith, J. R., Baker, J. H., Morgan, R. A., Eglitis, M. A., and Anderson, W. F., 1991, Expression of a foreign gene in cats reconstituted with retroviral vector infected autologous bone marrow, *Blood* **78:**230–237.

Lotze, M., 1991, Lymphocytes as cellular vehicles for gene therapy in mouse and man, *Proc. Natl. Acad. Sci. USA* **88:**3155–3159.

Lu, L., Xiao, M., Clapp, D. W., Li, Z.-H., and Broxmeyer, H. E., 1993, High efficiency retroviral mediated gene transduction into single isolated immature and replatable CD34^{3+} hematopoietic stem/progenitor cells from human umbilical cord blood, *J. Exp. Med.* **178:**2089–2096.

Luskey, B. D., Rosenblatt, M., Zsebo, K., and Williams, D. A., 1992, Stem cell factor, interleukin-3, and interleukin-6 promote retroviral-mediated gene transfer into murine hematopoietic stem cells, *Blood* **80:**396–402.

Marty, L., Roux, P., Royer, M., and Piechaczyk, M., 1990, MoMuLV-derived self-inactivating retroviral vectors possessing multiple cloning sites and expressing the resistance to either G418 or hygromycin B, *Biochimie* **72:**885–887.

Mauch, P., Ferrara, J., and Hellman, S., 1989, Stem cell self-renewal considerations in bone marrow transplantation, *Bone Marrow Transpl.* **4:**600–601.

Medin, J. A., Migita, M., Pawliuk, R., Jacobson, S., Amiri, M., Kluepfel-Stahl, S., Brady, R. O., Humphries, R. K., and Karlsson, S., 1996, A bicistronic therapeutic retroviral vector enables sorting of transduced CD34$^+$ cells and corrects the enzyme deficiency in cells of Gaucher patients, *Blood* **87:**1754–1762.

Merrouche, Y., Negrier, S., and Bain, C., 1995, Clinical application of retroviral gene transfer in oncology: Results of a French study with tumor infiltrating lymphocytes transduced with the gene of resistance to neomycin, *J. Clin. Onc.* **13:**410.

Miller, A. D., and Rosman, G. J., 1989, Improved retroviral vectors for gene transfer and expression, *BioTechniques* **7:**980–990.

Miller, A. D., 1990a, Retrovirus packaging cells, *Hum. Gene Ther.* **1:**5–14.

Miller, A. D., 1992a, Human gene therapy comes of age, *Nature* **357:**455–460.

Miller, A. D., 1992b, Retroviral vectors, *Curr. Top. Microbiol. Immunol.* **158:**1–24.

Miller, D. G., Adam, M. A., and Miller, A. D., 1990, Gene transfer by retrovirus vectors occurs only in cells that are actively replicating at the time of infection, *Mol. Cell. Biol.* **10:**4239–4242.

Miller, A. D., Garcia, J. V., von Suhr, N., Lynch, C. M., Wilson, C., and Eiden, M. V., 1991, Construction and properties of retrovirus packaging cells based on gibbon ape leukemia virus, *J. Virol.* **65:**2220–2224.

Miller, A. D., Miller, D. G., Garcia, J. V., and Lynch, C. M., 1993, Use of retroviral vectors for gene transfer and expression, *Methods Enzymol.* **217:**581–599.

Miller, A. R., Skotzko, M. J., Rhoades, K., Belldegrun, A. S., Tso, C. L., Kaboo, R., McBride, W. H., Jacogs, E., Kohn, D. B., Moen, R., and Economou, J. S., 1992, Simultaneous use of two retroviral vectors in human gene marking trials: Feasibility and potential applications, *Hum. Gene Ther.* **3:**619–624.

Mintz, B., Anthony, K., and Littwin, S., 1984, Monoclonal derivation of mouse myeloid and lymphoid lineage from totipotent hematopoietic stem cells experimentally engrafted in fetal hosts, *Proc. Natl. Acad. Sci. USA* **81:**7830–7835.

Mitani, K., Wakamiya, M., and Caskey, C. T., 1993, Long-term expression of retroviral transduced adenosine deaminase in human primitive hematopoietic progenitors, *Hum. Gene Ther.* **4:**9–16.

Moolten, F. L., and Cupples, L. A., 1992, A model for predicting the risk of cancer consequent to retroviral gene therapy, *Hum. Gene Ther.* **3:**479–486.

Moore, K. A., Scarpa, M., Kooyer, S., Utter, A., Caskey, C. T., and Belmont, J. W., 1991, Evaluation of lymphoid-specific enhancer addition or substitution in a basic retrovirus vector, *Hum. Gene Ther.* **2:**300–307.

Moore, K. A., Deisseroth, A. B., Reading, C. L., Williams, D. E., and Belmont, J. W., 1992, Stromal support enhances cell-free retroviral vector transduction of human bone marrow long-term culture initiating cells, *Blood* **79:**1393–1399.

Morecki, S., Karson, E., Cornetta, K., Kasid, A., Aebersold, P., Blaese, R. M., Anderson, W. F., and Rosenberg, S. A., 1991, Retrovirus-mediated gene transfer into CD4$^+$ and CD8$^+$ human T cell subsets derived from tumor-infiltrating lymphocytes and peripheral blood mononuclear cells, *Cancer Immunol. Immunother.* **32:**342–352.

Morgan, R. A., and Anderson, W. F., 1993, Human gene therapy, *Ann. Rev. Biochem.* **62:**191–217.

Morganstern, J. J. P., and Land, H., 1990, Advanced mammalian gene transfer: High titre retroviral vectors with multiple drug selection markers and a complementary helper-free packaging cell line, *Nucleic Acids Res.* **18:**3580–3587.

Moritz, T., Patel, V. P., and Williams, D. A., 1994, Bone marrow extracellular matrix molecules improve gene transfer into human hematopoietic cells via retroviral vectors, *J. Clin. Invest.* **93:**1451–1457.

Muench, M. O., Firpo, M. T., and Moore, M. A. S., 1993, Bone marrow transplantation with interleukin-1 plus *kit*-ligand ex vivo expanded bone marrow accelerates hematopoietic reconstitution in mice without the loss of stem cell lineage and proliferative potential, *Blood* **81:**3463–3473.

Mulligan, R. C., 1993, The basic science of gene therapy, *Science* **260:**926–932.

Murray, L., Chen, B., Galy, A., Chen, S., Tushinski, R., Uchida, N., Negrin, R., Tricot, G., Jagannath, S., Barlogie, B., Hoffman, R., and Tsukamoto, A., 1995, Enrichment of hematopoietic stem cell activity in the CD34+Thy-1 + Lin- subpopulation from mobilized peripheral blood, *Blood* **85:**368–378.

Murray, L. J., Bruno, E., Yeo, E. L., Tsukamoto, A., Hoffman, R., and Sutherland, D., 1994, CDw109 antibody 8A3 identifies a minor subset of CD34+ fetal bone marrow cells that includes multilineage and megakaryocyte progenitor cells as well as hematopoietic stem cells, *Blood* **84:**320–327.

Naldini, L., Blomer, U., Gallay, P., Ory, D., Mulligan, R., Gage, F. H., Verma, I. M., and Trono, D., 1996, In vivo gene delivery and stable transduction of nondividing cells by a lentiviral vector, *Science* **272:**263–267.

Neering, S. J., Hardy, S. F., Minamoto, D., Spratt, S. K., and Jordan, C. T., 1996, Transduction of primitive human hematopoietic cells with recombinant adenovirus vectors, *Blood*, in press.

Nienhuis, A. W., McDonagh, K. T., and Bodine, D. M., 1991, Gene transfer into hematopoietic stem cells, *Cancer* **67:**2700–2704.

Nolta, J. A., and Kohn, D. B., 1990, Comparison of the effects of growth factors on retroviral vector-mediated gene transfer and the proliferative status of human hematopoietic progenitor cells, *Hum. Gene Ther.* **1:**250–257.

Nolta, J. A., Sender, S. L., Barranger, J. A., and Kohn, D. B., 1990, Expression of human glucocerebrosidase in murine long-term bone marrow cultures after retroviral vector-mediated transfer, *Blood* **75:**780–787.

Nolta, J. A., Smogorzewska, E. M., and Kohn, D. B., 1995, Analysis of optimal conditions for retroviral-mediated transduction of primitive human hematopoietic cells, *Blood* **86:**101–110.

O'Shaughnessy, J. A., Cowan, K. H., and Neinhuis, A. W., 1994, Retroviral mediated transfer of the multi-drug resistanec gene (MDR-1) into hematopoietic cells during autologous transplantation after intensive chemotherapy for metastatic breast cancer, *Hum. Gene Ther.* **5:**890–891.

Ohashi, T., Boggs, S., Robbins, P., Bahnson, A., Patrene, K., Wei, F.-S., Wei, J.-F., Li, J., Lucht, L., Fei, Y., Clark, S., Kimak, M., He, H., Mowery-Rushton, P., and Barranger, J. A., 1992, Efficient transfer and sustained high expression of the human glucocerebrosidase gene in mice and their functional macrophages following transplantation of bone marrow transduced by a retroviral vector, *Proc. Natl. Acad. Sci. USA* **89:**11332–11336.

Osborne, W. R. A., Hock, F. A., Kaleko, M., and Miller, D. A., 1990, Long-term expression of human adenosine deaminase in mice after transplantation of bone marrow infected with amphotropic retroviral vectors, *Hum. Gene Ther.* **1:**30–31.

Peters, S. O., Kittler, E. L. W., Ramshaw, H. S., and Quesenberry, P. J., 1995, Murine marrow cells expanded in culture with IL-3, IL-6, IL-11 and SCF acquire an engraftment defect in normal hosts, *Exp. Hematol.* **23:**461–466.

Reems, J. A., and Torok-Storb, B., 1995, Cell cycle and functional differences between $CD34^{+}/CD38^{hi}$ and $CD34^{+}/CD38^{lo}$ human marrow cells after in vitro cytokine exposure, *Blood* **85:**1480–1487.

Reincke, U., Hannon, E. C., Rosenblatt, M., and Hellman, S., 1982, Proliferative capacity of murine hematopoietic stem cells in vitro, *Science* **215:**1610–1619.

Riddell, S. R., Elliott, M., Lewinsohn, D. A., Gilbert, M. J., Wilson, L., Manley, S. A., Lupton, S. D., Overell, R. W., Reynolds, T. C., Corey, L., and Greenberg, P. D., 1996, T-cell mediated rejection of gene-modified HIV-specific cytotoxic T lymphocytes in HIV-infected patients, *Nat. Med.* **2:**216–223.

Rill, D. E., Santana, V. M., Roberts, W. M., Nilson, T., Bowman, L. C., Krance, R. A., Heslop, H., Moen, R. C., Ihle, J. N., and Brenner, M. K., 1994, Direct demonstration that autologous bone marrow transplantation for solid tumors can return a multiplicity of tumorigenic cells, *Blood* **84:**380–383.

Rill, D. R., Buschle, M., Foreman, N. K., Bartholomew, C., Moen, R. C., Santana, V. M., Ihle, J. N., and Brenner, M. K., 1992, Retrovirus mediated gene transfer as an approach to analyze neuroblastoma relapse after autologous bone marrow transplantation, *Hum. Gene Ther.* **3:**120–129.

Roe, T. Y., Reynolds, T. C., Yu, G., and Brown, P. O., 1993, Integration of murine leukemia virus DNA depends on mitosis, *EMBO J.* **12:**2099–2108.

Rooney, C. M., Smith, C. A., Ng, C. Y. C., Loftin, S., Li, C., Krance, R. A., Brenner, M. K., and Heslop, H. E., 1995, Use of gene modified virus specific T lymphocytes to control Epstein–Barr virus related lymphoproliferation, *Lancet* **345:**9–13.

Rosenberg, S. A., 1991, Immunotherapy and gene therapy of cancer, *Cancer Res.* **51:**5074–5079.

Rosenberg, S. A., Aebersold, P., Cornetta, K., Kasid, A., Morgan, R. A., Moen, R., Karson, E. M., Lotze, M. T., Yang, J. C., Topalian, S. L., Merino, M. J., Culver, K., Miller, A. D., Blaese, R. M., and Anderson, W. F., 1990, Gene transfer into humans: Immunotherapy of patients with advanced melanoma, using tumor-infiltrating lymphocytes modified by retroviral gene transduction, *N. Engl. J. Med.* **323:**570–578.

Russell, S. J., Hawkins, R. E., and Winter, G., 1993, Retroviral vectors displaying functional antibody fragments, *Nucleic Acids Res.* **21:**1081–1085.

Schiller, G., Vescio, R., Freytes, C., Spitzer, G., Sahebi, F., Lee, M., Wu, C. H., Cao, J., Lee, J. C., Hong, C. H., Lichtenstein, A., Lill, M., Hall, J., Berenson, R., and Berenson, J., 1995, Transplantation of $CD34^+$ peripheral blood progenitor cells after high-dose chemotherapy for patients with advanced multiple myeloma, *Blood* **86:**390–397.

Schnierle, B. S., Moitz, D., Jeschke, M., and Groner, B., 1996, Expression of chimeric envelope proteins in helper cell lines and integration into Moloney murine leukemia virus particles, *Gene Ther.* **3:**334–342.

Schuening, F., Miller, A. D., Torok-Storb, B., Bensinger, W., Storb, R., Reynolds, T., Fisher, L., Buckner, C. D., and Appelbaum, F. R., 1994, Study on contribution of genetically marked peripheral blood repopulating cells to hematopoietic reconstitution after transplantation, *Hum. Gene Ther.* **5:**1523–1534.

Schuening, F. G., Storb, R., Stead, R. B., Goehle, S., Nash, R., and Miller, A. D., 1989, Improved retroviral transfer of genes into canine hematopoietic progenitor cells kept in long-term marrow culture, *Blood* **74:**150–152.

Schuening, F. G., Kawahara, K., Miler, A. D., To, R., Goehle, S., Steward, D., Mullally, K., Fisher, L., Graham, T. C., Appelbaum, F. R., Hackman, R., Osborne, W. R. A., and Storb, R., 1991a, Retrovirus-mediated gene transduction into long-term repopulating marrow cells of dogs, *Blood* **78:**2560–2568.

Schuening, F. G., Kawahara, K., Miller, A. D., To, R., Goehle, S., Stewart, D., Mullally, K., Fisher, L., Graham, T. C., Appelbaum, F. R., *et al.*, 1991b, Retrovirus-mediated gene transduction into long-term repopulating marrow cells of dogs, *Blood* **78:**2568–2576.

Shimada, T., Fujii, H., Mitsuya, H., and Nienhuis, A. W., 1991, Targeted and highly efficient gene transfer into $CD4^+$ cells by a recombinant human immunodeficiency virus retroviral vector, *J. Clin. Invest.* **88:**1043–1047.

Sirard, C., Lapidot, T., Vormoor, J., Cashman, J. D., Doedens, M., Murdoch, B., Jamal, N., Messner, H., Addey, L., Minden, M., Laraya, P., Keating, A., Eaves, A., Lansdorp, P. M., Eaves, C. J., and Dick, J. E., 1996, Normal and leukemic SCID-repopulating cells (SRC) coexist in the bone marrow and peripheral blood from CML patients in chronic phase, whereas leukemic SRC are detected in blast crisis, *Blood* **87:**1539–1548.

Smith, L. A., Weissman, I. L., and Heimfeld, S., 1991, Clonal analysis of hematopoietic stem-cell differentiation in vivo, *Proc. Natl. Acad. Sci. USA* **88:**2780–2788.

Snodgrass, R., and Keller, G., 1987, Clonal fluctuation within the haematopoietic system of mice reconstituted with retrovirus-infected stem cells, *EMBO J.* **6:**3950–3955.

Somia, N. V., Zoppe, M., and Verma, I. M., 1995, Generation of targeted retroviral vectors by using single-chain variable fragment: An approach to *in vivo* gene delivery, *Proc. Natl. Acad. Sci. USA* **92:**7570–7574.

Sorrentino, B. P., Brandt, S. J., Bodine, D., Gottesman, M., Pastan, I., Cline, A., and Nienhuis, A. W., 1992, Selection of drug resistant bone marrow cells in vivo after retroviral transfer of human MDR, *Science* **257:**90–99.

Stead, R. B., Kwok, W. W., Storb, R., and Miller, A. D., 1988, Canine model for gene therapy: Inefficient gene expression in dogs reconstituted with autologous marrow infected with retroviral vectors, *Blood* **71:**740–742.

Stewart, A. K., Dubé, I. D., Kamel-Reid, S., and Keating, A., 1995, A phase I study of autologous bone marrow transplantation with stem cell gene marking in multiple myeloma, *Hum. Gene Ther.* **6:**107–119.

Sutherland, D. R., Watt, S. M., Dowden, G., Karhi, K., Baker, M. A., Greaves, M. F., and Smart, J. E., 1988, Structural and partial amino acid sequence analysis of the human hemopoietic progenitor cell antigen CD34, *Leukemia* **2:**793–803.

Sutherland, D. R., Yeo, E., Ryan, A., Mills, G. B., Bailey, D., and Baker, M. A., 1991, Identification of a cell-surface antigen associated with activated T lymphoblasts and activated platelets, *Blood* **77:**84–93.

Sutherland, D. R., and Keating, A., 1992, The CD34 antigen: Structure, biology, and potential clinical applications, *J. Hematother.* **1:**115–129.

Sutherland, H. J., Lansdorp, P. M., Henkelman, D. H., Eaves, A. C., and Eaves, C. J., 1990, Functional characterization of individual human hematopoietic stem cells cultured at limiting dilution on supportive marrow stromal layers, *Proc. Natl. Acad. Sci. USA* **87:**3584–3588.

Szilvassy, S. J., Fraser, C. C., Eaves, C. J., Lansdorp, P. M., Eaves, A. C., and Humphries, R. K., 1989, Retrovirus-mediated gene transfer to purified hemopoietic stem cells with long-term lymphomyelopoietic repopulating ability, *Proc. Natl. Acad. Sci. USA* **86:**8790–8798.

Szilvassy, S. J., and Cory, S., 1994, Efficient retroviral gene transfer to purified long-term repopulating hematopoietic stem cells, *Blood* **84:**74–83.

Toksoz, D., Zsebo, K. M., Smith, K. A., Hu, S., Brankow, D., Suggs, S. V., Martin, F. H., and Williams, D. A., 1992, Support of human hematopoiesis in long-term bone marrow cultures by murine stromal cells selectively expressing the membrane-bound and secreted forms of the human homolog of the steel gene product, stem cell factor, *Proc. Natl. Acad. Sci. USA* **89:**7350–7354.

Valsesia-Wittmann, S., Morling, F. J., Nilson, B. H. K., Takeuchi, Y., Russell, S. J., and Cosset, F.-L., 1996, Improvement of retroviral retargeting by using amino acid spacers between an additional binding domain and the N-terminus of Moloney murine leukemia virus SU, *J. Virol.* **70:**2059–2064.

van Beusechem, V. W., Bakx, T. A., Kaptein, L. C. M., Bart-Baumeister, J. A. K., Kukler, A., Braakman, E., and Valerio, D., 1993, Retrovirus-mediated gene transfer into rhesus monkey hematopoietic stem cells: The effect of viral titers on transduction efficiency, *Hum. Gene Ther.* **4:**230–239.

Van Zant, G., Chen, J. J., and Scott-Micus, K., 1991, Developmental potential of hematopoietic stem cells determined using retrovirally marked allogeneic marrow, *Blood* **77:**750–756.

Vescio, R. A., Hong, C. H., Cao, J., Kim, A., Schiller, G. J., Lichtenstein, A. K., Berenson, R. J., and Berenson, J. R., 1994, The hematopoietic stem cell antigen, CD34, is not expressed on the malignant cells in multiple myeloma, *Blood* **84:**3283–3290.

von Kalle, C., Kiem, H.-P., Goehle, S., Darovsky, B., Heimfeld, S., Torok-Storb, B., Storb, R., and Schuening, F. G., 1994, Increased gene transfer into human hematopoietic progenitor cells by extended in vitro exposure to a pseudotyped retroviral vector, *Blood* **84:**2890–2897.

Ward, M., Richardson, C., Pioli, P., Smith, L., Podda, S., Goff, S., Hesdorffer, C., and Bank, A., 1994, Transfer and expression of the human multiple drug resistance gene in human CD34+ cells, *Blood* **84:**1408–1414.

Weider, R., Cornetta, K., Kessler, S. W., and Anderson, W. F., 1991, Increased efficiency of retroviral-mediated gene transfer and expression in primate bone marrow progenitors after 5-fluorouracil-induced hematopoietic supression and recovery, *Blood* **77:**440–448.

Weinthal, J., Nolta, J. A., Yu, X. J., Lilley, J., Uribe, L., and Kohn, D. B., 1991, Expression of human glucocerebrosidase following retroviral vector-mediated transduction of murine hematopoietic stem cells, *Bone Marrow Transpl.* **8:**400–403.

Weiss, R. A., and Tailor, C. S., 1995, Retrovirus receptors, *Cell* **82:**531–533.

Wieder, R., 1991, Cryopreserved primate bone marrow cells can be used for retroviral-mediated gene transfer, *Hum. Gene Ther.* **2:**320–323.

Williams, D. A., 1990, Expression of introduced genetic sequences in hematopoietic cells following retroviral-mediated gene transfer, *Hum. Gene Ther.* **1:**20–22.

Xu, L.-C., Kluepfel-Stahl, S., Blanco, M., Schiffmann, R., Dunbar, C., and Karlsson, S., 1995, Growth factors and stromal support generate very efficient retroviral transduction of peripheral blood $CD34^+$ cells from Gaucher patients, *Blood* **86:**141–146.

Yan, X.-Q., Lacey, D., Fletcher, F., Hartley, C., McElroy, T., Sun, Y., Xia, M., Mu, S., Saris, C., Hill, D., Hawley, R. G., and McNiece, I. K., 1995, Chronic exposure to retroviral vector encoded MGDF (*mpl*-ligand) induces lineage-specific growth and differentiation of megakaryocytes in mice, *Blood* **86:**4025–4033.

Chapter 10

Antisense Strategies to Leukemia

Stephen G. O'Brien

1. INTRODUCTION

In the 43 years since publication of the first description of the structure of DNA (Watson and Crick, 1953) our understanding of the molecular pathogenesis of malignant disease has developed at a remarkable rate. However, the potential of exploiting this knowledge in disrupting molecular genetic processes for experimental or therapeutic purposes has been disappointing. Antisense technology offers this possibility and the hope of highly specific anti-leukemia/lymphoma therapy, but the development of this technology has been somewhat problematic. In 1978 Zamecnick *et al.* published a paper describing the effects of a tridecamer oligonucleotide complementary to the 3′ and 5′ reiterated terminal sequences of Rous sarcoma virus 35S RNA on the production of virus. This was probably the first antisense experiment, and the elegance of the principle of antisense technology has attracted many academic and commercial research groups to investigate antisense as an experimental and therapeutic tool. In the early 1980s little further work was conducted mainly because of the difficulties in reliably synthesizing adequate quantities of DNA oligonucleotides. However, innovative biotechnology companies developed DNA synthesis technology to a high standard in the mid to late 1980s allowing the reliable production of μg to mg quantities of pure unmodified DNA and nuclease-resistant DNA analogs. This development fueled an exponential growth of antisense publications but many of the published experiments have been difficult to reproduce. In recent years the complex interactions of oligonucleotides with pro-

Stephen G. O'Brien Department of Haematology, University of Wales College of Medicine, Cardiff CF4 4XN, Wales, United Kingdom.

Blood Cell Biochemistry, Volume 8: Hematopoiesis and Gene Therapy, edited by Fairbairn and Testa. Kluwer Academic/Plenum Publishers, New York, 1999.

teins and nucleic acids has highlighted the need for carefully controlled experiments, and many previous publications were not optimal in this regard. However, among the many conflicting and irreproducible published results, carefully controlled data indicate that true antisense effects can be achieved, although conditions probably have to be carefully tailored to individual experimental systems. This review describes the concepts and supporting data underlying the mechanisms of action of antisense and ribozymes and examines some of the available experimental systems and clinical data applied to hematology, before attempting a prediction of the role of antisense and other synthetic nucleic acids as future therapies for hematological malignancy. Antisense oligomers cannot be adopted unquestioningly as simple tools to disrupt gene expression, and the reader is encouraged to question constantly whether observed effects are truly caused by antisense inhibition of the production of a specific gene product.

2. ANTISENSE AND RIBOZYMAL DESIGN AND MECHANISMS OF ACTION

Antisense oligomers are short synthetic sequences of DNA or RNA, usually composed of between 15 to 30 bases. By designing an oligomer to be antiparallel or "antisense" to a specific sequence (Figure 1a) it is possible to inhibit transcription, if DNA is targeted, or translation if mRNA is the target. There is good evidence that antisense RNA plays an important role in regulating gene expression in prokaryotic organisms (Nellen and Lichtenstein, 1993; Wagner and Simons, 1994). Given the estimated size of the human genome, the minimum number of bases that should theoretically define a unique mRNA sequence is, on average, 13. For DNA the figure is 17. In principle, by designing antisense oligomers longer than this, the genetic machinery of a cell can be specifically disrupted at these various levels (Figure 1b): transcription (so-called "triple-helix" interactions), pre-mRNA splicing, nuclear and cytoplasmic mRNA "capping," and/or degradation and cytoplasmic translation. Oligomer length is an important determinant of specificity but making oligomers longer does not necessarily increase specificity. Evidence from a *Xenopus* oocyte system indicates that increasing oligomer length may exacerbate the problems of nonspecific cleavage by virtue of the increasing number of internal shorter sequences that can partially hybridize and direct cleavage (Woolf *et al.*, 1992). The vast majority of experiments have used exogenously introduced molecules, but it is feasible to use a gene transfer approach to incorporate vectors into genomic DNA that continually produce antisense RNA or ribozymes (Noonberg *et al.*, 1994; Cameron and Jennings, 1989, 1991; Martiat *et al.*, 1993). The usual major limitation of transfer efficiency still applies, however. Another, far less common oligonucleotide intervention is using an oligomer whose sequence is homologous to regions of genomic DNA that are known binding sites for transcription factors. Thus such oligomers act as "decoys" for known factors that regulate transcription (Harel Bellan *et al.*, 1989). To be effective, antisense and ribozyme molecules need to remain stable both extra- and intracellularly, cross cell membranes, be localized to their site of

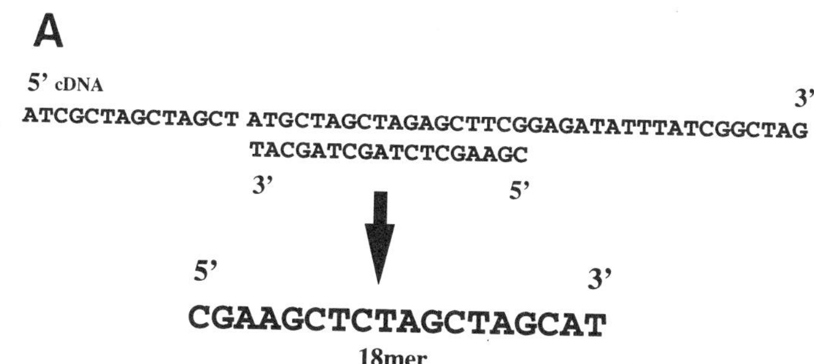

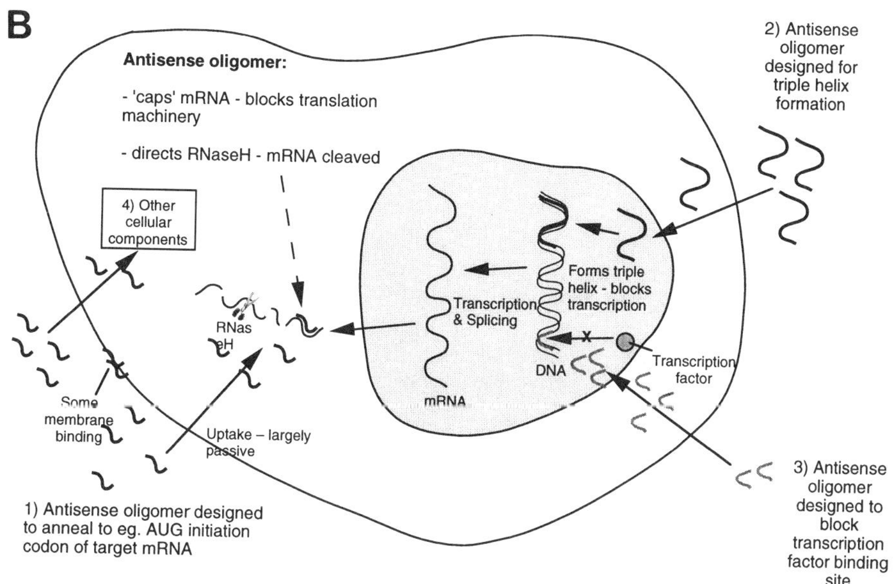

FIGURE 1. Schematic diagram of design and mechanisms of action of antisense oligonucleotides. A: Antisense design. The design of most antisense effectors is based on the known cDNA (and hence mRNA) sequence of a target gene. These molecules are designed to disrupt translation in the cytoplasm. The example shows a putative gene that is targeted at the AUG initiation codon. The antisense oligomer has the same sequence reading from 5′ to 3′ as the antiparallel or antisense strand of the cDNA. B: Mechanisms of action. Antisense oligomers can be designed to act at various levels in disrupting gene expression. In addition it has become evident that oligonucleotides interact with a variety of cell surface and intracellular proteins via a mechanism that has nothing to do with "classical antisense." In some circumstances these so-called aptameric effects may be operative at the same time as an antisense effect, making experimental interpretation particularly difficult.

action and effectively destroy only their intended target. Can these criteria be achieved?

2.1. Oligonucleotide Analogs and Stability

Naturally occurring phosphodiester DNA is inherently sensitive to degradation by nucleases in serum, which greatly limits its utility as an antisense effector.

Accordingly considerable effort has gone into developing DNA analogs that demonstrate enhanced nuclease resistance, high binding affinity, good transfer as cross cell membranes, and site specific cleavage of targets. Modifications to phosphodiester DNA can be made to one of three groups within nucleosides and internucleoside linkages, (1) the phosphodiester linkage; (2) the heterocyclic group; and (3) the deoxyribose sugar group. Some comparative studies exist (Morvan *et al.*, 1993). However phosphorothioate analogs are the most extensively evaluated, and more than 30 other analogs combine modifications of one or more of the above groups (Milligan *et al.*, 1993). Some analogs completely replace the usual phosphodiester internucleoside linkage with a peptide (Hanvey *et al.*, 1992; Nielsen *et al.*, 1991). These peptide nucleic acids are usefully active, but certain physicochemical constraints may limit their biological utility. As can be surmised by the plethora of analogs, the ideal molecule has not yet been defined.

2.2. Cellular Uptake

As with most areas of antisense research, there is some controversy over the mechanisms by which oligonucleotides enter cells and even whether they enter at all. There is some evidence for a receptor-mediated endocytic mechanism (Loke *et al.*, 1989), although this is not clear cut (Zamecnik *et al.*, 1994), and potential specific receptors have been characterized (Yakubov *et al.*, 1989). Following uptake into the endosomal compartment, oligomers may become trapped or rapidly removed from the cell (Gao *et al.*, 1993; Geselowitz and Neckers, 1992), and in effect a very small proportion of available oligomer may reach the intended site of action. In some studies, the efficiency of uptake is related to the differentiation state of the target cells (Zhao *et al.*, 1994) and depends on protein kinase C (PKC) (Stein *et al.*, 1993). Paradoxically, phosphorothioate oligomers inhibit PKC, and other proteins and therefore may inhibit their own uptake. Once inside the, cell oligomer that escapes the endosomal compartment moves to the nucleus (Beltinger *et al.*, 1995), an observation confirmed in microinjection experiments (Leonetti *et al.*, 1991; Wagner *et al.*, 1993), and there is some evidence of a specific oligomer degradation machinery within cells (Ryte *et al.*, 1993). Methods to enhance uptake have included electroporation (Bergan *et al.*, 1993), conjugation with poly-L-lysine, transferrin or other moieties (Citro *et al.*, 1992, 1994), and using various lipid preparations (Thierry and Dritschilo, 1992; Akhtar *et al.*, 1991; Lappalainen *et al.*, 1994; Bennett *et al.*, 1992; Capaccioli *et al.*, 1993). Lipid formulations have been useful, but many such preparations exhibit inherent toxicity that confounds the interpretation of antisense effects (Yeoman *et al.*, 1992). Some authors contend that oligomers gain access to cells without lipid facilitation (Nestle *et al.*, 1994). Lately some groups have been using listeriolysin and streptolysin O to introduce oligomers into cells with promising results (Barry *et al.*, 1993; Spiller and Tidd, 1995).

2.3. Mechanisms of Target Inactivation by Antisense Oligomers

In general the utility of antisense is predicated on the ability to specifically down-regulate a gene product. This must conceptually limit applications to situations where overexpression of a single gene is pathogenetically important. Loss of expression of genes, such as p53, may be as important as overexpression of a particular gene in certain circumstances, and malignant transformation is probably a multistep process in many diseases. With these provisos, how do antisense oligomers disrupt gene expression?

Oligomers can be designed to bind within the minor groove of nuclear DNA by Hoogsteen base pairing to form a triple helix and disrupt transcription (Helene *et al.*, 1992) (Figure 1). Triple-helix formation is conventionally limited to homopurine–homopyrimidine sequences within the target DNA which currently limits possible targets. However, this target sequence requirement may not be as stringent as once thought because some mixed sequence sites are recognized by oligomers in which G-residues of the incoming third strand form stable base triplets with T-A base pairs on the target DNA. This occurs where the T residues interrupt a homopurine site (Griffin and Dervan, 1989). Benzol(e)pyridoindol triplex oligomer derivatives greatly enhance inhibition of transcription initiation (Mergny *et al.*, 1992), but the triplex approach generally has not been widely adopted. In the nucleus, oligomers also act as decoys for characterized transcription factors (Harel Bellan *et al.*, 1989) or disrupt RNA splicing (Kulka *et al.*, 1989).

Oligomers of appropriate sequence can be designed to anneal to specific spliced mRNA species in the cytoplasm. This interaction may inhibit translation by steric hindrance (Agarwal *et al.*, 1988) or may direct the cleavage of the target mRNA molecule by inducing one or more of the RNAseH group of enzymes (Chiang *et al.*, 1991; Giles and Tidd, 1992a; Giles *et al.*, 1995b; Walder and Walder, 1988). A paradoxical feature of phosphorothioates is that they directly inhibit RNAseH (Gao *et al.*, 1992). Curiously reduced gene expression can sometimes be elucidated by using sense molecules (Cameron and Jennings, 1991). As discussed in more detail later, oligomers bind to certain proteins *via* a so-called aptameric effect (Ellington and Szostak, 1990) which profoundly affects the function of a given protein but has nothing to do with "classical" antisense mechanisms.

2.4. Ribozymal Principles and Design

Ribozymes are a unique class of catalytic RNA molecules, first described in the early 1980s in *Tetrahymena* group I intron pre-mRNA splicing and in the ribozymal component of ribonuclease P, that recognize and cleave specific mRNA sequences (Cech, 1987; Guerrier-Takada *et al.*, 1983). The ability of RNA to act enzymatically in this way depends on the presence of a 2′-OH group on the ribose sugar, which is not present in DNA, and on the single-stranded nature of the RNA which allows forming complex structures stabilized by complementary base-pairing and in other ways (Kiehntopf *et al.*, 1995). Depending on their secondary conformation, ribozymes have been variously designated as "hammerhead," "hairpin," or "axehead," and these molecules recycle mRNA in normal cellular physiology. They can be introduced exogenously into cells although they are even less stable than DNA oligonucleotides and are generally larger molecules. Alternatively, ribozymes can be encoded by retroviral vectors that are introduced into cells by gene therapy. They have received less investigation than antisense oligomers, largely because of the difficulties in synthesis, stability, and handling, but have been usefully employed in several experimental systems (Kiehntopf *et al.*, 1995). Intriguingly, in addition to blocking gene expression similarly to antisense oligomers, they can also be designed to repair defective mRNA (Sullenger and Cech, 1994). One day it may be possible to correct mutations in tumor suppressor genes, such as p53 by using this technology although this is a long way into the future. Many of the considerations of stability and uptake discussed in relation to antisense oligomers are also applicable to ribozymes.

3. CONTROLS, EXPERIMENTAL SYSTEMS, AND DIFFICULTIES IN INTERPRETATION

Early antisense publications and some current papers have assumed that an antisense oligomer does what it is intended to do. This makes the reliable interpretation of many published studies very difficult, if not impossible, because now it is very clear that certain oligonucleotides affect cellular processes by means other than "classical" antisense effects (Stein and Cheng, 1993). The end points most commonly evaluated have been the analysis of (1) target RNA by Northern blotting or reverse transcriptase—polymerase chain reaction (RT-PCR); (2) protein product of the target gene; and (3) biological effect—usually by morphology or proliferation assay. All of these methods are legitimate if used in the correct context but often data have been derived from these analyses using only one control oligomer. Therefore, firm conclusions could not be drawn (Wagner, 1994). Furthermore, each of these analytical methods has individual problems. For example, short-lived target RNA species expressed at a relatively low level are often compared with β actin mRNA whose constitutive expression is at much higher levels. It is entirely possible that an antisense oligomer may disrupt, nonspecifically, several RNA species expressed at low level although still permitting significant expression of β actin. A directly comparable RNA species should therefore be evaluated, for example, ABL for comparison with BCR-ABL (Cross *et al.*, 1994). Another compounding factor is that on occasion RNA but not protein levels are affected and significant biological effects occur (Smetsers *et al.*, 1995), emphasizing the need for both analyses. Biological effect endpoints are of limited value but allow the initially assessing of nonspecific toxicities (O'Brien *et al.*, 1994; Vaerman *et al.*, 1995). So, is it possible to demonstrate a true antisense effect conclusively? The answer to this question carries legal connotations in that although there is no definitive procedure to prove that antisense exists, carefully conducted investigations and newer detection methods can prove the case beyond reasonable doubt. Optimally designed antisense experiments comprise two broad components: appropriate test and control oligomers and appropriate test systems.

3.1. Controls

It is probably inadequate to design antisense experiments with one test oligomer and one control. A recent leader in *antisense research and development* suggested that, given realistic practical constraints, at least two controls should be incorporated (Stein and Krieg, 1994). What those controls should be is the subject of much debate but sequences to be considered are sense; reverse antisense; totally random oligomers of the same length and chemistry; random oligomers of the same length and chemistry but with the same base composition as test antisense oligo; mismatched antisense; antisense against another specific mRNA target; and oligomers that control for known troublesome motifs (see section 3.3). Good experiments will have a crossover design where two different targets are assessed by using appropriate antisense and control oligomers (e.g., Wagner *et al.*, 1993).

3.2. Test Systems

Newer test systems have been developed recently that provide more compelling evidence of antisense effects. Protein assays and RT-PCR continue to be useful, but reverse ligase-mediated PCR (RL-PCR) (Bertrand *et al.*, 1993) has recently been applied to antisense research and has extended the ways of looking at RNA degradation products. RT-PCR in combination with RL-PCR (Figure 2) provides compelling evidence that a target RNA molecule has been cleaved at a specific site and is a useful method for assessing oligomer specificity (Giles *et al.*, 1995b). *In vitro* transcription systems (Giles and Tidd, 1992b) also provide valuable data on cleavage specificity before moving into cellular assays, but findings are not always consistent among such basic *in vitro* systems and more complex cellular assays. Finally, retroviral vectors have been constructed that contain a short cDNA sequence, homologous to the intended target mRNA, upstream of a reporter construct, for example, chlomamphenicol acetyl transferase or luciferase. Oligomer treatment of cells transfected with such constructs facilitate the definition of specific antisense effectors and the system is readily adapted to any target sequence (O'Brien *et al.*, 1995a).

3.3. Difficulties in Interpretation

The nonspecific interactions of oligomers have already been briefly alluded to, and new observations are constantly being described. A number of biological effects have been ascribed to certain motifs within oligomers (Yaswen *et al.*, 1993). For example, a simple CpG motif modulates immune function. When injected intraperitoneally, phosphorothioates that contain the CpG motif stimulate a dramatic increase in immunoglobulin secretion within 24 hours and increased expression of activation markers, such as MHC class II (Krieg, 1995). The same motif also induces interferon production and NK cell activation (Tamamoto *et al.*, 1994). A 3′ TAT motif is inhibitory in CML cell lines (Vaerman *et al.*, 1995), and Bergan and colleagues have determined that GGC motifs within what were originally thought to be BCR-ABL antisense oligomers directly inhibit the tyrosine kinase activity of $p210^{BCR\text{-}ABL}$ protein by an aptameric interaction (Bergan *et al.*, 1995). Curiously, the effects of motifs, such as the well-known G quartet may depend on flanking sequences (Maltese *et al.*, 1995), but as yet the rules governing this effect have not been elucidated. Many nonspecific effects have been described with phosphorothioate oligomers. However, the scale of problems associated with

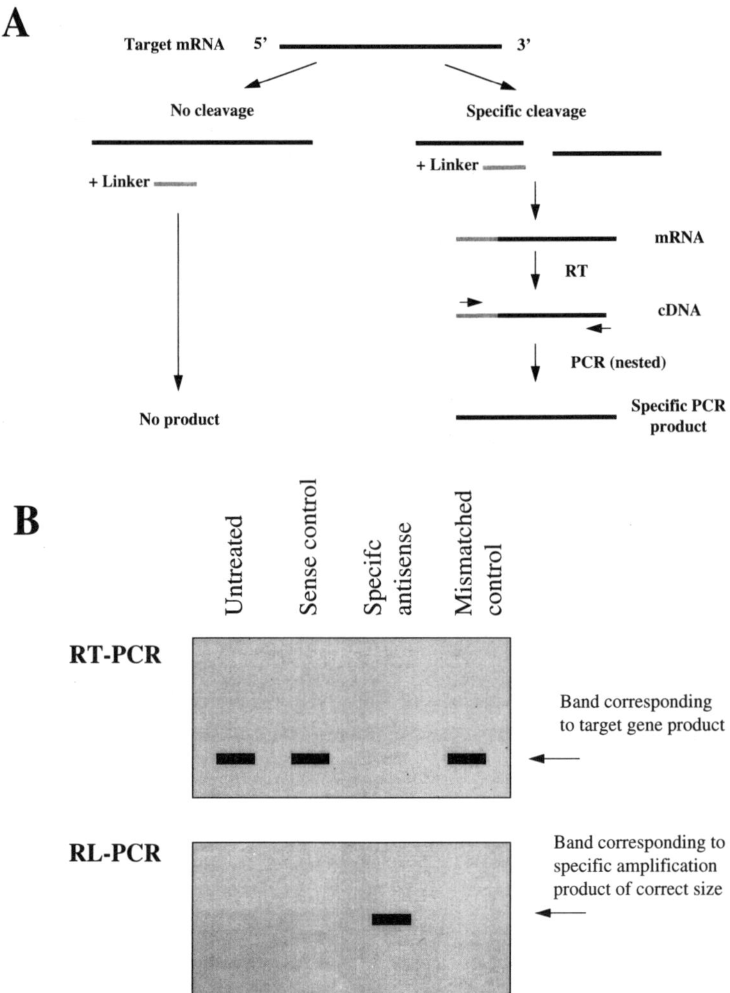

FIGURE 2. Reverse ligase-mediated polymerase chain reaction. A: The RL-PCR procedure generates a PCR product of predicted length when the initial target mRNA species has been cleaved in the expected location. If no cleavage or nonspecific cleavage has occured, either no PL-PCR product or products of unexpected size, respectively, are generated. B: In conjunction with reverse transcriptase polymerase chain reaction (RT-PCR) corroborative data can be generated to determine the specificity of a given antisense oligomer. In this schematic example the specific antisense oligomer has cleaved its target mRNA resulting in the disappearance of the RT-PCR band and a specific cleavage product of appropriate size has been generated in the RL-PCR reaction. (For example, see Giles *et al.*, 1995b.)

these oligomers, compared to those oligomers incorporations other chemistries, may be somewhat exaggerated by virtue of the widespread availability of the former corpared with the latter technologies. A number of groups have observed nonspecific effects (Ho *et al.*, 1991; Reed *et al.*, 1990), and some workers have directly attributed the degree of nonspecific protein binding to the phosphorothioate component of the oligomer (Brown *et al.*, 1994). Sometimes the effects may be nonantisense yet sequence specific (Bennett *et al.*, 1994). The fact that oligomers are polyanions may be part of the answer. In their induction of the Sp1 transcription factor (Perez *et al.*, 1994) and their binding to basic fibroblast growth factor (bFGF), acidic fibroblast growth factor (FGF-4), platelet-derived growth factor (PDGF), and vascular endothelial growth factor (VEGF; Guvakova *et al.*, 1995), phosphorothioate oligomers behave like the polyanions suramin and pentosan polysulphate. These observations and the ability of phosphorothioates to bind to heparin-binding proteins may be critical determinants of their biological behavior. Other analogs are not without blame, and even more unusual oligomer structures, such as some self complementary 3′ cholesterol-modified oligomers cause sequence specific, nonantisense effects (Zhou *et al.*, 1994a).

4. ANTISENSE AND RIBOZYMES IN EXPERIMENTAL HEMATOLOGY

Table I provides an overview of areas where antisense has been applied to hematologically relevant molecular targets (for a review, see Kirkland *et al.*, 1994). Many of these targets have obvious therapeutic potential, but a handful of targets have attracted the most attention.

The MYB gene, located on chromosome 6 (q22–24), is the human homologue of the viral v-myb gene that gives rise to avian myeloblastosis. MYB encodes a nuclear DNA-binding protein that plays a role in regulating the growth and differentiation of hemopoietic progenitors (Caracciolo *et al.*, 1990). Preliminary studies have shown that a 24-mer antisense oligonucleotide, complementary to codons 2 to 7 of the MYB gene, inhibits the formation of CFU-GM and BFU-E from patients who have AML and CML to a significantly greater extent than it forms colonies from normal marrow (Calabretta *et al.*, 1991). Furthermore, the same antisense molecule, used systemically in a SCID mouse model of blast crisis CML, significantly prolongs survival compared with control oligomers and untreated animals (Ratajczak *et al.*, 1992b). About 75% of chronic phase CML patients demonstrate apparently sequence-specific inhibition of CFU-GM growth which is also associated with down-regulation of the BCR-ABL message (Ratajczak *et al.*, 1992a). It is possible that BCR-ABL expression may be indirectly regulated by MYB *via* a pathway involving MYC (Cogswell *et al.*, 1993), but details of such a mechanism have not been formally established. These preliminary data were the basis of the first human trials using the 24-mer phosphorothioate MYB antisense compound, LR 3001 (Lynx Therapeutics Inc., Hayward, CA) described later.

Because of the ubiquitous nature of the BCR-ABL fusion gene in patients who have chronic myeloid leukemia (CML), a number of studies have attemped to block the expression of $p210^{BCR\text{-}ABL}$ by using antisense and ribozymal strategies. As can be seen from Table I, numerous oligomer chemistries and lengths and different experimental systems have been evaluated. Most groups have designed their oligomers to be symmetrically antiparallel to junctional sequences in BCR-ABL, targeting one of the two common chimeric mRNAs—either b2a2 or b3a2. The seminal BCR-ABL antisense study was done by Szczylik *et al.* in 1991. In this study it was observed that

Table I
Some Examples of Antisense Applications in Experimental Hematology

Molecular target	Oligomer chemistry/comments[a]	Reference
ABL	PO. Human BM progenitors. Inhibition of colony formation.	(Rosti *et al.*, 1992)
Acetylcholinesterase	PO. Murine bone marrow cells.	(Patinkin *et al.*, 1994)
BCL2	PS. Human follicular small cleaved-cell lymphoma/SCID mice.	(Abubakr *et al.*, 1994)
	PS and chemotherapy. Normal CD34+ cells. BCL2 positive myeloid cell lines.	(Campos *et al.*, 1994)
	PS capped. DoHH2 B cell lymphoma line/SCID mice.	(Cotter *et al.*, 1994)
	PO and Ara C. AML blasts.	(Keith *et al.*, 1995)
	PO. Human lymphoma line SU-DHL4.	(Kitada *et al.*, 1993)
	PO. B-cell lymphoma line DHL4.	(Ryte *et al.*, 1993)
	PS. Follicular lymphoma **Clinical trial**.	(Webb *et al.*, 1996)
BCR	PO to upstream BCR.	(McGahon *et al.*, 1994)
	PO. K562 cell line.	(Taj *et al.*, 1990)
BCR-ABL	PO. Junctional sequences.	(Bedi *et al.*, 1994)
	PS. Junctional. **Clinical trial** of autograft purging in CML.	(de Fabritiis *et al.*, 1993, 1994, 1995a)
	PS. Specificity seen with certain culture conditions.	(Maekawa *et al.*, 1995)
	MP/PO/PS chimeric oligomers. Streptolysin O.	(Giles *et al.*, 1995a)
	PO. No suppression.	(Kabisch *et al.*, 1994)
	PO/PS. CML-CP cells. Nonspecific effects.	(Kirkland *et al.*, 1993)
	PS. CML-CP cells.	(Mahon *et al.*, 1993)
	RV-encoded RNA antisense.	(Martiat *et al.*, 1993)
	PS/PO. Nonspecific effects.	(O'Brien *et al.*, 1994)
	PS and mafosfamide. Mouse model.	(Skorski *et al.*, 1993)
	PS. Infusion protocol in SCID mice.	(Skorski *et al.*, 1994b)
	PS. Effects of BCR-ABL antisense on GAP expression.	(Skorski *et al.*, 1994a)
	PS. Effects on PI3 kinase expression.	(Skorski *et al.*, 1995)
	PO/PS. Decreased mRNA but not protein.	(Smetsers *et al.*, 1994, 1995; Smetsers and Mensink, 1995)
	PO. CML-BC. Seminal BCR-ABL	(Szczylik *et al.*, 1991)
	MP/lipid facilitation. Cell lines—selective.	(Tari *et al.*, 1994)
	5′ and 3′ capped—enhances antiproliferative capacity. Antisense paper.	(Thomas *et al.*, 1994)
	PO/PS. 3′ TAT is the inhibitory motif.	(Vaerman *et al.*, 1995)
BLK	PS. B-cell NHL—CH31.	(Yao and Scott, 1993)
CD23	PO/PS. Human tonsillar B-cells, B-CLL cells.	(Fournier *et al.*, 1994)
DEF	PO. Murine erythroleukemia lines—N23, N3.17.	(Sparatore *et al.*, 1993)
EGR-1	PS capped. Murine myeloid leukemia M1. Normal myeloblasts.	(Nguyen *et al.*, 1993)
FES	PO. HL60/promyeloctic leukemia cell lines.	(Ferrari *et al.*, 1994)
GM-CSF	PS. AML blasts.	(Rogers *et al.*, 1994)
HOX-3.3	PO. Murine erythroleukemia.	(Takeshita *et al.*, 1993)
IL-11	PO. Human megakaryocytes.	(Kobayashi *et al.*, 1993)

Table I (*Continued*)

Molecular target	Oligomer chemistry/comments[a]	Reference
IL-2	PO. Human PBMCs	(Kato *et al.*, 1994)
IL-4	PO. Murine lymphoma line CH12.LX.	(Louie *et al.*, 1993)
IL-6	PO. Hairy cell leukemia cells.	(Barut *et al.*, 1993)
Ki-67	PO. Multiple myeloma line IM9.	(Schülter *et al.*, 1993)
LYN	PS. 5′ cholesterol capped. Murine B-cell lymphoma line BCL1. Human Burkitt's lymphoma line—Daudi.	(Scheuermann *et al.*, 1994)
MDR-1	PS and adriamycin. Murine lymphoid leukemia P338/ADR.	(Azuma *et al.*, 1994)
	PS. Multiple myeloma line 8226/DOX.	(Kay *et al.*, 1994)
Mn superoxide dismutase	PO. HL60 & K562.	(Kizaki *et al.*, 1993)
MPL	PO. Blood CD34+ cells. Effect on megakaryopoiesis.	(Methia *et al.*, 1993)
MYB	PS. HL60, ML3, KG1 lines.	(Anfossi *et al.*, 1989)
	PO +/− folic acid-poly-l-lysine. HL60.	(Citro *et al.*, 1992, 1994)
	PS. CML patient material. K562/SCID mice.	(Calabretta *et al.*, 1993; Gewirtz and Calabretta, 1991; Ratajczak *et al.*, 1992a)
	PS. **Clinical trial** of autograft purging in CML.	(Luger *et al.*, 1994; O'Brien *et al.*, 1995b)
MYC	PS (electroporated). U937 cell line.	(Bergan *et al.*, 1993)
	Triplex strategy	(Cooney *et al.*, 1988)
	PO/PS. Murine leukemia P388—cell free RNA system.	(Dewangee *et al.*, 1994)
	PS. Murine B-cell lymphoma. WEHI 231.	(Fischer *et al.*, 1994)
	PO. HL60—causes inhibition and differentiation.	(Holt *et al.*, 1988)
	PO. PBMCs—induction of cell cycle synchronization	(Kato *et al.*, 1994)
	PO. Murine T cells.	(Kim *et al.*, 1994)
	PO/PS/end capped. U937 cells.	(Rosolen *et al.*, 1993)
	PO. T-ALL. CEM-C7 cells.	(Thulasi *et al.*, 1993)
NF-kB	PS. HL60.	(Sokoloski *et al.*, 1993)
p53	PS. **Clinical trial** in AML and MDS.	(Bayever *et al.*, 1993)
	PS capped. Various CML cell lines.	(Bi *et al.*, 1993)
	PS. Normal and CML-CP CD34 cells.	(Bi *et al.*, 1994)
	PS. AML blasts.	(Zhu *et al.*, 1994)
PIM1	Chimeric αβ anomeric. Cell-free system.	(Gottich *et al.*, 1994)
PKCβ1	PO/PS. HL60—effect on differentiation.	(Gamard *et al.*, 1994)
RAF-1	PS. Human megakaryocytic leukemia line MO7.	(Brennscheidt *et al.*, 1994)
SRC	RV encoded antisense RNA. U937 line.	(Waki *et al.*, 1994)
Transferrin receptor	HL60/K562/BV173.	(Guimaraes *et al.*, 1994)
	Human PBMCs.	(Kato *et al.*, 1994)

[a] Ara C—cytosine arabinoside; BC—blast crisis; BM—bone marrow; CP—chronic phase; MP—methylphosphonate; NHL—non-Hodgkin's lymphoma; PBMCs—peripheral blood mononuclear cells; PO—phosphodiester; PS—phosphorothioate; RV—retroviral.

BCR-ABL antisense phosphodiester treatment specifically inhibits cells taken from CML patients in blast crisis. The end points examined were CFU-GM and BFU-E assays and analysis of BCR-ABL mRNA. In these experiments the oligomers did not affect normal cells. At the time these observations were very exciting and provoked a flurry of activity among many groups, both academic and commercial, to reproduce and extend these data. However subsequent studies yielded conflicting results, and it is still difficult to say confidently that, in the context of BCR-ABL, true antisense effects have been achieved.

In our own laboratory, apparently specific antisense effects were achieved when using a test antisense oligomer and one sense control. However, when a more extensive panel of control oligomers was employed (i.e., b2a2 sense and antisense oligomers employed in experiments with b3a2-expressing cells and *vice versa*), similar degrees of inhibition were seen (O'Brien *et al.*, 1994). As described elsewhere in this chapter, the interactions between so-called antisense effectors and a variety of functionally important cellular proteins may be as important as, if not more important than, any interactions with BCR-ABL mRNA.

The ubiquitous problems of oligomer uptake and specificity have plagued BCR-ABL as much as any other antisense target. These problems have been addressed very elegantly by Tidd and colleagues who, in addition to adopting the streptolysin O transient permeabilization method for introducing DNA into cells (Barry *et al.*, 1993; Spiller and Tidd, 1995), have thoroughly evaluated so-called chimeric oligonucleotides which consist of a variable number of flanking nucleosides linked, for example, with methylphosphonate linkages (residues that do not direct RNaseH cleavage) surrounding a central portion of either phosphodiester or phosphorothioate DNA. By altering the relative composition of these linkages in such chimeric oligomers it is possible to define oligomers that effectively and specifically cleave BCR-ABL mRNA in both cell-free *in vitro* transcription systems and cellular systems (Giles *et al.*, 1992b, 1995a). So, although historically BCR-ABL antisense has been problematic, the development of more elegant assay systems and newer oligomer analogs may still allow this area of antisense research to bear fruit.

BCR-ABL directed ribozymes have been employed with good results so far (James *et al.*, 1996; Kearney *et al.*, 1995; LeoPold *et al.*, 1995; Pachuk *et al.*, 1994; Snyder *et al.*, 1993), but because they are composed of RNA, these molecules are more difficult to handle and have not been as widely adopted as DNA oligomers.

5. CLINICAL TRIALS IN HEMATOLOGY

Probably the first attempt at treating human disease using antisense was pioneered by the Omaha group (Bayever *et al.*, 1992). In June of 1992, under emergency FDA arrangements, the first systemic administration of an antisense oligonucleotide directed against the p53 gene was given to a 19-year-old man who had relapsed acute myeloid leukemia (AML). Although no useful clinical effect was observed, there was some *in vitro* inhibition of proliferation of blast cells taken from the patient on days 6 and 11 postinfusion. The Omaha group extended this study to evaluate 17 patients who had resistant AML or myelodysplasia. Again no significant clinical responses were observed but escalating doses of the antisense agent were well tolerated (Bayever *et al.*, 1993). This group has since extended its studies using antisense in combination with other chemotherapeutic agents. So far no major drug-related adverse events have been reported in any of the human antisense trials, although in primates given particularly high doses, some adverse events and even deaths have been reported (Cornish *et al.*, 1993; Galbraith *et al.*, 1994). The mechanism involved widespread complement activation and this may becaused in part by the motif-dependent effects on the immune system described previously.

In a study conducted jointly by the Hammersmith Hospital in London and the University of Pennsylvania in Philadelphia, autologous bone marrow cells were collected from patients who had CML and subjected to an *in vitro* purging procedure using a 24mer phosphorothioate antisense oligomer directed against codons 2–7 of the human MYB gene. The design of the study is shown in Figure 3. So far, 13 patients have been recruited for this study, and four were either entirely or predominantly Ph-negative at the three-month postautograft assessment. This Ph-negativity has been transient in all cases, but one patient has been followed up for move than a year without requiring any further therapy, and the study is ongoing (Luger *et al.*, 1994; O'Brien *et al.*, 1995b).

In a companion study, Gewirtz and colleagues have been evaluating the effects of intravenously administering the same MYB oligonucleotide to patients who have advanced phases of CML. The agent has been well tolerated, and some hematological responses have been observed. Both the *in vitro* and *in vivo* studies are ongoing.

In Rome, eight patients who have advanced phase CML (seven accelerated phase, one second chronic phase) have been treated with a 26mer phosphorothioate oligomer directed symmetrically at the BCR-ABL junction in a study conducted in collaboration with Lynx Therapeutics (Hayward, CA). In this study, similarly to the MYB study, autologous stem cells were purged *in vitro* before being returned to the patient as an autograft (de Fabritiis *et al.*, 1995b). The purging procedure did not have an adverse effect on engraftment (de Fabritiis *et al.*, 1995a). Thirty to one-hundred percent of cells were Ph-negative after the purging procedure, and in two patients complete Ph-negativity was achieved postautograft, albeit transiently. Two

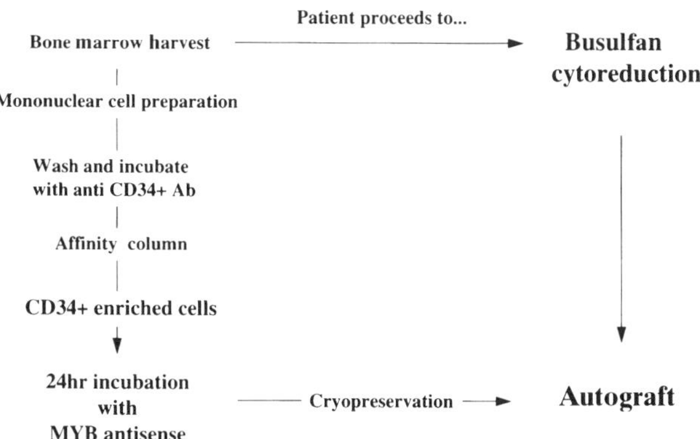

FIGURE 3. Purging of autologous stem cells prior to autografting in chronic myeloid leukemia using an antisense MYB oligomer.

other patients achieved a major cytogenetic response which again was transient. Six patients received interferon postautograft, but it is not possible to make any meaningful comment now about the impact of this procedure on survival.

Follicular lymphoma (FL) is characterized by the t(14;18) translocation which leads to increased expression of the BCL2 gene product. It is thought that BCL2 is prolongs the survival of the malignant cell by its effects on the inhibition of apoptosis. In many ways, therefore, BCL2 is an ideal paradigm for antisense studies because of the clear mechanism by which the inhibition of a particular gene product directly triggers cell death. In a phase I study at the Royal Marsden Hospital in London, nine patients who have FL have been treated with a two week course of a subcutaneously administered 18mer phosphorothioate oligomer directed against the initiation codon of BCL2 mRNA. The study is being conducted in collaboration with Genta Inc. (San Diego, CA). These patients had all previously been unresponsive to conventional therapies. One patient achieved a complete response, two a partial response, and most patients experienced a useful degree of symptomatic relief. Given the apparently resistant nature of the disease in these cases, the preliminary results are encouraging and the study is ongoing (Webb *et al.*, 1996).

6. FUTURE PROSPECTS

In view of the often conflicting published (and unpublished) antisense and ribozymal data, what predictions can be made for the future of these technologies? Antisense and nonantisense oligomers do have a future although developments are likely to be very different from what one may have predicted during the infancy of these technologies. At the same time alternative approaches are emerging, such as the development of "designer" DNA-binding proteins that affect transcription (Choo *et al.*, 1994) and may allow the disruption of specific molecular genetic mechanisms. Stem cell gene marking technology (Brenner *et al.*, 1993; Deisseroth *et al.*, 1994) will allow more accurate assessment of the efficiency of antisense purging techniques, and there are probably five main areas where other significant developments will be made.

First, it is likely that new DNA and RNA analogs will be developed that may overcome some of the problems of specificity, efficiency, and uptake encountered with "first-generation" oligomers. 2'O-methylribose, C5 propyne (Wagner *et al.*, 1993), αβ anomeric (Gottich *et al.*, 1994), phosphoramidate, and formacetal oligonucleotides seem promising. Appropriately designed chimeric oligomers, particularly those that contain some methylphosphonate residues (Zhou *et al.*, 1994b; Larrouy *et al.*, 1992), are particularly promising in directing specific target cleavage. Biotechnology companies are busy producing a considerable number of new DNA and RNA analogs, and more than 30 have been evaluated.

Secondly, there are likely to be developments in technologies to enhance the uptake of oligomers into cells. A number of lipid formulations have been used historically to this end, but none of these compounds has emerged as clearly superior. The more traditional methods of introducing genetic material into cells, such as electroporation and calcium phosphate precipitation, have major limitations in technical optimization and transfer efficiency, and it is unlikely that there will be significant further developments with these methods. Likewise, until major breakthroughs are made in virallymediated gene transfer, the prospects for antisense/ribozyme-encoding shuttle vectors are equally limited. Recently evaluated bacterial products, such as listeriolysin and streptolysin O (Barry *et al.*, 1993), are very promising. With streptolysin O, once conditions have been optimized for a particular experiment, oligomers are introduced into up to 85% of cells with minimal toxicity (Spiller and Tidd, 1995). For *in vivo* use, although both experimental animals and humans have received intravenous infusions of oligonucleotides, few if any convincing data to demonstrate cellular uptake in this setting. It will probably be quite some time before any significant advance is made in improving such uptake and for the foreseeable future useful clinical applications will be mainly found in *in vitro* manipulating/autografting.

Thirdly, more relevant targets for antisense intervention will probably be discovered. To date many of the targets that have been evaluated in hematological malignancies have not been expressed solely in the malignant cell. Rather the differential dependence of the malignant versus normal cell on a particular gene product has been exploited. This is essentially the same principle for conventional chemotherapy and does not fully exploit the potential specificity of antisense. It is likely that new targets for genetic interventions will be defined in due course which will further expand the scope of the antisense approach more specifically if truly specific oligomers are applied.

Fourth, it may well be that therapeutic antisense or aptameric oligomers will have to be employed as adjuvants to conventional treatment, in the context of minimal disease load or early relapse. There has been an unrealistic expectation of what may be achieved therapeutically using antisense technology in isolation, and it is not surprising that there have been many technical hurdles for this new technology, which promises to switch off gene expression with pinpoint accuracy and dramatic effects. It is possible that multiple genetic lesions could be targeted with a cocktail of antisense oligomers with or without chemotherapy. The investigation of antisense in combination with other treatment and in particular disease contexts will be an important area of development but clinical trials will take some time and will have to be carefully designed and analyzed to evaluate whether antisense adjuvant therapy improves on the results of conventional chemotherapy.

Finally, the "unwanted" side effects of so-called antisense molecules will probably be increasingly exploited in the area of aptamer development. The finding that certain oligonucleotides bind with high affinity to some proteins by virtue of certain sequence motifs within the oligomer (Ellington and Szostak, 1990) is being actively investigated by a number of research groups. The nature of the sequence motifs that direct this so-called sequence-dependent but not sequence-specific binding is not currently well understood. It is likely that oligomer secondary structure is an important factor but to date most studies of aptameric effects have been largely empiric.

For example, by repeated selection and PCR amplification of an oligonucleotide library, Gilead Sciences Inc. (Foster City, CA) developed a 15-mer oligonucleotide aptamer (5′-GGTTGGTGTGGTTGG-3′) which binds specifically to and inhibits thrombin (Bock *et al.*, 1992). It has been shown by solution NMR that this intriguing oligomer studies adopts a compact, symmetrical structure consisting of two guanine tetrads and three loops. This throne-like structure binds with high affinity to thrombin and exhibits anticoagulant activity in animal models with a rapid onset and short half-life. If the issue of cost can be addressed, which may only be a matter of time, this molecule could become a very valuable anticoagulant, for example, in cardiac bypass surgery.

NexStar (Boulder, CO) has been developing its proprietary "Selex" technology using similar principles. In this system a "target" protein is bound to a column and a large number (10^{11}–10^{13}) of oligomers of random sequence, in this case usually modified RNA species, are run through the column repeatedly. The final stage is eluting and sequencing the oligomer(s) with highest affinity and honing down the candidates until a single oligomer of defined sequence and high protein-binding affinity is derived. This process is laborious and time-consuming, and a considerable number of technical variables have to be optimized, such as oligomer length, stability, and purity and the number of randomers put into the system. In addition there is no guarantee that the aptamer will bind to a functionally important site on the target protein. However, although this technology is still in its infancy, impressive results have been obtained in targeting cell surface molecules, such as the selectins and receptors for growth factor, such as EGF and PDGF. A clinical application of this technology, for example, could be installing into the diabetic eye an aptameric oligonucleotide that binds to and inhibits the vascular endothelial growth factor (VEGF) receptor. This might reduce the hypoxic retinal neovascularization that is so troublesome in these patients.

Newer technical approaches, such as surface plasma resonance and evanescent wave technology, should make selecting aptamers quicker and more efficient and should facilitate the development of "nucleic acid therapeutics." Although extracellular/cell surface proteins are clearly the most obvious targets of aptamer strategies in the immediate future, it is possible that intracellular proteins relevant in malignant disease could also be targeted. The technology already exists for generating the required quantities of purified transcription factor proteins by using baculovirus systems.

To conclude, antisense research is a field where collaborations between groups that would not usually be brought together is becoming increasingly important if not essential. Hence the skills of organic chemists and biochemists in producing pure oligomers by stringent quality control are as critical to antisense projects as the skills of molecular and cell biologists and clinical scientists. Likewise, collaborations between academia and industry are increasingly important for the scientific and commercial viability of research programs. Although the influence of the biotechnology industry has not always been beneficial because of a certain amount of 'hype' and selective reporting of positive data, one must appreciate that many of the important developments in antisense research would not have been made without their innovation. Recently the antisense community has realized that rather than trying to play down or frankly ignore difficulties with antisense, carefully definiting and evaluating these problems allows important new breakthroughs—some quite unexpected (Stein, 1995; Wagner, 1995). Based on this more realistic view of what can be expected from antisense, ribozymal, and aptamer technology, one can be fairly optimistic that useful experimental and therapeutic niches can be found for these intriguing nucleic acid molecules.

7. REFERENCES

Abubakr, Y. A., Mohammed, R., Maki, A., Dan, M., Du, W., Smith, M. R., and Al-Katib, A., 1994, Effectiveness of bcl-2 antisense oligodeoxynucleotides against human follicular small-cleaved cell lymphoma (FSCCL)-SCID mice xenograft model, *Blood* **84:**374a (abstract).

Agarwal, S., Goodchild, J., Civeira, M. P., Thornton, A. T., Sarin, P. M., and Zamecnik, P. C., 1988, Oligodeoxynucleoside phosphoramidates, and phosphorothioates as inhibitors of human immunodeficiency virus, *Proc. Natl. Acad. Sci. USA* **85:**7079–7083.

Akhtar, S., Basu, S., Wickstrom, E., and Juliano, R. L., 1991, Interactions of antisense DNA oligonucleotide analogs with phospholipid membranes (liposomes), *Nucleic Acids Res.* **19:**5551–5559.

Anfossi, G., Gewirtz, A. M., and Calabretta, B., 1989, An oligomer complementary to c-myb-encoded mRNA inhibits proliferation of human myeloid leukemia cell lines, *Proc. Natl. Acad. Sci. USA* **86:**3379–3383.

Azuma, E., Hiratake, S., Nishiguchi, Y., Etoh, M., Nagai, M., Ohkubo, T., Umemoto, M., Zhang, X. L., Cao, D. C., Komada, Y., and Sakurai, M., 1994, In vivo treatment of multidrug-resistant murine leukemia with antisense MDR1 oligodeoxynucleotides, *Blood* **84**(Suppl. 1)**:**43a (abstract).

Barry, E. L., Gesek, F. A., and Friedman, P. A., 1993, Introduction of antisense oligonucleotides into cells by permeabilization with streptolysin O, *Biotechniques* **15:**1016–1018, 1020.

Barut, B., Chauhan, D., Uchiyama, H., and Anderson, K. C., 1993, Interleukin-6 functions as an intracellular growth factor in hairy cell leukemia in vitro, *J. Clin. Invest.* **92:**2346–2351.

Bayever, E., Iversen, P., Smith, L., Spinolo, J., and Zon, G., 1992, Systemic human antisense therapy begins [editorial], *Antisense Res. Dev.* **2:**109–110.

Bayever, E., Iversen, P. L., Bishop, M. R., Sharp, J. G., Tewary, H. K., Arneson, M. A., Pirruccello, S. J., Ruddon, R. W., Kessinger, A., and Zon, G., 1993, Systemic administration of a phosphorothioate oligonucleotide with a sequence complementary to p53 for acute myelogenous leukemia and myelodysplastic syndrome: Initial results of a phase I trial, *Antisense Res. Dev.* **3:**383–390.

Bedi, A., Zehnbauer, B. A., Barber, J. P., Sharkis, S. J., and Jones, R. J., 1994, Inhibition of apoptosis by BCR-ABL in chronic myeloid leukemia, *Blood* **83:**2038–2044.

Beltinger, C., Saragovi, H. U., Smith, R. M., LeSauteur, L., Shah, N., DeDionisio, L., Christensen, L., Raible, A., Jarett, L., and Gewirtz, A. M., 1995, Binding, uptake, and intracellular trafficking of phosphorothioate-modified oligodeoxynucleotides, *J. Clin. Invest.* **95:**1814–1823.

Bennett, C. F., Chiang, M. Y., Chan, H., Shoemaker, J. E., and Mirabelli, C. K., 1992, Cationic lipids enhance cellular uptake and activity of phosphorothioate antisense oligonucleotides, *Mol. Pharmacol.* **41:**1023–1033.

Bennett, C. F., Chiang, M. Y., Wilson-Lingardo, L., and Wyatt, J. R., 1994, Sequence specific inhibition of human type II phospholipase A2 enzyme activity by phophorothioate oligonucleotides, *Nucleic Acids Res.* **22:**3202–3209.

Bergan, R. C., Connell, Y., Fahmy, B., and Neckers, L., 1993, Electroporation enhances c-myc antisense oligodeoxynucleotide efficacy, *Nucleic Acids Res.* **21:**3567–3573.

Bergan, R. C., Kyle, E., Connell, Y., and Neckers, L., 1995, Inhibition of protein-tyrosine kinase activity in intact cells by the aptameric action of oligodeoxynucleotides, *Antisense Res. Dev.* **5:**33–38.

Bertrand, E., Fromont Racine, M., Pictet, R., and Grange, T., 1993, Visualization of the interaction of a regulatory protein with RNA in vivo, *Proc. Natl. Acad. Sci. USA* **90:**3496–3500.

Bi, S., Lanzn, F., and Goldman, J. M., 1993, The abnormal p53 protein expressed in CML cell lines are non-functional, *Leukemia* **7:**1840–1846.

Bi, S., Lanza, F., and Goldman, J. M., 1994, The involvement of "tumor suppressor" p53 in normal and chronic myelogenous leukemia hemopoiesis. AU: Bi-S; Lanza-F; Goldman-JM, *Cancer Res.* **54:**582–586.

Bock, L. C., Griffin, L. C., and Latham, J. A., 1992, Selection of single stranded DNA molecules that bind and inhibit human thrombin, *Nature* **355:**564–566.

Brenner, M. K., Rill, D. R., Moen, R. C., Krance, R. A., Mirro, J., Jr., Anderson, W. F., and Ihle, J. N., 1993, Gene marking to trace origin of relapse after autologous bone-marrow transplantation, *Lancet* **341:**85–86.

Brennscheidt, U., Riedel, D., Kölch, W., Bonifer, R., Brach, M. A., Ahlers, A., Mertelsmann, R. H., and Herrman, F., 1994, Raf-1 is a necessary component of the mitogenic response of the human megakaryoblastic leukemia cell line MO7 to human stem cell factor, granulocyte-macrophage colony stimulating factor, interleukin 3 and interleukin 9, *Cell Growth and Differentiation* **5:**367–372.

Brown, D. A., Kang, S. H., Gryaznov, S. M., DeDionisio, L., Heidenreich, O., Sullivan, S., Xu, X., and Nerenberg, M. I., 1994, Effects of phosphorothioate modification of oligonucleotides on specific protein binding, *J. Biol. Chem.* **269:**26801–26808.

Calabretta, B., Sims, R. B., Valtieri, M., Caracciolo, D., Szczylik, C., Venturelli, D., Ratajczak, M., Beran, M., and Gewirtz, A. M., 1991, Normal and leukemic hematopoietic cells manifest differential sensitivity to inhibitory effects of c-myb antisense oligodeoxynucleotides: An in vitro study relevant to bone marrow purging, *Proc. Natl. Acad. Sci. USA* **88:**2351–2355.

Calabretta, B., Venturelli, D., and Gewirtz, A. M., 1993, Functional significance of c-myb expression in normal and leukemic hematopoiesis, *Cancer Invest.* **11:**191–197.

Cameron, F. H., and Jennings, P. A., 1989, Specific gene suppression by engineered ribozymes in monkey cells, *Proc. Natl. Acad. Sci. USA* **86:**9139–9143.

Cameron, F. H., and Jennings, P. A., 1991, Inhibition of gene expression by a short sense fragment, *Nucleic Acids Res.* **19:**469–475.

Campos, L., Sabido, O., Rouault, J. P., and Guyotat, D., 1994, Effects of BCL-2 antisense oligodeoxynucleotides on in vitro proliferation and survival of normal marrow progenitors and leukemic cells, *Blood* **84:**595–600.

Capaccioli, S., Di Pasquale, G., Mini, E., Mazzei, T., and Quattrone, A., 1993, Cationic lipids improve antisense oligonucleotide uptake and prevent degradation in cultured cells and in human serum, *Biochem. Biophys. Res. Commun.* **197:**818–825.

Caracciolo, D., Venturelli, D., Valtieri, M., Peschle, C., Gewirtz, A. M., and Calabretta, B., 1990, Stage-related proliferative activity determines c-myb functional requirements during normal human hematopoiesis, *J. Clin. Invest.* **85:**55–61.

Cech, T. R., 1987, The chemistry of self-splicing RNA and RNA enzymes, *Science* **236:**1532–1539.

Chiang, M. Y., Chan, H., Zounes, M. A., Freier, S. M., Lima, W. F., and Bennett, C. F., 1991, Antisense oligonucleotides inhibit ICAM-1 expression by two distinct mechanisms, *J. Biol. Chem.* **266:**18162–18167.

Choo, Y., Sanchez-Garcia, I., and Klug, A., 1994, In vivo repression by a site-specific DNA-binding protein designed against an oncogenic sequence, *Nature* **372:**642–645.

Citro, G., Perrotti, D., Cucco, C., D'Agnano, I., Sacchi, A., Zupi, G., and Calabretta, B., 1992, Inhibition of leukemia cell proliferation by receptor-mediated uptake of c-myb antisense oligodeoxynucleotides, *Proc. Natl. Acad. Sci. USA* **89:**7031–7035.

Citro, G., Szczylik, C., Ginobbi, P., Zupi, G., and Calabretta, B., 1994, Inhibition of leukaemia cell proliferation by folic acid-polylysine-mediated introduction of c-myb antisense oligodeoxynucleotides into HL-60 cells, *Br. J. Cancer* **69:**463–467.

Cogswell, J. P., Cogswell, P. C., Kuehl, W. M., Cuddihy, A. M., Bender, T. M., Engelke, U., Marcu, K. B., and Ting, J. P., 1993, Mechanism of c-myc regulation by c-Myb in different cell lineages, *Mol. Cell Biol.* **13:**2858–2869.

Cooney, M., Czernuszewicz, G., Postal, E. H., Flint, S. J., and Hogan, M. E., 1988, Site-specific oligonucleotide binding represses transcription of the human c-myc gene in vitro, *Science* **241:**456–459.

Cornish, K. G., Iversen, P. L., Smith, L., Arneson, M. A., and Bayever, E., 1993, Cardiovascular effects of a phosphorothioate oligonucleotide with sequence antisense to p53 in the conscious Rhesus monkey, *Pharmacol. Commun.* **3:**239–247.

Cotter, F. E., Johnson, P., Hall, P., Pocock, C., Mahdi, N., Cowell, J. K., and Morgan, G., 1994, Antisense oligonucleotides suppress B-cell lymphoma growth in a SCID-hu mouse model, *Oncogene* **9:**3049–3055.

Cross, N. C., Lin, F., and Goldman, J. M., 1994, Appropriate controls for reverse transcription polymerase chain reaction (RT-PCR), *Br. J. Haematol.* **87:**218.

de Fabritiis, P., Amadori, S., Calabretta, B., and Mandelli, F., 1993, Elimination of clonogenic

Philadelphia-positive cells using BCR-ABL antisense oligodeoxynucleotides, *Bone Marrow Transplant.* **12:**261–265.

de Fabritiis, P., Lisci, E., Montefusco, M., Mancini, S., Buffolino, P., Pontis, P., Amadori, B., Calabretta, B., and Mandelli, F., 1994, Autograft after in vitro purging with BCR-ABL antisense oligonucleotides for patients with CML in advanced phase, *Bone Marrow Transplant.* **14**(Suppl. 3)**:**S80.

de Fabritiis, P., Amadori, S., Petti, M. C., Mancini, M., Montefusco, E., Picardi, A., Geiser, T., Campbell, K., Calabretta, B., and Mandelli, F., 1995a, In vitro purging with BCR-ABL antisense oligodeoxynucleotides does not prevent haematologic reconstitution after autologous bone marrow transplantation, *Leukemia* **9:**662–664.

de Fabritiis, P., Montefusco, M., Avvisati, G., Sala, R., Mancini, M., Lisci, A., Geiser, T. G., Calabretta, B., and Mandelli, F., 1995b, Bone marrow purging with BCR-ABL antisense oligonucleotides and autograft for patients with chronic myelogenous leukaemia, *Bone Marrow Transplant.* **15**(Suppl. 2)**:**S107.

Deisseroth, A. B., Zu, Z., Claxton, D., Hanania, E. G., Fu, S., Ellerson, D., Goldberg, L., Thomas, M., Janicek, K., and Anderson, W. F., 1994, Genetic marking shows that Ph+ cells present in autologous transplants of chronic myelogenous leukemia (CML) contribute to relapse after autologous bone marrow in CML, *Blood* **83:**3068–3076.

Dewangee, M. K., Ghafouripour, A. K., Kapadvanjwala, M., and Samy, A. T., 1994, Kinetics of hybridisation of mRNA of c-myc oncogene with ^{111}In-labelled antisense oligodeoxynucleotide probes by high-pressure liquid chromatography, *Biotechniques* **16:**844–849.

Ellington, A. D., and Szostak, J. W., 1990, In vitro selection of RNA molecules that bind specific ligand, *Nature* **346:**818–822.

Ferrari, S., Manfredini, R., Tagliafica, E., Grande, A., Barbien, D., Balestri, R., Pizzanelli, M., Zucchini, P., Citro, G., Zupi, G., Franceschi, C., and Torelli, U., 1994, Antiapoptotic effect of c-fes protooncogene during granulocytic differentiation, *Leukemia* **8**(Suppl. 1)**:**S91 (abstract).

Fischer, G., Kent, S. C., Joseph, L., Green, D. R., and Scott, D. W., 1994, Lymphoma models for B cell activation and tolerance. X. Anti-m-mediated growth arrest and apoptosis of murine B cell lymphomas is prevented by the stabilisation of myc, *J. Exp. Med.* **179:**221–227.

Fournier, S., Rubio, M., Delespesse, G., and Sarfati, M., 1994, Role for low-affinity receptor for IgE (CD23) in normal and leukemic B-cell proliferation, *Blood* **84:**1881–1886.

Galbraith, W. M., Hobson, W. C., Giclas, P. C., Schecter, P. J., and Agarwal, S., 1994, Complement activation and hemodynamic changes following administration of phosphorothioate oligonucleotides in the monkey, *Antisense Res. Dev.* **4:**201–207.

Gamard, C. J., Blobe, G. C., Hannun, Y. A., and Obeid, L. M., 1994, Specific role for protein kinase C beta in cell differentiation, *Cell Growth and Differentiation* **5:**495–412.

Gao, W. Y., Han, F. S., Storm, C., Egan, W., and Cheng, Y. C., 1992, Phosphorothioate oligonucleotides are inhibitors of human DNA polymerases and RNase H: Implications for antisense technology, *Mol. Pharmacol.* **41:**223–229.

Gao, W. Y., Storm, C., Egan, W., and Cheng, Y. C., 1993, Cellular pharmacology of phosphorothioate homooligodeoxynucleotides in human cells, *Mol. Pharmacol.* **43:**45–50.

Geselowitz, D. A., and Neckers, L. M., 1992, Analysis of oligonucleotide binding, internalization, and intracellular trafficking utilizing a novel radiolabeled crosslinker, *Antisense Res. Dev.* **2:**17–25.

Gewirtz, A. M., and Calabretta, B., 1991, Role of the c-myb and c-abl protooncogenes in human hematopoiesis, *Ann. N.Y. Acad. Sci.* **628:**63–73.

Giles, R. V., and Tidd, D. M., 1992a, Enhanced RNase H activity with methylphosphonodiester/phosphodiester chimeric antisense oligodeoxynucleotides, *Anti cancer Drug Des.* **7:**37–48.

Giles, R. V., and Tidd, D. M., 1992b, Increased specificity for antisense oligodeoxynucleotide targeting of RNA cleavage by RNase H using chimeric methylphosphonodiester/phosphodiester structures, *Nucleic Acids Res.* **20:**763–770.

Giles, R. V., Spiller, D. G., Green, J. A., Clark, R. E., and Tidd, D. M., 1995a, Optimization of antisense oligodeoxynucloetide structure for targeting BCR-ABL mRNA, *Blood* **86:**744–754.

Giles, R. V., Spiller, D. G., and Tidd, D. M., 1995b, Detection of ribonuclease H-generated mRNA fragments in human leukemia cells following reversible membrane permeabilization in the presence of antisense oligodeoxynucleotides, *Antisense Res. Dev.* **5:**23–31.

Gottich, M., Baud-Demattei, M. V., Lescot, E., Giorgi-Renault, S., Shabarova, Z., Dautry, F., Malvy, C., and Bertrand, J. R., 1994, In vitro inhibition of the pim-1 protooncogene by chimeric oligodeoxyribonucleotides composed of alpha and beta anomeric fragments, *Gene* **149:**5–11.

Griffin, L. C., and Dervan, P. B., 1989, Recognition of thymidine:adenine base pairs by guanine in a pyrimidine triple helix motif, *Science* **245:**967–971.

Guerrier-Takada, C., Gardiner, K., Marsch, T., Pace, N., and Altman, S., 1983, The RNA moiety of ribonuclease P is the catalytic subunit of the enzyme, *Cell* **35:**849–857.

Guimaraes, J. E. T., Szczylik, C., Koziolkiewicz, M., Moreira, I., and Ramos, J. P., 1994, An antisense oligonucleotide to the transferrin receptor inhibits proliferation of leukemic cells in vitro, *Blood* **84**(Suppl. 1)**:**607a (abstract).

Guvakova, M. A., Yabukov, L. A., Vlodavsky, I., Tonkinson, J. L., and Stein, C. A., 1995, Phosphorothioate oligodeoxynucleotides bind to basic fibroblast growth factor, inhibiting its binding to cell surface receptors, and remove it from low affinity binding sites on extracellular matrix, *J. Biol. Chem.* **270:**2620–2627.

Hanvey, J. C., Peffer, N. J., Bisi, J. E., Thomson, S. A., Cadilla, R., Josey, J. A., Ricca, D. J., Hassman, C. F., Bonham, M. A., Au, K. G., Carter, S. G., Bruckenstein, D. A., Boyd, A. L., Nobel, S. A., and Babiss, L. E., 1992, Antisense and antigene properties of peptide nucleic acids, *Science* **258:**1481–1485.

Harel Bellan, A., Brini, A., Ferris, D. F., Robin, P., and Farrar, W. L., 1989, In situ detection of a heat-shock regulatory element binding protein using a soluble short synthetic enhancer sequence, *Nucleic Acids Res.* **17:**4077–4087.

Helene, C., Thuong, N. T., and Harel Bellan, A., 1992, Control of gene expression by triple helix-forming oligonucleotides. The antigene strategy, *Ann. N.Y. Acad. Sci.* **660:**27–36.

Ho, P. T., Ishiguro, K., Wickstrom, E., and Sartorelli, A. C., 1991, Non-sequence-specific inhibition of transferrin receptor expression in HL-60 leukemia cells by phosphorothioate oligodeoxynucleotides, *Antisense Res. Dev.* **1:**329–342.

Holt, J. T., Redner, R. L., and Neinhuis, A. W., 1988, An oligomer complementary to c-myc mRNA inhibits proliferation of HL60 promyelocytic cells and induces differentiation, *Mol. Cell Biol.* **8:**963–973.

James, H., Mills, K., and Gibson, I., 1996, Investigating and improving the specificity of ribozymes directed against the BCR-ABL translocation, *Leukemia* **10:**1054–1064.

Kabisch, A., Perenyi, L., Seay, U., Lohmeyer, J., and Pralle, H., 1994, Unmodified phosphodiester antisense oligodeoxynucleotides to the BCR-ABL junction do not suppress Philadelphia-positive clonogenic cells, *Acta Haematol.* **92:**190–196.

Kato, J., Kogho, Y., Kondo, H., Saski, K., and Nitsu, Y., 1994, Antisense oligodeoxynucleotides for IL-2, c-myc and transferrin receptor synchronise mitogen-activated lymphocytes in the G1 phase, *Scand. J. Immunol.* **39:**499–505.

Kay, H. D., Tarantolo, S., and Smith, L. J., 1994, Antisense oligonucleotides inhibit the expression of human multi-drug resistance (MDR-1) gene and dramatically increase in vitro chemosensitivity of human multiple myeloma cells, *Blood* **84**(Suppl. 1)**:**39a (abstract).

Kearney, P., Wright, L. A., Milliken, S., and Biggs, J. C., 1995, Improved specificity of ribozyme-mediated cleavage of BCR-ABL mRNA, *Exp. Hematol.* **23:**986–989.

Keith, F. J., Bradbury, D. A., Zhu, Y. M., and Russell, N. H., 1995, Inhibition of bcl-2 with antisense oligonucleotides induces apoptosis and increases the sensitivity of AML blasts to Ara-C, *Leukemia* **9:**131–138.

Kiehntopf, M., Esquivel, E. L., Brach, M. A., and Herrmann, F., 1995, Clinical applications of ribozymes, *Lancet* **345:**1027–1031.

Kim, Y. H., Bucholz, M. A., Chrest, F. J., and Nordin, A. A., 1994, Up-regulation of c-myc induces the gene expression of the murine homologues of p34cdc2 and cyclin dependent kinase-2 in T lymphocytes, *J. Immunol.* **152:**4328–4333.

Kirkland, M. A., O'Brien, S. G., McDonald, C., Davidson, R. J., Cross, N. C., and Goldman, J. M., 1993, BCR-ABL antisense purging in chronic myeloid leukaemia [letter], *Lancet* **342:**614.

Kirkland, M. A., O'Brien, S. G., and Goldman, J. M., 1994, Antisense therapeutics in haematological malignancies, *Br. J. Haematol.* **87:**447–452.

Kitada, S., Miyashita, T., Tanaka, S., and Reed, J. C., 1993, Investigations of antisense oligonucleotides targeted against bcl-2 RNAs, *Antisense Res. Dev.* **3:**157–163.

Kizaki, M., Sakashita, A., Karmakar, A., Lin, C. W., and Koeffler, H. P., 1993, Regulation of manganese superoxide dismutase and other antioxidant genes in normal and leukemic hematopoietic cells and their relationship to cytotoxicity by tumour necrosis factor, *Blood* **82:**1142–1147.

Kobayashi, S., Teramura, M., Sugawara, I., Oshimi, K., and Mizoguchi, H., 1993, Interleukin-11 acts as an autocrine growth factor for human megakaryocyte cell lines, *Blood* **81:**889–895.

Krieg, A., 1995, CpG motifs in bacterial DNA trigger B-cell activation, *Nature* **374:**546–549.

Kulka, M., Smith, C., Aurelian, L., Fishelevich, R., Meade, K., Miller, P., and Ts'o, P., 1989, Site specificity of the inhibitory effects of oligo (nucleoside methylphosphonates) complementary to the acceptor splice junction of herpes simplex virus type I immediate early mRNA, *Proc. Natl. Acad. Sci. USA* **86:**6868–6873.

Lappalainen, K., Urtti, A., Jaaskelainen, I., Syrjanen, K., and Syrjanen, S., 1994, Cationic liposomes mediated delivery of antisense oligonucleotides targeted to HPV 16 E7 mRNA in CaSki cells, *Antiviral Res.* **23:**119–130.

Larrouy, B., Blonski, C., Boiziau, C., Stuer, M., Moreau, S., Shire, D., and Toulme, J. J., 1992, RNase H-mediated inhibition of translation by antisense oligodeoxyribonucleotides: Use of backbone modification to improve specificity, *Gene* **121:**189–194.

Leonetti, J. P., Mechti, N., Degols, G., and Lebleu, B., 1991, Nuclear accumulation of microinjected antisense oligonucleotides, *Nucleosides and Nucleotides* **10:**537–539.

Leopold, L. H., Shore, S. K., Newkirk, T. A., Reddy, R. M. V., and Reddy, E., 1995, Multi-unit ribozyme-mediated cleavage of bcr-abl mRNA in myeloid leukemias, *Blood* **85:**2162–2170.

Loke, S. L., Stein, C. A., Zhang, X. H., Mori, K., Nakanishi, M., Subasinghe, C., Cohen, J. C., and Neckers, L. M., 1989, Characterization of oligonucleotide transport into living cells, *Proc. Natl. Acad. Sci. USA* **86:**3474–3478.

Louie, S. W., Ramirez, L. M., Krieg, A. M., Maliszewski, C. R., and Bishop, G. A., 1993, Endogenous secretion of IL-4 maintains growth and Thy-1 expression of a transformed B cell clone, *J. Immunol.* **150:**399–405.

Luger, S. M., Ratajczak, M. Z., Stadtmauer, E. A., Mangan, P., Magee, D., Silberstein, L., Edelstein, M., Nowell, P., and Gewirtz, A. M., 1994, Autografting for chronic myeloid leukemia (CML) with C-MYB antisense oligodeoxynucleotide purged bone marrow: A preliminary report, *Blood* **84**(Suppl. 1)**:**151a (abstract).

Maekawa, T., Kimura, S., Hirakawa, K., Murakami, A., Zon, G., and Abe, T., 1995, Sequence specificity on the growth suppression and induction of apoptosis of chronic myeloid leukemia cells by BCR-ABL antisense oligodeoxynucleoside phosphorothioates, *Int. J. Cancer* **62:**63–69.

Mahon, F. X., Belloc, F., and Reiffers, J., 1993, Antisense oligomers in chronic myeloid leukaemia [letter; comment], *Lancet* **341:**566.

Maltese, J., Sharma, H., Vassilev, L., and Narayanan, R., 1995, Sequence context of antisense RelA/NF-kappa B phosphorothioates determines specificity, *Nucleic Acids Res.* **23:**1146–1151.

Martiat, P., Lewalle, P., Taj, A. S., Philippe, M., Larondelle, Y., Vaerman, J. L., Wildmann, C., Goldman, J. M., and Michaux, J. L., 1993, Retrovirally transduced antisense sequences stably suppress P210BCR-ABL expression and inhibit the proliferation of BCR/ABL-containing cell lines, *Blood* **81:**502–509.

McGahon, A., Bissonnette, R., Schmitt, M., Cotter, K. M., Green, D. R., and Cotter, T. G., 1994, BCR-ABL maintains resistance of chronic myelogenous leukemia cells to apoptotic cell death, *Blood* **83:**1179–1187.

Mergny, J. L., Duval-Valentin, G., Nguyen, C. H., Perrouault, L., Faucon, B., Rougee, M., Montenay-Garestier, T., Bisagni, E., and Helene, C., 1992, Triple helix specific ligands, *Science* **256:**1681–1684.

Methia, N., Louache, F., Vainchenker, W., and Wendling, F., 1993, Oligodeoxynucleotides antisense to the proto-oncogene c-mpl specifically inhibit in vitro megakaryocytopoiesis, *Blood* **82:**1395–1401.

Milligan, J. F., Matteucci, M. D., and Martin, J. C., 1993, Current concepts in antisense drug design, *J. Med. Chem.* **36:**1923–1937.

Morvan, F., Porumb, H., Degols, G., Lefebvre, I., Pompon, A., Sproat, B. S., Rayner, B., Malvy, C., Lebleu, B., and Imbach, J. L., 1993, Comparative evaluation of seven oligonucleotide analogues as potential antisense agents, *J. Med. Chem.* **36:**280–287.

Nellen, W., and Lichtenstein, C., 1993, What makes an mRNA anti-sense-itive? *Trends. Biochem. Sci.* **18:**419–423.

Nestle, F. O., Mitra, R. S., Bennett, C. F., Chan, H., and Nickoloff, B. J., 1994, Cationic lipid is not required for uptake and selective inhibitory activity of ICAM-1 phosphorothioate antisense oligonucleotides in keratinocytes, *J. Invest. Dermatol.* **103:**569–575.

Nguyen, H. Q., Hoffman-Liebermann, B., and Liebermann, D. A., 1993, The zinc finger transcription factor Egr-1 is essential for and restricts differentiation along the macrophage lineage, *Cell* **72:**197–203.

Nielsen, P. E., Egholm, M., Berg, R. H., and Buchhardt, O., 1991, Sequence-selective recognition of DNA by strand displacement with a thymidine-substituted polyamide, *Science* **254:**1497–1500.

Noonberg, S. B., Scott, G. K., Garovoy, M. R., Benz, C. C., and Hunt, C. A., 1994, In vivo generation of highly abundant sequence-specific oligonucleotides for antisense and triplex gene regulation, *Nucleic Acids Res.* **22:**2830–2835.

O'Brien, S. G., Kirkland, M. A., Melo, J. V., Rao, H. M., Davidson, R. J., McDonald, C., and Goldman, J. M., 1994, Antisense BCR-ABL oligomers cause non-specific inhibition of chronic myeloid leukemia cell lines, *Leukemia* **8:**2156–2162.

O'Brien, S. G., Cross, N. C., Kirkland, M. A., and Goldman, J. M., 1995a, A novel BCR-ABL/CAT reporter construct system can define the functional specificity of BCR-ABL antisense, *Blood* **86:**737a (abstract).

O'Brien, S. G., Gewirtz, A. M., Rule, S. A., Hawkins, T. E., Ratajczak, M. Z., Savage, D., Luger, S. M., and Goldman, J. M., 1995b, Autografting for CML using bone marrow purged with MYB antisense oligonucleotide, *Exp. Hematol.* **23:**804 (abstract).

Pachuk, C. J., Yoon, K., Moelling, K., and Coney, L. R., 1994, Selective cleavage of bcr-abl chimeric RNAs by a ribozyme targeted to non-contiguous sequences, *Nucleic Acids Res.* **22:**301–307.

Patinkin, D., Lev-Lehman, E., Ginzburg, D., Zakut, H., Eckstein, F., and Soreq, H., 1994, Antisense acetylcholinesterase oligonucleotide promotes stem cell expansion and suppresses hematopoietic apoptosis, *Blood* **84**(Suppl. 1)**:**574a (abstract).

Perez, J. R., Li, Y. L., Stein, C. A., Majumder, S., van Oorschot, A., and Narayanan, R., 1994, Sequence-independent induction of Sp 1 transcription factor activity by phosphorothioate oligonucleotides, *Proc. Natl. Acad. Sci. USA* **91:**5957–5963.

Ratajczak, M. Z., Hijiya, N., Catani, L., DeRiel, K., Luger, S. M., McGlave, P., and Gewirtz, A. M., 1992a, Acute- and chronic-phase chronic myelogenous leukemia colony-forming units are highly sensitive to the growth inhibitory effects of c-myb antisense oligodeoxynucleotides, *Blood* **79:**1956–1961.

Ratajczak, M. Z., Kant, J. A., Luger, S. M., Hijiya, N., Zhang, J., Zon, G., and Gewirtz, A. M., 1992b, In vivo treatment of human leukemia in a scid mouse model with c-myb antisense oligodeoxynucleotides, *Proc. Natl. Acad. Sci. USA* **89:**11823–11827.

Reed, J. C., Stein, C., Subasinghe, C., Haldar, S., Croce, C. M., Yum, S., and Cohen, J., 1990, Antisense mediated inhibition of BCL2 protooncogene expression and leukemic cell growth and survival: Comparisons of phosphodiester and phosphorothioate oligodeoxynucleotides, *Cancer Res.* **50:**6565–6570.

Rogers, S. Y., Bradbury, D., Kozolwski, R., and Russell, N. H., 1994, Evidence for internal autocrine regulation of growth in acute myeloblastic leukemia cells, *Exp. Hematol.* **22:**593–597.

Rosolen, A., Kyle, E., Chavany, C., Bergan, R. C., Kalman, E. T., Crouch, R., and Neckers, L., 1993, Effect of over-expression of bacterial ribonuclease H on the utility of antisense MYC oligodeoxynucleotides in the monocytic leukemia cell line U937, *Biochemistry* **75:**79–85.

Rosti, V., Bergamaschi, G., Ponchio, L., and Cazzola, M., 1992, c-abl function in normal and chronic myelogenous leukemia hematopoiesis: In vitro studies with antisense oligomers, *Leukemia* **6:**1–7.

Ryte, A. S., Morelli, S., Mazzei, M., Alama, A., Franco, P., Canti, G. F., and Nicolin, A., 1993, Oligonucleotide degradation contributes to resistance to antisense compounds, *Anticancer Drugs* **4:**197–200.

Scheuermann, R. H., Racila, E., Tucker, T., Yefenof, E., Street, N. E., Vitetta, E. S., Picker, L. J., and Uhr, J. W., 1994, *Proc. Natl. Acad. Sci. USA* **91:**4048–4054.

Schülter, C., Duchrow, M., Wohlenberg, C., Becker, M. H. G., Key, G., Flad, H. D., and Gerdes, J., 1993, The cell proliferation-associated antigen of antibody Ki-67: A very large, ubiquitous nuclear protein with numerous repeated elements, representing a new kind of cell cycle-maintaining protein, *J. Cell. Biol.* **123:**513–519.

Skorski, T., Nieborowska Skorska, M., Barletta, C., Malaguarnera, L., Szczylik, C., Chen, S. T., Lange, B., and Calabretta, B., 1993, Highly efficient elimination of Philadelphia leukemic cells by exposure to bcr/abl antisense oligodeoxynucleotides combined with mafosfamide, *J. Clin. Invest.* **92:**194–202.

Skorski, T., Kanakaraj, P., Ku, D. H., Nieborowska Skorska, M., Canaani, E., Zon, G., Perussia, B., and Calabretta, B., 1994a, Negative regulation of p120GAP GTPase promoting activity by p210bcr/abl: Implication for RAS-dependent Philadelphia chromosome positive cell growth, *J. Exp. Med.* **179:**1855–1865.

Skorski, T., Nieborowska Skorska, M., Nicolaides, N. C., Szczylik, C., Iversen, P., Iozzo, R. V., Zon, G., and Calabretta, B., 1994b, Suppression of Philadelphia1 leukemia cell growth in mice by BCR-ABL antisense oligodeoxynucleotide, *Proc. Natl. Acad. Sci. USA* **91:**4504–4508.

Skorski, T., Kanakaraj, P., Nieborowska Skorska, M., Ratajczak, M. Z., Wen, S., Zon, G., Gewirtz, A. M., Perussia, B., and Calabretta, B., 1995, Phosphatidylinositol-3 kinase activity is regulated by BCR-ABL and is required for the growth of Ph chromosome-positive cells, *Blood* **86:**726–736.

Smetsers, T. F., Skorski, T., van de Locht, L. T., Wessels, H. M., Pennings, A. H., de Witte, T., Calabretta, B., and Mensink, E. J., 1994, Antisense BCR-ABL oligonucleotides induce apoptosis in the Philadelphia chromosome-positive cell line BV173, *Leukemia* **8:**129–140.

Smetsers, T. F., and Mensink, E. J., 1995, Specificity of BCR-ABL antisense oligonucleotides [letter], *Blood* **85:**597–598.

Smetsers, T. F., van de Locht, L. T., Pennings, A. H., Wessels, H. M. C., de Witte, T., and Mensink, E. J., 1995, Phosphorothioate BCR-ABL antisense oligonucleotides induce cell death, but fail to reduce cellular BCR-ABL protein levels, *Leukemia* **9:**118–130.

Snyder, D. S., Wu, Y., Wang, J. L., Rossi, J. J., Swiderski, P., Kaplan, B. E., and Forman, S. J., 1993, Ribozyme-mediated inhibition of bcr-abl gene expression in a Philadelphia chromosome-positive cell line, *Blood* **82:**600–605.

Sokoloski, J. A., Sartorelli, A. C., Rosen, C. A., and Narayanan, R., 1993, Antisense oligonucleotides to the p65 subunit of NF-kappa B block CD11b expression and alter adhesion properties of differentiated HL-60 granulocytes, *Blood* **82:**626–631.

Sparatore, B., Patrone, M., Passalacqua, M., Pessino, A., Falchetto, R., Melloni, E., and Pontremoli, S., 1993, Characterization of the biological role of murine erythroleukemia cells ‘differentiation enhancing factor’ using antisense oligodeoxynucleotides, *Biochem. Biophys. Res. Commun.* **193:**941–946.

Spiller, D. G., and Tidd, D. M., 1995, Nuclear delivery of antisense oligodeoxynucleotides through reversible permeablization of human leukemia cells with streptolysin O, *Antisense Res. Dev.* **5:**13–21.

Stein, C. A., and Cheng, Y. C., 1993, Antisense oligonucleotides as therapeutic agents—is the bullet really magical? *Science* **261:**1004–1012.

Stein, C. A., Tonkinson, J. L., Zhang, L. M., Yakubov, L. A., Gervasoni, J., Taub, R., and Rotenberg, S. A., 1993, Dynamics of the internalization of phosphodiester oligodeoxynucleotides in HL60 cells, *Biochemistry* **32:**4855–4861.

Stein, C. A., and Krieg, A. M., 1994, Problems in interpretation of data derived from in vitro and in vivo use of oligodeoxynucleotides, *Antisense Res. Dev.* **4:**67–69.

Stein, C. A., 1995, Does antisense exist? *Nat. Med.* **1:**1119–1121.

Sullenger, B. A., and Cech, T. R., 1994, Ribozyme-mediated repair of defective mRNA by targeted trans-splicing, *Nature* **371:**619–622.

Szczylik, C., Skorski, T., Nicolaides, N. C., Manzella, L., Malaguarnera, L., Venturelli, D., Gewirtz, A. M., and Calabretta, B., 1991, Selective inhibition of leukemia cell proliferation by BCR-ABL antisense oligodeoxynucleotides, *Science* **253:**562–565.

Taj, A. S., Martiat, P., Dhut, S., Chaplin, T. L., Dowding, C., Th'ng, K. H., Goldstein, I., Daley, G. Q., Young, B. D., and Goldman, J. M., 1990, Inhibition of $p210^{BCR/ABL}$ expression in K562 cells by electroporation with an antisense oligonucleotide, *Leukemia and Lymphoma* **3:**201–208.

Takeshita, K., Bollekens, J. A., Hijaya, N., Ratajczak, M. Z., Ruddle, F. H., and Gewirtz, A. M., 1993, A homeobox gene of the antennapedia class is required for human adult erythropoiesis, *Proc. Natl. Acad. Sci. USA* **90:**3535–3540.

Tamamoto, T., Yamamoto, S., Kataoka, T., and Tokunaga, T., 1994, Ability of oligonucleotides with certain palindromes to induce interferon production and augment natural killer cell activity is associated with their base length, *Antisense Res. Dev.* **4:**119–122.

Tari, A. M., Tucker, S. D., Deisseroth, A., and Lopez Berestein, G., 1994, Liposomal delivery of methylphosphonate antisense oligodeoxynucleotides in chronic myelogenous leukemia, *Blood* **84:**601–607.

Thierry, A. R., and Dritschilo, A., 1992, Intracellular availability of unmodified, phosphorothioated and liposomally encapsulated oligodeoxynucleotides for antisense activity, *Nucleic Acids Res.* **20:**5691–5698.

Thomas, M., Kosciolek, B., Wang, N., and Rowley, P., 1994, Capping of bcr-abl antisense oligonucleotides enhances antiproliferative activity against chronic myeloid leukemia cell lines, *Leukemia Res.* **18:**401–408.

Thulasi, R., Harbour, D. V., and Thompson, E. B., 1993, Suppression of c-myc is a critical step in glucocorticoid-induced human leukemic cell lysis, *J. Biol. Chem.* **268:**18306–18311.

Vaerman, J. L., Lammineur, C., Moureau, P., Lewalle, P., Deldime, F., Blumenfeld, M., and Martiat, P., 1995, BCR-ABL antisense oligodeoxyribonucleotides suppress the growth of leukemic and normal hematopoietic cells by a sequence-specific but nonantisense mechanism, *Blood* **86:**3891–3896.

Wagner, E. G., and Simons, R. W., 1994, Antisense RNA control in bacteria, phages, and plasmids, *Annu. Rev. Microbiol.* **48:**713–742.

Wagner, R. W., Matteucci, M. D., Lewis, J. G., Gutierrez, A. J., Moulds, C., and Froehler, B. C., 1993, Antisense gene inhibition by oligonucleotides containing C-5 propyne pyrimidines, *Science* **260:**1510–1513.

Wagner, R. W., 1994, Gene inhibition using antisense oligodeoxynucleotides, *Nature* **372:**333–335.

Wagner, R. W., 1995, The state of the art in antisense research, *Nat. Med.* **1:**1116–1118.

Waki, M., Kitanaka, A., Kamano, H., Tanaka, T., Kubota, Y., Ohnishi, H., Takahara, J., Irino, S., Thomas, M., Kosciolek, B., Wang, N., and Rowley, P., 1994, Antisense src expression inhibits U937 human leukemia cell proliferation in conjunction with reduction of c-myb expression, *Biochem. Biophys. Res. Commun. Leukemia Res.* **18:**401–408.

Walder, R. Y., and Walder, J. A., 1988, Role of RNaseH in hybrid-arrested translation by antisense oligonucleotides, *Proc. Natl. Acad. Sci. USA* **85:**5011–5015.

Watson, J. D., and Crick, F. H. C., 1953, A structure for deoxyribose nucleic acid, *Nature* **171:**737–738.

Webb, A., Cunningham, D., Cotter, F., Hill, M., Clark, P., di Stefano, F., Viner, C., Preneville, J., Rahl, S., and Dziewanowska, Z., 1996, Follicular lymphoma BCL2 antisense trial: Preliminary results, *Ann. Oncol.* **7**(Suppl. 3)**:**32 (abstract).

Woolf, T. M., Melton, D. A., and Jennings, C. G., 1992, Specificity of antisense oligonucleotides in vivo, *Proc. Natl. Acad. Sci. USA* **89:**7305–7309.

Yakubov, L. A., Deeva, E. A., Zarytova, V. F., Ivanova, E. M., Ryte, A. S., Yurchenko, L. V., and Vlassov, V. V., 1989, Mechanism of oligonucleotide uptake by cells: Involvement of specific receptors? *Proc. Natl. Acad. Sci. USA* **86:**6454–6458.

Yao, X. R., and Scott, D. W., 1993, Antisense oligodeoxynucleotides to the blk tyrosine kinase prevent anti-m-chain-mediated growth inhibition and apoptosis in a B-cell lymphoma, *Proc. Natl. Acad. Sci. USA* **90:**7946–7951.

Yaswen, P., Stampfer, M. R., Ghosh, K., and Cohen, J. S., 1993, Effects of sequence of thioated oligonucleotides on cultured human mammary epithelial cells, *Antisense Res. Dev.* **3:**67–77.

Yeoman, L. C., Danels, Y. J., and Lynch, M. J., 1992, Lipofectin enhances cellular uptake of antisense DNA while inhibiting tumor cell growth, *Antisense Res. Dev.* **2:**51–59.

Zamecnik, P. C., Aghajanian, J., Zamecnik, M., Goodchild, J., and Witman, G., 1994, Electron micrographic studies of transport of oligodeoxynucleotides across eukaryotic cell membranes, *Proc. Natl. Acad. Sci. USA* **91:**3156–3160.

Zamecnik, P. C., and Stephenson, M. L., 1978, Inhibition of Rous sarcoma virus replication and cell transformation by a specific oligodeoxynucleotide, *Proc. Natl. Acad. Sci. USA* **75:**280–284.

Zhao, Q. Y., Waldschmidt, T., Fisher, E., Herrera, C. J., and Krieg, A. M., 1994, Stage-specific oligonucleotide uptake in murine bone marrow B-cell precursors, *Blood* **84:**3660–3665.

Zhou, J. H., Pai, B. S., Reed, M. W., Gamper, H. B., Lukhtanov, E., Podyminogin, M., Meyer, R. B., and Cheng, Y. C., 1994a, Discovery of short, 3′-cholesterol-modified DNA duplexes with unique antitumor cell activity, *Cancer Res.* **54:**5783–5711.

Zhou, L., Morocho, A. M., Chen, B. C., and Cohen, J. S., 1994b, Synthesis of phosphorothioate-methylphosphonate oligonucleotide co-polymers, *Nucleic Acids Res.* **22:**453–456.

Zhu, Y. M., Bradbury, D. A., and Russell, N. H., 1994, Wild-type p53 is required for apoptosis induced by growth factor deprivation in factor-dependent leukaemic cells, *Br. J. Cancer* **69:**468–472.

Chapter 11

Transfer of Drug Resistance Genes into Bone Marrow Stem and Progenitor Cells:

Implications for Cancer Chemotherapy

J. A. Rafferty and L. J. Fairbairn

1. INTRODUCTION

Administering chemotherapy is a major frontline approach in treating many cancers. Now a large number of agents used alone, but more often in combination, exert cytotoxic effects on tumor cells when delivered systemically. The general effectiveness of antitumor drugs is a function of dose (intended versus actual), scheduling, and the inherent relative resistance of tumor versus normal cells to some or all components of the chemotherapeutic cocktail. Although alterations in the dose and particularly the drug delivery schedule can favorably effect the balance between acceptable tumor kill and the side effects of therapy, the dose-limiting toxicities of anticancer drugs remain a major problem.

The normal tissues most susceptible to collateral toxic effects are those with a high mitotic index, such as the hematopoietic system and the gastrointestinal tract, although significant pulmonary, nephro- and neurotoxicities are also frequently observed. Thus, in the hematopoietic system chemotherapy is often associated with myelosuppression, with episodes of neutropenia leaving patients prone to infection, and thrombocytopenia leading to problems of hemorrhage. The clinical result of such effects can themselves be fatal but most often result in modifications to the

J. A. Rafferty and L. J. Fairbairn Paterson Institute for Cancer Research, Christie Hospital (NHS) Trust, Manchester M20 4BX, United Kingdom.

Blood Cell Biochemistry, Volume 8: Hematopoiesis and Gene Therapy, edited by Fairbairn and Testa. Kluwer Academic/Plenum Publishers, New York, 1999.

dose and/or frequency of chemotherapy and may even lead to the complete cessation of treatment. The direct consequence of this is likely to be an adverse effect on the outcome of therapy as a result of suboptimal tumor cytoreduction. The development of various supportive measures, especially for the hematopoietic system, has been an important step forward. These strategies range from administering antibiotics and nutrient support to overcome infection as a result of febrile neutropenia to the supply of bone marrow and peripheral blood stem cells to reestablish hematopoiesis. Indeed the use and success of supportive care for acute hematological toxicity has allowed high-dose, intensive chemotherapy to become more commonplace for some malignancies. However, as patient survival from the acute effects of chemotherapy increases, it seems likely that the frequency of longer term side effects of treatment, including therapeutically related malignancy, will increase.

In this article we briefly review the current procedures for overcoming myelosuppression as a consequence of chemotherapy and examine the prospect of using gene therapy as an alternative to protecting normal hematopoietic stem cells from dose-limiting toxicity. We also consider the potential of this approach to spare target cell populations from the mutagenic effects of many chemotherapeutic regimens which in turn could reduce the risk of therapeutically related malignancy. We focus on the hematopoietic system because (1) myelosuppression is often the principal dose-limiting toxicity of many antitumor drugs; (2) this tissue is amenable to *ex vivo* manipulation and gene transfer; and (3) protecting this system will serve as a paradigm for protecting stem cell populations in other drug-sensitive tissues.

2. CURRENT STRATEGIES FOR HAEMOPOIETIC SUPPORT DURING CHEMOTHERAPY

These approaches can be broadly categorized as (1) administration of blood and associated products; (2) the use of peptide factors which can stimulate or inhibit hematopoiesis; and (3) bone marrow or peripheral blood stem/progenitor cell transplantation.

2.1. Blood and Associated Products

Prophylactic platelet transfusions are used to counteract thrombocytopenia, a condition in which the risk of hemorrhage increases directly with a fall in platelet count (Newland, 1995). Although this approach clearly increases the efficacy of chemotherapy, intensive platelet replacement regimes risk exposure to infection and alloimmunization. In certain circumstances both red cell and granulocyte transfusions can be considered, particularly in patients with evident cardiopulmonary and vascular disease or bacterial/fungal infections, respectively.

However, in all instances the increased use of these products has health and financial implications. It is also reasonable to conclude that the eventual widespread use of recombinant human hematopoietic growth factors may circumvent the need for direct cell transfusion or blood-derived products.

2.2. Peptide Factors

2.2.1. Stimulatory Factors

Now, a large number of glycoproteins that regulate hematopoietic progenitor cell proliferation and differentiation have been identified. Consequently, these factors are increasingly used to support and assist the recovery of bone marrow during and postchemotherapy. Indeed it is conceivable that these drugs will eventually supplant blood-derived products. For example, the use of recombinant human granulocyte colony-stimulating factor to enhance myelopoietic recovery reduces the severity and extent of neutropenia, hence decreases the frequency of secondary infections and thereby the need for further intensive, hospital-based support (Testa and Dexter, 1992; Van Hoef *et al.*, 1994). Similarly, growth factors including the platelet growth factor thrombopoietin, that stimulate the magakaryocyte lineage may be able to reduce the risk of hemorrhage significantly by decreasing clotting times (Foster *et al.*, 1995).

Growth factors have also been used to support myelopoiesis during conventional cycles of chemotherapy and also to allow intensifying therapy. In one study, dose intensification using granulocyte macrophage-colony-stimulating Factor (GM-CSF) in combination with vincristine, ifosfamide, carboplatin, and etoposide indicated that three-weekly rather than four-weekly scheduling was tolerated in patients receiving GM-CSF. Further, although the incidence of febrile neutropenia, antibiotic use, and hospitalization or transfusion requirements was independent of GM-CSF use, the two-year survival for patients receiving this agent every three weeks was 32% compared with 25% for those on a four-weekly schedule versus 15% for the non-GM-CSF treated group (Ranson and Thatcher, 1995).

It is to be anticipated that the use of combined growth factors should ultimately allow a broader range of antitumor agents to be tolerated. However, there is little definitive evidence of the effects of hematopoietic growth factors on stem cells and the response of this cell population could be a major determinant of the future usefulness of the cytokines. If cytokine-mediated expansion of hematopoietic progenitors occurs at the cost of stem cell self-renewal capacity, then the possibility of longer term marrow failure has to be considered. Finally, the costs of using these currently expensive recombinant proteins may also limit their usefulness.

2.2.2. Inhibitory Factors

There are a number of naturally occurring cytokines produced by macrophages, fibroblasts, and T cells that inhibit the cell cycle of primitive hematopoietic cells. Among these, macrophage inflammatory protein 1alpha (MIP-1α) is currently in clinical trials. This 96 amino acid peptide is a reversible inhibitor of CFU-S proliferation and *in vitro* and *in vivo* protects hematopoietic cells from a variety of cycle-active antitumor agents, such as hydroxyurea and cytosine arabinoside (Graham *et al.*, 1990; Lord *et al.*, 1992). The cell-cycle inhibitory action of MIP-1α is abrogated in the progenitor cells of chronic myelogenous leukemia and thus presents the possibility of sparing normal hematopoietic cells from toxicity without affecting the sensitivity of the tumor cells. However, as MIP-1 α provides protection only against the cytotoxic effects of cell-cycle-active agents, its use may be limited to regimens containing such drugs.

2.3. Bone Marrow and Peripheral Blood Progenitor Cell Transplantation

The use of allogenic bone marrow transplantation allows giving more intense courses of chemotherapy, particularly for refractory or relapsed disease, as compromised hematopoietic function is reconstituted from the normal donor graft. In leukemic patients this may give the added advantage of a graft versus disease effect. However, because a minority of patients have eligible donors, the infusion of autologous marrow is also used to assist recovery post-chemotherapy (Shpall *et al.*, 1994).

Peripheral blood progenitor cells (PBPC), as an alternative to marrow, are now widely used to assist hematopoietic recovery and are often used as an alternative to bone marrow transplantation. These cells are mobilized into circulation by administering cytotoxic drugs and hematopoietic growth factors. There is a wealth of data suggesting that they sustain short to medium term hematopoiesis and therefore are of major use in combating the acute effects of myelosuppression (Van Hoef *et al.*, 1994a; Pettengell *et al.*, 1995). Encouraging data also suggest that PBPC may reconstitute long-term hematopoietic recovery (Dunbar *et al.*, 1995). The combined importance of bone marrow and PBPC transplantation, combined with hematopoietic growth factor treatments, is that they have allowed using high-dose therapy as a component of first-line treatment for a number of cancers. In some instances this strategy is producing higher response and survival rates (Leonard, 1997).

Although these techniques are effective in overcoming acute myelosuppression in many instances, they are not helpful in overcoming the long-term, particularly the leukemogenic effects, of chemotherapy on the hematopoietic system. Indeed the high-dose strategies that they have helped to become more commonplace may result in an increased incidence of long-term, therapeutically related disease.

2.4. Perspective

The previous protocols (except for the proposed use of MIP-1α) emphasis the rescue of already damaged marrow postchemotherapy. But the long term effects of residual damage in surviving (stem) cells are not addressed, and it is anticipated that the chronic effects of such damage will in fact be exacerbated because cells survive otherwise lethal levels of toxic insult. In addition, the resistance of tumor cells, especially after high-dose therapy, still remains a major problem. Therefore a treatment regimen that protects sensitive cells from the acute and chronic effects of chemotherapy and which also incorporates a tumour sensitization strategy could dramatically increase the efficacy of many antitumor drugs. One approach to achieving this would be to use gene transfer technology to express drug resistance functions in the stem/early progenitor cells of dose-limiting organs and thereby to render them less sensitive to the toxic effects that lead to acute and chronic tissue injury (Baum *et al.*, 1996; Rafferty *et al.*, 1996). An ideal and elegant extension of this concept is to incorporate mutations into the resistance gene, so that its product retains full functional activity against primary substrates, but becomes insensitive to inhibition/inactivation by pseudosubstrates that normally reverse resistance. This raises the prospect of circumventing the resistance of tumor cells and simultaneously affording protection against collateral toxicity to normal (mutant-expressing) cells. Now, protecting the more primitive cells of the hematopoietic system is a sensible first objective which would serve as the archetypical study for protecting other drug-sensitive sites. Following we review the current status of a number of gene-based strategies that use drug resistance functions to augment the therapeutic index of anticancer agents.

3. GENE TRANSFER, EXPRESSION, AND STEM CELL PROTECTION

The success of any approach of this nature is a function of the vector used for transfer, the target cell population, and the level and duration of expression required of the therapeutic gene.

3.1. Gene Transfer into Hematopoietic Cells

Currently, the most widely used and efficient method for introducing genetic material into hematopoietic cells exploits the natural ability of viruses, and particularly retroviruses, to infect and express their genomes in a variety of cells (Ali *et al.*, 1995; Miller *et al.*, 1993; and see Chapters 3 and 4). Now large number of retroviral genomes have been modified to constrain their pathogenicity and limit their replicative competence in target cells thereby making them safer to handle and use in humans (Miller *et al.*, 1993; Russell and Miller, 1996). Removing such deleterious sequences has also created space for inserting exogenous gene sequences that may be of therapeutic value and which can be expressed under the control of viral or nonviral promoters, as appropriate. A number of additional features make the retroviruses useful as gene therapy vectors including their capacity to integrate into the host genome. The significance of this is that the recombinant viral genome, including the therapeutic cassette, is inherited by the progeny of infected cells. In hematopoietic cells, infection of stem cells would result in the mature cells of this system inheriting the gene and potentially its capacity to be expressed.

The actual cellular target for gene delivery depends on the desired clinical outcome of the therapeutic strategy. It could be argued that if acute myelosuppression is to be overcome, expression of resistance genes in mature progenitors would be sufficient. This, however, is likely to have a number of shortcomings, principally because most (although not all) mature hematopoietic cells have a relatively short life span (Dexter and Spooncer, 1987). Thus, because chemotherapy is usually a series of successive treatments, it is likely that the duration of the therapeutic regimen would exceed that of any protective period, resulting in only a partial alleviation of myelosuppression. Similarly if a patient relapsed and required further chemotherapy, it would be ideal not to have to carry out a second round of gene transfer. Finally, the protection of committed progenitor cells would do little to combat therapeutically related hematopoietic malignancy (Boffetta and Kaldor, 1994; Najean, 1987). Because genetic changes in hematopoietic stem cells are considered a major etiological component of these disorders, then the most primitive cell population must be targets for expression (Dexter and Spooncer, 1987). Notwithstanding this, it is not unreasonable to consider that the descendants of these cells will also express resistance functions and will also be protected from the collateral toxic effects of chemotherapy.

However, as targets for gene transfer, the pluripotent stem cell population poses a number of difficulties (Dunbar and Young, 1996). They are difficult to maintain in culture without undergoing differentiation or apoptosis and this, taken together with their rarity (<0.01% of the total hematopoietic compartment), represents a major challenge in terms of gene delivery to and expression in hematopoietic stem cells. An additional impediment to gene transfer into these cells, at least using vectors, such as retroviruses that require dividing cells as targets, is that stem cells are largely proliferatively quiescent. Nevertheless, these problems are not insurmountable. Growth factors have been used to maintain the survival of hematopoietic stem cell populations *ex vivo* and to explore ways for inducing them to proliferate (Luskey *et al.*, 1992). Under these circumstances there is, of course, the risk that the self-renewal capacity of the stem cell is jeopardized. When these *ex vivo* manipulations are used as a component of a gene therapy protocol, any commitment to differentiation would be accompanied by eventual clonal extinction and the loss of the therapeutic gene. One way to compensate for this outcome is to culture bone marrow in close association with the stromal elements in which the hematopoietic stem and progenitor cells normally reside and function. Cells maintained in such long-term bone marrow cultures can be used to reestablish hematopoiesis in experimental animals and humans during bone marrow transplantation and thus to retain pluripotent characteristics (Dexter *et al.*, 1977). Additionally, the stem cell component of these cultures are more readily transduced by retroviruses if they are in a stromal environment (Moore *et al.*, 1992). Thus further understanding the self-renewal and repopulating abilities of the cells in these conditions is likely to lead to more efficient gene delivery protocols. This will be especially true if protocols for enriching early hematopoietic cells (*e.g.*, sorting using antibodies to CD34 or by functional selection for proliferative quiescence) do not overwhelmingly abrogate their capacity to behave as stem cells (Berardi *et al.*, 1995).

3.2. Genes Conferring Drug Resistance

A large number of gene products confer cellular drug resistance, and many of these have been identified as major factors that influence the responsiveness of tumors to a variety of antitumor agents (Table I; Gottesman *et al.*, 1995; Margison and O'Connor, 1990; Moscow and Dixon, 1993). It is also clear from correlative measurements of resistance functions and particularly from gene transfer experiments that otherwise sensitive cells are (often dramatically) protected from the myriad biological effects of clinically active agents by enhanced expression of such resistance factors (Gottesmann *et al.*, 1994). As a result, many avenues of research

Table I
Some Resistance Factors that Could Be Useful for Gene-Based Approaches to Stem Cell Protection

Resistance function	Agent(s) protected against
Multidrug resistance 1 (MDR-1)	Anthracyclins (adriamycin, daunorubicin) Vinca alkaloids (vincristine, vinblastine)
(Mutant) O^6-alkylguanine-DNA-alkyltransferase	O^6-Alkylating agents (dacarbazine, temozolomide, BCNU)
Mutant dihydrofolate reductase	Methotrexate
Aldehyde dehydrogenase	Cyclophosphamide
Thymidylate synthase	5-Fluoracil
Glutathione-based detoxifying enzymes	Anthracyclins
Metallothioien	Cisplatin, chlorambucil

now focus on enhancing the resistance level of bone marrow using these types of genes, but here we review the progress of work with multidrug resistance gene (MDR-1) and O^6-alkylguanine-DNA alkyltransferase (ATase) encoded resistance (Gottesman *et al.*, 1995; Margison and O'Connor, 1990).

3.2.1. MDR-1

The MDR-1 gene is probably the most obvious candidate to use for stem cell protection because of the broad substrate specificity of this mechanism (Gottesman *et al.*, 1995). The product of the MDR-1 gene, a 170-kDa plasma-membrane-associated p-glycoprotein (P-gp), functions as an ATP-dependent drug efflux pump that prevents the intracellular accumulation of agents to detrimental concentrations (Juliano and Ling, 1976). Intriguingly, P-gp confers resistance to a wide range of unrelated agents, such as anthracyclins, podophyllotoxins, vinca alkaloids, actinomycin D, and taxol. Resistance is often acquired and may be the result of an amplified MDR-1 locus or may reflect more subtle transcriptional controls (Van der Bliek, 1988). Whichever, the expression of this protein may be a key determinant of successful chemotherapy involving these agents, and there is intense interest in developing agents that act as pseudosubstrates and could be used to saturate P-gp-mediated tumor resistance before conventional chemotherapy (Gottesman *et al.*, 1995; Kessel, 1986). However, unless these agents are tumor-specific, there is a risk that their use will exacerbate the collateral toxic effects of agents in normal cells.

Experiments in mice that overexpress P-gp in bone marrow have shown that it is possible to overcome leucopenia and other features of myelosuppression after exposure to a number of appropriate agents. In those studies that involve retroviruses, the transduction of early progenitor cells has been demonstrated and resistance to appropriate agents shown (Licht, 1995; Richardson and Bank, 1995; Sorrentino *et al.*, 1992). Importantly, it was also possible to show resistance to taxol-induced myelosuppression in mice which had received modified marrow from previously transplanted primary recipients, indicating transduction and expression in hematopoietic stem cells (Hanania and Deisseroth, 1994). *In vitro* studies using human CD34$^+$ cells from either marrow, peripheral, or cord blood as targets for P-gp transduction have also demonstrated the potential efficacy of this approach. In one case 25% of viable CD34$^+$ cells had detectable levels of P-gp after two weeks in culture, although the transduced protein was localized to the nuclear and the plasma membrane (Bertolini *et al.*, 1994). It is not yet clear what effect, if any, this will have on the normal function of the nuclear membrane but it is important to consider potentially adverse disturbances in normal cellular physiology as a consequence of gene transfer. The functional status of P-gp in these studies was determined by analyzing the efflux of the fluorescent substrate rhodamine 123 (Rh123) or by the resistance to taxol of transduced versus untransduced CD34$^+$ selected cells. Transduced cells did not accumulate Rh123 and were more resistant to taxol than untransduced cells. Importantly, it has been recently demonstrated that expression of P-gp as a result of retroviral gene transfer can protect CD34$^+$ cells *in vitro* against doses of taxol corresponding to the levels seen in human serum during chemotherapy (Baum *et al.*, 1995). Phase 1 clinical trials of MDR-1 transduction into human bone marrow are now in progress or planned (Hesdorffer *et al.*, 1994; O'Shaughnessy *et al.*, 1994).

The use of the MDR-1 gene in cell protection protocols has also led to the use of P-gp expression as a dominant selectable marker to identify cells that are transduced with an otherwise unselectable gene (Licht *et al.*, 1997). This sort of strategy has taken two approaches. The first of these used chimeric P-gp fusion proteins with, for example, adenosine deaminase or alpha-galactosidase (Germann *et al.*, 1990; Sugimoto *et al.*, 1995). In both cases it was possible to select cells that express the unselected function based on increased colchicine or vincristine resistance. As an alternative, coexpression of a second protein along with P-gp was achieved by utilizing internal ribosomal entry signals to allow translating both proteins from a single bicistronic messenger RNA (Metz *et al.*, 1996). Thus, the use of a single promoter element to drive expression of both genes avoids the problem of promoter silencing relative to the unselected gene function. Although it may be desirable or even essential in some cases, to have some means of selecting cells that express "passenger" genes of interest, it is worth considering what hazards are associated with using P-gp substrates, many of which are probably human carcinogens (Tinwell and Ashby, 1994), as selective agents. In clinical gene therapy, selecting of cells that have escaped toxicity risks returning to patients cells that may carry mutagenic levels of DNA damage. Furthermore, if selection is to be carried out *in vivo* (*i.e.*, following reinfusion of transduced cells), adverse short-term and long-term effects on other tissues would be anticipated.

3.2.2. ATase

The ATase protein repairs O^6-alkylguanine (O^6-alkG) adducts in DNA, which may be toxic, mutagenic, transforming, carcinogenic, clastogenic, and teratogenic, if allowed to persist (Margison and O'Connor, 1990; Pegg, 1990). Agents that typically introduce this type of damage into DNA are the chloroethylnitrosoureas (*e.g.*, 1,3,bis (2-chloroethyl)1-nitrosourea (BCNU), mitozolomide) and related methylating agents (*e.g.*, DTIC, temozolomide), collectively known as the O^6-alkylating agents. Because of the toxicity of this group, they are often used as antitumor treatments (D'Incalci *et al.*, 1988). The toxic effects of O^6-chloroethylguanine probably result as a consequence of interstrand cross-links forming *via* the cyclic intermediate *N*1, O^6-ethanoguanine (Tong *et al.*, 1982). There is evidence that this latter adduct forms a covalent complex with ATase and this may in itself be significantly toxic (Gonzaga *et al.*, 1992). It is less clear how O^6-methylguanine (O^6-MeG) mediates a toxic effect. It may be that it relates to the ability of O^6-MeG to mismatch with thymine. This mispair is a substrate for DNA mismatch repair mechanisms which attempt to excise the thymine residue. The mispair is regenerated following DNA replication, and attempts at repair again ensue, generating a potentially lethal, effectively permanent strand break (Ceccotti *et al.*, 1996). However, a recent report indicates that O^6-MeG in DNA arrests the replicative apparatus *in vitro* (Voigt and Topal, 1995). Such events *in vivo* could prove cytotoxic. The O^6-alkylating agents are also carcinogenic and this most likely results from the miscoding potential of O^6-alkG as described previously (Saffhill *et al.*, 1985).

Now a large body of data show that overexpression of ATase in cells otherwise sensitive to O^6-alkylating agents confers protection against the toxic, mutagenic, carcinogenic, clastogenic, and transforming effects of these agents (reviewed in Margison and O'Connor, 1990; Pegg, 1990). Furthermore, overexpression of human or bacterial ATases in the tissues of transgenic mice protects them from the induction of thymic lymphoma (Dumenco *et al.*, 1993) and hepatocellular carcinoma (Nakatsuru *et al.*, 1993) by *N*-methyl-*N*-nitrosourea (MNU) and *N*-nitrosodimethylamine respectively. The bone marrow of mice that are homozygous for targeted mutations in both ATase alleles is characterized by hypersensitivity to MNU, suggesting that functional ATase expression is a critical determinant of the outcome of exposure of normal cells to this class of DNA damaging agents (Tsuzuki *et al.*, 1996). The role of ATase as a potential resistance factor in tumors has also been established in a number of experimental studies in which the levels of ATase correlate with the response of human tumor xenografts to O^6-alkylating agents (Brent *et al.*, 1993). These and related studies have stimulated interest in approaches to surmounting the resistance provided by ATase in tumor cells (Margison *et al.*, 1996). Recent efforts to improve the chemotherapeutic efficacy of O^6-alkylating agents have centered on attempts to deplete the ATase protein. One such approach is to use alkyl analogs of free base guanine, such as O^6-benzylguanine (O^6-beG), which is a potent inactivator of mammalian ATase (Elder *et al.*, 1994) and often dramatically potentiates drug toxicity *in vitro* and *in vivo* (Baer *et al.*, 1993; Dolan *et al.*, 1990, 1991). Although such treatments increase the tumour kill by BCNU in xenograft-bearing animals, a concomitant increase in nonspecific toxicity of the agent has also been reported (Dolan *et al.*, 1993). Further, exposure of human primary bone marrow to O^6-beG at concentrations that would be expected to deplete ATase activity in many tumors renders hematopoietic cells more sensitive to being killed by the methylating agent temozolomide (Fairbairn *et al.*, 1995). In a subsequent analysis we have shown that O^6-beG also increases the *in vivo* toxicity and clastogenicity of BCNU and temozolomide (Chinnasamy *et al.*, 1997). Based on these findings, it is anticipated that the frequency of mutation may also increase as a result of ATase depletion by this means. Clearly, caution is required in the current clinical trials if the problem of cytotoxicity and therapeutically related secondary malignancy are not to be exacerbated.

The use of ATase depleting agents is also significant in any gene therapy strategy aimed at overcoming O^6-alkylating-agent-induced acute and long-term bone marrow damage. Because the human ATase protein (in common with all its mammalian homologues) is very sensitive to O^6-beG depletion at levels likely to be physiologically achieved in humans, it is reasonable to conclude that any degree of protection bestowed on bone marrow by the product of a transduced ATase cDNA would be reduced or even totally abolished. Studies of the comparative reactivity of bacterial ATase homologues with O^6-beG have indicated that both the *E.coli ogt* and *ada* protein are more resistant to inactivation by this agent (Elder *et al.*, 1994). Indeed the *ada* protein is effectively refractory to reaction with O^6-beG. Thus, the use of *ada* in any transduction protocol would provide a system whereby bone marrow could be protected even in the presence of inactivators. However, the *in vivo* expression of a bacterial protein in human cells could have an immunological consequences (Harris *et al.*, 1995; Rafferty *et al.*, 1996). An alternative strategy to expressing *E.coli* proteins became available with the reports that the sensitivity of the human ATase (hAT) to O^6-beG is altered by mutating of key amino acid residues that may be critical in determining access of inactivator substances to the ATase active centre (Crone *et al.*, 1994). Thus alteration of proline$_{140}$ to alanine (hATPA mutant) results in a 16-fold increase in resistance to O^6-beG relative to wild-type hAT, as determined by IC_{50} measurements (the concentration of O^6-beG needed to achieve a 50% reduction in ATase activity, Table II). A more dramatic effect is achieved by further mutating of the hATPA protein. Changing glycine$_{156}$ to alanine increases the IC_{50} >1000-fold above the native protein. Clearly, expressing the hATPA/GA mutant in gene therapy could potentially protect bone marrow from the acute and longer term effects of the O^6-alkylating agents while allowing the concurrent use of ATase inactivators, such as O^6-beG. However, as a prelude to initiating extensive studies with this mutant, we further evaluated the characteristics of the PA and the PA/GA mutants (Hickson *et al.*, 1996). Many reported mutants of

Table II
Concentrations of O^6-beG Required to Achieve 50% Inactivation (IC_{50}) of Various ATases

ATase origin	O^6-beG IC_{50}(μM)
Human wild-type (hAT)	0.04
Mutant hAT (hATPA)	2.5
Mutant hAT (hATPA/GA)	>500
E. coli ada	>500

hAT are characterized by increased lability. In a gene therapy context, this would result in decreased protective capacity but might also result in enhanced immunogenicity because of increased degradation. In this respect, a small number of amino acid changes substantially alter the immunogenic profiles of a number of proteins (Ngo Giang Huong *et al.*, 1995). Concerns over the *in vitro* stability of the hATPA and hATPA/GA mutants were somewhat allayed by our observation that they are substantially stabilized in the presence of DNA and that the kinetics of methyl group transfer from MNU-treated calf thymus DNA is not significantly different relative to hAT. In the presence of added calf thymus DNA the IC_{50} for the hATPA/GA mutant is about 1200-fold higher than hAT (Figure 1). As a final test of the efficacy of the function of these mutants, both were expressed in a mammalian cell line that is normally highly sensitive to the toxic effects of O^6-alkylating agents (Hickson *et al.*, 1996). These experiments definitively demonstrate that although expression of both mutants and the wild-type hAT protein protect these cells from toxicity, this effect is abolished in the presence of physiologically relevant doses of O^6-beG in all cases except for the hATPA/GA mutant (Figure 2).

A number of studies that involve the expression of wild-type hAT or *ada* protein in primary murine bone marrow have been carried out by way of proof of principle (Allay *et al.*, 1995; Harris *et al.*, 1995; Jelinek *et al.*, 1996; Maze *et al.*, 1996; Moritz *et al.*, 1995). In mice reconstituted with hAT transduced bone marrow, several reports indicate a small to modest survival of hematopoietic progenitors to BCNU. In one of these studies it was possible to demonstrate hematopoietic protection over a five week period. Because committed progenitor cells were used as

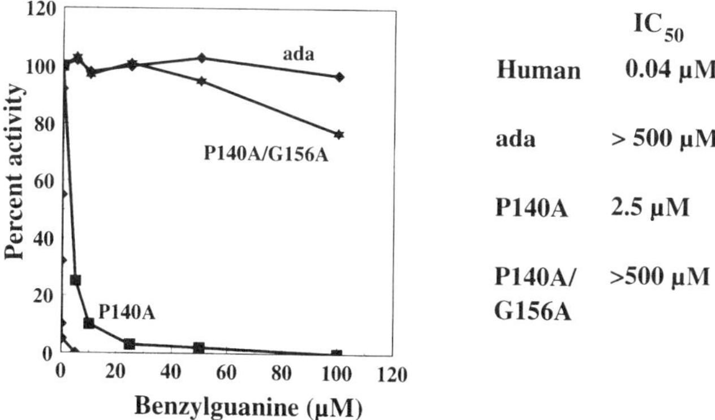

FIGURE 1. Residual activity of ATase proteins following preincubation with varying concentrations of O^6-beG for 1 hr at 37°C. Extracts from bacterial cells expressing wild-type or either of the mutant ATases were preincubated with increasing concentrations of O^6-beG for 1 hr in the presence of CT DNA. Then the ATase activities of the extracts were determined by adding [^{3}H]-MNU treated DNA substrate to measure the residual methyl transfer capacity. The hAT protein was inactivated by very low concentrations of O^6-beG ($IC_{50} = 0.16\,\mu M$). The hATPA protein was ~16 times ($IC_{50} = 2.5\,\mu M$) and the hATPA/GA protein >3000 times ($IC_{50} > 500\,\mu M$) more resistant to O^6-beG inactivation than the wild-type hAT protein. (For comparison, the depletion profiles of the bacterial *ada* ($IC_{50} > 500\,\mu M$) are included in the figure.)

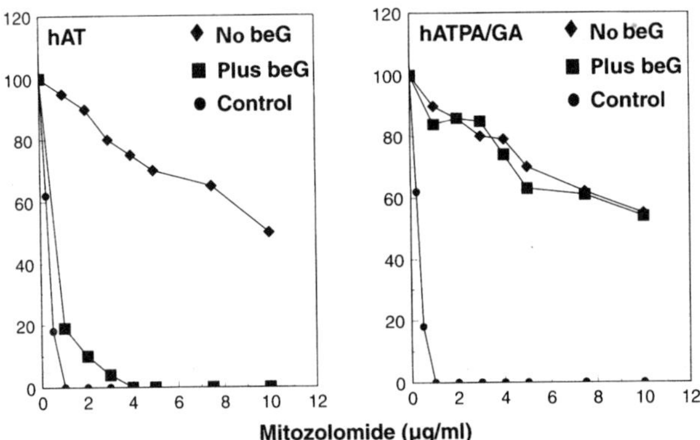

FIGURE 2. Survival of control, hAT (a,b), and hATPA/GA (c,d) that express RJKO cells after exposure to increasing concentrations of mitozolomide in the presence or absence of 20 µM O^6-beG. The results of an MTT-based assay for analyzing the growth inhibitory effects of mitozolomide are shown as percentage survival versus mitozolomide dose, and the points are the means of triplicate experiments. O^6-beG (20 µM) or vehicle control was added 2 hr before adding a range of doses of mitozolomide (0–10 µg/ml). Then the cells were incubated for five days (near confluence) before MTT assay. As predicted from their extremely low (negligible) levels of ATase, control RJKO cells are extremely sensitive to the toxic effects of mitozolomide. Expression of either the wild-type or double mutant ATase protein in these cells conferred significant resistance ($p < 0.001$) to the toxic effects of mitozolomide. Treatment with O^6-beG had no significant effect on the sensitivity of control cells to mitozolomide-induced toxicity. However, O^6-beG dramatically sensitize cells that express wild-type ATase to the cytotoxic effect of mitozolomide ($p < 0.001$). In contrast, cells that express the hATPA/GA protein retain their resistance to mitozolomide in the presence of 20 µM O^6-beG.

targets in these studies and not stem cells, the restricted timescale of protection is expected (Moritz *et al.*, 1995). In the other study, resistance of GM-CFC isolated from reconstituted mice to BCNU was demonstrated *in vitro*, although the effect of pretreatment with O^6-beG on progenitor survival was not reported. Experiments in mice carrying *ada*-reconstituted marrow has also demonstrated increased hematopoietic progenitor cell survival, depending on the dose of BCNU given. Some protection against anemia and thrombocytopenia but not neutropenia was observed (Harris *et al.*, 1995). Cell survival advantage was evident for at least 30 days and was also observed in the presence of O^6-beG as would be predicted. Although encouraging, it is still not possible to comment on the efficacy of long-term protection from myelosuppression by ATase gene transfer from these models.

Until now, our own studies have focused on using long-term murine bone marrow cultures to demonstrate the potential of stem cell protection (Jelinek *et al.*, 1996). After transducing primary cultures with the hAT cDNA, it was possible to demonstrate levels of ATase more than 100 times above those of controls in the nonadherent cells of the long-term cultures as long as four months posttransduction. This enhanced ATase level correlates with a threefold increase in the survival of GM-CFC to the toxic effects (LD37) of MNU. This protection was long-term and effective against three serial doses of MNU, indicating that very primitive cells had been transduced. It is clearly important to demonstrate this level and duration of protection *in vivo*, particularly to doses of O^6-alkylating agent that restrict the growth of human tumor xenografts.

4. FURTHER CONSIDERATIONS

4.1. General Advantages

The gene-based stem cell protection approach outlined has a number of potentially attractive features that might make it advantageous compared with existing protocols. Although initially small numbers of target cells might be transduced, it is anticipated that the frequency of drug-resistant cells will increase with each round of chemotherapy. Thus this particular application may be well suited to selection where dose intensification is a clinical option. Additionally, although long-term expression of drug resistance is desirable, it is not essential because the protective period need last only as long as the duration of chemotherapy, and thus many of the problems that hamper other gene therapy strategies as a consequence of gene silencing (Challita and Kohn, 1994) may not impinge to the same extent on stem cell protection.

The potential to generate resistance to a broad range of antitumor agents could become a major advantage of this strategy (*e.g.*, Doroshow *et al.*, 1995), thus using novel combinations of drugs to more efficiently effect tumor kill. Without a protective regimen, such novel drug cocktails might be prohibited because of their extreme myelotoxicity. Eventually the ability to determine "tumor drug-resistance profiles" would indicate which agents should be most active against the tumor, and then the choice of protective genes could be tailored for optimal chemotherapy.

Finally, for those antitumor drugs that are carcinogenic and cytotoxic, gene-based stem cell protection might also offer the hope of decreasing the frequency of therapeutically related malignancy by reducing the level of subtoxic damage in the hematopoietic stem cell compartment.

4.2. The Next Dose-Limiting Toxicities

A fairly self-evident criticism of any strategy for hematopoietic stem/progenitor cell protection, including any gene-based approach, relates to how much therapeutic advantage is gained from protection before the next dose-limiting toxicity level is reached. This relates in part to the inherent sensitivity of the tumor. In some cases small increases in dose might deliver a substantial tumor response. The use of agents, such as O^6-beG, might tip the balance in favor of enhanced tumor kill using nitrosoureas, but it is equally possible that collateral damage in other dose-limiting tissues might be exacerbated by using tumor sensitizers. The scale of this problem depends initially on how readily the toxicity in nonprotected tissues could be contained during periods of dose intensification.

A longer term prospect would be to use gene-based protection strategies for other drug-sensitive tissues. To achieve this it would mean that efficient *in vivo* delivery systems would have to be available, and a much clearer picture of the characteristics of stem cells in organs, such as gut, lung, and kidney, would need to be available. Although the technology for gene delivery to and expression at these sites is relatively new, reports are continually emerging with respect to targeting these tissues (Crystal *et al.*, 1995; Goldman *et al.*, 1995; Westbrook *et al.*, 1994). Therefore there is reason for cautious optimism, especially as vector systems, including nonviral methods, continue to evolve. Efforts to safeguard hematopoietic stem cells, although worthy in their own right, must thus be seen as a paradigm for protecting at-risk stem cells in other drug-sensitive tissues.

4.3. Target-Cell Selectability

Two separate issue relate to target cell selectability. The first of these is the need to transduce and to maintain appropriate levels of transgenic expression in the correct normal cell population. Thus identifying and using viral or mammalian gene promoters that are less likely to be constitutively down-regulated in early hematopoietic cells as a result of hypermethylation (Challita and Kohn, 1994) would overcome one of the most common technical obstacles encountered in situations where long term expression is desirable. To this end the development of vectors from viruses that replicate and sustain expression in embryonic stem cells and primitive haemopoietic stem cells may begin to settle some of these issues (Grez *et al.*, 1990). These problems, however, are not unique to the stem cell protection field but relate to nearly all gene therapy strategies.

A second issue associated with cell selectability is more specific to the chemoprotection approach and concerns the potentially catastrophic possibility of transducing drug resistance genes into tumor cells that may be contaminating bone marrow or peripheral blood samples due for transduction. There is now good evidence that such metastatic tumor cells contribute significantly to the tumor mass in patients who have received autologous bone marrow grafts and thus the risk of generating a drug-resistant tumor must be considered (Brenner *et al.*, 1993; Rill *et al.*, 1994). The level of risk initially depends on the origins of the primary disease. Hence, marrow contamination with metastases is generally more common in breast or prostate cancer compared with ovarian carcinoma in which such involvement is rare. However, it is important to use additional levels of control irrespective of the natural history of the primary disease. A number of options are possible. Purging strategies, either as positive selection for normal cells, negative selection against malignant cells, or a combination of both, are the most obvious approach to pursue (Negrin, 1992). Thus positive selection for the presence of CD34 cell surface marker would eradiate many tumor cells but is unlikely to be totally effective in purging because tumors derived from epithelia may express CD34 (Monihan *et al.*, 1994). This technique is more likely to be effective if combined with additional measures, such as the use of vectors that are more selective in transducing target cells by virtue of antibody- or ligand-mediated specificity (Buschle *et al.*, 1995; Han *et al.*, 1995; Kasahara *et al.*, 1994; Somia *et al.*, 1995; Wagner *et al.*, 1992) or that use tissue specific promoters to drive transgenic expression (Burn *et al.*, 1992; Dziennis *et al.*, 1995; Sun *et al.*, 1995; Yamaguchi *et al.*, 1994). The experimental experience with such vectors is that selectivity for transduction of or expression in the intended target cells is not always absolute. Still further alternatives include the coexpression of any one of a number of prodrug activating genes which could allow the ablation of all transduced cells. A variation on this theme is to use a mutant form of a drug-resistance gene which does not confer resistance to at least one type of antitumour cytotoxic agent which would again allow all transduced cells to be killed. Again the most useful strategy will likely result from combinating these techniques but until their general efficacy is established it will be critical to maintain a backup, unmanipulated marrow for an autologous graft.

4.4. Therapy-Related Malignancy

The prospect for reducing the frequency of therapeutically related malignancy by enhanced expression of drug-resistance functions in hematopoietic stem cells has already been alluded to. Certainly, in murine model systems the expression of ATase is important in modifying target tissue response to carcinogenic doses of appropriate alkylating agents. If a similar effect were realized in bone marrow transduced with and expressing one or more drug-resistance genes, then the impact of this strategy for stem cell protection could be immense. However, the indications from carcinogenesis studies may not be the best guide for what to expect clinically. During chemotherapy, higher, more intentionally toxic doses of drug are given and thus much higher levels of DNA damage are likely to accumulate. One impact of enhanced DNA repair gene expression would be a reduced level of damage in a proportion of cells to subtoxic but not necessarily submutagenic levels. This would result in the survival of a population of cells that would otherwise have died, and expansion of these survivors could result in an enhanced mutational frequency that could give rise to a malignant clonal population. Clearly a much more careful evaluation of the effectiveness of enhanced DNA repair in providing long-term protection *in vivo* against the myriad effects of O^6-alkylating agents is necessary.

5. CONCLUDING REMARKS

Current data suggest that, given adequate gene transfer and expression in target cells, hematopoietic stem cell protection during chemotherapy should certainly provide protection against the toxic side effects of drug treatment. The combination of this with tumor sensitization offers exciting prospects for significant increases in the therapeutic results to be achieved with current treatment schedules and holds out hopes for developing new, more effective schedules. However, issues surrounding late effects, damage at sites other than the bone marrow, and the transduction of metastatic tumor cells remain to be addressed.

6. REFERENCES

Ali, M., Lemoine, N. R., and Ring, C. J., 1994, The use of DNA viruses as vectors for gene therapy, *Gene Therapy* **1**:367–384.

Allay, J. A., Dumenco, L. L., Koc, O. N., Liu, L., and Gerson, S. L., 1995, Retroviral transduction and expression of the human alkyltransferase cDNA provides nitrosourea resistance to haematopoietic cells, *Blood* **85:**3342–3351.

Baer, J. C., Freeman, A. A., Newlands, E. S., Watson, A. J., Rafferty, J. A., and Margison, G. P., 1993, Depletion of O^6-alkylguanine-DNA alkyltransferase correlates with potentiation of temozolomide and CCNU toxicity in human tumour cells, *Br. J. Cancer* **67:**1299–1302.

Baum, C., Hegewisch Becker, S., Eckert, H. G., Stocking, C., and Ostertag, W., 1995, Novel retroviral vectors for efficient expression of the multidrug resistance (mdr-1) gene in early haematopoietic cells, *J. Virol.* **69:**7541–7547.

Baum, C., Margison, G. P., Eckert, H-G., Fairbairn, L. J., Ostertag, W., and Rafferty, J. A., 1996, Gene transfer to augment the therapeutic index of anticancer chemotherapy, *Gene Therapy* **3:**1–3.

Berardi, A. C., Wang, A., Levine, J. D., Lopez, P., and Scadden, D. T., 1995, Functional isolation and characterization of human haematopoietic stem cells, *Science* **267:**104–108.

Bertolini, F., de Monte, L., Corsini, C., Lazzari, L., Lauri, E., Soligo, D., Ward, M., Bank, A., and Malavasi, F., 1994, Retrovirus-mediated transfer of the multidrug resistance gene into human haemopoietic progenitor cells, *Br. J. Haematol.* **88:**318–324.

Boffetta, P., and Kaldor, J. M., 1994, Secondary malignancies following cancer chemotherapy, *Acta Oncol.* **33:**591–598.

Brenner, M. K., Rill, D. R., Moen, R. C., Krance, R. A., Mirro, J. Jr., Anderson, W. F., and Ihle, J. N., 1993, Gene-marking to trace origin of relapse after autologous bone-marrow transplantation, *Lancet* **341:**85–86.

Brent, T. P., von Wronski, M. A., Edwards, C. C., Bromley, M., Margison, G. P., Rafferty, J. A., Pegram, C. N., and Bigner, D. D., 1993, Identification of nitrosourea-resistant human rhabdomyosarcomas by *in situ* immunostaining of O^6-methylguanine-DNA methyltransferase, *Oncol. Res.* **5:**83–86.

Burn, T. C., Satterthwaite, A. B., and Tenen, D. G., 1992, The human CD34 haematopoietic stem cell antigen promoter and a 3′ enhancer direct haematopoietic expression in tissue culture, *Blood* **80:**3051–3059.

Buschle, M., Cotten, M., Kirlappos, H., Mechtler, K., Schaffner, G., Zauner, W., Birnstiel, M. L., and Wagner, E., 1995, Receptor-mediated gene transfer into human T lymphocytes via binding of DNA/CD3 antibody particles to the CD3 T cell receptor complex, *Hum. Gene Ther.* **6:**753–761.

Ceccotti, S., Aquilina, G., Macpherson, P., Yamada, M., Karran, P., and Bignami, M., 1996, Processing of O^6-methylguanine by mismatch correction in human cell-extracts, *Curr. Biol.* **6:**1528–1531.

Challita, P. M., and Kohn, D. B., 1994, Lack of expression from a retroviral vector after transduction of murine haematopoietic stem cells is associated with methylation *in vivo*, *Proc. Natl. Acad. Sci. USA* **91:**2567–2571.

Chinnasamy, N., Rafferty, J. A., Hickson, I., Ashby, J., Tinwell, H., Margison, G. P., Dexter, T. M., and Fairbairn, L. J., 1997, O^6-benzylguanine potentiates the *in vivo* toxicity and mutagenicity of temozolomide and BCNU in mouse bone marrow, *Blood* **89:**1566–1573.

Crone, T. M., Goodtzova, K., Edara, S., and Pegg, A. E., 1994, Mutations in human O^6-alkylguanine-DNA alkyltransferase imparting resistance to O^6-benzylguanine, *Cancer Res.* **54:**6221–6227.

Crystal, R. G., Jaffe, A., Brody, S., Mastrangeli, A., McElvaney, N. G., Rosenfeld, M., Chu, C. S., Danel, C., Hay, J., and Eissa, T., 1995, A phase 1 study, in cystic fibrosis patients, of the safety, toxicity, and biological efficacy of a single administration of a replication deficient, recombinant adenovirus carrying the cDNA of the normal cystic fibrosis transmembrane conductance regulator gene in the lung, *Hum. Gene Ther.* **6:**643–666.

Dexter, T. M., Allen, T. D., and Lajtha, L. G., 1997, Conditions controlling the proliferation of haemopoietic stem cells in vitro, *J. Cell Physiol.* **91:**335–344.

Dexter, T. M., and Spooncer, E., 1987, Growth and differentiation in the hemopoietic system, *Annu. Rev. Cell Biol.* **3:**423–441.

D'Incalci, M., Citti, L., Taverna, P., and Catapona, C. V., 1988, Importance of the DNA repair enzyme O^6-alkyltransferase (AT) in cancer chemotherapy, *Cancer Treat. Rev.* **15:**5723–5727.

Dolan, M. E., Moschel, R. C., and Pegg, A. E., 1990, Depletion of mammalian O^6-alkylguanine-DNA alkyltransferase activity by O^6-benzylguanine provides a means to evaluate the role of this protein in protection against carcinogenic and therapeutic alkylating agents, *Proc. Natl. Acad. Sci. USA* **87:**5368–5372.

Dolan, M. E., Mitchell, R. B., Mummert, C., Moschel, R. C., and Pegg, A. E., 1991, Effect of O^6-benzylguanine analogues on sensitivity of human tumour cells to the cytotoxic effects of alkylating agents, *Cancer Res.* **51:**3367–3372.

Dolan, M. E., Pegg, A. E., Moschel, R. C., and Grindey. G. B., 1993, Effect of O^6-benzylguanine on the sensitivity of human colon tumour xenografts to 1,3-bis(2-chloroethyl)-1-nitrosourea (BCNU). *Biochem. Pharmacol.* **46:**285–290.

Doroshow, J. H., Metz, M. Z., Matsumoto, L., Winters, K. A., Sakai, M., Muramatsu, M., and Kane, S. E., 1995, Transduction of NIH 3T3 cells with a retrovirus carrying both human MDR1 and glutathione *S*-transferase pi produces broad-range multidrug resistance, *Cancer Res.* **55:**4073–4078.

Dumenco, L. L., Allay, E., Norton, K., and Gerson, S. L., 1993, The prevention of thymic lymphomas in transgenic mice by human O^6-alkylguanine-DNA alkyltransferase, *Science* **259:**219–222.

Dunbar, C. E., Cottler Fox, M., Ja, O. S., Doren, S., Carter, C., Berenson, R., Brown, S., Moen, R. C., Greenblatt, J., Stewart, F. M., Berenson, R., Brown, S., Moen, R. C., Greenblatt J., Stewart, F. M., Leitman, S. F., Wilson, W. H., Cowan, K., Young, N. S., and Nienhuis, A. W., 1995, Retrovirally marked CD34-enriched peripheral blood and bone marrow cells contribute to long-term engraftment after autologous transplantation, *Blood* **85:**3048–3057.

Dunbar, C. E., and Young, N. S., 1996, Gene marking and gene therapy directed at primary haemopoietic stem cells, *Curr. Opinion Haematol.* **3:**430–437.

Dziennis, S., Van Etten, R. A., Pahl, H. L., Morris, D. L., Rothstein, T. L., Blosch, C. M., Perlmutter, R. M., and Tenen, D. G., 1995, The CD11b promoter directs high-level expression of reporter genes in macrophages in transgenic mice [published erratum appears in 1995, *Blood* **85**(7):1983], *Blood* **85:**319–329.

Elder, R. H., Margison, G. P., and Rafferty, J. A., 1994, Differential inactivation of mammalian and *Escherichia coli* O^6-alkylguanine-DNA alkyltransferases by O^6-benzylguanine, *Biochem. J.* **298:**231–235.

Fairbairn, L. J., Watson, A. J., Rafferty, J. A., Elder, R. H., and Margison, G. P., 1995, O^6-benzylguanine increases the sensitivity of human primary bone marrow cells to the cytotoxic effects of temozolomide, *Exp. Hematol.* **23:**112–116.

Foster, D. C., Sprecher, C. A., Grant, F. J., Kramer, J. M., Kuijper, J. L., Holly, R. D., Whitmore, T. E., Heipel, M. D., Bell, L. A., Ching, A. F., McGrane, V., Hart, C., Ohara, P. J., and Lok, S., 1995, Human thrombopoietin: Gene structure, cDNA sequence, expression, and chromosomal localization, *Proc. Natl. Acad. Sci. USA* **91:**13023–13027.

Germann, U. A., Chin, K. V., Pastan, I., and Gottesman, M. M., 1990, Retroviral transfer of a chimeric multidrug resistance-adenosine deaminase gene, *FASEB J.* **4:**1501–1507.

Goldman, M. J., Litzky, L. A., Engelhardt, J. F., and Wilson, J. M., 1995, Transfer of the CFTR gene to the lung of nonhuman primates with E1-deleted, E2a-defective recombinant adenoviruses: A preclinical toxicology study, *Hum. Gene Ther.* **6:**839–851.

Gonzaga, P. E., Potter, P. M., Niu, T. Q., Yu, D., Ludlum, D. B., Rafferty, J. A., Margison, G. P., and Brent, T. P., 1992, Identification of the cross-link between human O^6-methylguanine-DNA methyltransferase and chloroethylnitrosourea-treated DNA, *Cancer Res.* **52:**6052–6058.

Gottesman, M. M., Germann, U. A., Aksentijevich, I., Sugimoto, Y., Cardarelli, C. O., and Pastan, I., 1994, Gene transfer of drug resistance genes. Implications for cancer therapy, *Ann. N.Y. Acad. Sci.* **716:**126–138.

Gottesman, M. M., Hrycyna, C. A., Schoenlein, P. V., Germann, U. A., and Pastan, I., 1995, Genetic analysis of the multidrug transporter, *Ann. Rev. Genet.* **29:**607–649.

Graham, G. J., Wright, E. G., Hewick, R., Wolpe, S. D., Wilkie, N. M., Donaldson, D., Lorimore, S., and Pragnell, I. B., 1990, Identification and characterization of an inhibitor of haemopoietic stem cell proliferation, *Nature* **344:**442–444.

Grez, M., Akgun, E., Hilberg, F., and Ostertag, W., 1990, Embryonic stem cell virus, a recombinant murine retrovirus with expression in embryonic stem cells, *Proc. Natl. Acad. Sci. USA* **87:**9202–9206.

Han, X., Kasahara, N., and Kan, Y. W., 1995, Ligand-directed retroviral targeting of human breast cancer cells, *Proc. Natl. Acad. Sci. USA* **92:**9747–9751.

Hanania, E. G., and Deisseroth, A. B., 1994, Serial transplantation shows that early haematopoietic precursor cells are transduced by MDR-1 retroviral vector in a mouse gene therapy model, *Cancer Gene Ther.* **1:**21–25.

Harris, L. C., Marathi, U. K., Edwards, C. C., Houghton, P. J., Srivastava, D. K., Vanin, E. F., Sorrentino, B. P., and Brent, T. P., 1995, Retroviral transfer of a bacterial alkyltransferase gene into murine bone marrow protects against chloroethylnitrosourea cytotoxicity, *Clin. Cancer Res.* **1:**1359–1368.

Hesdorffer, C., Antman, K., Bank, A., Fetell, M., Mears, G., and Begg, M, 1994, Human MDR gene transfer in patients with advanced cancer, *Hum. Gene Ther.* **5:**1151–1160.

Hickson, I., Fairbairn, L. J., Chinnasamy, N., Margison, G. P., Dexter, T. M., and Rafferty, J. A., 1996, Protection of mammalian cells against chloroethylating agent toxicity by an O^6-benzylguanine-resistant mutant of human O^6-alkylguanine-DNA-alkyltransferase, *Gene Ther.* **3:**868–877.

Jelinek, J., Fairbairn, L. J., Dexter, T. M., Rafferty, J. A., Stocking, C., Ostertag, W., and Margison, G. P., 1996, Long-term protection of haematopoiesis against the cytotoxic effects of multiple doses of nitrosourea by retrovirus-mediated expression of human O^6-alkylguanine DNA-alkyltransferase, *Blood* **87:**1957–1961.

Juliano, R. L., and Ling, V., 1976, A surface glycoprotein modulating drug permeability in Chinese hamster ovary cell mutants, *Biochim. Biophys. Acta* **455:**152–162.

Kasahara, N., Dozy, A. M., and Kan, Y. W., 1994, Tissue-specific targeting of retroviral vectors through ligand-receptor interactions [see comments], *Science* **266:**1373–1376.

Kessel, D., 1986, Circumvention of resistance to anthracyclines by calcium antagonists and other membrane-perturbing agents, *Cancer Surv.* **5:**109–127.

Leonard, R. C., 1997, The advancement of high dose chemotherapy and dose intensification schedules, *Ann. Oncol.* Suppl **8:**S3–8.

Licht, T., Aksentijevich, I., Gottesman, M. M., and Pastan, I., 1995, Efficient expression of functional human MDR1 gene in murine bone marrow after retroviral transduction of purified haematopoietic stem cells, *Blood* **86:**111–121.

Licht, T., Herrmann, F., Gottesman, M. M., and Pastan, I., 1997, *In vivo* drug-selectable genes: A new concept in gene therapy, *Stem Cells* **15:**104–111.

Lord, B. I., Dexter, T. M., Clements, J. M., Hunter, M. A., and Gearing, A. J., 1992, Macrophage inflammatory protein protects multipotent haematopoietic cells from the cytotoxic effects of hydroxyurea *in vivo*, *Blood* **79:**2605–2609.

Luskey, B. D., Rosenblatt, M., Zsebo, K., and Williams, D. A., 1992, Stem cell factor, interleukin-3, and interleukin-6 promote retroviral-mediated gene transfer into murine haematopoietic stem cells, *Blood* **80:**396–402.

Margison, G. P., and O'Connor, P. J. 1990, Biological consequences of reactions with DNA: Role of specific lesions, in *Handbook of Experimental Pharmacology* 94/1 (C. S. Cooper, and P. L. Grover, eds.), Springer, Berlin, Heidelberg, pp. 547–571.

Margison, G. P., Rafferty, J. A., Elder, R. H., Kelly, J., Watson, A. J., Willington, M. A., Hickson, I., Fairbairn, L. J., Dexter, T. M., Jelinek, J., Stocking, C., Baum, C., Ostertag, W., Eghhazi, S., Hansson, J., Ringborg, U., Donnelly, D., McMurry, T. B. H., McCormick, J., and McElhinney, R. S., 1996, Modulating nitrosourea response in tumours and normal tissue: Application to Muphoran, *Drugs of Today* **32:**51–59.

Maze, R., Carney, J. P., Kelley, M. R., Glassner, B. J., Williams, D. A., and Samson, L., 1996, Increasing DNA repair methyltransferase levels via bone marrow stem cell transduction rescues mice from the toxic effects of 1,3-bis(2-chloroethyl)-1-nitrosourea, a chemotherapeutic alkylating agent, *Proc. Natl. Acad. Sci. USA* **93:**206–210.

Metz, M. Z., Matsumoto, L., Winters, K. A., Doroshow, J. H., and Kane, S. E., 1996, Bicistronic and 2-gene retroviral vectors for using MDR1 as a selectable marker and a therapeutic gene, *Virology* **217:**230–241.

Miller, A. D., Miller, D. G., Garcia, J. V., and Lynch, C. M., 1993, Use of retroviral vectors for gene transfer and expression, *Methods Enzymol.* **217:**581–599.

Monihan, J. M., Carr, N. J., and Sobin, L. H., 1994, CD34 immunoexpression in stromal tumours of the gastrointestinal tract and in mesenteric fibromatoses, *Histopathology* **25:**469–473.

Moore, K. A., Deisseroth, A. B., Reading, C. L., Williams, D. E., and Belmont, J. W., 1992, Stromal support enhances cell-free retroviral vector transduction of human bone marrow long-term culture-initiating cells, *Blood* **79:**1393–1399.

Moritz, T., Mackay, W., Glassner, B. J., Williams, D. A., and Samson, L., 1995, Retrovirus-mediated expression of a DNA repair protein in bone marrow protects haematopoietic cells from nitrosourea-induced toxicity *in vitro* and *in vivo*, *Cancer Res.* **55:**2608–2614.

Moscow, J. A., and Dixon, K. H., 1993, Glutathione-related enzymes, glutathione and multi-drug resistance, *Cytotechnology* **12:**155–170.

Najean, Y., 1987, The iatrogenic leukaemias induced by radio- and/or chemotherapy, *Med. Oncol. Tumour Pharmacother* **4:**245–257.

Nakatsuru, Y., Matsukuma, S., Nemoto, N., Sugano, H., Sekiguchi, M., and Ishikawa, T., 1993, O^6-methylguanine-DNA methyltransferase protects against nitrosamine-induced hepatocarcinogenesis, *Proc. Natl. Acad. Sci. USA* **90:**6468–6472.

Negrin, R. S., 1992, Use of the polymerase chain reaction for the detection of tumour cell involvement of bone marrow and peripheral blood: Implications for purging, *J. Hematother* **1:**361–368.

Newland, A. C., 1995, The problem of thrombocytopenia and its management, *Anticancer Drugs* **6**(S5):65–73.

Ngo Giang Huong, N., Kayibanda, M., Deprez, B., Levy, J. P., Guillet, J. G., and Tilkin, A. F., 1995, Mutations in residue 61 of H-Ras p21 protein influence MHC class II presentation, *Int. Immunol.* **7:**269–275.

O'Shaughnessy, J. A., Cowan, K. H., Nienhuis, A. W., McDonagh, K. T., Sorrentino, B. P., Dunbar, C. E., Chiang, Y., Wilson, W., Goldspiel, B., Kohler, D., Cottlerfox, M., Leitman, S., Gottesman, M., Pastan, I., Denicoff, A., Noone, M., and Gress, R., 1994, Retroviral mediated transfer of the human multidrug resistance gene (MDR-1) into haematopoietic stem cells during autologous transplantation after intensive chemotherapy for metastatic breast cancer, *Hum. Gene Ther.* **5:**891–911.

Pegg, A. E., 1990, Mammalian O^6-alkylguanine-DNA alkyltransferase: Regulation and importance in response to alkylating carcinogenic and therapeutic agents, *Cancer Res.* **50:**6119–6129.

Pettengell, R., Woll, P. J., Thatcher, N., Dexter, T. M., and Testa, N. G., 1995, Multicyclic, dose-intensive chemotherapy supported by sequential reinfusion of haematopoietic progenitors in whole blood, *J. Clin. Oncol.* **13:**148–156.

Rafferty, J. A., Hickson, I., Chinnasamy, N., Lashford, L. S., Margison, G. P., Dexter, T. M., and Fairbairn, L. J., 1996, Chemoprotection of normal tissues by transfer of drug resistance genes, *Cancer Metastasis Rev.* **15:**365–383.

Ranson, M., and Thatcher, N., 1995, The importance of dose and schedule in chemotherapy for small-cell lung cancer, *Anticancer Drugs* **6**(S5):53–63.

Richardson, C., and Bank, A., 1995, Preselection of transduced murine haematopoietic stem cell populations leads to increased long-term stability and expression of the human multiple drug resistance gene, *Blood* **86:**2579–2589.

Rill, D. R., Santana, V. M., Roberts, W. M., Nilson, T., Bowman, L. C., Krance, R. A., Heslop, H. E., Moen, R. C., Ihle, J. N., and Brenner, M. K., 1994, Direct demonstration that autologous bone marrow transplantation for solid tumours can return a multiplicity of tumorigenic cells, *Blood* **84:**380–383.

Russell, D. W., and Miller, A. D., 1996, Foamy virus vectors. *J. Virol.* **70:**217–222.

Saffhill, R., Margison, G. P., and O'Connor, P. J., 1985, Mechanisms of carcinogenesis induced by alkylating agents, *Biochim. Biophys. Acta* **823:**111–145.

Shpall, E. J., Jones, R. B., and Bearman, S., 1994, High-dose therapy with autologous bone marrow transplantation for the treatment of solid tumours, *Curr. Opinion Oncol.* **6:**135–138.

Somia, N. V., Zoppe, M., and Verma, I. M., 1995, Generation of targeted retroviral vectors by using single-chain variable fragment: An approach to *in vivo* gene delivery, *Proc. Natl. Acad. Sci. USA* **92:**7570–7574.

Sorrentino, B. P., Brandt, S. J., Bodine, D., Gottesmann, M., Pastan, I., Cline, A., and Nienhuis, A. W., 1992, Selection of drug resistant bone marrow cells in vitro after retroviral transfer of human mdr-1, *Science* **257:**99–103.

Sugimoto, Y., Aksentijevich, I., Murray, G. J., Brady, R. O., Pastan, I., and Gottesman, M. M., 1995, Retroviral coexpression of a multidrug resistance gene (MDR1) and human alpha-galactosidase A for gene therapy of Fabry disease, *Hum. Gene Ther.* **6:**905–915.

Sun, Z., Yergeau, D. A., Tuypens, T., Tavernier, J., Paul, C. C., Baumann, M. A., Tenen, D. G., and Ackerman, S. J., 1995, Identification and characterization of a functional promoter region in the human eosinophil IL-5 receptor alpha subunit gene, *J. Biol. Chem.* **270:**1462–1471.

Testa, N. G., and Dexter, T. M., 1992, Colony-stimulating factors in the clinic, *Curr. Opinion Biotechnol.* **3:**687–692.

Tinwell, H., and Ashby, J., 1994, Genetic toxicity and potential carcinogenicity of taxol, *Carcinogenesis* **15:**1499–1501.

Tong, W. P., Kirk, M. C., and Ludlum, D. B., 1982, Formation of the crosslink 1-(*N*3-deoxycytidyl)-2-(*N*1-deoxyguanosinyl)-ethane in DNA treated with *N,N*-bis(2-chloroethyl)-*N*-nitrosourea, *Cancer Res.* **42:**3102–3105.

Tsuzuki, T., Sakumi, K., Shiraishi, A., Kawate, H., Igarashi, H., Iwakuma, T., Tominaga, Y., Zhang, S. M., Shimizu, S., and Ishikawa, T., 1996, Targeted disruption of the DNA-repair methyltransferase gene renders mice hypersensitive to alkylating agent, *Carcinogenesis* **17:**1215–1220.

Van der Bliek, A. M., Baas, F., Van der Velde, M., Koerts, T., Biedler, J. L., Meyers, M. B., Ozols, R. F., Hamilton, T. C., Joenje, H., and Borst, P., 1988, Genes amplified and overexpressed in human multidrug-resistant cell lines, *Cancer Res*, **48:**5927–5932.

Van Hoef, M. E., Baumann, I., Lange, C., Luft, T., de Wynter, E. A., Ranson, M., Morgenstern, G. R., Yvers, A., Dexter, T. M., Testa, N. G., and Howell, A., 1994a, Dose-escalating induction chemotherapy supported by lenograstim preceding high-dose consolidation chemotherapy for advanced breast cancer. Selection of the most acceptable regimen to induce maximal tumour response and investigation of the optimal time to collect peripheral blood progenitor cells for haematological rescue after high-dose consolidation chemotherapy, *Ann. Oncol.* **5:**217–224.

Van Hoef, M. E., Ranson, M., Morgenstern, G. R., Baumann, I., Lange, C., de Wynter, E. A., Testa, N. G., and Howell, A., 1994b, Rapid haematological recovery after high-dose consolidation chemotherapy with peripheral blood progenitor cells (PBPC) as sole source of support collected at a single apheresis [letter], *Bone Marrow Transplant.* **13:**839–840.

Voigt, J. M., and Topal, M. D., 1995, O^6-methylguanine-induced replication blocks, *Carcinogenesis* **16:**1775–1782.

Wagner, E., Zatloukal, K., Cotten, M., Kirlappos, H., Mechtler, K., Curiel, D. T., and Birnstiel, M. L., 1992, Coupling of adenovirus to transferrin-polylysine/DNA complexes greatly enhances receptor-mediated gene delivery and expression of transfected genes, *Proc. Natl. Acad. Sci. USA* **89:**6099–6103.

Westbrook, C. A., Chmura, S. J., Arenas, R. B., Kim, S. Y., and Otto, G., 1994, Human APC gene expression in rodent colonic epithelium in vivo using liposomal gene delivery, *Hum. Mol. Genet.* **3:**2005–2010.

Yamaguchi, Y., Zhang, D. E., Sun, Z., Albee, E. A., Nagata, S., Tenen, D. G., and Ackerman, S. J., 1994, Functional characterization of the promoter for the gene encoding human eosinophil peroxidase, *J. Biol. Chem.* **269:**19410–19419.

Chapter 12

HIV Gene Therapy Using Hairpin Ribozymes in Hematopoietic Stem/Progenitor Cells

Xinqiang Li, Flossie Wong-Staal, Anthony D. Ho, and Ping Law

1. RIBOZYME FOR GENE THERAPY OF AIDS

1.1. Ribozymes

Ribozymes are a class of small metalloenzymes composed entirely of RNA which cleave specific RNA sequences (Christoffersen and Marr, 1995; Kiehntopf *et al.*, 1995; Pyle, 1993). Different natural ribozymal structures have been isolated from such diverse sources as tetrahymena, tobacco ringspot virus, plant viroids, virusoids, and satellite viruses; and hepatitis delta virus (Michel *et al.*, 1989; Pyle, 1993). According to their molecular structures, the natural ribozymes are classified into at least six different groups: Group I introns (Cech, 1987), Group II introns (Michel *et al.*, 1989), the M1 RNA subunit of the ribonucleoprotein enzyme RNase P (Guerrier-Takada, *et al.*, 1983), hammerhead (Uhlenbeck, 1987), hairpin (Hampel and Tritz, 1989), and hepatitis δ RNA (Sharmeen *et al.*, 1988; Wu *et al.*, 1989). Members of the first three classes are typically larger (>200 nucleotides) and cleave RNA to produce a 3′ hydroxyl group (Cech, 1992; Michel *et al.*, 1989). The latter three classes are typically smaller (30–80 nucleotides), cleave RNA by

Xinqiang Li, Flossie Wong-Staal, Anthony D Ho, and Ping Law Blood and Marrow Transplant Program, Department of Biology and Medicine, University of California, San Diego, La Jolla, California 92093.

Blood Cell Biochemistry, Volume 8: Hematopoiesis and Gene Therapy, edited by Fairbairn and Testa. Kluwer Academic/Plenum Publishers, New York, 1999.

transesterification, and produce a 2′-, 3′-cyclic phosphate and a 5′ hydroxyl terminus (Cech, 1992). Definitive triplet RNA sequences are required to bind and cleave hammerhead and hairpin ribozymes. The hammerhead ribozyme recognizes an NUX-triplet, where N is any nucleotide and X represents A, C, or U, and cleaves at 3′ to the N residue (Ruffner *et al.*, 1990). The hairpin ribozyme recognizes a GNZ-triplet, where Z is either U or C, and cleaves 5′ to the G residue (Chowrira *el al.*, 1991). A GUC triplet is required for efficient trans cleavage of the hairpin ribozyme (Ojwang *et al.*, 1992). Because of their relatively small sizes and minimal substrate sequence requirements, both hairpin and hammerhead ribozymes can be engineered to bind to specific RNA molecules by attaching sequences complementary to the nucleotides near the cleavage site of the target.

1.2. Factors Affecting Ribozymal Gene Therapy

AIDS may be particularly amenable to ribozyme-based therapeutic strategies. Because HIV infection requires reverse transcription of RNA, ribozymes directed against the viral genome could potentially lead to degradation of viral RNA before reverse transcription (thus preventing infection) and inhibition of mRNA expression after HIV integration into the human genome (thus suppressing viral propagation). Binding of ribozyme to RNA is similar to the use of antisense oligonucleotides, but ribozymes degrade the target RNA, which prevents viral reactivation if the antisense oligo/target complex is denatured. Because it is truly catalytic, one ribozyme molecule can bind and inactivate numerous molecules of substrate RNA.

The efficacy of ribozyme-mediated cleavage of HIV RNA *in vivo* is affected by several factors: levels of intracellular ribozyme expression; the compartmentalization of ribozymes and HIV RNA; the stability of ribozyme transcripts; and the accessibility of the embedded target sequence. We have chosen the hairpin system because of its potential stability due to a high degree of intrinsic secondary structure and its highly efficient cleavage under physiological conditions (Ojwang *et al.*, 1992). The catalytic core of the hairpin ribozyme is only 55–60 base pairs, in the size range of naturally occurring, ubiquitous, small RNA molecules, such as tRNA, small nuclear RNA (snRNA, U1 and U6), and virally expressed RNA (virally-associated RNA of adenovirus) which are transcribed by the pol III promotor. We engineered a hairpin ribozyme to recognize and cleave at the U5 region of HIV, a sequence that is highly conserved among different variants of HIV-1 (Yu *et al.*, 1993). To ensure a high level of intracellular expression, different ribozyme constructs were produced using the pol III promoter of either the internal A and B box of the $tRNA^{val}$ (Cotten and Birnstiel, 1989) or the adenovirus VA1 gene (Jennings and Molley, 1987). Both forms of ribozyme have comparable functional capacity (Yu *et al.*, 1993). These expression cassettes were further cloned into murine retrovirus vectors. HIV replication, measured by the production of p24, is markedly inhibited by the vectors in transiently transfected (Yu *et al.*, 1993) or stably transduced T cell lines (Yamada *et al.*, 1994a,b) and in primary lymphocytes from normal and HIV-infected donors (Leavitt *et al.*, 1994). To minimize further the potential of target virus escaping from inactivation by the ribozymes, we produced another construct encoding ribozymes that targeted the pol region of HIV-1 and the U5 region, described previously, in a single vector (Leavitt *et al.*, unpublished data). This double-ribozyme vector, designated MY-2, is more effective than previous constructs that contain a single ribozyme. Colocalization of the ribozyme and its target RNA were reported by Sullenger and Cech (1993) in a study where the ribozyme transcript included a packaging signal such that, the probability of contact between the ribozyme and the target RNA sequence was increased. As a result, the effectiveness of target degradation was enhanced. We designed a chimeric RNA decoy-ribozyme molecule by fusing the U5 ribozyme to the stem loop II (SLII) region of HIV Rev response element (RRE) which binds to Rev, permitting efficient splicing and cytoplasmic translocation of HIV mRNA (Yamada *et al.*, 1996). An SLII-U5 ribozyme RNA would be expected to display a dual function of inhibiting HIV replication through its ribozymal cleavage and its decoy effect. The activity of this fusion molecule was further facilitated because of several reasons: an increased association of ribozyme and HIV mRNA by binding the Rev protein; an increase in the turnover of the ribozyme by binding Rev to the ribozyme–RRE complex, resulting in enhanced catalytic activity; and an increase in the stability of the ribozyme RNA by protecting it from nuclease degradation by a highly folded, secondary structure of SLII. Indeed, Yamada *et al.* (1996) showed that the SLII-U5 ribozyme is persistently expressed in stable cell lines over a 25-week period and that the construct is more effective in HIV inhibition than the ribozyme alone or the SLII structure linked with a disabled ribozyme. Combining all of these parameters, we have designed a vector that contains two copies of the SLII-U5 ribozyme cassette inserted in both LTR regions of a retroviral vector, plus an SLII-env ribozyme cassette, which is expressed from an internal promoter and targets the conserved envelope region of HIV-1 (Gervaix *et al.*, 1997). Preliminary experiments have shown that this "triple copy" vector is extremely efficient in inhibiting the replication of all five classes (A-E) of phylogenetically diverse strains of HIV-1, isolated from different geographical locations and transmitted by different paths of infection. By coexpressing a combination of different small therapeutic RNAs (ribozymes and decoys) that have additive or synergistic activities to target multiple conserved regions of the HIV-1 genome, it is conceivable that virus escape through mutations can be prevented during long-term *in vivo* therapy.

2. GENE THERAPY USING HEMATOPOIETIC STEM/PROGENITOR CELLS

Although hematopoietic stem cells represent ideal targets for gene therapy, major obstacles have to be resolved. The pluripotent hematopoietic stem cells (PHSC) responsible for long-term engraftment in bone marrow transplantation have yet to be identified. Various assays have been developed to measure the function and frequency of these cells, but all have remained controversial. The majority of PHSC are noncycling, hence their susceptibility to retroviral transduction is limited. The proportion of the PHSC is rare among hematopoietic tissues (<1 in 10^4), and hence the probability of contact between PHSC and vectors is small.

2.1. Identification of Stem/Progenitor Cells

With the development of antibodies against the cell-surface CD34 marker, it has been shown by flow cytometric techniques that the stem/progenitor cells are contained within the $CD34^+$ cell populations (Civin *et al.*, 1984; Kraus *et al.*, 1996; Strauss *et al.*, 1986; Sutherland and Keating 1992). The proportion of $CD34^+$ cells is 1 to 5% in normal marrow (Stauss *et al.*, 1986), <0.5% in peripheral blood under steady-state hematopoiesis (Bender *et al.*, 1991), and ~0.5% to 5% in peripheral blood progenitor cell collections of patients or normal donors after mobilization using growth factors with or without chemotherapy (Haas *et al.*, 1990; Ho *et al.*, 1993; Huhn *et al.*, 1996; Kessinger *et al.*, 1988; Korbling *et al.*, 1995; Lane *et al.*, 1995; Siena *et al.*, 1989; To *et al.*, 1984). Other surface markers have been used to characterize the early or primitive hematopoietic cells versus lineage-committed progenitor cells. Current understanding identifies the primitive cells as $CD45^{dim/positive}$; negative for all differentiation or mature leukocyte markers (such as CD33, CD71, CD10, CD19, CD2, CD3, CD8, CD14, CD15, and CD56, etc.) (lineage negative) (Baum *et al.*, 1992; Bender *et al.*, 1991; Huang and Terstappen 1994a; Krause *et al.*, 1996; Murray *et al.*, 1995; Terstappen *et al.*, 1991); $CD38^-$ (Ho *et al.*, 1996; Terstappen *et al.*, 1991), Thy-1^+ (CD90) (Baum *et al.*, 1992); rhodamine 123^{dull} (Srour *et al.*, 1991a; Traycoff *et al.*, 1994); and with low expression of growth factor receptors for IL-3 (CD123) (Sato *et al.*, 1993) and stem cell factor (Kawashima *et al.*, 1996). There is some controversy regarding the presence of surface HLA-DR, but most studies demonstrate that the primitive cells are HLA-$DR^{dim/positive}$ (Huang and Terstappen, 1994a,b; Saeland *et al.*, 1992; Srour *et al.*, 1991b; Traycoff *et al.*, 1994). The proportion of primitive cells thus identified is <1% of the $CD34^+$ cell populations. The surface-marker expression pattern of primitive stem cells has been confirmed by complex *in vitro* culture techniques, such as single cell sorting and blast cell colony assays (Brandt *et al.*, 1988; Huang and Terstappen 1992; Leary and Ogawa 1987), and by implantation of human hematopoietic cells into immune-tolerant animals, such as fetal sheep (Zanjani *et al.*, 1992) and SCID mice (Lapidot *et al.*, 1992; Torbett *et al.*, 1995). However, the ultimate demonstration of the PHSC still rests in the long-term, durable, engraftment of patients. Taken together with the fact the $CD34^+$ cells constitute about 1% of marrow or mobilized blood, the most commonly utilized sources for hematopoietic cells, the frequency of PHSC, containing the primitive cell populations, is estimated to be $<10^{-4}$.

2.2. Enrichment of Stem/Progenitor Cells

Recently, cell enrichment systems have been developed for clinical applications of $CD34^+$ cells (Berenson *et al.*, 1991; Ishizawa *et al.*, 1993; Miltenyi *et al.*, 1990; Okarma *et al.*, 1992; Papadimitriou *et al.*, 1995; Shpall *et al.*, 1994; Strauss *et al.*, 1991). At least three large-scale systems are in various stages of clinical trials. The CellPro system uses a biotinylated-IgM CD34 antibody (12.8) to capture the target cells onto an avidin column and releases the $CD34^+$ cells by mechanical disruption (Berenson *et al.*, 1991). The Baxter system uses an IgG1 CD34 (9C5) antibody and Dynal paramagnetic microspheres to rosette and capture of the target cells on permanent magnets. The rosetted $CD34^+$ cells are released by enzymatic digestion using chymopapain (Ishizawa *et al.*, 1993; Strauss *et al.*, 1991), or competitive displacement (Tseng-Law *et al.*, 1995). The Applied Immune Sciences (AIS) system uses lectins for an initial debulking step, and then captures the target cells on flasks or large surfaces coated with the anti-CD34 antibody, ICH3. The $CD34^+$ cells are released by mechanical disruption (Okarma *et al.*, 1992). The final enriched product from all of these systems, using marrow or mobilized peripheral blood as a starting material, typically retains 1 to 5% of leukocytes contains 30 to 95% $CD34^+$ cells, and yields 25 to 75%.

Transplantation of the cells has resulted in durable engraftment of hematopoiesis, similar to that obtained after infusing unmanipulated marrow or mobilized blood progenitor cells. Recently, Systemix has initiated a Phase I clinical trial in multiple myeloma patients using $CD34^+CD90^+$ (Thy-1^+) cells produced by high speed sorting (Tricot *et al.*, 1995). In addition, AmCell (Bridell *et al.*, 1995) has developed a large-scale version of a system, originally invented by Miltenyi *et al.*, (1990) using iron-containing microbeads. The target cells are captured on a column, and the microbeads are not released from the cells. The system is not yet in clinical trial. The manufacturers of all of the aforementioned systems have commercialized smaller scale research devices based on the same principles.

With these systems as a preliminary step, further purification of the primitive hematopoietic cells by sorting or other methods becomes simpler and less time-consuming. The need for large quantities of viral supernatant containing high titers of infectious particles is reduced because of the reduction in the total cell number, and hence the reaction volume during transduction. It has also encouraged the first generation of gene therapy trials using enriched $CD34^+$ cells (Hanania *et al.*, 1995; Hoogerbrugge *et al.*, 1996; Kohn *et al.*, 1995).

2.3. Stimulation of Stem/Progenitor Cells for Transduction

Retroviral vectors can be incorporated only into cells that are actively replicating (Miller *et al.*, 1992). Because PHSC are predominantly quiescent and mitotically inactive, different strategies have been developed to induce PHSC into cell cycle. Using flow cytometric techniques, we have studied the cell-cycle kinetics of enriched $CD34^+$ cells from mobilized peripheral blood for three generations under a variety of cytokine combinations, such as stem cell factor (SCF), IL-1, IL-3, IL-6, IL-11, G-CSF, GM-CSF, and flk2/flt3 ligand (Agrawal *et al.*, 1996). After 48 hr of incubation, the best cytokines for inducing mitosis are SCF + IL-1, SCF + IL-3, SCF + G-CSF, and SCF + GM-CSF. The cells remain in a noncycling state without added cytokines. After 72 hr, although most cells have divided once and some cells are in the third cell cycle, ~20 to 30% of the $CD34^+$ cells remain quiescent. Under the same stimulating conditions, the $CD34^+CD38^-$ cells, the subsets containing the more primitive stem/progenitor cells are quiescent for 72 hr. These results are similar to other published reports (Nolta *et al.*, 1995; Young *et al.*, 1996). Using a prolonged exposure to tritiated thymidine (suicide assay), Ponchio *et al.* (1996) demonstrated that most of the long term culture initiating cells (LTCIC) in peripheral blood are quiescent. Knaan-Shanzer *et al.* (1996) confirmed that although marrow $CD34^+$ cells are transduced by single incubation with retroviral supernatant, the more primitive CD34^{bright} lineage negative subset contains relatively few cells in active cycle, and the cells are refractory to transduction. These studies indicate that retroviral transfection of the pluripotent stem/progenitor cells may be problematic because of the noncycling status of the target cells.

Hematopoietic cells of different origins (marrow, cord blood, or peripheral blood) respond differently to growth factor stimulation. Shah *et al.* (1996) recently reported that the flk2/flt3 ligand combined with IL-3 and IL-6 induces higher proliferation of CD34^{+}CD38^{-} cells than SCF. The expansion of long-term culture cinitiating cells (LTCIC) is also enhanced. However, the effects are more pronounced with marrow CD34^{+}CD38^{-} cells than with the same subset from cord blood. The thymidine suicide study of Ponchio *et al.* (1995) demonstrated that the LTCIC from marrow are in a more proliferative state than those in peripheral blood. These studies suggest that the optimal conditions for stimulation and retroviral transduction may differ depending on the source of the hematopoietic cells.

Various cytokines have been studied to determine the optimal *in vitro* conditions for retroviral transduction of the progenitor cells. A combination of IL-3, IL-6 and SCF is the most efficient in transfecting marrow-derived stem/progenitor cells (Lu *et al.*, 1993, 1994). The use of irradiated stroma increases transduction of stem/progenitor cells from marrow but not the same cell population from peripheral blood (Lu *et al.*, 1994; Nolta *et al.*, 1995). The following explanations, singly or together, might account for the observation: (1) Colocalization allows the retroviruses to adhere to the stromal elements, which facilitates entry into stem/progenitor cells via the adhesion molecule systems. Using culture flasks coated with fibronectin, Moritz *et al.* (1994) showed that gene transfer into progenitor cells is as efficient as using stroma. (2) Stem/Progenitor cells would be directly stimulated into mitosis after attachment onto stroma via the integrin system (Moritz *et al.*, 1994). (3) Production of cytokines, known or unknown, by the stromal layer induces the quiescent stem/progenitor cells into cycling, thus increasing the possibility of integrating retroviral vectors (Moritz *et al.*, 1994). Using cord blood CD34^{+} cells, Hatzfield *et al.* (1996) found that blocking transforming growth factor (TGF)-β1 increases transduction efficiency. The TGF-β1 blocking is especially effective for transducing the more primitive progenitor cells. It is possible that removing inhibitory factor(s) is as important for achieving a high efficiency of transduction as providing sufficient stimulatory factor(s) or an appropriate microenvironment such as a stromal layer.

2.4. Preparation of Vectors and Hematopoietic Stem Cells

Retroviral vectors have to the bind to the cell surface and be transported into the cell before integrating into DNA. Increasing the contact of vectors with hematopoietic cells increases transduction. Repeated incubation of hematopoietic cells with high-titer vectors (Kohn *et al.*, 1995; Kotani *et al.*, 1994; Paul *et al.*, 1993), and the use of polycations to modify the electrostatic properties of the cell surface, have been studied and reported to be effective to various extents (Aubin *et al.*, 1994; Cornetta and Anderson, 1989). Physical parameters, such as Brownian motion and the decay of the viral particles at culture conditions, become limiting factors in bringing the vectors into contact with the target cells. Recently, Chuck and Palsson (1996), proposed a "flow-through" technique to increase the contact between vector and targets. Passing the cell/vector suspension slowly through a filter enables trapping the (larger) cells onto filters, while allowing the (smaller) viral particles that have not made contact with cells to pass through. Circulating the vector-containing medium repeatedly *via* the filter produces high efficiency transduction of cell lines. Now, studies using hematopoietic cells in similar conditions have been initiated.

Vectors constructed from adeno-associated virus (AAV) can potentially transfect nondividing cells (Shaughnessy *et al.*, 1996). Indeed, AAV vectors have been successfully used to introduce various genes into human marrow progenitor cells (Wang *et al.*, 1995), erythroid progenitor cells (Goodman *et al.*, 1994; Miller, *et al.*, 1994; Zhou, *et al.*, 1996), and mature and immature cord blood stem cells (Broxmeyer *et al.*, 1995; Zhou *et al.*, 1994). Contrary to the use of retroviral vectors, growth factor stimulation of the target cells is necessary for high efficiency transduction (Chatterjee *et al.*, 1995; Zhou *et al.*, 1994). A trans-gene has been detected in colony-forming committed progenitor cells and LTCIC, indicating that early hematopoietic cells are transduced (Chatterjee *et al.*, 1995; Zhou *et al.*, 1994). It is not yet known whether the PHSC are transduced by AAV vectors. Because high-titer stocks of AAV vector are required, the presence of replication-competent viruses (RCV), and hence the detection of RCV using sensitive methods (1 or 2 RCV in 10^{12} vectors), has been the major hindrance in therapeutic trials using AAV vectors (Smith *et al.*, 1996).

2.5. Expression in Progeny Cells

Another potential hurdle in using primitive hematopoietic stem cells as targets for gene therapy is obtaining sustained expression of the trans-gene in progeny cells. Using neomycin resistance gene transfer and G418 selection, transduction efficiencies of enriched $CD34^+$ cells were low (Brenner *et al.*, 1993). However, if gene incorporation into single progenitor colony was measured using DNA PCR, >75% of all CFU-GM contained the neo-marker (Lu *et al.*, 1993, 1994). It is possible that the promoter of the transfected gene is not effective in the progeny cells. Equally possible is the hypothesis that as the primitive cells differentiate into mature compartments, those regions of the chromosomes containing the trans-gene are deactivated, terminating the expression of the neomycin resistance protein and leading to poor colony formation in the presence of G418. Thus, the transduction of primitive hematopoietic stem/progenitor cells faces two major problems: (1) inducing the primitive cells to replicate, but not differentiate to facilitate retroviral genetransfer and (2) maintaining the expression of the trans-gene in the progeny cells to facilitate retroviral genetransfer.

2.6. Clinical Gene Marking/Gene Therapy Trials

Despite all the obstacles, transplantation of genetically marked or transduced stem/progenitor cells into patients has been partially successful. Brenner *et al.* (1993)

showed that transplantation of marrow incubated with growth factor combination (without CD34$^+$ cell enrichment) and transduced using retroviral vectors produces progeny cells marked with the trans-gene. In a different study, Dunbar *et al.* (1995), using similar transduction conditions, demonstrated that the genetically modified cells could originate from mobilized peripheral blood and marrow. In the first gene therapy trial using gene transfer into hematopoietic stem cells to correct adenosine deaminase (ADA) deficiency, Kohn *et al.* (1995) transduced autologous cord blood CD34$^+$ cells (enriched with the CellPro System) with a functional ADA sequence in a retroviral vector. Low level of cells carrying the ADA trans-gene (10^{-4} to 10^{-5}) was detected in the peripheral blood of recipients two years after infusion. Preliminary results have shown an increase in the proportion of cells that express the ADA gene, suggesting a selective advantage for the genetically corrected stem/progenitor cells. In a different trial to correct ADA deficiency, Hoogerbrugge *et al.* (1996) enriched marrow CD34$^+$ cells by the AIS system and cocultured the cells in IL-3 with an irradiated virus-producing cell line. Transduction efficiency, measured in the colony-forming progenitor cells, was low (<15%). Upon reinfusion, the trans-gene was found in only one out of three patients for a short period of three months, and expression was not detected. The differing results reported in the two ADA trials could reflect important differences in selecting the source of stem cells, and the stimulation conditions for transduction. A gene therapy approach for cancer was proposed by Deisseroth *et al.* (Hanania *et al.*, 1995). The multidrug-resistance gene was introduced into the stem/progenitor cells to induce protection of the hematopoietic system against the toxic effects of escalating doses of taxol. Preliminary results are encouraging, although an assessment of the efficacy of the treatment is not available yet. Other diseases targeted for gene therapy trials using hematopoietic stem cells include chronic granulomatous disease (Porter *et al.*, 1996; Sekhsaria *et al.*, 1993) and Gaucher disease (Fink *et al.*, 1990; Nolta *et al.*, 1992). One common finding of the clinical trials reported to date is the small proportion (<0.1%) of transfected progeny cells and the low level of gene expression detected. This confirms the *in vitro* difficulties of transducing primitive stem/progenitor cells.

3. TRANSDUCTION OF STEM/PROGENITOR CELLS USING RIBOZYMAL CONSTRUCTS

Previous attempts to treat AIDS patients with marrow transplantation were not successful (Contu *et al.*, 1993; Torlontano *et al.*, 1992). Although engraftment was detected and did not differ from that in patients without HIV infection, the patients did not survive long enough to draw definitive conclusions. In one case, no active HIV-1 infection was detected (Contu *et al.*, 1993), while in another case, persistent HIV-1 positivity was reported after marrow transplantation (Torlontano *et al.*, 1992). If the stem/progenitor cells could be transfected with anti-HIV ribozymes, the progeny cells might be protected against HIV. We have initiated a series of preclinical studies to evaluate this possibility. CD34$^+$ cells, isolated from cord blood of normal infants using the Baxter ISOLEX system, were transduced with hairpin ribozyme constructs (Yu *et al.*, 1995). After culturing in growth factors

(SCF + IL3 + IL-6) for three weeks, the progeny monocytes/macrophages were challenged with HIV-bal, a monocyte-tropic strain of HIV. Production of p24 was inhibited in those cells transduced with the vectors carrying the ribozyme gene, whereas cells transduced with a control vector were infected by HIV-bal, as evidenced by the production of p24. A different study using CD34$^+$ cells from the cord blood of normal, HIV-exposed, and HIV-infected infants showed that the *in vitro* cloning efficiency of the CD34$^+$ cells was not affected by transfection with retroviral vectors that contain the hairpin ribozymal constructs (Li *et al.*, 1998). When cord blood CD34$^+$ cells from HIV-infected infants are transfected with the ribozymal gene and cultured, the progeny monocytes/macrophages are protected from HIV infection by using both the HIV-bal and the maternal HIV strain. These studies showed that *in vitro* protection from HIV-infection is achieved by following transduction of stem/progenitor cells with the ribozymal gene constructs.

4. TOWARD CLINICAL TRIALS

4.1. HIV Infection of Stem/Progenitor Cells

It is controversial whether human stem/progenitor cells are targets of HIV. The heterogeneity of the CD34$^+$ cells and of the functional assays to measure the PHSC account for part of the confusion. Studies using hematopoietic cells from HIV-infected patients were inconclusive. One report showed that 14 to 37% of the CD34$^+$ cells from patients were infected by HIV and that as much as 0.2% of the CD34$^+$ cells were positive by PCR or after coculturing (Stanley *et al.*, 1992). The proportions were higher than those of lymphocytes in the same patients. Others have demonstrated the presence of viral DNA in hematopoietic progenitor colonies (Kaczmarkski *et al.*, 1992). However, conflicting results have been reported in a number of studies. Davis *et al.* (1991) showed that no proviral DNA was detected in CFU-GM generated from the marrow of HIV-seropositive subjects. Von Laer *et al.* (1990) and Molina *et al.* (1990) also failed to detect infected cells in the CD34$^+$ cell population enriched from the marrow of HIV-infected subjects. Using *in situ* hybridization and immunocytochemical techniques, Ganser *et al.* (1990) did not locate RNA or protein from single colonies derived from the marrow of three AIDS patients. Negative PCR was also reported by De Luca *et al.* (1993), using CD34$^+$ cells and CFU-GM, with or without suspension cultures, from six AIDS patients. Our own results, using CD34$^+$ cells from an HIV-infected infant, showed that a small fraction of the CD34$^+$ cells also express p24 (Li *et al.*, submitted manuscript). The observation was subsequently confirmed by the fact that colonies from the cord blood sample are positive by PCR using HIV-specific primers. It is also unclear whether PHSC from normal individuals are infected by HIV. The viral replication and infection detected in the CD34$^+$ cell population might simply reflect infection of the progeny monocyte/macrophages generated by the culturing of CD34$^+$ cells. Some reports have indicate that the cells with detectable virus are CD4$^+$CD34$^-$ and showed positive esterase staining, indicative of monocytes (Folks *et al.*, 1988; Kitano *et al.*, 1991). Even if HIV-infected stem/progenitor cells are present in AIDS patients, the proportion of such a cell population is small compared to the whole $CD34^+$ population, and most of the $CD34^+$ cells are not targets of HIV infections.

4.2. Mobilization of Peripheral Blood Stem Cells from AIDS Patients

Compared to bone marrow harvests, peripheral blood stem/progenitor cells (PBSC) collected by apheresis procedures would be an easier source of $CD34^+$ cells for HIV-gene therapy. Studies on mobilizing PBSC of normal subjects for allogeneic transplantation indicated that administering G-CSF (at 10μg/kg/d for four or more days) is safe and has minor side effects (Korbling *et al.*, 1995; Lane *et al.*, 1995). Sufficient quantities of $CD34^+$ cells are collected in one to two leukaphaeresis sessions in most cases. Using GM-CSF and G-CSF, either combined or sequentially, the same quantities of $CD34^+$ cells are harvested as in G-CSF alone (Lane *et al.*, 1995). Analysis of $CD34^+$ subsets, however, revealed that the proportions of primitive hematopoietic cells ($CD34^+CD38^-$) are higher in donors receiving G-CSF and GM-CSF (Ho *et al.*, 1996). In one instance, a peripheral blood stem cell allograft donor was not adequately mobilized with G-CSF, but repeated mobilization using a combination of GM-CSF and G-CSF was successful (Corringham, 1995). Little information regarding the mobilization of peripheral blood stem cells from AIDS patients is currently available. It is possible that the response of AIDS patients to G-CSF and/or GM-CSF may be quite different from that of normal individuals. In addition, antiviral treatments, such as AZT, may also suppress marrow function and lead to inferior mobilization. Administration of GM-CSF and/or G-CSF might even induce activation of HIV. However, no such activation has so far been reported from studies using G-CSF or GM-CSF for treating HIV-related or introgenic neutropenia in AIDS patients (Kimura *et al.*, 1990; Sloand *et al.*, 1993). Growth factors have also been used during chemotherapy for AIDS-related malignancies (Krown *et al.*, 1992). Although GM-CSF increases HIV production *in vitro* by infected leukocyte populations, such as T cells and monocytes/macrophages, administering GM-CSF to patients did not produce any demonstrable viral stimulation (Koyangi *et al.*, 1988; Perno *et al.*, 1992). However, one report has shown that p24 antigen concentration increases by more than two-fold in lymphoma patients after the second cycle of chemotherapy (Kaplan *et al.*, 1991). G-CSF, on the other hand, does not increase virus production *in vitro* (Davison *et al.*, 1994; Kimura *et al.*, 1990). When G-CSF was administered to AIDS patients for neutropenia induced by zidovudine treatment, AIDS related malignancies, bacterial sepsis, aphthous ulcers, or refractory fungal infections, no increase in p24 or viremia was attributable to G-CSF (Manders *et al.*, 1995; Vecchiarelli *et al.*, 1995). It remains unclear, however, whether the side effects of G-CSF in asymptomatic HIV seropositive patients can be tolerated or what the response to G-CSF would be in this patient population. Preclinical evaluation of G-CSF mobilization of stem/progenitor cells from HIV-infected patients is currently underway.

4.3. Clinical Trials and Further Developments

Mobilized peripheral blood stem cells are ideal targets for HIV gene therapy, especially in adult patients. Large number of $CD34^+$ cells are collected in multiple leukaphaeresis sessions with minimal discomfort to the patients. The initial protocol includes mobilizing peripheral blood stem cells, enriching CD34$^+$ cells, transducing the cells under stimulation of growth factor combinations, and reinfusing the genetically modified cells. Useful information, such as the kinetics of the transduced stem/progenitor cells and the expression of the trans-gene, will be collected. Eventually, myeloablation may be required to allow engrafting the transduced CD34$^+$ cells. It is possible that myeloablation can be achieved by using a combination of antiviral drugs. Whether it is necessary to increase the frequency of genetically modified cells *in vitro*, such as by selection with G418 remains unclear. Once infused, the cells expressing the trans-gene, and therefore resistant to HIV, are expected to have a survival advantage over the unmanipulated cells.

The use of cord blood stem cells is an attractive strategy for pediatric patients. Infusion transduced stem cells from either autologous or allogeneic sources would probably require manipulating cryopreserved samples. Because the rate of HIV infections in infants born to HIV-positive mothers could be as low as 5% under AZT prophylaxis (Kuhn and Stein, 1995), collection and cryopreservation of cord blood stem cells at the time of delivery can yield the required quantities CD34$^+$ cells for ribozymal gene therapy if the newborns subsequently prove to be HIV-infected. In the allogeneic setting, HLA-matching and other logistical considerations render working with fresh cells practically impossible. We have demonstrated that enriching CD34$^+$ cells from thawed mobilized peripheral blood stem cell collections is possible (Law *et al.*, 1993). However, it is not clear whether sufficient quantities of cord blood CD34$^+$ cells can be selected from cryopreserved samples in matched unrelated transplants.

Despite the uncertainties of clinical trials and the difficulties in transducing mitotically inactive pluripotent stem cells, gene therapy represents one of the best options for HIV-infected individuals. In contrast to the use of mature lymphocytes as targets, successful engraftment of genetically modified PHSC may have a durable effect. With recent developments, it is likely that this treatment modality will become a reality within the next few years.

ACKNOWLEDGEMENT. The research is supported in part by NIH grants no. 1-R01-DK49619 and 5-U19-AI3662) and by the Pediatric AIDS Foundation. The expert editorial assistance of Barbara Vickers is gratefully acknowledged.

5. REFERENCES

Agrawal, Y. P., Agrawal, R. S., Sinclair, A. M., Young, D., Maruyama, M., Levine, F., and Ho, A. D., 1996, Cell cycle kinetics and VSV-G pseudotyped retrovirus mediated gene transfer in blood-derived CD34$^+$ cells, *Exp. Hematol.* **24:**738–747.

Aubin, R. A., Weinfeld, M., Mirzayans, R., and Paterson, M. C., 1994, Polybrene/DMSO-assisted gene transfer, *Mol. Biotechnol.* **1:**29–48.

Baum, C. M., Weissman, I. L., Tsukamoto, A. S., Buckle, A. M., and Peault, B., 1992, Isolation of a candidate human hematopoietic stem-cell population, *Proc. Natl. Acad. Sci. USA* **89:**2804.

Bender, J. G., Unverzagt, K. L., Walker, D. E., Lee, W., Van Epps, D. E., Smith, D. H., Stewart, C. C., and To, L. B., 1991, Identification and comparison of CD34-positive cells and their subpopulations from normal peripheral blood and bone marrow using multicolor flow cytometry, *Blood* **77:**2591–2596.

Berenson, R. J., Bensinger, W. I., Hill, R. S., Andrews, R. G., Garcia-Lopez, J., Kalamasz, D. F., Still, B. J., Spitzer, G., Buckner, C. D., Bernstein, I. D., and Thomas, E. D., 1991, Engraftment after infusion of CD34⁺ marrow cells in patients with breast cancer or neuroblastoma, *Blood* **77:**1717.

Brandt, J., Baird, N., Lu, L., Srour, E., and Hoffman, R., 1993, Characterization of a human hematopoietic progenitor cell capable of forming blast cell containing colonies *in vitro*, *J. Clin. Invest.* **82:**1017.

Brenner, M. K., Rill, D. R., Holladay, M. S., Heslop, H. E., Moen, R. C., Buschle, M., Krance, R. A., Santana, V. M., Anderson, W. F., and Ihle, J. N., 1993, Gene marking to determine whether autologous marrow infusion restores long-term haemopoiesis in cancer patients, *Lancet* **342:**1134–1137.

Briddell, R., Zilm, K., Kern, B., Stoney, G., Harding, F., Recktenwald, D., Miltenyi, S., and McNiece, I., 1995, Depletion of t-lymphocyte subsets in peripheral blood apheresis harvests from normal donors by purification of cells expressing the CD34 antigen, *Blood* **86**(10)(Suppl. 1)**:**223a.

Broxmeyer, H. E., Cooper, S., Etienne-Julan, M., Wang, X. S., Ponnazahagan, S., Braun, S., Lu, L., and Srivastava, A., 1995, Cord blood transplantation and the potential for gene therapy. Gene transduction using a recombinant adeno-associated viral vector, *Ann. N.Y. Acad. Sci.* **770:**105–115.

Cech, T. R., 1987, The chemistry of self-splicing RNA and RNA enzymes, *Science* **236:**1532–1539.

Cech, T. R., 1992, Ribozyme engineering, *Curr. Opinion Struct. Biol.* **2:**605–609.

Chatterjee, S., Lu, D., Podsakoff, G., and Wong, K. K. Jr., 1995, Strategies for efficient gene transfer into hematopoietic cells; the use of adeno-associated virus vectors in gene therapy, *Ann. N.Y. Acad. Sci.* **770:**79–90.

Chowrira, B. M., Berzal, H.A., and Burke, J. M., 1991, Novel guanosine requirement for catalysis by the hairpin ribozyme, *Nature* **354:**320–322.

Christoffersen, R. E., and Marr, J. J., 1995, Ribozymes as human therapeutic agents, *J. Med. Chem.* **38**(12)**:**2023–2037.

Chuck, A. S., and Palsson, B. O., 1996, Consistent and high rates of gene transfer can be obtained using flow-through transduction over a wide range of retroviral titers, *Hum. Gene Ther.* **7:**743–750.

Civin, C. I., Strauss, L. C., Brovall, C., Fackler, M. J., Schwartz, J. F., and Shaper, J. H., 1984, Antigenic analysis of hematopoiesis III. A hematopoietic progenitor cell surface antigen defined by a monoclonal antibody raised against KG-1a cells, *J. Immunol.* **133:**157–165.

Contu, L., La Nasa, G., Arras, M., Pizzati, A., Vacca, A., Carcassi, C., Ledda, A., Boero, R., Orru, S., Pintus, A., Schivo, L., Faa, G., Costa, V., and Pitzus, F., 1993, Allogeneic bone marrow transplantation combined with multiple anti-HIV-1 treatment in a case of AIDS, *Bone Marrow Transplant.* **12**(6)**:**669–671.

Cornetta, K., and Anderson, W. F., 1989, Protamine sulfate as an effective alternative to polybrene in retroviral-mediated gene transfer: Implications for human gene therapy, *J. Virol. Methods* **23:**1187–1194.

Corringham, R. E. T., 1995, Rapid and sustained allogeneic transplantation using immunoselected CD34⁺-selected peripheral blood progenitor cells mobilized by recombinant granulocyte- and granulocyte-macrophage colony-stimulating factors (letter), *Blood* **86:**2052–2054.

Cotten, M., and Birnstiel, M. L., 1989, Ribozyme mediated destruction of RNA *in vivo*, *EMBO J.* **8:**3861–3866.

Davis, B. R., Schwartz, D. H., Marx, J. C., Johnson, C. E., Berry, J. M., Lyding, J., Merigan, T. C., and Zander, A., 1991, Absent or rare human immunodeficiency virus infection of bone marrow stem/progenitor cells *in vivo*, *J. Virol.* **65**(4)**:**1985–1990.

Davison, F. D., Kaczmarski, R. S., Pozniak, A., Mufti, G. J., and Sutherland, S., 1994, Quantification of HIV by PCR in monocytes and lymphocytes in patients receiving antiviral treatment and low dose recombinant human granulocyte macrophage colony stimulating factor, *J. Clin. Path.* **47**(9)**:**855–857.

De Luca, A., Teofill, L., Antinori, A., Iovino, M. S., Mencarini, P., Visconti, E., Tamburrini, E., Leone, G., and Ortona, L., 1993, Haemopoietic CD34⁺ progenitor cells are not infected by HIV-1 *in vivo* but show impaired clonogenesis, *Br. J. Haematol.* **85:**20–24.

Dunbar, C. E., Cottler-Fox, M., O'Shaugnessy, J. A., Doren, S., Carter, C., Berenson, R., Brown, S., Moen, R. C., Greenblatt, J., Stewart, F. M., Leitman, S. F., Wilson, W. H., Cowan, K., Young, N. S., and Nienhuis, A. W., 1995, Retrovirally marked CD34-enriched peripheral blood and bone marrow cells contribute to long-term engraftment after autologous transplantation, *Blood* **85**(11)**:**3048–3057.

Fink, J. K., Correll, P. H., Perry, L. K., Brady, R. O., and Karlsson, S., 1990, Correction of glucocerebrosidase deficiency after retroviral-mediated gene transfer into hematopoietic progenitor cells from patients with Gaucher disease, *Proc. Natl. Acad. Sci. USA* **87:**2334.

Folks, T. M., Kessler, S. W., Orenstein, J. M., Justement, J. S., Jaffe, E., and Fauci, A. S., 1988, Infection and replication of HIV-1 in purified progenitor cells of normal human bone marrow, *Science* **242:**919–922.

Ganser, A., Ottman, O. C., von Briesen, H., Volkers, B., Rubsamen-Waigmann, H., and Hoelzer, D., 1990, Changes in the haematopoietic progenitor cell compartment in the acquired immunodeficiency syndrome, *Res. Virol.* **141:**185.

Gervaix, A., Schwarz, L., Law, P., Ho, A. D., Loonex, D., Lane, T. A., and Wong-Staal, F., 1997, Gene therapy targeting peripheral blood $CD34^+$ hematopoietic stem cells of HIV-infected individuals, *Human Gene Therapy* **8:**2229–2238.

Goodman, S., Xiao, X., Donahue, R. E., Moulton, A., Miller, J., Walsh, C., Young, N. S., Samulski, R. J., and Nienhuis, A. W., 1994, Recombinant adeno-associated virus-mediated gene transfer into hematopoietic progenitor cells, *Blood* **84**(5)**:**1492–1500.

Guerrier-Takada, C., Cardiner, K., Marsh, T., Pace, N., and Altman, S., 1983, The RNA moiety of ribonuclease P is the catalytic subunit of the enzyme, *Cell* **35:**849–857.

Haas, R., Ho, A. D., Bredthauer, U., Cayeux, S., Egerer, G., Knauf, W., and Hunstein, W., 1990, Successful autologous transplantation of blood stem cells mobilized with recombinant human granulocyte-macrophage colony-stimulating factor, *Exp. Hematol.* **18:**94.

Hampel, A., and Tritz, R., 1989, RNA catalytic properties of the minimum (–) sTRSV sequence, *Biochemistry* **28:**4929–4933.

Hanania, E. G., Kavanagh, J., Giles, R. E., Kudelka, A., Rahman, Z., Holmes, F., Hortobagyi, G., Hamer, J., Calvert, L., Finnegan, M. B., Mante, R., Ellerson, D., Geisler, D., Wang, T., Su, Y., Zu, Z., Chen, N., Berenson, R., Heimfeld, S., Claxton, D., Mechetner, E., Holzmayer, T., Mehra, R., Cote, R., Champlin, R., and Deisseroth, A. B., 1995, Rapid neutrophil recovery in autologous transplants using cells that have been exposed to multiple drug resistance (MDR-1) retroviral vector, *Blood* **86**(10)(Suppl. 1)**:**462a.

Hatzfeld, A., Batard, P., Panterne, B., Taieb, F., and Hatzfeld, J., 1996, Increased stable retroviral gene transfer in early hematopoietic progenitors released from quiescence, *Hum. Gene Ther.* **7:**207–213.

Ho, A. D., Glück, S., Germond, C., Sinoff, C., Dietz, G., Maruyama, M., and Corringham, R. E. T., 1993, Optimal timing for collections of blood progenitor cells following induction chemotherapy and granulocyte-macrophage colony-stimulating factor for autologous transplantation in advanced breast cancer, *Leukemia* **17**(11)**:**1738–1746.

Ho, A. D., Young, D., Maruyama, M., Corringham, R. E. T., Mason, J. R., Thompson, P., Grenier, K., Law, P., Terstappen, L. W. M. M., and Lane, T., 1996, Pluripotent and lineage-committed $CD34^+$ subsets in leukapheresis products mobilized by G-CSF, GM-CSF versus a combination of both, *Exp. Hematol.* in press.

Hoogerbrugge, P. M., van Beusechem, V. W., Fischer, A., Debree, M., le Deist, F., Perignon, J. L., Morgan, G, Gaspar, G., Fairbanks, L. D., Skeoch, C. H., Moseley, A., Harvey, M., Levinsky, R. J., and Valerio, D., 1996, Bone marrow gene transfer in three patients with adenosine deaminase deficiency, *Gene Ther.* **3:**179–183.

Huang, S., and Terstappen, L. W. M. M., 1992, Formation of hematopoietic microenvironment and hematopoietic stem cells from single human bone marrow stem cells, *Nature* **360:**745–749.

Huang, S., and Terstappen, L. W., 1994a, Formation of haematopoietic microenvironment and hematopoietic stem cells from single human bone marrow stem cells [retraction of Huang, S., and Terstappen, L. W. M. M., 1992, *Nature*, **360**(6406)**:**745–749], *Nature* **368:**664.

Huang, S., and Terstappen, L. W. M. M., 1994b, Lymphoid and myeloid differentiation of single human $CD34^+$, $HLA\text{-}DR^+$, $CD38^-$ hematopoietic stem cells, *Blood* **83:**1515–1526.

Huhn, R. D., Yurkow, E. J., Tushinski, R., Clarke, L., Sturgill, M. G., Hoffman, R., Sheay, W., Cody, R., Philipp, C., Resta, D., and George, M., 1996, Recombinant human interleukin-3 (rhIL-3) enhances the mobilization of peripheral blood progenitor cells by recombinant human granulocyte colony-stimulating factor (rhG-CSF) in normal volunteers, *Exp. Hematol.* **24:**839–847.

Ishizawa, L., Hangoc, G., Van De Ven, C., Cairo, M., Burgess, J., Mansour, V., Gee, A., Hardwick, A., Traycoff, C., Srour, E., Hoffman, R., and Law, P., 1993, Immunomagnetic separation of $CD34^+$ cells from human bone marrow, cord blood, and mobilized peripheral blood, *J. Hematother.* **2:**333–338.

Jennings, P. A., and Molley, R. L., 1987, Inhibition of SV40 replicon function by engineered antisense RNA transcribed by RNA polymerase III, *EMBO J.* **6:**3043–3047.

Kaczmarski, R. S., Davison, F., Blair, E., Sutherland, S., Moxham, J., McManus, T., and Mufti, G. J., 1992, Detection of HIV in haemopoietic progenitors, *Br. J. Haematol.* **82**(4)**:**764–769.

Kaplan, L. D., Kahn, J. O., Crowe, S., Northfelt, D., Neville, P., Grossberg, H., Abrams, D. I., Tracey, J., Mills, J., and Volberding, P. A., 1991, Clinical and virologic effects of recombinant human granulocyte-macrophage colony-stimulating factor in patients receiving chemotherapy for human immunodeficiency virus-associated non-Hodgkin's lymphoma: Results of a randomized trial, *J. Clin. Oncol.* **9**(6)**:**929–940.

Kawashima, I., Zanjani, E. D., Graca, A.-P., Flake, A. W., Zeng, H. Q., and Ogawa, M., 1996, $CD34^+$ human marrow cells that express low levels of kit protein are enriched for long-term marrow-engrafting cells, *Blood* **87:**4136–4142.

Kessinger, A., Armitage, J. O., and Landmark, J. D., 1988, Autologous peripheral hematopoietic stem cell transplantation restores hematopoietic function following marrow ablative therapy, *Blood* **71:**723.

Kiehntopf, M., Esquivel, E. L., Brach, M. A., and Herrmann, F., 1995, Ribozymes: Biology, biochemistry, and implications for clinical medicine, *J. Mol. Med.* **73:**65–71.

Kimura, S., Matsuda, J., Ikematsu, S., Miyazono, K., Ito, A., Nakahata, T., Minamitani, M., Shimada, K., Shiokawa, Y., and Takaku, F., 1990, Efficacy of recombinant human granulocyte colony-stimulating factor on neutropenia in patients with AIDS, *AIDS* **4:**1251–1255.

Kitano, K., Abboud, C. N., Ryan, D. H., Quan, S. G., Baldwin, G. C., and Golde, D. W., 1991, Macrophage-active colony-stimulating factors enhance human immunodeficiency virus type 1 infection in bone marrow stem cells, *Blood* **77**(8)**:**1699–1705.

Knaän-Shanzer, S., Valerio, D., and van Beusechem, V. W., 1996, Cell cycle state, response to hemopoietic growth factors and retroviral vector-mediated transduction of human hemopoietic stem cells, *Gene Ther.* **3:**323–333.

Kohn, D. B., Weinberg, K. I., Nolta, J. A., Heiss, L. N., Lenarsky, C., Crooks, G. M., Hanley, M. E., Annett, G., Brooks, J. S., el-Koureiy, A., Lawrence, K., Wells, S., Moen, R. C., Bastian, J., Williams-Herman, D. E., Elder, M., Wara, D., Bowen, T., Hershfield, M. S., Mullen, C. A., Blaese, R. M., and Parkman, R., 1995, Engraftment of gene-modified umbilical cord blood cells in neonates with adenosine deaminase deficiency, *Nat. Med.* **1**(10)**:**1017–1023.

Korbling, M., Przepiorka, D., Huh, Y. O., Engel, H., van Besien, K., Giralt, S., Andersson, B., Kleine, H. D., Seong, D., Deisseroth, A. B., Andreeff, M., and Champlin, R., 1995, Allogeneic blood stem cell transplantation for refractory leukemia and lymphoma: Potential advantage of blood over marrow allografts, *Blood* **85:**1659.

Kotani, H., Newton, P. B. III, Zhang, S., Chiang, Y. L., Otto, E., Weaver, L., Blaese, R. M., Anderson, W. F., and McGarrity, G. J., 1994, Improved methods of retroviral vector transduction and production for gene therapy, *Hum. Gene Ther.* **5:**19–28.

Koyangi, Y., O'Brien, W. A., Zhao, J. Q., Golde, D. W., Gassen, J. C., and Chen, I. S., 1988, Cytokines alter production of HIV-1 from primary mononuclear phagocytes, *Science* **241:**1673–1675.

Krause, D. S., Fackler, M. J., Civin, C. I., and May, W. S., 1996, CD34: Structure, biology, and clinical utility, *Blood* **87**(1)**:**1–13.

Krown, S. E., Paredes, J., Bundow, D., Polsky, B., Gold, J. W., and Flomenberg, N., 1992, Interferon-alpha, zidovudine, and granulocyte-macrophage colony-stimulating factor: A phase I AIDS Clinical Trials Group study in patients with Kaposi's sarcoma associated with AIDS, *J. Clin. Oncol.* **10**(8)**:**1344–1351.

Kuhn, L., and Stein, Z. A., 1995, Mother to infant HIV transmission: Timing, risk factors and prevention, *Paediatr. Perinat. Epidemiol.* **9**(1)**:**1.

Lane, T. A., Law, P., Maruyama, M., Young, D., Burgess, J., Mullen, M., Mealiffe, M., Terstappen, L. W. M. M., Hardwick, A., Moubayed, M., Oldham, F., Corringham, R. E. T., and Ho, A. D., 1995, Harvesting and enrichment of hematopoietic progenitor cells mobilized into the peripheral blood of normal donors by granulocyte-macrophage colony-stimulating factor (GM-CSF) or G-CSF: Potential role in allogeneic marrow transplantation, *Blood* **85:**275.

Lapidot, T., Pflumio, F., Doedens, M., Murdoch, B., Williams, D. E., and Dick, J. E., 1992, Cytokine stimulation of multilineage hematopoiesis from immature human cells engrafted in SCID mice, *Science* **255:**1137–1141.

Law, P., Ishizawa, L., Burgess, J., Mansour, V., Hangoc, G., Lazarus, H., Ho, A. D., Bender, J., Smith, S., Shilling, M., and Gee, A. P., 1992, High purity immunomagnetic selection of CD34+ cells from fresh and frozen mobilized peripheral blood stem cell (M-PBSC) collections, *Blood* **80**(10)(Suppl. 1)**:**261a.

Leary, A. G., and Ogawa, M., 1987, Blast cell colony assay for umbilical cord blood and adult bone marrow progenitors, *Blood* **69:**953.

Leavitt, M. C., Yu, M., Yamada, O., Kraus, G., Looney, D., Poeschla, E., and Wong-Staal, F., 1994, Transfer of an anti-HIV-1 ribozyme gene into primary human lymphocytes, *Hum. Gene Ther.* **5:**1115–1120.

Li, Y., Gervaix, A., Larg, D., Law, P., Spector, S., Ho, A. D., and Wong-Staal, F., 1998, Gene therapy targeting cord blood derived CD34+ cells from HIV-exposed infants: preclinical studies, *Gene Therapy* **5:**233–239.

Lu, L., Xiao, M., Clapp, D. W., Li, Z-H., and Broxmeyer, H. E., 1993, High efficiency retroviral mediated gene transduction into single isolated immature and replatable CD34+ hematopoietic stem/progenitor cells from human umbilical cord blood, *J. Exp. Med.* **178:**2089–2096.

Lu, M., Maruyama, M., and Zhang, N., 1994, High efficiency retroviral-mediated gene transduction into CD34+ cells purified from peripheral blood, *Hum. Gene Ther.* **5:**203–208.

Manders, S. M., Kostman, J. R., Mendez, L., and Russin, V. L., 1995, Thalidomide-resistant HIV-associated aphthae successfully treated with granulocyte colony-stimulating factor, *J. Am. Acad. Dermatol.* **33**(2 Pt 2)**:**380–382.

Michel, F., Umesono, K., and Ozeki, H., 1989, Comparative and functional anatomy of group II catalytic introns—a review, *Gene* **82:**5–30.

Miller, D. G., Adam, M. A., and Miller, A. D., 1992, Gene transfer by retrovirus vectors occurs only in cells that are actively replicating at the time of infection, *Mol. Cell. Biol.* **10:**4239–4242.

Miller, J. L., Donahue, R. E., Sellers, S. E., Samulski, R. J., Young, N. S., and Nienhuis, A. W., 1994, Recombinant adeno-associated virus (rAAV)-mediated expression of a human γ-globin gene in human progenitor-derived erythroid cells, *Proc. Natl. Acad. Sci. USA* **91:**10183–10187.

Miltenyi, S., Müller, W., Weichel, W., and Radbruch, A., 1990, High gradient magnetic cell separation with MACS, *Cytometry* **11:**231–238.

Molina, J. M., Scadden, D. T., Sakaguchi, M., Fuller, B., Woon, A., and Groopman, J. E., 1990, Lack of evidence for infection of or effect on growth of hematopoietic progenitor cells after *in vivo* or *in vitro* exposure to human immunodeficiency virus, *Blood* **76**(12)**:**2476–2482.

Moritz, T., Patel, V. P., and Williams, D. A., 1994, Bone marrow extracellular matrix molecules improve gene transfer into human hematopoietic cells via retroviral vectors, *J. Clin. Invest.* **93:**1451–1457.

Murray, L., Chen, B., Galy, A., Chen, S., Tushinski, R., Uchida, N., Negrin, R., Tricot, G., Jagannath, S., Vesole, D., Barlogie, B., Hoffman, R., and Tsuiamoto, A., 1995, Enrichment of human hematopoietic stem cell activity in the CD34+Thy-1+Lin− subpopulation from mobilized peripheral blood, *Blood* **85:**368.

Nolta, J. A., Yu, X. J., Bahner, I., and Kohn, D. B., 1992, Retroviral-mediated transfer of the human glucocerebrosidase gene into cultured Gaucher bone marrow, *J. Clin. Invest.* **90:**342.

Nolta, J. A., Smogorzewska, E. M., and Kohn, D. B., 1995, Analysis of optimal conditions for retroviral-mediated transduction of primitive human hematopoietic cells, *Blood* **86**(1)**:**101–110.

Ojwang, J. O., Hampel, A., Looney, D. J., Wong-Staal, F., and Rappaport, J., 1992, Inhibition of human immunodeficiency virus type 1 expression by a hairpin ribozyme, *Proc. Natl. Acad. Sci. USA* **89**(22)**:**10802–10806.

Okarma, T., Lebkowski, J., Schain, L., Harvey, M., Tricot, G., Srour, E., Meyers, W. G., Burnett, A., Sniecinski, I., and O'Reilly, R. J., 1992, The AIS cellector: A new technology for stem cell purification, In *Advances in Bone Marrow Purging and Processing*, (D. A. Worthington-White, A. P. Gee, and S. Gross, eds.), Wiley-Liss, New York, pp. 475–486.

Papadimitriou, C. A., Roots, A., Koenigsmann, M., Koenigsmann, M., Mücke, C., Oelmann, E., Oberberg, D., Reufi, B., Thiel, E., and Berdel, W. E., 1995, Immunomagnetic selection of CD34+ cells from fresh peripheral blood mononuclear cell preparations using two different separation techniques, *J. Hematol.* **4:**539–544.

Paul, R. W., Morris, D., Hess, B. W., Dunn, J., and Overell, R. W., 1993, Increased viral titer through concentration of viral harvests from retroviral packaging cell lines, *Hum. Gene Ther.* **4:**609–615.

Perno, C. F., Cooney, D. A., Gao, W. Y., Hao, Z., Johns, D. G., Foli, A., Hartman, N. R., Calio, R., Broder, S., and Yarchoan, R., 1992, Effects of bone marrow stimulatory cytokines on human immunodeficiency virus replication and the antiviral activity of dideoxynucleosides in cultures of monocyte/macrophages, *Blood* **80:**995–1003.

Ponchio, L., Conneally, E., and Eaves, C., 1995, Quantitation of the quiescent fraction of long-term culture-initiating cells in normal human blood and marrow and the kinetics of their growth factor-stimulated entry into S-phase *in vitro*, *Blood* **86**(9)**:**3314–3321.

Porter, C. D., Parkar, M. H., Collins, M. K. L., Levinsky, R. J., and Kinnon, C., 1996, Efficient retroviral transduction of human bone marrow progenitor and long-term culture-initiating cells: Partial reconstitution of cells from patients with X-linked chronic granulomatous disease by gp^{91}-*phox* expression, *Blood* **87:**3722–3730.

Pyle, A. M., 1993, Ribozymes: A distinct class of metalloenzymes, *Science* **261:**708–714.

Ruffner, D. E., Stormo, G. D., and Uhlenbeck, O. C., 1990, Sequence requirements of the hammerhead RNA self-cleavage reaction, *Biochemistry* **29:**10695–10702.

Saeland, S., Duvert, V., Caux, D., Pandrau, D., Favre, C., Valle, A., Durand, I., Charbord, P., deVries, J., and Banchereau, J., 1992, Distribution of surface-membrane bound molecules on bone marrow and cord blood $CD34^+$ hematopoietic cells, *Exp. Hematol.* **20:**24.

Sato, N., Caux, C., Kitzamura, T., Watanabe, Y., Arai, K., Banchereau, J., and Miyajima, A., 1993, Expression and factor-dependent modulation of the interleukin-3 receptor subunits on human hematopoietic cells, *Blood* **82**(3)**:**752–761.

Sekhsaria, S., Gallin, J. I., Linton, G. F., Mallory, R. M., Mulligan, R. C., and Malech, H. L., 1993, Peripheral blood progenitors as a target for genetic correction of $p47^{phox}$-deficient chronic granulomatous disease, *Proc. Natl. Acad. Sci. USA* **90:**7446.

Shah, A. J., Smogorzewska, E. M., Hannum, C., and Crooks, G. M., 1996, Flt3 ligand induces proliferation of quiescent human bone marrow $CD34^+CD38^-$ cells and maintains progenitor cells *in vitro*, *Blood* **87**(9)**:**3563–3570.

Sharmeen, L., Kuo, M. Y. P., Dinter-Gottlieb, G., and Taylor, J., 1988, Antigenomic RNA of human hepatitis delta virus can undergo self-cleavage, *J. Virol.* **62:**2674–2679.

Shaughnessy, E., Lu, D., Chatterjee, S., and Wong, K. K., 1996, Parvoviral vectors for the gene therapy of cancer, *Semin. Oncol.* **23**(1)**:**159–171.

Shpall, E. J., Jones, R. B., Bearman, S. I., Franklin, W. A., Archer, P. G., Curiel, T., Bitter, M., Clamman, H. N., Stemmer, S. M., Purdy, M., Myers, S. E., Hami, L., Taffs, S., Heimfeld, S., Hallagan, J., and Berenson, R. J., 1994, Transplantation of enriched CD34-positive autologous marrow into breast cancer patients following high-dose chemotherapy: Influence of CD34-positive peripheral-blood progenitors and growth factors on engraftment, *J. Clin. Oncol.* **12:**28.

Siena, S., Bregni, M., Brando, B., Ravagnani, F., Bonadonna, G., and Gianni, A. M., 1989, Circulation of $CD34^+$ hematopoietic stem cells in the peripheral blood of high-dose cyclophosphamide treated patients: Enhancement by intravenous recombinant human granulocyte-macrophage colony stimulating factor, *Blood* **74:**1905.

Sloand, E., Kumar, P. N., and Pierce, P. F., 1993, Chemotherapy for patients with pulmonary Kaposi's sarcoma: Benefit of filgrastim (G-CSF) in supporting dose administration, *South. Med. J.* **86**(11)**:**1219–1224.

Smith, K. T., Shepherd, A. J., Boyd, J. E., and Lees, G. M., 1996, Gene delivery systems for use in gene therapy: An overview of quality assurance and safety issues, *Gene Ther.* **3:**190–200.

Srour, E. F., Leemhuis, T., Brandt, J. E., van Besien, K., and Hoffman, R., 1991a, Simultaneous use of rhodamine 123, phycoerythrin, Texas red, and allophycocyanin for the isolation of human hematopoietic progenitor cells, *Cytometry* **12:**179.

Srour, E. F., Brandt, J. E., Briddell, R. A., Leemhuis, T., van Besien, K., and Hoffman, R., 1991b, Human $CD34^+HLA\text{-}DR^-$ bone marrow cells contain progenitor cells capable of self-renewal, multilineage differentiation, and long-term *in vitro* hematopoiesis, *Blood Cells* **17:**287.

Stanley, S. K., Kessler, S. W., Justement, J. S., Schnittman, S. M., Greenhouse, J. J., Brown, C. C., Musongela, L., Musey, K., Kapita, B., and Fauci, A. S., 1992, $CD34^+$ bone marrow cells are infected with HIV in a subset of seropositive individuals, *J. Immunol.* **149:**689–697.

Strauss, L. C., Rowley, S. D., LaRussa, V. F., Sharkis, S. J., Stuart, R. K., and Civin, C. I., 1986, Antigenic analysis of hematopoiesis V: Characterization of My-10 antigen expression by normal lymphohematopoietic progenitor cells, *Exp. Hematol.* **14:**878–886.

Strauss, L. C., Trischmann, T. M., Rowley, S. D., Wiley, J. M., and Civin, C. L., 1991, Selection of normal human hematopoietic stem cells for bone marrow transplantation using immunomagnetic microspheres and CD34 antibody, *Am. J. Pediatr. Hematol./Oncol.* **2:**217.

Sullenger, B. A., and Cech, T. R., 1993, Tethering ribozymes to a retroviral packaging signal for destruction of viral RNA, *Science* **262:**1566–1569.

Sutherland, D. R., and Keating, A., 1992, The CD34 antigen: Structure, biology, and potential clinical applications, *J. Hematol.* **1:**115–129.

Terstappen, L. W. M. M., Huang, S., Safford, M., Lansdorp, P. M., and Loken, M. R., 1991, Sequential generations of hematopoietic colonies derived from single nonlineage-committed $CD34^+/CD38^-$ progenitor cells, *Blood* **77:**1218–1227.

To, L. B., Haylock, D. N., Kimber, R. J., and Juttner, C. A., 1984, High levels of circulating haematopoietic stem cells in very early remission from acute non-lymphoblastic leukaemia and their collection and cryopreservation, *Br. J. Haematol.* **58:**399.

Torbett, B. E., Conners, K., Shao, L. E., Mosier, D. E., and Yu, J., 1995, High level multilineage engraftment of human hematopoietic cells is maintained in NOC/SCID mice, *Blood* **86**(10)(Suppl. 1)**:**112a.

Torlontano, G., Di Bartolomeo, P., Di Girolamo, G., Angrilli, F., Verani, P., Maggiorella, M. T., Dragani, A., Iacone, A., Papalinetti, G., Olioso, P., Cosentino, L., and Dantonio, D., 1992, AIDS-related complex treated by antiviral drugs and allogeneic bone marrow transplantation following conditioning protocol with busulphan, cyclophosphamide, and cyclosporin, *Haematologica* **77**(3)**:**287–290.

Traycoff, C. M., Abboud, M. R., Laver, J., Brandt, J. E., Hoffman, R., Law, P., Ishizawa, L., and Srour, E. F., 1994, Evaluation of the *in vitro* behavior of phenotypically defined populations of umbilical cord blood hematopoietic progenitor cells, *Exp. Hematol.* **22:**215–222.

Tricot, G., Gazitt, Y., Jagannath, S., Vesole, D., Reading, C., Juttner, C., Hoffman, R., and Barlogie, B., 1995, $CD34^+THY^+LIN^-$ peripheral blood stem cells (PBSC) effect timely trilineage engraftment in multiple myeloma (MM), *Blood* **86**(10)(Suppl. 1)**:**293a.

Tseng-Law, J., Curtis, J., Kobori, J., and Deans, R., 1995, Peptide epitopes of anti-CD34 monoclonal antibodies which function as release reagents for $CD34^+$ cell selection *Blood* **86**(10)(Suppl. 1)**:**490a.

Uhlenbeck, O. C., 1987, A small catalytic oliogoribonucleotide, *Nature* **328:**596–500.

Vecchiarelli, A., Monari, C., Baldelli, F., Pietrella, D., Retini, C., Tascini, C., Francisci, D., and Bistoni, F., 1995, Beneficial effect of recombinant human granulocyte colony-stimulating factor on fungicidal activity of polymorphonuclear leukocytes from patients with AIDS, *J. Infect. Dis.* **171**(6)**:**1448–1454.

von Laer, D., Hufert, F. T., Fenner, T. E., Schwander, S., Dietrich, M., Schmitz, H., and Kern, P., 1990, $CD34^+$ hematopoietic progenitor cells are not a major reservoir of the human immunodeficiency virus, *Blood* **76**(7)**:**1281–1286.

Wang, X. S., Yoder, M. C., Zhou, S. Z., and Srivastava, A., 1995, Parvovirus B19 promoter at map unit 6 confers autonomous replication competence and erythroid specificity to adeno-associated virus 2 in primary human hematopoietic progenitor cells, *Proc. Natl. Acad. of Sci. USA* **92**(26)**:**12416–12420.

Wu, H. N., Lin, Y. J., Lin, F. P., Makino, S., Chang, M. F., and Lai, M. M. C., 1989, Human hepatitis delta virus RNA subfragments contain an autocleavage activity, *Proc. Natl. Acad. Sci. USA* **86:**1831–1835.

Yamada, O., Yu, M., Yee, J. K., Kraus, G., Looney, D. J., and Wong-Staal, F., 1994a, Intracellular immunization of human T-cells with a hairpin ribozyme against human immunodeficiency virus type 1, *Gene Ther.* **1:**39–45.

Yamada, O., Kraus, G., Leavitt, M. C., Yu, M., and Wong-Staal, F., 1994b, Activity and cleavage site specificity of an anti-HIV-1 hairpin ribozyme in human T-cells, *Virology* **205:**121–126.

Yamada, O., Kraus, G., Luznik, L., Yu, M., and Wong-Staal, F., 1996, A chimeric HIV-1 minimal RRE/ribozyme molecule exhibits dual antiviral function and inhibits cell–cell transmission of HIV-1, *J. Virol.* **70:**1596–1901.

Young, J. C., Varma, A., DiGiusto, D., and Backer, M. P., 1996, Retention of quiescent hematopoietic cells with high proliferative potential during *ex vivo* stem cell culture, *Blood* **87:**545–556.

Yu, M., Ojwang, J., Yamada, O., Hampel, A., Rapapport, J., Looney, D., and Wong-Staal, F., 1993, A hairpin ribozyme inhibits expression of diverse strains of human immunodeficiency virus type 1, *Proc. Natl. Acad. Sci. USA* **90:**6340–6344.

Yu, M., Leavitt, M. C., Maruyama, M., Yamada, O., Young, D., Ho, A. D., and Wong-Staal, F., 1995, Intracellular immunization of human fetal cord blood stem/progenitor cells with a ribozyme against human immunodeficiency virus type 1, *Proc. Natl. Acad. Sci. USA* **92:**699–703.

Zanjani, E. D., Pallavicini, M. G., Ascensao, J. L., Flake, A. W., Langlois, R. G., Reitsma, M., MacKintosh, F. R., Stutes, D., Harrison, M. R., and Tavassoli, M., 1992, Engraftment and long-term expression of human fetal hemopoietic stem cells in sheep following transplantation *in utero*, *J. Clin. Invest.* **89:**1178.

Zhou, S. Z., Cooper, S., Kang, L. Y., Ruggieri, L., Heimfeld, S., Srivastava, A., and Broxmeyer, H. E., 1994, Adeno-associated virus 2-mediated high efficiency gene transfer into immature and mature subsets of hematopoietic progenitor cells in human umbilical cord blood, *J. Exp. Med.* **179:**1867–1875.

Zhou, S. Z., Li, Q., Stamatoyannoupoulas, G., and Srivastava, A., 1996, Adeno-associated virus 2-mediated transduction and erythroid cell-specific expression of a human β-globin gene, *Gene Ther.* **3:**223–229.

Chapter 13

Molecular Immunotherapy by Gene Transfer

Rosa Maria Diaz and Richard G. Vile

1. INTRODUCTION

An attractive approach to cancer gene therapy is to deliver genes that enhance the immunogenicity of tumor cells, thereby augmenting the immune response against them (Nabel *et al.*, 1992, Rosenberg *et al.*, 1993, Tepper and Mule, 1994). Using the immune system presents three major theoretical advantages for cancer gene therapy:

1. If it can be activated to recognize tumor-specific antigens on tumor cells, the *specificity* of the immune response should mean that systemic toxicity is re-duced to a minimum because only tumor cells that express the antigens will be killed;
2. Once activated, immune responses have a natural *response amplification* mechanism so that only a small stimulus (low levels of gene transfer) is required to produce a large response. That response should, in theory, be bodywide and protect against the recurrence of the disease.
3. Recruiting the body's own immunity to recognize and destroy the tumor cells should be far less toxic than current treatments, such as chemotherapy and radiotherapy.

There is good evidence now that at least some tumors express tumor antigens which are recognized under certain circumstances by the immune system (Boon *et*

Rosa Maria Diaz Richard Dimbleby/ICRF Department of Cancer Research, Rayne Institute, St. Thomas' Hospital, London SE1 7EH, United Kingdom. **Richard G. Vile** Molecular Medicine Program, Guggenheim 18, Mayo Clinic, Rochester, Minnesota 55905.

Blood Cell Biochemistry, Volume 8: Hematopoiesis and Gene Therapy, edited by Fairbairn and Testa. Kluwer Academic/Plenum Publishers, New York, 1999.

al., 1994). Therefore, it has been proposed that expressing various types of immunostimulatory molecules in tumor cells might enhance immune recognition, possibly by overcoming intrinsic defects in the pathways of antigen presentation by tumor cells (Pardoll, 1993). The hope is that tumor cells engineered to express such molecules, either *ex vivo* as vaccines or directly by *in vivo* gene delivery, will generate long lasting immunity to unmodified tumor cells that grow at distant sites in the body. Encouraging results have been obtained from animal models that use tumor cells modified to express cytokines (*e.g.*, IL-2, IL-4, GM-CSF, IFN; Gilboa and Kim Lyerly, 1994; Tepper and Mule, 1994); costimulatory molecules (*e.g.*, members of the B7 family; Ramarathinam *et al.*, 1994; Townsend and Allison, 1993); MHC molecules (Browning and Bodmer, 1992); allogeneic antigens (Plautz *et al.*, 1993); and syngeneic tumor antigens (Hawkins *et al.*, 1993). Human clinical trials are underway to see if these results translate into clinical gains in humans (Gilboa and Kim Lyerly, 1994; Tepper and Mule, 1994). However, the mass of preclinical data from animal models threatens to swamp a rational translation of gene transfer protocols into patient trials, and a clear understanding of the mechanisms by which gene transfer might be used to stimulate antitumor immunity is required.

2. ARE TUMORS ANTIGENIC?

For immune control of tumors, in whatever form to be possible, tumor cells must express determinants which, at least potentially, can be recognized by components of the immune system. In addition, these determinants must qualitatively or quantitatively differ enough from normal cellular determinants to ensure that any subsequent immunity raised against them does not lead to autoimmune destruction of normal cells (Golumbek *et al.*, 1993).

The early work on transplantation of tumors between syngeneic hosts demonstrated the existence of transplantation antigens on tumor cells. When seen as a vaccinating challenge, these antigens, lead to the stimulation of immune responses that mediate rejection of secondary challenges of immunogenic tumor cells. Such animal data led to and continues to provoke hopes that tumor cell preparations might be used as cancer vaccines to stimulate antitumor immunity in patients who have established disease (Bystryn, 1990; Morton *et al.*, 1993a; Oettgen and Old, 1991). Recently, however, molecular techniques have been used to identify and clone individual genes whose products fulfill some of the criteria of tumor antigens. This has only been achieved for a limited range of human tumors (Boon *et al.*, 1992; Houghton, 1994) and has led to a new era of tumor vaccination trials. However, in addition to generating new hopes for the use of "molecular vaccines" in cancer therapy, these results have also highlighted complex paradoxes which must also be confronted.

Classes of Tumor Antigens

Several classes of molecules have now been identified at a molecular level which might act as tumor antigens and even perhaps as tumor immunogens (Boon *et al.*, 1994; Houghton, 1994; Pardoll, 1994; Table I).

Table I
Human Tumor Antigens[a]

Viral antigens derived from genes of HPV; EBV; HTLV-1; HBV
Differentiation antigens: Tyrosinase, gp75/TRP-1, gp100/Pmel17, Melan-A/MART-1
Tumor-specific antigens: Mutated CDK4, Mutated β-Catenin; MUM-1
Antigens shared between tumor types: MAGE, GAGE, BAGE, MUC-1, Her-2neu; intronic sequence of GnT-V; mutated oncogene products

[a] Reviewed in Boon and van der Bruggen, 1996.

2.1.1. Non-Self Tumor Antigens

The most obvious types of determinants that could act as rejection antigens on tumor cells are viral proteins which derive from an oncogenic virus. These proteins may be those derived directly from the transforming proteins themselves, such as the human papilloma virus E6 or E7 proteins (Chen *et al.*, 1991), or they may be other viral antigens not directly involved in the process by which the virus transforms the cell, for instance, the viral structural proteins. In fact, it is thought that only between 15–25% of human cancers have a viral etiologies (Schulz and Vile, 1992), and even then there is good evidence that virally induced tumor cells very often down-regulate expression of the most immunogenic viral proteins (such as envelope proteins; Klein and Boon, 1993). This probably represents a form of immunosurveillance because virally infected cells that express foreign antigens will be rapidly selected out: Only infected cells that lose or down-regulate expression of these proteins survive immune clearance long enough to become transformed by the action of the viral-transforming proteins. Nonetheless, this still leaves the transforming proteins as potential targets for T cell and humoral immune responses (see later), and considerable research effort is currently directed to determine the most immunogenic parts of proteins, such as the papilloma virus E6 and E7 proteins, which are maintained in transformed cells in cervical neoplasia (Chen *et al.*, 1991).

The other class of "non-self" antigens which might be available to signal an emerging tumor population to the immune system is the mutated cellular proteins whose mutation is integral to the transformation process. Mutations to proto-oncogenes or tumor suppressor genes are essential to the genesis of all human tumors (Vogelstein and Kinzler, 1993). As a result of these genetic mutations, oncogenes and mutated tumor-suppressive genes produce protein products that differ from normal proteins by one or a few amino acid residues. There is growing evidence that cytotoxic T cells can be detected, from both animal models and patient populations, which react against mutated regions of oncoproteins, such as RAS and tumor-suppressive proteins, such as p53, although they have minimal reactivity against their normal conterparts (Chen *et al.*, 1992; Jung and Schluesener, 1991; Nijman *et al.*, 1994; Schlichtholz *et al.*, 1992; Skipper and Stauss, 1993). Therefore, even though these "antigens" are derived from host-cell-encoded self genes (as opposed to virally encoded "foreign" genes), they may serve as immunogenic targets for the immune system, provided that the appropriate peptides can pass successfully through the proteasome processing pathway and be presented by Class I MHC molecules on the surface of tumor cells.

2.1.2. Self Tumor Antigens

Within the last few years, molecular biology has been used to clone a new set of potential human tumor antigens. These studies have revealed that proteins that are neither foreign (non-self) nor mutated versions of normal cellular proteins can serve as targets for cytotoxic T cell responses against tumor cells.

The first class of such genes were cloned from human melanomas using a biological assay in which cytolytic T cell (CTL) clones derived from a patient are used to identify a specific molecule expressed by the melanoma cells from the same patient (Gaugler *et al.*, 1994; Van der Bruggen *et al.*, 1991). The MAGE family of genes are *unmutated* versions of a cellular gene which is expressed in early ontogeny but not normally in mature tissues other than the testes. In addition, screening of other tumor types shows that MAGE is expressed on a variety of tumor cells (Brasseur *et al.*, 1992) but not on their corresponding normal cellular counterparts. Similar biological assays based on the use of patient CTL have also been used to clone other antigens, including the melanocyte-specific enzyme tyrosinase (Brichard *et al.*, 1993) and MART protein (Kawakami *et al.*, 1994b). These differ from the MAGE family of antigens in that they are normally expressed on melanocytes but are expressed in greater quantities in patients with melanoma, partly because of the large numbers of cells that express the proteins.

The CTL response to these antigens is specific based on two related observations:

1. Melanoma cells that do not express the antigens are not killed by the respective patient CTL (Boon *et al.*, 1994; Brichard *et al.*, 1993);
2. The antigenic peptides must be presented in the context of specific MHC molecules, *i.e.*, melanoma cells that express the antigen but lack the appropriate MHC Class I molecule are not lysed by the patient CTL (Kawakami *et al.*, 1994a).

This property of tumor antigen presentation has recently been used to identify an antigenic epitope in human melanoma (Cox *et al.*, 1994). Peptides were eluted from MHC Class I molecules on tumor cells, fractionated by chromatography, and analyzed by tandem mass spectromoetry. A peptide epitope was identified which, when complexed with the appropriate MHC Class I molecule, was recognized by CTLs derived from the same patient and from five other melanoma patients. This peptide forms part of a previously unidentified protein that is specific to melanocytes and melanoma cells.

These classes of antigens have the hallmarks of being recognized in *specific, MHC restricted, T-cell-mediated immune responses*. This has been used to argue that such antigens could be used as vaccines in patients whose tumors express the antigen and who have the correct MHC haplotype to ensure that the antigen is correctly presented to the immune system (Marchand *et al.*, 1993; Traversari *et al.*, 1992).

In contrast, a population of T lymphocytes has also been identified that partly resembles NK cells in that they lyse their targets in an MHC unrestricted fashion, but also resembles CTL in that they are specific for the target antigen encoded by the MUC-1 gene that is expressed on the surface of breast and pancreatic tumors (Barnd *et al.*, 1989; Taylor-Papadimitriou *et al.*, 1993). MUC-1 does not have to be processed *via* the proteasome pathway typical of MHC Class I presentation but is recognized by its cell-surface expression by a mechanism which is still unclear.

3. ANTIGEN PRESENTATION PATHWAYS

The molecular identification of tumor antigens has provided a welcome boost to the long-standing dreams of tumor immunologists to activate tumor-specific immune reactivity that recognizes and eradicates metastatic deposits throughout the body (Kedar and Klein, 1992). The attraction of the immune system in cancer therapy is that, once appropriately activated against tumor-specific determinants, it has both very high levels of antigen specificity and built-in response amplification so that, in theory, only a small activation signal produces long-lasting, bodywide protection.

These properties make the immune system the most attractive target for current attempts at gene therapy of cancer because no gene delivery system, or even chemotherapeutic drug, currently has the required specificity or efficiency to target all of the tumor cells in the bodies of most cancer patients (Vile and Russell, 1994).

Generation of an antitumor immune response depends on the existence of tumor antigens that are recognized by the immune system. The endogenously synthesized antigen is processed intracellularly within the proteasome into short peptides (typically about nine amino acids long) selected for binding into the molecular "groove" formed at the surface of a molecule of the Class I major histocompatibility complex (MHC). Then, the MHC-peptide complex is transported to the cell surface for antigen presentation to T cells (Neefjes and Momburg, 1993). The tumor antigen-MHC Class I complex is recognized by a high-affinity binding reaction to a T cell receptor (TCR) of a CD8+ cytolytic T cell (CTL). Complexing of the TCR with antigen initiates intracellular signalling to the nucleus of the CTL that stimulates the expression of the effector functions of the T cell—in this case, killing the target (tumor) cell (Janeway and Bottomly, 1994). However, for the CD8+ cell to become fully activated for killing, it must also receive additional stimulatory signals provided by binding cytokines to their receptors on the T cell surface. In turn, the cytokines are, secreted by CD4+ T helper cells that have been activated by the presentation of the tumor antigen by a professional antigen-presenting cell (APC), such as a dendritic cell or a macrophage (Paul and Seder, 1994). These APC must take up shed antigen, proteolyticaly process it *via* a separate endosomal antigen-processing pathway, and present antigenic peptides complexed with an MHC Class II molecule (Neefjes & Momburg, 1993). In addition to the MHC-antigen complexes on the tumor and APC cell surface binding to the TCR on the T cells, full activation also requires the complexing of other surface molecules at the opposing cell surfaces. One such interaction, increasingly recognized as important in tumor rejection, is the binding of the costimulatory molecule B7.1 or B7.2 (on the APC) to its ligand CD28 (on the T cell; Allison, 1994; June *et al.*, 1994).

Therefore, an MHC-restricted cytolytic T cell response to generate to a specific tumor antigen, both presentation of the antigenic peptide by the tumor cell (MHC Class I) and cytokine "help" produced by presentation of the antigen to CD4+ helper T cells are required.

Following successful activation, the CTL will divide so that many daughter clones are produced, all with identical antigen specificity (the same TCR). In addition, certain types of helper T cells that persist in the periphery will recognize any future challenge from tumor cells that express the same antigen. Ideally, this will provide a pool of effector CD8+ T cells, which circulate through the body and destroy any tumor cells that have metastasized, and a pool of memory cells that in the future can initiate an attack on any cells that express the same tumor antigen.

4. IMMUNOTHERAPY BY GENE TRANSFER

The endogenous immune response outlined previously does not operate optimally, if at all, in patients who develop cancer. This failure could result from for a variety of causes. For example, many tumor cells down-regulate or lose expression of MHC Class I molecules, so that antigens cannot be presented (Browning and Bodmer, 1992; Restifo *et al.*, 1993; Vegh *et al.*, 1993). The lack of immunogenicity of tumor cells may also be result from the absence of effective operation of the CD4+ T helper arm of the presentation pathway (Pardoll, 1992). For instance, shedding of tumor antigens and their uptake by APC may be very ineffective in the patient so that full activation of tumor-specific CD4+ helper cells is prevented and complete activation of the CTL fails because of a lack of cytokine secretion from the helper cells (Figure 1A).

These considerations have led to the suggestion that transfer of appropriate genes directly into tumor cells or into other cell types may bypass defects in the antigen-presentation pathways of the immune response to tumor cells (Colombo & Forni, 1994; Pardoll, 1992; Tepper and Mule, 1994) (Figure 1B). This was the theory behind the first experiments in which cytokine genes were transferred into tumor cells to create gene-modified vaccines. Thus, for example, tumor cells modified by gene transfer to express the helper cytokine interleukin-2 act more effectively as antigen-presenting cells and fulfill the both functions of direct antigen presentation to CD8+ cells and cytokine activation of the same cells by local secretion of the cytokine gene (Dranoff *et al.*, 1993; Figure 1B). Since the first such studies of gene transfer to tumor cells in rodent models in the 1980s, a wide variety of immunomodulatory genes successfully used to induce antitumor responses in rodent models have led to the initiation of clinical trials in humans. In addition to many cytokines, gene transfer of accessory molecules, such as MHC genes (Tanaka *et al.*, 1988), or costimulatory molecules, such as B7 (Ramarathinam *et al.*, 1994; Townsend and Allison, 1993) may also enhance the antigen-presenting nature of the tumor cells and generate tumor-specific CTL responses. Because of the diversity of the data on different genes in different experimental models, it seems at first

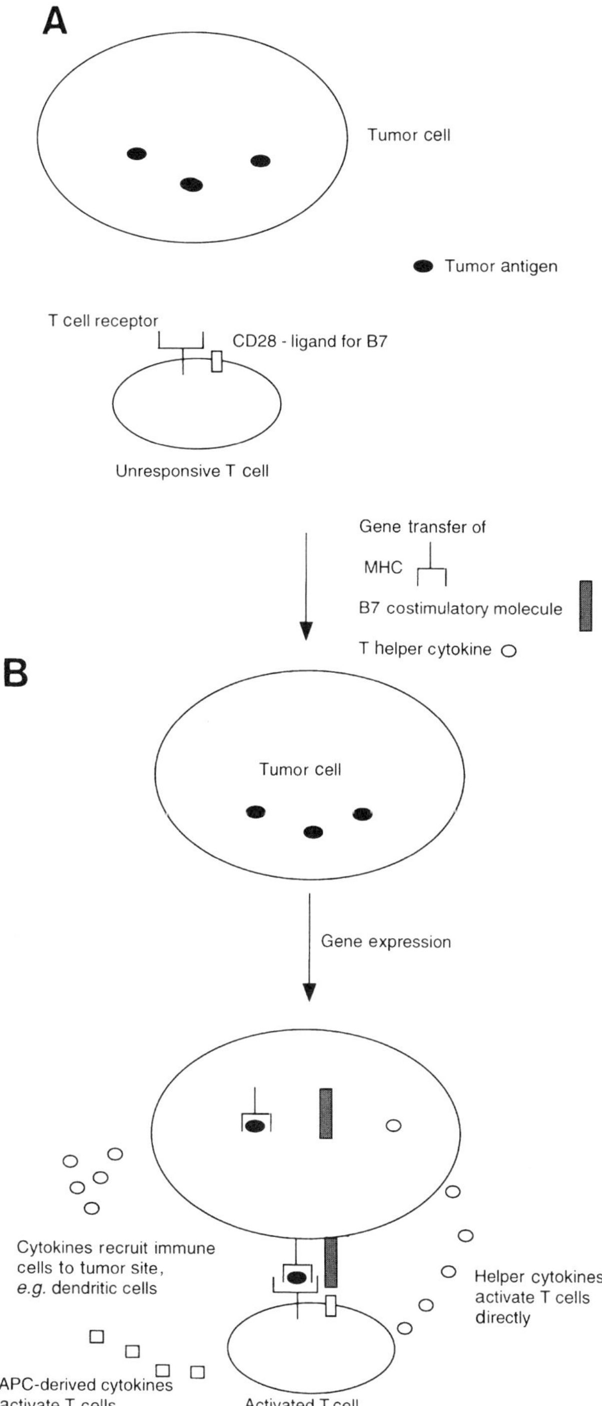

FIGURE 1. A. Tumor cell cannot present antigen to the immune system because it lacks antigen-presentation machinery, for example, MHC, costimulatory molecule or adequate T cell helper cytokine production. B. Gene transfer converts a tumor cell of low intrinsic antigen-presenting capability (see A) to a cell of high intrinsic antigen-presenting capability which can activate a tumor-specific T cell response. C. Gene transfer induces release of tumor antigens that, after uptake and presentation by professional antigen-presenting cells, activate a tumor-specific T cell response.

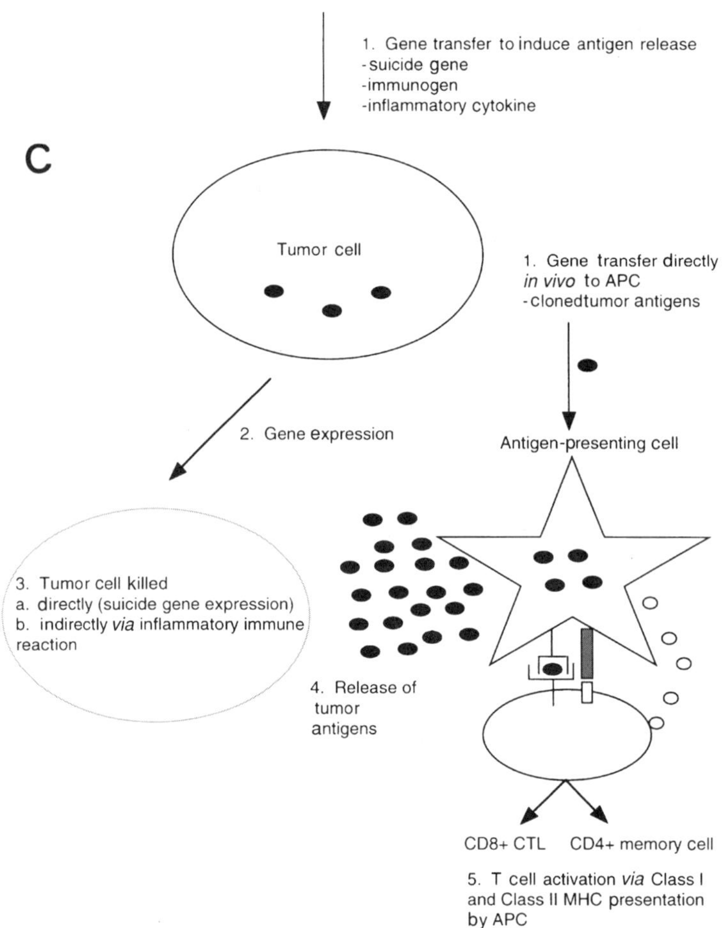

FIGURE 1. (*Continued*)

inspection that the final choice may be somewhat of a lottery which will only be characterization of alternative cytokines with other pleiotropic properties, suggesting that better choices may be possible (see later and Table II).

Other cytokine genes have proved potent in several independent studies, and these activities indicate their ability to activate specific immune functions (Table II), especially those effectivee in recruiting and activating the antigen-presentation pathways. For example, GM-CSF has well described properties as a maturation factor for early human and mouse bone marrow progenitors of dendritic cells (Inaba *et al.*, 1992), and given the scheme described previously for the mechanisms of antigen presentation, it would be most attractive to be able to recruit antigen-presenting cells to the site of a tumour so that they might receive shed tumor antigens. This theoretical attraction of GM-CSF is also supported by several experimental studies (Berns *et al.*, 1995; Carducci *et al.*, 1995; Dranoff *et al.*, 1993, Saito *et al.*, 1994; Stoppacciaro *et al.*, 1993). In a comparison of the ability of genetically

Table II
Examples of Cytokines that Successfully Generate Antitumor Immune Responses Following Gene Transfer in Animal Models[a]

Cytokine	Principal immune cell mediator
IL-2	CB8+, CD4+ T cells, NK cells
IL-4	Macrophages, eosinophils
IL-6	Non T cells, macrophages
IL-7	CD4+, CD8+ T cells
IL-12	Macrophages, dendritic cells, CD4+,CD8+ T cells
GM-CSF	Dendritic cells, macrophages, CD4/8+ T cells
IFN-g	CD8+ T cells, macrophages
TNF-a	CD4+, CD8+ T cells
Costimulatory molecules (B71/2)	CD8+ T cells

[a] Reviewed in Forni *et al.*, 1995; Tepper and Mule, 1994.

engineered, irradiated cells, GM-CSF expression consistently proved the most effective way to generate long lasting systemic immunity against a number of tumor cells, including melanoma, colon carcinoma, renal sarcoma, lung carcinoma, and two fibrosarcomas lines. Similarly, GM-CSF transduced melanoma cells are completely reliant on tumor presentation by bone-marrow-derived dendritic cells (rather than the tumor cells) for the rejection responses seen in this system (Huang *et al.*, 1994). This underscores the importance of APC in generating effective immmune memory.

It should be stressed, however, that not all studies which have compared different cytokines show that GM-CSF is the superior cytokine (Allione, 1994; Saito *et al.*, 1994; Vieweg *et al.*, 1994). Furthermore, the effects of dosage of GM-CSF are still unclear. No dose threshold was seen with GM-CSF, in contrast with IL-2, in one study (Schmidt *et al.*, 1995), although a separate group has reported that a threshold level of GM-CSF secretion can be reached (Abe *et al.*, 1995).

Clearly, other genes could equally well be the candidate of choice. In particular, cytokines could be chosen for their ability to divert T helper cell responses into the Th1 pathway, which is believed important for generating cell-mediated immunity (Dallman, 1995; Kelso, 1995; Paul and Seder, 1994; Zitvogel *et al.*, 1996). In this respect, cytokine gene transfer of IL-2, IFN-g or IL-12 may be useful (Paul and Seder, 1994). IL-12 also has stimulatory effects on antigen-presenting pathways and may be equally valuable in this respect (Banks *et al.*, 1995; Tahara and Lotze, 1995; Tahara *et al.*, 1995). Conversely, other studies have shown the efficacy of Th2 helper cytokines (Gerard *et al.*, 1996; Giovarelli *et al.*, 1995; Pericle *et al.*, 1994).

In summary, a broad spectrum of cytokines is efficacious in animal models. Our ability to deliver several genes simultaneously to tumor cells *in vivo* is clearly limited (maybe currently two or three), and we lack a clear understanding of how multiple genes would interact *in vivo*. Hence, our ability for effective predictions of the optimal cytokine(s) for gene transfer remains limited. Theoretical considerations, based on identifying common themes emerging from the literature, followed by eventual empirical determination in limited clinical trials seems to be the best way forward.

4.1. Gene Transfer of Components of the Antigen-Presentation Apparatus

Gene transfer into tumor cells, using genes encoding MHC (Tranaka *et al.*, 1988) or B7 (Allison, 1994), for example, might be used to overcome defects in the antigen-presenting pathways *in vivo* (Figure 1B). Such molecular therapies aim to transform the tumor cell into as effective an antigen-presenting cell as possible. In particular, much enthusiasm has been generated for transfer of genes that encode the costimulatory molecules of the B7 family. For complete activation, a T cell requires the antigen-specific signal provided by antigen bound to an MHC molecule and also a second, costimulatory signal provided by B7 which binds to a receptor on the T cell surface, known as CD28. Gene transfer of members of the B7 family into tumor cells initially gave rise to optimism that tumor cells might be made to function as effective antigen-presenting cells *in vivo* (Hellstrom *et al.*, 1995). However, more recently it has become clear that B7 can deliver positive activation signals to T cells (*via* ligation of CD28) and also negative signals *via* ligation of a second resolved following clinical trials in patients. However, a careful review of the literature may reveal some common principles which allow translation into rational human trials.

4.2. Cytokines

Cytokines that have proved successful in generating local and/or systemic responses *in vivo* have been characterized in various model systems (Cavallo *et al.*, 1992,1993, Dranoff *et al.*, 1993; Hock *et al.*, 1993a) reviewed in (Forni *et al.*, 1995; Tepper and Mule, 1994). In a few cases, some of these cytokines also lead to the generation of specific responses directed against tumor cells (Cavallo *et al.*, 1993; Giovarelli *et al.*, 1995; Pericle *et al.*, 1994; Porgador *et al.*, 1993). Of these cytokines, IL-2 has received the most attention and in different systems has been successful in generating local inflammation and subsequently giving rise to systemic immunity via tumor-specific immune responses (Cavallo *et al.*, 1993; Connor *et al.*, 1993; Porgador *et al.*, 1993; Visseren *et al.*, 1994). However, other groups have distinguished between the ability of this cytokine to generate local tumor rejection and subsequent protection, especially in nonimmunogenic tumors (Dranoff *et al.*, 1993; Karp *et al.*, 1993).

In addition, the levels of IL-2 secreted by the modified cells can affect the nature of the response (Fakhrai *et al.*, 1995; Schmidt *et al.*, 1995). If the initial inflammatory reaction is very aggressive, it can lead to rapid disappearance of the incipient tumor before the antigen load is suffient to trigger any tumor-specific component of the immune response (Colombo *et al.*, 1992). There is also a balance *in vivo* between the immune system's ability to exert inhibitory effects on tumor growth (*via* activation of tumoricidal immune cells) and stimulatory effects (*via* activation of tumor cell growth direct; Prehn, 1994; Seung *et al.*, 1995).

In summary, IL-2 can act as a potent inducer of nonspecific inflammation and, in some cases, may promote specific antitumor responses. Therefore, it was one of the earliest cytokine genes used in clinical trials (Foa *et al.*, 1992). However, the ligand CTLA-4 (Krummel and Allison, 1995; Walunas *et al.*, 1994). In addition, an incomplete understanding of the accessory signals required for optimally costimulating and activating effective memory responses to unmodified tumor cells has recently suggested that gene transfer of B7 may not be an ideal way to stimulate antitumor immunity and may even be deleterious (Chong *et al.*, 1996).

4.3. Gene Transfer of Nonspecific Immunogens

Various types of cancer vaccines, either oncolysates of cancer cells or intact cells in autologous or allogeneic settings, have incorporated adjuvants, such as BCG, Freund's complete adjuvant, or any of the more recent formulations. Such trials have all produced responses which have been sporadically impressive but often difficult to replicate (Dalgleish, 1996). The best results from such trials have come from allogeneic melanoma cell vaccines (Morton *et al.*, 1993a, b). The allogeneic component of these vaccines has undoubtedly also added to their immune stimulatory effects, and it is thought that they enhance the subsequent tumor-specific immune reaction by generating an initially high level of inflammation.

Allogeneic and autologous tumor cell vaccines have been tried seriously since the turn of the century (Dalgleish, 1996). Somewhat ironically, ninety years later the power and elegance of molecular biology has led to trying very similar approaches in gene therapy. Thus, Nabel and colleagues have initiated clinical trials, in which a plasmid encoding an allogeneic MHC molecule, HLA-B7, is injected directly into HLA-B7 negative tumor nodules (Nabel *et al.*, 1992). This protocol is effectively autologous cell vaccination (using the patient's own preexisting tumor for injection) coupled with allogeneic vaccination (by introducing an allo-MHC). The allo-MHC is provided as a powerful adjuvant to induce immunologic inflammation/activation at the site of the tumor. It is hoped tumor-specific immune reactivity can be generated as a by-product of the inflammation and leads to systemic clearance of distant unmodified tumor cells (Figure 1C). This is effective in rodent models (Nabel *et al.*, 1992; Plautz *et al.*, 1993), and preliminary reports suggest that tumor-specific immune responses are generated in human patients (Nabel *et al.*, 1993).

4.4. Direct Cell Killing

Studies from several laboratories, including our own, have recently shown that a strategy designed initially to treat localized tumors may have wider applicability in activating antitumor immune responses, in part by inducing of localized inflammation (Barba *et al.*, 1994; Caruso *et al.*, 1993; Consalvo *et al.*, 1995; Mullen *et al.*, 1994; Vile *et al.*, 1994). In our studies with the B16 melanoma, expression of the HSVtk gene combined with administering the prodrug gancicolvir causes cell death and a bystander immune protective effect against unmodified parental cells (Vile *et al.*, 1994). The B16 cells die predominantly by necrosis rather than apoptosis (Melcher *et al.*, 1998). As a result of these observations, we have proposed a two-step model by which an antitumor immune response might be generated against a normally nonimmunogenic tumor. Because leads to significant inflammatory responses *in vivo*, it may be that the rapid, high-evel, necrotic cell death of B16 cells provides an initial (nonspecific) stimulus for recruiting immune cells to the dying tumors. This is consistent with our observation that inflammatory cytokines (such as IL-2 and TNFa) are induced at the tumor site. Apoptotic cell death, on the other hand, is not usually sociated with inflammatory responses (Wyllie, 1993). The inflammatory response, produced by necrotic cell killing may also provide a "danger" signal to the immune system, which, it has been suggested, is critical for promoting immune responses and overcoming tolerance to tumor cells (Ridge *et al.*, 1996).

The subsequent generation of tumor-specific immunity (Vile *et al.*, 1994) may stem from the fact that cell killing *in situ* increases the availability of tumor antigens, both quantitatively and/or qualitatively, to the immune system in a form in which they can be readily processed, whereas in parental tumors they remain immunologically hidden (Figure 1C). This localized, rapid release of a high concentration of tumor cell debris and antigens may activate an antitumor immune response *via* the uptake and presentation of the antigens by antigen-presenting cells (APC) in the tumor itself or following their migration to the lymph nodes (Colombo and Forni, 1994; Dranoff *et al.*, 1993; Huang *et al.*, 1994; Maass *et al.*, 1995). The detection of mRNA encording GM-CSF and a macrophage infiltrate in the dying tumors may reflect a role for APCs in enhanced antigen presentation, consistent with reports that expression of GM-CSF in melanoma cells is effective in generating immunity by recruiting APC to the tumor site (Armstrong *et al.*, 1996, Dranoff *et al.*, 1993).

4.5. Gene Transfer of Cloned Tumor Antigens

The molecular characterization of tumor antigens has also opened the possibility of direct DNA vaccination against cancer. Intramuscular injection of naked DNA that encodes antigens has been proposed as a safe, inexpensive means of stimulating specific immunologic responses in cancer (Bright *et al.*, 1996; Hawkins *et al.*, 1993; Wang *et al.*, 1995) and other diseases (Ulmer *et al.*, 1993). For example, rapid screening of patient tumor biopsies can identify which of the spectrum of known tumor antigens is being expressed and, if the patient is of an MHC haplotype known to present peptides of a given antigen, vaccination with the gene for the antigen may be effective in protecting against metastases that express the antigen. Clinical trials of DNA vaccination against specific antigens in certain cancers is already underway, especially for melanomas that expressing MAGE genes (see previous) and for B cell lymphomas that express unique, easily clonable idiotypic antigens (Hawkins *et al.*, 1993).

The mechanisms by which DNA vaccination actually works is still unclear because the mechanisms of presentation have not been fully elucidated. However, increasingly it seems apparent that intramuscular DNA vaccinations with defined antigens may be effective because the relevant expression of the encoded antigens may not occur in the myocytes themselves but in dendritic cells infiltrating the site of injection (Pardoll and Beckerleg, 1995; Figure 1C).

5. AIMS, GOALS, AND TARGETS FOR GENE TRANSFER IN IMMUNOTHERAPY

The early studies of gene transfer for immunotherapy centred around using the tumor cells themselves as the target for gene transfer (of cytokines or costimulatory molecules), to augment their antigen-presenting capabilities (Table IIIA, Figure 1B). However, from the previous discussion, it has become clear that strategies in which the target antigens are themselves released from the tumor cells and are presented by other cell types, may generate superior immune responses against tumor antigens (Table IIIB, Figure 1C). In some ways this is self-evident because there are many cell types, such as dendritic cells or other professional antigen presenting cells (APC), which are much better qualified to present antigens than most epithelial tumor cells.

For example, recent studies have shown that bone-marrow-derived APC (rather than the tumor cells themselves) may be the principal cell type responsible for tumor antigen presentation to CD8+ T cells in a class I MHC-restricted manner (Huang *et al.*, 1994). APC can present tumor antigens to both CD8+ and CD4+ lymphocytes *in vivo* leading to the simultaneous priming of separate subsets of antitumor effector cells (Levitsky *et al.*, 1994). Therefore, any procedures which make the antigens more accessible to the relevant APC might be expected to augment the efficacy of vaccination.

In support of this model, it has been shown that antitumor vaccination can be achieved by fusing tumor cells (the source of the antigens) with autologous B cells (the source of fully functional antigen-presenting machinery; Guo *et al.*, 1994). In contrast, the tumor cells alone are unable to elicit protective immunity. Similarly, B cells transfected with a known tumor antigen stimulate effective immune reactivity *in vivo* against the antigen (Pecher and Finn, 1996). In both of these cases, transferring the antigen to the cells most effective in presenting them gives superior results compared to antigen existence in their natural environment of the tumor cells. This is also consistent with generating antitumor immunity after transfer of some inflam-

Table III
Classes of Genes Used to Generate Antitumor Immune Mediated Responses in Animal Models

A. *To convert tumor cells from low to high antigen-presenting capability:*
   1. Cytokines (see Table II; Forni *et al.*, 1995; Tepper and Mule, 1994);
   2. Costimulatory genes (Hellstrom *et al.*, 1995);
   3. MHC molecules or other components of the antigen processing machinery (Browning and Bodmer, 1992; Neefjes and Momburg, 1993; Powis and Geraghty, 1995; Restifo *et al.*, 1993).

B. *To promote transfer of tumor antigens from tumor cells to professional APC:*
   1. Immunogenic molecules, such as allogeneic MHC molecules (Nabel *et al.*, 1992) or bacterial heat shock proteins (Lukacs *et al.*, 1993);
   2. Autologous heat shock proteins that can present tumor associated peptides directly to T cells (Udono *et al.*,1994);
   3. Cytotoxic ("suicide") genes (Moolten, 1994);
   4. Individual tumor antigens (Boon and van der Bruggen, 1996; Hawkins *et al.*, 1993).

matory cytokine genes, such as IL-2. IL-2-mediated tumor rejection is also often accompanied by large amounts of cell debris generated at the tumor site (Colombo *et al.*, 1992) and associated that high levels of infiltrating macrophages that migrate from the tumor to the draining lymph nodes (Cavallo *et al.*, 1992, 1993; Colombo *et al.*, 1992; Pardoll, 1995) (Figure 1C). The optimal environment for antigen presentation to naive T cells in found in these lymph nodes. The importance of lymphoid localization of the antigen and the antigen-presenting cell has been confirmed by the demonstration that even fibroblasts can present foreign viral antigens efficiently to T cells but only within the milieu of the lymphoid organs (Kundig *et al.*, 1995). *In vivo*, professional APC rapidly carries antigen from the local tumor site to the lymph nodes. In contrast, tumor cells are usually located in nonlymphoid sites. Although they eventually migrate to the lymph nodes (an important stage of the metastatic process), by the time this occurs the immune stimulatory effects are insufficient to generate effective antitumor immunity, particulary because most tumor cells have lower inherent ability to present antigen.

6. UNIFICATION OF DIVERSE RESULTS FROM GENE TRANSFER STUDIES

In some respects the field of molecular immunotherapy by gene transfer is in danger of becoming a victim of its own success, at least in terms of the preclinical data generated from animal models. Because so many immunomodulatory genes have been successfully used in different systems to produce local and/or systemic antitumor effects (Table III), the relevance of these models in which can tumor rejection is readily generated, merits examination. In addition, if such studies are to form the basis of progression to clinical trials, the underlying immune mechanisms which lead to tumor cell rejection must be understood and subsequently translated into the human context. Indeed, results are frequently highly model-dependent and contradictory. Therefore, it seems highly unlikely that all the approaches which have been efficacious in diverse animal models will be successful in heating human cancers. A direct comparison of the true efficacy of different approaches is almost impossible because of the variability among studies in the histological types of tumors, the cell lines used, the levels of gene expression obtained, the genetic backgrounds of the rodent model used, the experimental designs of *in vivo* tumor growth, the challenges and vaccination, and the criteria used to assess "protection," "cure," and "immunogenicity" (Prehn, 1993). More recently, controlled comparisons have been made among the efficacies of different genes within a single experimental system (*e.g.*, Allione, 1994; Dranoff *et al.*, 1993; Hock *et al.*, 1993b), as have recommendations for standardizing experimental approaches. Nonetheless, results obtained by different laboratories rarely agree and there is as yet no consensus on what should be the optimal immunotherapeutic gene(s) for use in patient trials.

Recently, to unify this diverse field, we have proposed that there are three principal goals to be achieved by gene transfer for effective immunotherapy of neoplastic disease (Vile and Chong, in press). We suggest that the nature of the particular gene—be it a cytokine, a costimulatory molecule, an immunogen, a cytotoxic gene, or even a defined tumor antigen, should be considered, *in the human situation*, for its tendency to induce any or all of the following:

1. **Inflammation**—attracting immune cells of diverse nature and functions to the site of the tumor,
2. **Release of tumor antigens**—for uptake and presentation by professional antigen presenting cells, and/or
3. **Activation of a specific subset of immune cells which are important in the generation of immunological memory**—in particular, T cells or dendritic cells.

Most of the genes which have been successful in animal models have one or all of these properties *in vivo*, and it is because of the mechanistic basis of their use, rather than the results of any single model system, that genes for immunotherapy should be selected for human trials.

7. REFERENCES

Abe, J., Wakimoto, H., Yoshida, Y., Aoyagi, M., Hirakawa, K., and Hamada, H., 1995, Antitumor effect induced by granulocyte/macrophage-colony-stimulating factor gene-modified tumor vaccination: Comparison of adenovirus- and retirovirus-mediated genetic transduction, *J. Cancer Res. Clin. Oncol.* **121:**587–592.

Allione, A., Consalvo, M., Nanni, P., Lollini, P. L., Cavallo, F., Giovarelli, M., Forni, M., Gulino, A., Colombo, M. P., Dallabona, P., Hock, H., Blankenstein, T., Rosenthal, F. M., Gansbacher, B., Bosco, M. C., Musso, T., Gusella, L., and Forni, G., 1994, Immunizing and curative potential of replicating and nonreplicating murine mammary adenocarcinoma cells engineered with interleukin (IL)-2, IL-4, IL-6, IL-7, IL-10, tumor necrosis factor alpha, granulocyte-macrophage colony-stimulating factor, and gamma interferon gene or admixed with conventional adjuvants, *Cancer Res.* **54:**6022–6026.

Allison, J. P., 1994, CD28-B7 interactions in T-cell activation, *Curr. Opinion Immunol.* **6:**414–419.

Armstrong, C. A., Botella, R., Galloway, T. H., Murray, N., Kramp, J. M., Song, I. S., and Ansel, J. C., 1996, Antitumor effects of granulocyte-macrophage colony-stimulating factor production by melanoma cells, *Cancer Res.* **56:**2191–2198.

Banks, R. E., Patel, P. M., and Selby, P. J., 1995, Interleukin 12: A new clinical player in cytokine therapy, *Br. J. Cancer* **71:**655–659.

Barba, D., Hardin, J., Sadelain, M., and Gage, F. H., 1994, Development of antitumor immunity following thymidine kinase-mediated killing of experimental brain tumors, *Proc. Natl. Acad. Sci. USA* **91:**4348–4352.

Barnd, D. L., Lan, M. S., Metzgar, R. S., and Finn, O. J., 1989, Specific tumor histocompatibility complex-unrestricted recognition of tumor-associated mucins by human cytotoxic T cells, *Proc. Natl. Acad. Sci. USA* **86:**7159–7163.

Berns, A. J., Clift, S., Cohen, L. K., Donehower, R. C., Dranoff, G., Hauda, K. M., Jaffee, E., Lazenby, A. J., Levitsky, H. I., Marshall, F. F., Mulligan, R. C., Nelson, W. G., Owens, A. H., Pardoll, D. M., Parry, G., Partin, A. H., Piantadosi, S., Simons, J. W., and Zabora, J. R., 1995, Clinical protocol: Phase I study of non-replicating autologous tumor cell injections using cells prepared with or without GM-CSF gene transduction in patients with metastatic renal cell carcinoma, *Hum. Gene Ther.* **5:**347–368.

Boon, T., Cerottini, J. C., Van den Eynde, B., van der Bruggen, P., and Van Pel, A., 1994, Tumor antigens recognised by T lymphocytes, *Annu. Rev. Immunol.* **12:**337–365.

Boon, T., De Plaen, E., Lurquin, C., Van Den Eynde, B., Van Der Bruggen, P., *et al.*, 1992, Identification of tumor rejection antigens recognised by T lymphocytes, *Cancer Surv.* **13:**23–37.

Boon, T., and van der Bruggen, P., 1996, Human tumor antigens recognized by T lymphocytes, *J. Exp. Med.* **183:**725–729.

Brasseur, F., Marchand, M., Vanwijck, R., Herin, M., Lethe, B., Chomez, P., and Boon, T., 1992, Human gene MAGE-1, which codes for a tumor-rejection antigen, is expressed by some breast tumors, *Int. J. Cancer* **52:**839–841.

Brichard, V., Van Pel, A., Wolfel, T., Wolfel, C., De Plaen, E., Lethe, B., Coulie, P., and Boon, T., 1993, The tyrosinase gene encodes for an antigen recognised by autologous cytolytic T lymphocytes on HLA-A2 melanomas, *J. Exp. Med.* **178:**489–495.

Bright, R. K., Beames, B., Shearer, M. H., and Kennedy, R. C., 1996, Protection against a lethal tumor challenge with SV40-transformed cells by the direct injection of DNA-encoding SV40 large tumor antigen, *Cancer Res.* **56:**1126–1130.

Browning, M. J., and Bodmer, W. F., 1992, MHC antigens and cancer: Implications for T-cell surveillance, *Curr. Opinion Immunol.* **4:**613–618.

Bystryn, J. C., 1990, Tumour vaccines, *Cancer Metastasis Rev.* **9:**81–91.

Carducci, M. A., Ayyagari, S. R., Sanda, M. G., and Simons, J. W., 1995, Gene therapy for human prostate cancer, *Cancer* **75:**2013–2020.

Caruso, M., Panis, Y., Gagandeep, S., Houssin, D., Salzmann, J. L., and Klatzmann, D., 1993, Regression of established macroscopic liver metastases after in situ transduction of a suicide gene, *Proc. Natl. Acad. Sci. USA* **90:**7024–7028.

Cavallo, F., Di Pierro, F., Giovarrelli, M., Gulino, A., Vacca, A., Stoppacciaro, A., Forni, M., Modesti, A., and Forni, G., 1993, Protective and curative potential of vaccination with interleukin-2-gene transfected cells from a spontaneous mouse mammary adenocarcinoma, *Cancer Res.* **53:**5067–5070.

Cavallo, F., Giovarrelli, M., Gulino, A., Vacca, A., Stoppacciaro, A., Modesti, A., and Forni, G., 1992, Role of neutrophils and CD4+ T lymphocytes in the primary and memory response to nonimmunogenic murine mammary adenocarcinoma made immunogenic by IL-2 gene transfer, *J. Immunol.* **149:**3627–3635.

Chen, L., Thomas, E. K., Hu, S. L., Hellstrom, I., and Hellstrom, K. E., 1991, Human papilloma virus type 16 nucleoprotein E7 is a tumor rejection antigen, *Proc. Natl. Acad. Sci. USA* **88:**110–114.

Chen, W., Peace, D. J., Rovira, D. K., *et al.*, 1992, T cell immunity to the joining region of p210-bcr-abl protein, *Proc. Natl. Acad. Sci. USA* **89:**1468–1472.

Chong, H., Hutchinson, G., Hart, I. R., and Vile, R. G., 1996, Expression of costimulatory molecules by tumor cells decreases tumorigenicity but may also reduce systemic anti-tumor immunity, *Hum. Gene Ther.*, in press.

Colombo, M. P., and Forni, G., 1994, Cytokine gene transfer in tumor inhibition and tumor therapy: Where are we now?, *Immunol. Today* **15:**48–51.

Colombo, M. P., Modesti, A., Parmiani, G., and Forni, G., 1992, Local cytokine availability elicits tumor rejection and systemic immunity through granulocyte-T-lymphocyte cross talk, *Cancer Res.* **52:**4853–4857.

Connor, J., Bannerji, R., Saito, S., Heston, W., Fair, W., and Gilboa, E., 1993, Regression of bladder tumors in mice treated with interleukin-2 gene-modified tumor cells, *J. Exp. Med.* **177:**1127–1134.

Consalvo, M., Mullen, C. A., Modesti, A., Musiani, P., Allione, A., Cavallo, F., Giovarelli, M., and Forni, G., 1995, 5-Fluorocytosine-induced eradication of murine adenocarcinomas engineered to express the cytosine deaminase suicide gene requires host immune competence and leaves an efficient memory, *J. Immunol.* **154:**5302–5312.

Cox, A. L., Skipper, J., Chen, Y., Henderson, R. A., Darrow, T. L., Shabanowitz, J., Engelhard, V. H., Hunt, D. F., and Slingluff, C. L., 1994, Identification of a peptide recognised by five melanoma-specific human cytotoxic T cell lines, *Science* **264:**716.

Dalgleish, A., 1996, The case for therapeutic vaccines, *Melanoma Res.* **6:**5–10.

Dallman, M. J., 1995, Cytokines and transplantation: Th1/Th2 regulation of the immune response to solid organ transplants in the adult, *Curr. Opinion Immunol.* **7:**632–638.

Dranoff, G., Jaffee, E., Lazenby, A., Golumbek, P., Levitsky, H., Brose, K., Jackson, V., Hamada, H., Pardoll, D., and Mulligan, R. C., 1993, Vaccination with irradiated tumor cells engineered to secrete murine granulocyte macrophage colony stimulating factor stimulates potent, specific, and long lasting anti-tumor immunity, *Proc. Natl. Acad. Sci. USA* **90:**3539–3543.

Fakhrai, H., Shawler, D. L., Gjerset, R., Naviaux, R. K., Koziol, J., Royston, I., and Sobol, R. E., 1995,

Cytokine gene therapy with interleukin-2-transduced fibroblasts: Effects of IL-2 dose on anti-tumor immunity, *Hum. Gene Ther.* **6:**591–601.

Foa, R., Guarini, A., and Gansbacher, B., 1992, IL-2 treatment for cancer: From biology to gene therapy, *Br. J. Cancer* **66:**992–998.

Forni, G., Cavallo, F., Consalvo, M., Allione, A., Dellabona, P., Casorati, G., and Giovarelli, M., 1995, Molecular approaches to cancer immunotherapy, *Cytokines Mol. Ther.* **1:**225–248.

Gaugler, B. B., Van den Eynde, B., van der Bruggen, P., Romero, P., Gaforio, J. J., De Plaen, E., Lethe, B., Brasseur, F., and Boon, T., 1994, Human gene MAGE-3 codes for an antigen recognised on a human melanoma by autologous cytolytic T lymphocytes, *J. Exp. Med.* **179:**921.

Gerard, C. M., Bruyns, C., Delavaux, A., Baduson, N., Dargent, J.-L., Goldman, M., and Velu, T., 1996, Loss of tumorigenicity and inceased immunogenicity induced by interleukin-10 gene transfer in B16 melanoma cells, *Hum. Gene Ther.* **7:**11–22.

Gilboa, E., and Kim Lyerly, H., 1994, Specific active immunotherapy of cancer using genetically modified tumor vaccines, *Biologic Therapy of Cancer* (V. T. De Vita, S. Hellman, and S. Rosenberg, eds.), Lippincott, Philadelphia, pp. 1–16.

Giovarelli, M., Musiani, P., Modesti, A., Dellabona, P., Casorati, G., Allione, A., Consalvo, M., Cavallo, F., di Pierro, F., De Giovanni, C., Musso, T., and Forni, G., 1995, Local release of IL-10 by transfected mouse mammary adenocarcinoma cells does not suppress but enhances antitumor reaction and elicits a strong cytotoxic lymphocyte and antibody-dependent immune memory, *Am. Assoc. Immunol.* **••:**3112–3123.

Golumbek, P., Levitsky, H., Jaffee, E., and Pardoll, D. M., 1993, The antitumor immune response as a problem of self-nonself discrimination: Implications for immunotherapy, *Immunol. Res.* **12:**183–192.

Guo, Y., Wu, M., Chen, H., Wang, X., Liu, G., Li, G., Ma, J., and Sy, M.-S., 1994, Effective tumor vaccine generated by fusion of hepatoma cells with activated B cells, *Science* **263:**518–520.

Hawkins, R. E., Winter, G., Hamblin, T. J., Stevenson, F. K., and Russell, S. J., 1993, A genetic approach to idiotypic vaccination, *J. Immunol.* **14:**273–278.

Hellstrom, K. E., Hellstrom, I., and Chen, L., 1995, Can co-stimulated tumor immunity be therapeutically efficacious?, *Immunol. Rev.* **145:**123–145.

Hock, H., Dorsch, M., Kunzendorf, U., Qin, Z., Diamantstein, T., and Blankenstein, T., 1993a, Mechanisms of rejection induced by tumor cell-targeted gene transfer of interleukin 2, interleukin 4, interleukin 7, tumor necrosis factor, or interferon gamma, *Proc. Natl. Acad. Sci. USA* **90:**2774–2778.

Hock, H., Dorsch, M., Kunzendorf, U., Uberla, K., Qin, Z., Diamanstein, T., and Blankenstein, T., 1993b, Vaccinations with tumor cells genetically engineered to produce different cytokines: Effectivity not superior to a classical adjuvant, *Cancer Res.* **53:**714–716.

Houghton, A. N., 1994, Cancer antigens: Immune recognition of self and altered self, *J. Exp. Med.* **180:**1–4.

Huang, A. Y. C., Golumbek, P., Ahmadzadeh, M., Jaffee, E., Pardoll, D., and Levitsky, H., 1994, Role of bone marrow derived cells in presenting MHC Class I-restricted tumor antigens, *Science* **264:**961–965.

Inaba, K., Inaba, M., Romani, M., *et al.*, 1992, Generation of large numbers of dendritic cells from mouse bone marrow cultures supplemented with granulocyte macrophage colony stimulating factor, *J. Exp. Med.* **176:**1693–1702.

Janeway, C. A., and Bottomly, K., 1994, Signals and signs for lymphocyte responses, *Cell* **76:**275–285.

June, C. H., Bluestone, J. A., Nadler, L. M., and Thompson, C. B., 1994, The B7 and CD28 receptor families, *Immunol. Today* **15:**321–331.

Jung, S., and Schluesener, H. J., 1991, Human T lymphocytes recognise a peptide of a single point mutated, oncogenic ras protein, *J. Exp. Med.* **173:**273–276.

Karp, S. E., Farber, A., Salo, J. C., Hwu, P., Jaffe, G., Asher, A. L., Shiloni, E., Restifo, N. P., Mule, J. J., and Rosenberg, S. A., 1993, Cytokine secretion by genetically modified non-immunogenic murine fibrosarcoma, *J. Immunol.* **150:**896–908.

Kawakami, Y., Eliyahu, S., Sakaguchi, K., Robbins, P. F., Rivoltini, L., Yannelli, J. R., Appella, E., and Rosenberg, S. A., 1994a, Identification of the immunodominant peptides of the MART-1 human melanoma antigen recognised by the majority of HLA-A2-restricted tumor infiltrating lymphocytes, *J. Exp. Med.* **180:**347–352.

Kawakami, Y., Eliyhu, S., Delgado, C. H., Robbins, P. F., Rivoltini, L., Topalian, S. L., Miki, T., and

Rosenberg, S. A., 1994b, Cloning of the gene coding for a shared human melanoma antigen recognised by autologous T cells infiltrating into tumor, *Proc. Natl. Acad. Sci. USA* **91:**3515–3519.

Kedar, E., and Klein, E., 1992, Cancer immunotherapy: Are the results discouraging? Can they be improved?, *Adv. Cancer Res.* **59:**245–322.

Kelso, A., 1995, Th1 and Th2 subsets: Paradigms lost?, *Immunol. Today* **16:**374–379.

Klein, G., and Boon, T., 1993, Tumor immunology: Present perspectives, *Curr. Opinion Immunol.* **5:**687–692.

Krummel, M. F., and Allison, J. P., 1995, CD28 and CTLA-4 have opposing effects on the response of T cells to stimulation, *J. Exp. Med.* **182:**459–465.

Kundig, T. M., Bachmann, M. F., DiPaolo, C., Simard, J. J. L., Battegay, M., Lother, H., Gessner, A., Kuhlcke, K., Ohashi, P. S., Hengartner, H., and Zinkernagel, R. M., 1995, Fibroblasts as efficient antigen-presenting cells in lymphoid organs, *Science* **268:**1343–1347.

Levitsky, H. I., Lazenby, A., Hayashi, R. J., and Pardoll, D., 1994, In vivo priming of two distinct antitumor effector populations: The role of MHC Class I expression, *J. Exp. Med.* **179:**1215–1224.

Lukacs, K. V., Lowrie, D. B., Stokes, R. W., and Colston, M. J., 1993, Tumor cells transfected with a bacterial heat-shock gene lose tumorigenicity and induce protection against tumors, *J. Exp. Med.* **178:**343–347.

Maass, G., Schmidt, W., Berger, M., Schilcher, F., Koszik, F., Schneeberger, A., Stingl, G., Birnstiel, M., and Schweighoffer, T., 1995, Priming of tumor specific T cells in the draining lymph nodes after immunization with interleukin 2-secreting tumor cells: Three consecutive stages may be required for successful tumor vaccination, *Proc. Natl. Acad. Sci. USA* **92:**5540–5544.

Marchand, M., Brasseur, F., Van der Bruggen, P., Coulie, P., and Boon, T., 1993, Perspectives for immunisation of HLA-A1 patients carrying a malignant melanoma expressing gene MAGE-1, *Dermatology* **186:**278–280.

Melcher, H. H., Todryk, S., Hardwick, N., Ford, M., Jacobson, M., and Vile, R. G., 1998, Tumor immunogenicity is determined by the mechanism of cell death via induction of heat shock protein expression, *Nature Medicine* **4:**581–587.

Moolten, F. L., 1994, Drug sensitivity ("suicide") genes for selective cancer chemotherapy, *Cancer Gene Ther.* **1:**279–287.

Morton, D. L., Foshag, L. J., Hoon, D. S. B., Nizze, J. A., Wanek, L. A., Chang, C., Davtyan, D. G., Gupta, R. K., Elashoff, R., and Irie, R. F., 1993a, Prolongation of survival in metastatic melanoma after active specific immunotherapy with a new polyvalent melanoma vaccine, *Ann. Surg.* **216:**463–482.

Morton, D. L., Hoon, D. S. B., Nizze, J., *et al.*, 1993b, Polyvalent melanoma vaccine improves survival of patients with metastatic melanoma, *Ann. N.Y. Acad. Sci.* **690:**120–134.

Mullen, C. A., Coale, M. M., Lowe, R., and Blaese, R. M., 1994, Tumors expressing the cytosine deaminase suicide gene can be eliminated in vivo with 5-fluorocytosine and induce protective immunity to wild type tumor, *Cancer Res.* **54:**1503–1506.

Nabel, G. J., Chang, A., Nabel, E. G., Plautz, G., Fox, B. A., Huang, L., and Shu, S., 1992, Clinical protocol: Immunotherapy of malignancy by in vivo gene transfer into tumors, *Hum. Gene Ther.* **3:**399–410.

Nabel, G. J., Nabel, E. G., Yang, Z. Y., Fox, B. A., Plautz, G. E., Gao, X., Huang, L., Shu, S., Gordon, D., and Chang, A. E., 1993, Direct gene transfer with DNA-liposome complexes in melanoma: Expression, biologic activity, and lack of toxicity in humans, *Proc. Natl. Acad. Sci. USA* **90:**11307–11311.

Neefjes, J. J., and Momburg, F., 1993, Cell biology of antigen presentation, *Curr. Opinion Immunol.* **5:**27–34.

Nijman, H. W., Van der Burg, S. H., Vierboom, M. P. M., Houbiers, J. G. A., Kast, W. M., and Melief, C. J. M., 1994, p53, a potential target for tumor-directed T cells, *Immunol. Lett.* **40:**171–178.

Oettgen, H. F., and Old, L. J., 1991, The history of cancer immunotherapy, in *Biologic Therapy of Cancer* (V. T. DeVita, S. Hellman, and S. A. Rosenberg, eds.), Lipincott, Philadelphia, pp. 87–119.

Pardoll, D., 1992, New strategies for active immunotherapy with genetically engineered tumor cells, *Curr. Opinion Immunol.* **4:**619–623.

Pardoll, D. M., 1993, Cancer vaccines, *Immunol. Today* **14:**310–316.

Pardoll, D. M., 1994, Tumour antigens: A new look for the 1990s, *Nature* **369:**357–358.

Pardoll, D. M., 1995, Paracrine cytokine adjuvants in cancer immunotherapy, *Ann. Rev. Immunol.* **13:**399–415.

Pardoll, D. M., and Beckerleg, A. M., 1995, Exposing the immunology of naked DNA vaccines, *Immunity* **3:**165–169.

Paul, W. E., and Seder, R. A., 1994, Lymphocyte responses and cytokines, *Cell* **76:**241–251.

Pecher, G., and Finn, O. J., 1996, Induction of cellular immunity in chimpanzees to human tumor-associated antigen mucin by vaccination with MUC-1 cDNA-transfected Epstein–Barr virus-immortalized autologous B cells, *Proc. Natl. Acad. Sci. USA* **93:**1699–1704.

Pericle, F., Giovarelli, M., Colombo, M. P., Ferrari, G., Musiani, P., Modesti, A., Cavallo, F., Di Pierro, F., Novelli, F., and Forni, G., 1994, An efficient Th2-type memory follows CD8+ lymphocyte-driven and eosinophil-mediated rejection of a spontaneous mouse mammary adenocarcinoma engineered to release IL-4+, *Am. Assoc. Immunol.* **••:**5659–5673.

Plautz, G. E., Yang, Z.-Y., Wu, B.-Y., Gao, X., Huang, L., and Nabel, G. J., 1993, Immunotherapy of malignancy by in vivo gene transfer into tumors, *Proc. Natl. Acad. Sci. USA* **90:**4645–4649.

Porgador, A., Gansbacher, B., Bannerji, R., Tzehoval, E., Gilboa, E., Feldman, M., and Eisenbach, L., 1993, Anti-metastatic vaccination of tumor bearing mice with IL-2-gene-inserted tumor cells, *Int. J. Cancer* **53:**471–477.

Powis, S. H., and Geraghty, D. E., 1995, What is the MHC?, *Immunol. Today* **16:**466–468.

Prehn, R. T., 1993, Two competing influences that may explain concomitant tumor resistance, *Cancer Res.* **53:**3266–3269.

Prehn, R. T., 1994, Stimulatory effects of immune reactions upon the growths of untransplanted tumors, *Cancer Res.* **54:**908–914.

Ramarathinam, L., Castle, M., Wu, Y., and Liu, Y., 1994, T cell co-stimulation by B7/BB1 induces CD8 T cell-dependent tumor rejection: An important role of B7/BB1 in the induction, recruitment, and effector function of antitumor T cells, *J. Exp. Med.* **179:**1205–1214.

Restifo, N. P., Esquivel, F., Kawakami, Y., Yewdell, J. W., Mule, J. J., Rosenberg, S. A., and Bennink, J. R., 1993, Identification of human cancers deficient in antigen processing, *J. Exp. Med.* **177:**265–272.

Ridge, J. P., Fuchs, E. J., and Matzinger, P., 1996, Neonatal tolerance revisited: Turning on newborn T cells with dendritic cells, *Science* **271:**1723–1726.

Rosenberg, S. A., French Anderson, W., Blaese, M., Hwu, P., Yannelli, J. R., Yang, J. C., Topalian, S., Schwartzentruber, D. J., Weber, J. S., Ettinghausen, S. E., Parkinson, D. N., and White, D. E., 1993, The development of gene therapy for the treatment of cancer, *Ann. Surg.* **218:**455–464.

Saito, S., Bannerji, R., Gansbacher, B., Rosenthal, F. M., Romanenko, P., Heston, W. D. W., Fair, W. R., and Gilboa, E., 1994, Immunotherapy of bladder cancer with cytokine gene modified tumor vaccines, *Cancer Res.* **54:**3516–3520.

Schlichtholz, B., Legros, Y., Gillet, D., Gaillard, C., Marty, M., Lane, D., Calvo, F., and Soussi, T., 1992, The immune response to p53 in breast cancer patients is directed against immunodominant epitopes unrelated to the mutational hot spot, *Cancer Res.* **52:**6380–6384.

Schmidt, W., Schweighoffer, T., Herbst, E., Maass, G., Berger, M., Schilcher, F., Schaffner, G., and Birnstiel, M. L., 1995, Cancer vaccines: The interleukin 2 dosage effect, *Proc. Natl. Acad. Sci USA* **92:**4711–4714.

Schulz, T. F., and Vile, R. G., 1992, Viruses in human cancer, in *Introduction to the Molecular Genetics of Cancer* (R. G. Vile, ed.), John Wiley and Sons, Chichester, pp. 137–176.

Seung, L. P., Seung, S. K., and Schrieber, H., 1995, Antigenic cancer cells that escape immune destruction are stimulated by host cells, *Cancer Res.* **55:**5094–5100.

Skipper, J., and Stauss, H. J., 1993, Identification of two cytotoxic T lymphocyte-recognised epitopes in the ras protein, *J. Exp. Med.* **177:**1493–1498.

Stoppacciaro, A., Melani, C., Parenza, M., Matracchio, A., Bassi, C., Baroni, C., Parmiani, G., and Colombo, M. P., 1993, Regression of an established tumor genetically modified to release granulocyte colony-stimulating factor requires granulocyte-T cell cooperation and T cell-produced interferon gamma, *J. Exp. Med.* **178:**151–161.

Tahara, H., and Lotze, M. T., 1995, Antitumor effects of interleukin-12 (IL-12): Applications for the immunotherapy and gene therapy of cancer, *Gene Ther.* **2:**96–106.

Tahara, H., Zitvogel, L., Strokus, W. J., Zeh, H. J. III, McKinney, T. G., Schreiber, R. D., Gubler, U.,

Robbins, P. D., and Lotze, M. T., 1995, Effective eradication of established murine tumors with 1L-12 gene therapy using a polycistronic retroviral vector, *J. Immunol.* **41:**6466–6474.

Tanaka, K., Gorelik, E., Watanabe, M., Hozumi, N., and Jay, G., 1988, Rejection of B16 melanoma induced by expression of a transfected major histocompatibility complex class I gene, *Mol. Cell. Biol.* **8:**1857–1861.

Taylor-Papadimitriou, J., Stewart, L., Burchell, J., and Beverley, P., 1993, The polymorphic epithelial mucin as a target for immunotherapy, *Ann. N.Y. Acad. Sci.* **7:**69–79.

Tepper, R. I., and Mule, J.J., 1994, Experimental and clinical studies of cytokine gene-modified tumor cells, *Hum. Gene Ther.* **5:**153–164.

Townsend, S. E., and Allison, J. P., 1993, Tumour rejection after direct co-stimulation of CD8+ T cells by B7-transfected melanoma cells, *Science* **259:**368–370.

Traversari, T., Van der Bruggen, P., Luescher, I. F., Lurquin, C., Chomez, P., Van Pel, A., De Plaen, E., Amar-Costesec, A., and Boon, T., 1992, A nonapeptide encoded by human gene MAGE-1 is recognised on HLA-A1 by cytolytic T lymphocytes directed against tumor antigen MZ2-E, *J. Exp. Med.* **176:**1453–1457.

Udono, H., Levey, D. L., and Srivastava, P. K., 1994, Cellular requirements for tumor-specific immunity elicited by heat shock proteins: Tumor rejection antigen gp96 primes CD8+ T cells in vivo, *Proc. Natl. Acad. Sci. USA* **91:**3077–3081.

Ulmer, J. B., Donnelly, J. J., Parker, S. E., Rhodes, G. H., Felgner, P. L., Dwarki, V. J., Gromkowski, S. H., *et al.*, 1993, Heterologous protection against influenza by injection of DNA encoding a viral protein, *Science* **259:**1745–1749.

Van der Bruggen, P., Traversari, C., Chomez, P., Lurquin, C., De Plaen, E., Van Den Eynde, B., Knuth, A., and Boon, T., 1991, A gene encoding an antigen recognised by cytolytic T lymphocytes on a human melanoma, *Science* **254:**1643–1647.

Vegh, Z., Wang, P., Vanky, F., and Klein, E., 1993, Selectively down regulated expression of major histocompatibilty complex class I alleles in human solid tumors, *Cancer Res.* **53:**2416–2420.

Vieweg, J., Rosenthal, F. M., Bannerji, R., Heston, W. D. W., Fair, W. R., Gansbacher, B., and Gilboa, E., 1994, Immunotherapy of prostate cancer in the Dunning rat model: Use of cytokine gene modified tumor vaccines, *Cancer Res.* **54:**1760–1765.

Vile, R. G., and Chong, H., 1996, Immunotherapy: Combinatorial molecular immunotherapy—a synthesis and suggestions, *Cancer Metastatis Reviews* **15:**351–364.

Vile, R. G., Nelson, J. A., Castleden, S., Chong, H., and Hart, I. R., 1994, Systemic gene therapy of murine melanoma using tissue specific expression of the HSVtk gene involves an immune component, *Cancer Res.* **54:**6228–6234.

Vile, R. G., and Russell, S. J., 1994, Gene transfer technologies for the gene therapy of cancer, *Gene Ther.* **1:**88–98.

Visseren, M. J. W., Koot, K. M., van der Voort, E., *et al.*, 1994, Production of interleukin-2 by EL-4 tumor cells induces natural killer cell- and T -cell mediated immunity, *J. Immunother.* **15:**119–128.

Vogelstein, B., and Kinzler, K. W., 1993, The multistep nature of cancer, *Trends Genet.* **9:**138–141.

Walunas, T. L., Lenschow, D. J., Bakker, C. Y., Linsley, P. S., Freeman, G. J., Green, J. M., Thompson, C. B., and Bluestone, J. A., 1994, CTLA-4 can function as a negative regulator of T cell activation, *Immunity* **1:**405–413.

Wang, B., Merva, M., Dang, K., Ugen, K. E., Williams, W. V., and Weiner, D. B., 1995, Immunization by direct DNA inoculation induces rejection of tumor cell challenge, *Hum. Gene Ther.* **6:**407–418.

Wyllie, A. H., 1993, Apoptosis (The 1992 Frank Rose Memorial Lecture), *Br. J. Cancer* **67:**205–208.

Zitvogel, L. J., Mayordomo, I., Tjanddrawan, T., DeLeo, A. B., Clarke, M. R., Lotze, M. T., and Storkus, W. J., 1996, Therapy of murine tumors with tumor-specific peptide pulsed dendritic cells: Dependence on T cells, B7 costimulation and Th1 associated cytokines, *J. Exp. Med.* **183:**87–97.

Chapter 14

DNA-Based Immunization

Heather L. Davis and Cynthia L. Brazolot Millan

1. INTRODUCTION

1.1. What is DNA-Based Immunization?

DNA vaccines belong to the new technology of nucleic acid-based immunization, also known as genetic immunization. This describes the induction of an immune response to an antigenic protein expressed *in vivo* after introducing its encoding polynucleotide. In theory, the encoding sequences can be in the form of either DNA or mRNA. However, in practice there are very few RNA vaccines (*e.g.*, Conry *et al.*, 1995a; Martinon *et al.*, 1993), probably because expression is too short-lived to be effective. Thus, most models of nucleic acid-based immunization described to date have used DNA, most often in the form of double-stranded, closed, circular plasmid DNA.

DNA-based immunization contrasts with classical immunization approaches where it is the antigen itself that is administered. Owing to certain unique features, DNA vaccines promise to overcome many of the disadvantages of current antigen-based vaccines. However, before discussing these, a brief overview of immune responses to immunization is presented.

1.2. Goals of Immunization

Two general types of immunity may be induced in response to an antigen (see Kuby, 1994): (1) humoral immunity, which is the production of antibodies by B cells,

Heather L. Davis Loeb Health Research Institute, Ottawa Civic Hospital, Ottawa, Ontario K1Y 4E9, Canada, and Faculties of Health Sciences and Medicine, University of Ottawa, Ottawa, Canada. **Cynthia L. Brazolot Millan** Loeb Health Research Institute, Ottawa Civic Hospital, Ottawa, Ontario K1Y 4E9, Canada.

Blood Cell Biochemistry, Volume 8: Hematopoiesis and Gene Therapy, edited by Fairbairn and Testa. Kluwer Academic/Plenum Publishers, New York, 1999.

and (2) cell-mediated immunity (CMI) which includes lytic (killing) or nonlytic effects on infected cells and helping B cells make antibodies. Induction of either type of immunity involves presentation of peptide components of the antigen by antigen-presenting cells (APC) (Figure 1).

B lymphocytes recognize and bind circulating soluble antigen *via* surface antibody receptors and thus become activated to differentiate into plasma cells that produce and secrete more antibodies. B cells also form memory cells that react quickly to a secondary challenge by an antigen, and produce higher and more sustained levels of antibody.

T lymphocytes play roles in developing both humoral and cellular immunity. T cells recognize antigen presented on cell surfaces *via* molecules encoded by the major histocompatibility complex of genes (MHC). Class I MHC presentation occurs on cells in which there is endogenous synthesis of antigen (*e.g.*, virally infected cells), whereas it is thought that class II MHC is associated only with APC (*e.g.*, macrophages, dendritic cells) which present exogenous antigen taken up by phagocytosis and digestion. T cells have traditionally been classified on the basis of their expression of clusters of differentiation (CD). All T cells are CD3+ and either CD4+ or CD8+, and they bind to MHC II and I, respectively. In general, CD8+ T cells are those that, when activated, differentiate into cytotoxic T lymphocytes (CTL). CTL act by both cytolytic and noncytolytic mechanisms on infected cells that present antigen *via* class I MHC. In contrast, CD4+ T cells generally act as T-helper

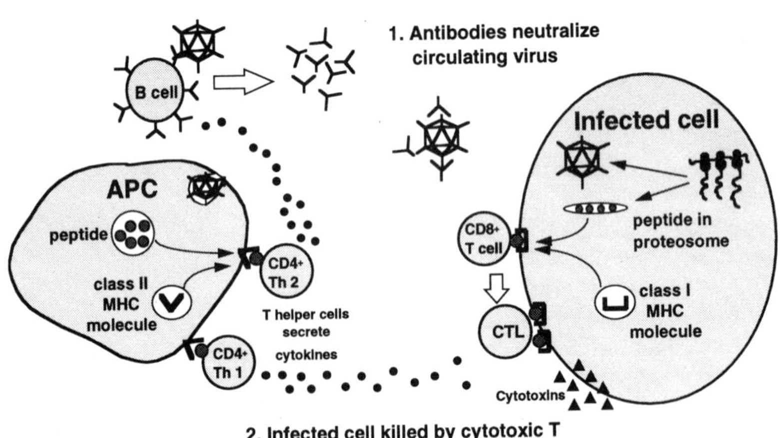

FIGURE 1. Humoral and cell-mediated immune responses against viral pathogens. Antibodies are produced by B cells after they are activated after interaction with circulating antigen. CD8+ T-cells are primed to become cytotoxic T lymphocytes (CTL) by recognizing peptides derived from foreign antigen synthesized in an infected cell and presented on the surface by class I major histocompatibility (MHC) molecules. CD4+ T-cells are stimulated to become T-helper (Th) cells by recognizing antigen presented by class II MHC on the surface of antigen-presenting cells (APC), such as macrophages, which phagocytose and process circulating viral particles. Cytokines secreted by Th2 cells further activate B cells to secrete more antibody whereas those secreted by Th1 cells permit complete activation of CTL. CTL can kill infected cells by release of cytotoxins, such as perforin.

cells (Th), which secrete cytokines. The two subclasses of Th cells, Th1 and Th2, facilitate cell-mediated and humoral immunity, respectively. Th1 cells secrete cytokines, such as interleukin-2 (IL-2), which stimulates CTL, and interferon-γ (IFN-γ), which inhibits Th2 cells. In contrast, Th2 cells secrete cytokines, such as IL-4, IL-5, IL-6, and IL-10 which stimulate B cells. IL-4 and IL-10 also act to inhibit Th1 cells. There is some overlap in function. Some CD4+ T cells act as CTL against target cells that present antigen *via* class II MHC. Other T cells (mostly CD8+) act as suppressor cells.

The interplay between humoral and cell-mediated immunity is complex, and involves simultaneous and sequential interactions between several cell types through cell–cell contact and/or mediation by secreted cytokines. For example, antibody is produced by activated B cells, which are further stimulated by cytokines secreted by Th2 cells, which themselves were activated by APC in the presence of antigen. Similarly, CD8+ cells are partially activated by recognizing antigen presented by MHC I on infected cells and, to become CTL are further stimulated by cytokines secreted by CD4+ Th cells, which themselves were previously stimulated by APC in lymphoid tissue by forming a trimolecular complex of antigen–MHC II–CD4+ (the cell–cell contact is essential).

Prophylactic vaccination is carried out to induce long-term protective immunity against a specific pathogen (*i.e.*, virus, bacterium, parasite) that is likely to be encountered at some time in the future. An ideal vaccine induces antibodies to neutralize circulating pathogen and CTL to kill (or affect by nonlytic mechanisms) infected cells. Although most antigen-based vaccination strategies induce humoral immunity, those processed solely as exogenous antigen (*i.e.*, whole killed and subunit vaccines) generally do not induce CMI, which is absolutely essential for protection against some diseases (*e.g.*, TB, malaria) (Figure 2). Even for those diseases where CTL are not essential for protection, it is generally thought that the presence of CMI offers greater protection than humoral immunity alone. In addition, vaccine strategies that induce CD8+ CTL might also be applicable to the immunotherapeutic treatment of chronically infected individuals or of diseases, such as cancer.

An ideal vaccine would have the following properties: (1) safe for all individuals, including those who are immunocompromised; (2) easily administered, preferably orally; (3) induces the full range of immune responses (*i.e.*, humoral and cell-mediated immunity); (4) long-lasting effect from a single dose (*i.e.*, no boosters); (5) easy and inexpensive to manufacture; (6) simplified yet rigorous quality assessment and control; and (7) heat stable. No vaccine meets all of these criteria now.

1.3. Shortcomings of Antigen-Based Vaccines

All vaccines used currently involve administering antigen, either as a whole pathogen (live or killed) or a component (subunit) thereof. Although such antigen-based vaccines have been spectacularly successful in reducing or completely eliminating the incidence of certain diseases, numerous diseases remain for which it has not been possible to produce an effective vaccine, largely because of the inherent limitations of these approaches (Lanzavecchia, 1993; WHO, 1990).

1.3.1. Live Attenuated Vaccines

Some pathogens (*e.g.*, viruses or bacteria) become attenuated (*i.e.*, nonpathogenic) when grown for prolonged periods under abnormal conditions. When used as vaccines (*e.g.*, measles, mumps, polio-Sabin), they usually induce excellent immunity by providing prolonged exposure to the immunogen and synthesis in self-cells (*i.e.*, endogenous antigen), thereby inducing CD8+ CTL function (Figure 2). More recently, live viral vaccines have become applicable to some diseases, for which the causative agent cannot be rendered nonpathogenic or cannot be grown in tissue culture (*e.g.*, hepatitis B virus = HBV), by cloning antigen-encoding sequences into established attenuated viral or bacterial cell lines (*e.g.*, vaccinia virus) to make recombinant vectors (WHO, 1990). The biggest disadvantage of the live attenuated vaccines, whether or not they carry a recombinant gene, is the possibility of reversion to a virulent form, especially in immunodeficient subjects (*e.g.*, neonates, HIV-infected, or malnourished individuals).

1.3.2. Whole Killed Pathogen Vaccines

These vaccines contain whole viruses (*e.g.*, rabies, polio-Salk) or bacteria that are killed by treatment with heat or chemicals (*e.g.*, formaldehyde, alkylating agents). In theory they have no risk of virulence although there have been incidents of infection due to incomplete inactivation and unexplained encephalitis reactions. Other disadvantages include loss of immunogenicity by denaturation (*i.e.*, with heat) and failure to induce CD8+ CTL because antigen is processed solely in an exogenous form.

1.3.3. Subunit Vaccines

Subunit vaccines involve administering only selected components of the pathogen (virus or bacterium). Some examples include synthetic peptides, recombinant

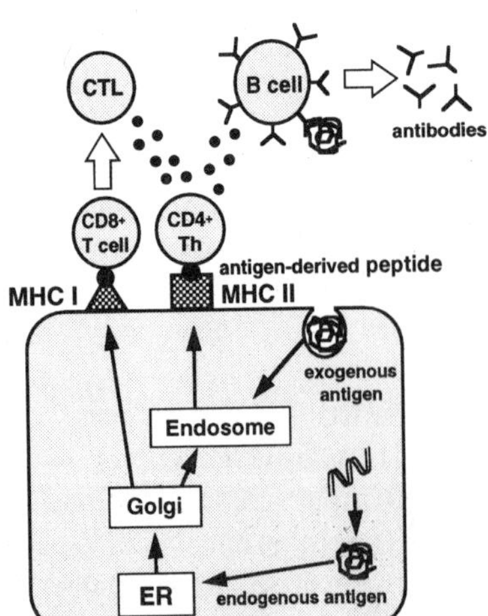

FIGURE 2. Processing of exogenous (circulating) antigen by APC usually results in presentation only by class II MHC and thus stimulates antibody production by B cells. In contrast, endogenous antigen (synthesized in a self-cell) is presented by both class I and II MHC and thus primes both humoral (antibodies) and cell-mediated (CTL) immune responses.

proteins purified from cell lines genetically engineered to produce the desired polypeptide or protein (*e.g.*, hepatitis B surface antigen = HBsAg), or purified macromolecules (*e.g.*, noninfectious subviral particles of HBsAg purified from the serum of chronically infected individuals). Although several kinds of injectable proteins have been developed and tested for immunization, they have not proven useful as vaccines against most diseases. For example, no peptide vaccine and only one recombinant protein vaccine (HBV) have been licensed for human use. Poor results with subunit vaccines most likely result from purely exogenous processing of antigen. In some cases (*e.g.*, where antigen is in the form of large particles) they may induce a CD4+ Th response, but their primary limitation is an inability to invoke a CD8+ CTL response. This is an important disadvantage because CMI is considered superior to humoral immunity alone and may even be essential for protection against certain pathogens. Another major disadvantage of subunit vaccines is that they induce only short-term immunity and thus there is a need for boosters. In addition, poor humoral responses are obtained with peptides that are too short to retain conformational determinants or with recombinant proteins that lack appropriate secondary modifications (*e.g.*, glycosylation) when produced in nonmammalian cells. Other drawbacks include limited supply (*e.g.*, purified macromolecules) and difficult and expensive production and purification (*e.g.*, recombinant protein vaccines). Thus, although subunit vaccines are generally safe and effective for inducing humoral immunity, they cannot be applied to many diseases, in particular those for which CMI is essential.

Therefore, there are still many diseases for which the classical antigen-based approaches cannot and are unlikely to provide safe and effective vaccines. In addition, none of the antigen-based vaccines are heat stable. This is an important factor for application in less developed countries because the requirement for refrigeration, frequently called the "cold-chain", adds considerably to the cost of vaccines. In an effort to overcome the limitations of antigen-based vaccines, novel alternative approaches to vaccination are currently being evaluated. For example anti-idiotype antibodies may serve as a template image of the antigen, and although these are expensive to produce, they may allow effective immunity against highly dangerous pathogens (*e.g.*, HIV). Another possibility is that of DNA-based vaccination, which offers many potential advantages over the antigen-based approach.

1.4. Unique Features of DNA-Based Immunization

DNA vaccines are an attractive alternative to the classical antigen-based vaccines for several reasons. First, they can be engineered to include only those genes that induce the desired immunity (*e.g.*, encoding polypeptides with identified B- and T-cell epitopes), while excluding those responsible for virulence and pathology. Because cloning vectors is relatively easy, one can make multivalent vaccines by including coding sequences for epitopes of more than one antigen. In contrast, it is not always possible to mix different proteins directly. In addition, DNA sequences can be modified to respond quickly to different or changing strains of pathogens (*e.g.*, for influenza). Furthermore the *in situ* production of the protein results in presentation of the antigen to the immune system via class I MHC which in turn induces CD8+ CTL. Thus, DNA vaccines have the efficacy of live (attenuated) vaccines but without the risk of inadvertent infection.

The use of plasmid DNA as the vaccinating molecule offers several other technical, economical, and logistical advantages that are particularly relevant to the urgent need for affordable and effective vaccines in the Third World. For example, continuously synthesizing low levels of antigen over at least several days promotes long-lasting immune responses which may preclude the requirement for booster immunization. This is of particular importance in developing regions of the world, where the cost of vaccine delivery is an important consideration and where about 20% of vaccinated individuals fail to return for booster injections (Kuby, 1994; WHO, 1991). In addition, DNA vaccines are easier and less expensive to manufacture than many of antigen-based vaccines, including recombinant proteins, and quality control is also easier. Finally, DNA is stable for years at ambient temperatures, a distinct advantage over the antigen-based vaccines where the need for a "cold-chain" adds considerably to the cost of vaccine delivery in areas of the world where refrigeration is not commonplace.

1.5. Potential Applications for DNA Vaccines

As outlined previously, DNA vaccines promise to overcome many of the shortcomings of classical antigen vaccines, providing that they do not present new safety or technical problems. For prophylactic purposes, they may allow developing vaccines against diseases for which it has not been previously possible to develop an antigen-based vaccine (*e.g.*, malaria). Even for those diseases for which antigen vaccines currently exist, the DNA approach potentially offers safe, efficacious, one-dose vaccines which are easy and inexpensive to manufacture and are heat stable. Such advantages are particularly attractive for application to the less developed areas of the world, but in addition are no less desirable for other areas of the world. The potential clinical interest of DNA vaccines has been indicated by several different animal models (see section 2), and several phase I human clinical trials have been initiated. Although potential safety issues may delay the use of DNA for large-scale vaccination of healthy people, the speed with which this technology has gone from initial discovery to human trials indicates that this may be sooner than originally envisioned.

DNA-based immunization also offers a unique opportunity to develop immunotherapeutic vaccines. Because of the endogenous synthesis of antigen and the induction of CD8+ CTL, it may be possible to use this strategy to treat chronically infected individuals or to induce specific immune responses against cancer cells.

1.6. History of DNA Vaccines

The possibility of using DNA to create safe and simple vaccines stems from the somewhat surprising discovery by Wolff *et al.* (1990) that a saline solution of pure plasmid DNA (sometimes called "naked" DNA to differentiate it from liposome-associated DNA) could, upon injection into muscles of mice, transfect some of the muscle fibers and result in long-term expression of a reporter gene.

DNA-based immunization against a recombinant protein expressed *in vivo* was first inadvertently demonstrated in 1992 by introducing plasmid DNA encoding human growth hormone (hGH) into the epidermis of mice, which subsequently exhibited circulating antibodies against hGH (Tang *et al.*, 1992). In this case, the DNA was coated onto gold particles which were introduced into the epidermis with a "gene-gun". Shortly thereafter, disease-specific DNA-based immunization against several viruses, including influenza A (Robinson *et al.*, 1993; Ulmer *et al.*, 1993), HIV (Wang *et al.*, 1993a,b), HBV (Davis *et al.*, 1993b), and rabies virus (Xiang *et al.*, 1994), and against one bacterial disease, tuberculosis (Lowrie *et al.*, 1994) and one parasitic disease, malaria (Sedegah *et al.*, 1994) was demonstrated in animal models. Since then, DNA vaccines have been developed against many more viral and other bacterial and parasitic diseases. Some of these, and the immune responses they induce, are discussed in greater detail in section 2.

1.7. Gene Transfer Methods for DNA-Based Immunization

DNA is introduced into cells of the body by a variety of means (see Miller, 1992), but only some of these are appropriate for immunization. For example, because prophylactic vaccination is almost always applied to a large population, only direct (*in vivo*) gene transfer could ever be envisioned for immunization. Furthermore, although direct gene transfer may be carried out using viral vectors or recombinant plasmid DNA (Davis *et al.*, 1993a), the use of viral vectors has the same limitations and disadvantages as classical vaccines based on attenuated viruses (see section 1.3.1) and are therefore of limited interest for immunization. Thus, plasmid DNA is the preferred vector for DNA-based immunization.

Pure plasmid DNA (*i.e.*, in an aqueous solution) transfects a variety of cells when injected directly into tissues, but the routes used most frequently for administering DNA vaccines are intramuscular (IM) and intradermal (ID). IM injection of plasmid DNA is used by many investigators because pure plasmid DNA transfects muscle fibers much more efficiently than other types of cells (Davis *et al.*, 1993c; Wolff *et al.*, 1990). On the other hand, efficient immunization is also obtained by ID injection of plasmid DNA, despite the fact that only a small number of cells are transfected (Raz *et al.*, 1994). In this case, efficient immunization may result from direct transfection of APC in the skin.

Another commonly used method for DNA-based immunization is the introduction of DNA-coated gold particles into the epidermis by a "gene-gun", which uses a particle accelerator or compressed helium to shoot the gold particles at high speed into the skin (Fynan *et al.*, 1993b; Tang *et al.*, 1992). This is particularly efficient for inducing CMI with extremely small quantities of DNA, probably because of direct penetration of some gold particles into APC (Fynan *et al.*, 1993b; Tang *et al.*, 1992).

The method of DNA delivery that gives the strongest immune responses depends on the antigen and the animal species. Generally, the IM route gives the best humoral response in mice, although this is not necessarily true in primates where skin routes are superior (Gramzinski *et al.*, 1998). All routes of vaccine introduction are generally efficient for inducing CTL, although much smaller doses of DNA are effective when a gene-gun is used for vaccination.

For the developing world, it would be highly desirable to administer DNA vaccines by easy and noninvasive means which do not require highly trained medical personnel. It is possible to induce humoral immunity in mice by intranasal instillation of antigen-encoding DNA formulated with cationic lipids (McCluskie and Davis, unpublished results). Several groups are also attempting to develop oral vaccines comprised of DNA encapsulated in biodegradable microspheres.

1.8. Design of Plasmid Vectors for DNA-Based Immunization

Plasmid vectors utilized for DNA-based immunization are similar to those used as general mammalian expression vectors, and therefore must contain a variety of discrete functional genes or sequences. Such plasmids typically include: (1) a bacterial origin of replication (*ori*); (2) a prokaryotic selectable marker gene; (3) antigen-coding sequences; (4) eukaryotic transcription regulatory elements (promoter ± enhancer and transcription termination sequences); and (5) RNA processing elements (polyadenylation signals and an optional intron element) (Figure 3).

The *ori* sequence preferably exhibits relaxed control over the number of plasmid copies existing in a bacterium, thereby making it easier to amplify large quantities of plasmid DNA before isolating it from the bacterial cells. Plasmids designed for DNA-based immunization specifically do not contain eukaryotic origins of replication to prevent the plasmids from amplifying in the eventual eukaryotic target cells. The selectable marker gene ensures that during bacterial and, therefore, plasmid amplification, only those bacteria that contain the recombinant plasmid survive and multiply. Selection markers are usually antibiotic resistance genes. Historically, the ampicillin resistance gene (coding for β-lactamase) has been most commonly used. However, intentionally introducing a gene into humans (the ultimate aim of most DNA-based immunization) that confers resistance to penicillin and its derivatives is highly undesirable. In contrast, the gene conferring resistance to the antibiotic kanamycin has been licensed for use in humans, so many current

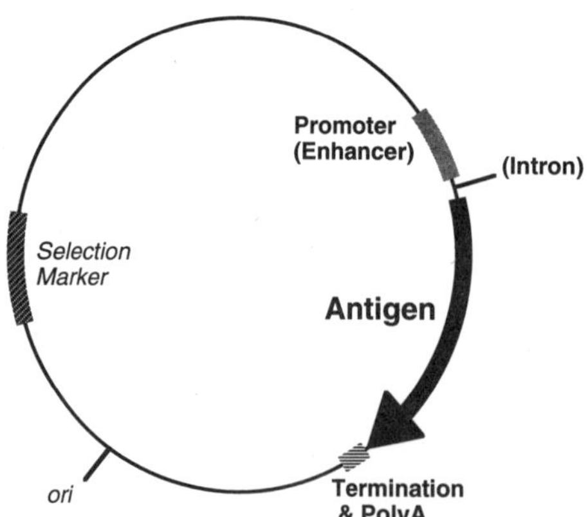

FIGURE 3. Elements required in a plasmid vector for DNA-based immunization. The plasmid must have a bacterial origin of replication (*ori*) and a marker gene for selection and specific amplification of the plasmid during growth of the bacterial host. Expression of the antigen-encoding sequences requires a promoter (enhancer optional) and termination elements and a polyadenylation signal (PolyA) for appropriate transcript processing. Inclusion of intron sequences is also optional. Elements that function in the prokaryotic host appear in italics. Eukaryotic-regulatory elements required for expression in the immunized host appear in bold.

plasmid vectors designed for DNA-based immunization contain this selection marker.

To allow for appropriate and efficient expression in the eventual immunized host, antigen-coding sequences must be inserted into the plasmid vector next to a eukaryotic promoter sequence, with or without enhancer sequences to augment expression. Such regulatory sequences can be chosen to try to control eventual expression in a tissue-specific or inducible manner. However, although it had been thought that tissue-specific promoters would ensure high levels of expression in specific cell-types, in reality, most tissue-specific promoters exhibit leaky expression. Furthermore, many tissue-specific promoters are derived from so-called "housekeeping" genes, and as such, regulate relatively low levels of expression. Therefore, the most common promoter elements employed are viral in origin [*e.g.*, the cytomegalovirus (CMV) promoter/enhancer] because many of these direct high levels of gene expression in a wide host-cell range. Transcription termination elements must be included downstream of the antigen-coding sequences to ensure appropriate termination of the expressed mRNA, and polyadenylation sequences are required for appropriate processing of the message. The inclusion of intron sequences is optional but may lead to enhanced levels of expression and/or transcript stability.

2. DNA VACCINES FOR PROTECTION AGAINST INFECTIOUS DISEASES

Animal Models of DNA Vaccines against Specific Diseases

Since the first demonstration of DNA-based immunization, direct gene transfer of plasmid DNA by various means has been used to immunize animals against many different viral, bacterial and parasitic antigens (see Davis and Whalen, 1995; Vogel and Sarver 1995). Several of these are summarized in Table I. In most cases a full range of immune responses has been obtained including antibodies, CTL, T-cell help and, where evaluation was possible, protection against challenge from the live pathogen. Furthermore, several different phase I human clinical trials of DNA vaccines have been undertaken in the USA and Sweden. Three of these trials are for HIV, and one is for influenza.

2.1.1. Humoral Responses

In most cases of immunization using plasmid expression vectors, antibodies have been found against the proteins produced. However the efficiency of inducing a humoral response varies considerably among models. In some cases a single injection of antigen-encoding DNA is sufficient to induce rapid, strong, and long-lasting antibody responses. In other cases, one or more booster injections of DNA are required to induce good or sustained levels of antibody. These differences are likely to be due at least partly to differences in the immunogenicity of the expressed antigen. However, because of the widely varying immunization schedules employed,

Table I
Summary of Disease Models for DNA-Based Immunization

Disease	Antigens	Species	Immune response	Protection	References
Viral					
SIV	gp110, gp130, gp160 (ene), gag	Monkeys	Ab, CTL	Partial (against lab isolates but not wild-type)	Lu *et al.*, 1996, Yasutomi *et al.*, 1996
AIDS (HIV-1)	gp120, gp140, gp160 (env), rev, gag, tat, nef	Mice, monkeys, chimpanzees, humans, rabbits, guinea pigs	Ab, CTL	ND	Barnett *et al.*, 1996; Hinkula *et al.*, 1997; Lu *et al.*, 1995; Okuda *et al.*, 1995; Shiver *et al.*, 1996; Ugen *et al.*, 1997; Wang *et al.*, 1993a,b, 1995; Williams *et al.*, 1993
African horsesickness virus	VP2 (capsid protein)	Horse	Ab	ND	Romito *et al.*, 1996
Dengue 2 virus	Envelope (E) glycoprotein premembrane (M) glycoprotein	Mice	Ab, CTL		Pardo *et al.*, 1996; Sariol *et al.*, 1996
St. Louis encephalitis virus	prM/E protein	Mice	Ab, CTL	Yes	Phillpotts *et al.*, 1996
HBV	HBsAg	Mice, monkeys, chimpanzees	Ab, CTL	ND	Davis *et al.*, 1993b, 1996b; Michel *et al.*, 1995; Prince *et al.*, 1996; Schirmbeck et al., 1995
HCV	Core protein (nucleocapsid)	Mice, monkeys	Ab, CTL	ND	Inchauspé *et al.*, 1996; Lagging *et al.*, 1995; Major *et al.*, 1995

HCV	cDNA- viral d Particle	Mice	Ab	ND	Polo *et al.*, 1995
HSV-1	gB and gD glycoproteins	Mice	Ab, CTL	Partial to complete	Ghiasi *et al.*, 1995; Manickan *et al.*, 1995
HSV-2	gB and gD Glycoprotein	Mice, guinea pigs	Ab	>90–100%	Bourne *et al.*, 1995; McClements *et al.*, 1996
Herpes-bovine type I	Glycoproteins	Mice, cows	Ab	Partial	Cox *et al.*, 1993; Iwasaki *et al.*, 1997
Rotavirus (group A)	VP4, VP6 or VP7 proteins	Mice	Ab, CTL	Yes	Herrmann *et al.*, 1996
LCMV lymphocytic choriomeningitis virus	Nucleoprotein	Mice	Ab, CTL	Partial (50%)	Martins *et al.*, 1995; Yokoyama *et al.*, 1995; Zarozinski *et al.*, 1995;
HTLV-1 Human T-cell Leukemia virus	env glycoprotein	Rat, rabbits	Ab		Ugen *et al.*, 1996
Human influenza virus	Hemagglutinin (HA) Nucleoprotein (NP)	Mice, ferrets, monkeys, chickens	Ab, CTL	Complete (even heterologous strain)	Donnelly *et al.*, 1995; Fynan *et al.*, 1993a,b, 1995; Justewicz *et al.*, 1995; Montgomery *et al.*, 1993; Pertmer *et al.*, 1995; Robinson *et al.*, 1993; Ulmer *et al.*, 1993, 1996; Yankauckas *et al.*, 1993
Swine influenza virus	HA	Pigs	Ab		Fynan *et al.*, 1993b
HPV (human papilloma virus	Major viral capsid protein L1	Rabbits	Ab	Yes (protection from warts)	Donnelly *et al.*, 1996
Measles	Hemagglutinin Glycoprotein	Mice, rabbits	Ab	Complete	Yang *et al.*, 1996
Rabies	Glycoprotein (G protein) or nucleoprotein	Mice	Ab, CTL	80–90% (G only, not NP)	Ray *et al.*, 1997; Xiang and Ertl, 1995; Xiang *et al.*, 1994, 1995

(continued)

Table I (*continued*)

Disease	Antigens	Species	Immune response	Protection	References
Bacterial					
Enteritis (porcine proliferative)	hsp60	Pigs	Ab, CTL	Reduced infection with live bacterial challenge	Dale *et al.*, 1996
Chlamydia trachomatis	L2 CTP synthetase gene	Mice	Ab	Partial	Brunham *et al.*, 1996
Mycoplasma pulmonis	Partial expression library	Mice	Ab, CTL	Yes	Barry *et al.*, 1995; Lai *et al.*, 1995
Tetanus	Fragment C of tetanus toxin	Mice	Ab	Yes	Anderson *et al.*, 1996
Tuberculsis—*Myocobacterium tuberculosis*	Proteins Ag85 (A,B,C) hsp65	Mice	Ab, CTL	Yes	Lowrie *et al.*, 1996; Lozes *et al.*, 1997
Parasites					
Malaria—*Plasmodium yoelli*	Circum sporozoite protein (PsCSP)	Mice, monkeys	Ab, CTL	>80%	Gramzinski *et al.*, 1996; Hoffman and Miller, 1996; Mor *et al.*, 1995; Sedegah *et al.*, 1994
Onchocerca volvulus	OvB20	Mice, birds, cattle	Ab, CTL	Reduced worm burden with challenge	Harrison and Bianco, 1996
Schistosomiasis—*S. mansoni* and *S. japonicum*	*S. mansoni* antigen (Sm23) *S. japonicum* paramyosin (Sj97) protein	Mice	Ab, CTL	Partial (Sm23) to none (Sj97)	Harn *et al.*, 1996; Waine *et al.*,1996; Yang *et al.*, 1995

it is difficult to assess the relative efficacy of the individual expression systems and the immunogens used. Differences in immune responses may also be attributed to the use of different animal models and different routes of administration.

With a potent immunogen (*e.g.*, HBsAg) and an efficient route of DNA administration (IM injection of pure plasmid DNA in mice), antibodies are detected as early as one week after injection of DNA and peak titers ($>10^5$) are obtained by four to eight weeks. Very high levels of antibody are detected for at least 17 months without a boost (Davis *et al.*, 1996a; Michel *et al.*, 1995). Potent and long-lasting humoral responses have also been obtained in mice by a single IM injection of DNA that expresses influenza nucleoprotein (NP) (Ulmer *et al.*, 1993). The earliest antibodies detected are primarily the IgM isotype, but shortly thereafter the IgG isotype predominate (Michel *et al.*, 1995). Such an IgM to IgG class shift strongly indicates T-helper function.

The humoral response to DNA vaccines is dose-dependent (Davis *et al.*, 1994). However, in contrast to the administration of proteins, the response depends on the absolute amount of DNA injected and also on the number of sites into which the dose is introduced (Brazolot Millan, Comanita and Davis, unpublished results). The doses most commonly used in mice range from 1–100 μg given at one to four sites. To immunize larger animals, it is not necessary to increase the dose proportionate to the body size. For example, Cox *et al.* (1993) obtained antibodies against bovine herpes virus glycoprotein in calves with only a fivefold higher dose of DNA than they used in mice. In addition, a chimpanzee attained equally high titers of anti-HBs when immunized with only a 20-fold higher dose of HBsAg-expressing DNA than used in mice despite a 500-fold difference in body weight (Davis *et al.*, 1996b).

The immune responses obtained with DNA-based immunization are faster and stronger than those obtained by an antigen-based approach (Figure 4). For example, anti-HBs antibodies appeared three weeks earlier and reached 100 fold higher titers after IM injection of HBsAg-expressing DNA than after injection of recombinant HBsAg protein, even though the amount of injected protein was at least 1000 times more than that which would have been expressed *in vivo* in the DNA-immunized animals (Davis *et al.*, 1996a).

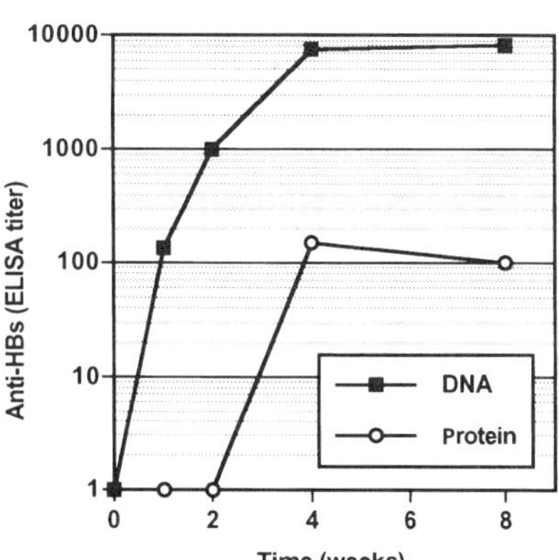

FIGURE 4. Anti-HBs humoral response in male C57BL/6 mice after immunization with HBsAg-expressing DNA (100 μg) or with recombinant HbsAg (4 μg). Each point is the mean end-point dilution titer for eight animals.

The efficiency of DNA-based immunization in inducing humoral responses is also demonstrated by the ability to overcome haplotype-restricted hyporesponsiveness to HBsAg in mice. Poorly-responding strains of mice (Milich, 1989) immunized with recombinant HBsAg protein had no detectable anti-HBs antibodies until after a boost. Yet when immunized with a single injection of HBsAg-expressing DNA, they developed anti-HBs antibodies as early as the good-responding strain of mice (Michel, Mancini, Whalen and Davis, unpublished results).

Other studies have shown that DNA vaccines result in efficient priming even if only a weak humoral response is detected. In the studies of Fynan *et al.* (1993a,b) which used DNA vectors that encode influenza hemagglutinin, antibodies were present only occasionally and only after a second DNA injection. Nonetheless, when influenza virus was used to challenge mice or chickens, antibody levels increased more rapidly (although not to higher levels) in animals inoculated with DNA expression vectors than in those treated with control DNA plasmids.

2.1.2. Cytotoxic T-Cell Responses

A corollary of DNA-based immunization is that the antigenic protein is necessarily synthesized *in vivo*. This results in the presentation of protein-derived peptides by MHC class I surface molecules, which should lead to the induction of CD8+ CTL. Indeed, this is the case because potent CTL have been detected in virtually all models where it has been evaluated (Table I).

As an example, after IM injection of mice with HBsAg-expressing plasmid DNA, strong CTL activity was detected in splenocytes as early as six days after DNA injection, and this persisted for at least several months (Davis *et al.*, 1995). Large numbers of CTL precursors were induced because specifically restimulated splenocytes exhibited extremely high specific lysis values (>80% at effector to target ratios as low as 5:1) after injection of 100 μg of HBsAg-expressing DNA. Furthermore, there were also fully competent primary CTL because high levels of specific lysis were also detected, even when the spleen cells were not specifically restimulated. In contrast, after injecting a large dose of recombinant HBsAg (equivalent to 1000 times more than would be synthesized *in situ* from the DNA), the specific lysis after specific restimulation was considerably less than induced by DNA (<50% at a 5:1 effector to target ratio), and no CTL were detected with nonspecific restimulation (Davis *et al.*, 1995). CTL activity in the absence of specific restimulation has also been detected in spleen cells of mice previously inoculated with influenza NP-expressing DNA constructs (Montgomery *et al.*, 1993; Ulmer *et al.*, 1993; Yankauckas *et al.*, 1993).

As with the humoral response, the induction of CTL is dose-dependent. After IM injection of pure plasmid DNA, CTL is detected with a dose as low as 1 μg DNA (Davis *et al.*, 1995, 1996c). Induction of CTL is particularly efficient when the gene-gun is used to deliver DNA-coated gold particles into the epidermis. In this case, potent CTL is detected with doses of DNA as low as 40 ng (Fynan *et al.*, 1993a,b). The high efficiency of this route is likely to be the result of direct penetration of some gold beads into professional APC in the skin (*e.g.*, Langerhans cells).

2.1.3. Cytokines and T-Helper Responses

Results from early studies indicated that DNA-based immunization primarily induces a Th1 response. However it now appears that, even though some responses are almost exclusively Th1, in most cases there is a mixed Th1 and Th2 response, and one of the two responses predominates. The identity of the Th response is usually determined by the cytokines secreted by splenocytes upon specific restimulation or by the isotypes of antigen-specific antibodies induced. Whether a Th1 or Th2 response occurs is determined by (1) the antigen; (2) the dose of antigen; (3) whether the antigen is secreted, cytoplasmic, or membrane-bound; (4) the route of administration; (5) the haplotype of the mouse immunized; and (6) whether or not adjuvant was also used. For example, with expression of α-1-antitrypsin, low doses of DNA administered IM or into the epidermis (gene-gun) led to a combined Th1/Th2 response with both IgG1 and IgG2a. However, high IM doses of DNA gave a predominantly Th1 response (IgG2a) (Barry and Johnston, 1996). In contrast, expression of influenza NP by plasmid DNA delivered in saline gives predominantly IgG2a (Th1, complement-dependent) but, following gene-gun gold particle delivery, gives predominantly IgG1 (Th2, complement-independent) (H. Robinson, University of Massachusetts, personal communication). DNA vaccination against bovine herpes virus induces predominantly IgG1 when a plasmid that encodes the secreted form of antigen is used but induces IgG2a with one that encodes the membrane-anchored form, even though both forms of antigen primarily induce IFN-γ (Iwasaki *et al.*, 1997). Regardless of the Th1/Th2 situation, almost all disease models result in coexistence of strong humoral and cellular immunity.

2.1.4. Protection against Disease

To consider DNA-based immunization a viable approach to vaccination, it must be demonstrated that the immune response obtained is sufficient to protect against infection by a pathogen. Challenge studies on animals in several of the DNA-based immunization models (see Table 1), have shown that such protection is obtained against viral, bacterial, and parasitic pathogens.

3. DNA VACCINES FOR IMMUNOTHERAPY

3.1. Treatment of Chronic Viral Infections

Because CD8+ CTL are efficiently induced, DNA vaccines might also be useful for treating established chronic viral infections. Evidence for this has been provided by studies on a mouse model of the HBV chronic carrier.

Transgenic (Tg) mice that constitutively express HBsAg in the liver are a model of the HBV chronic carrier because they tolerate the high levels of circulating antigen and do not produce any anti-HBs antibodies (Babinet *et al.*, 1985). DNA-based immunization of HBsAg-transgenic mice by IM injection of HBsAg-expressing DNA results in rapid appearance of anti-HBs antibodies and a concomitant loss of circulating antigen (Michel *et al.*, 1996). The antibody isotype (predominantly IgG2) and the profile of cytokines secreted by spleen-derived cells (predominantly IFN-γ) indicate that a primarily Th1 response is induced in these mice. The decrease in circulating antigen results from neutralization by antibodies and also from down-regulation of transgene expression in the liver because there is long-term disappearance of HBsAg mRNA. HBsAg-specific T-cells are responsible for the down-regulation of transgene expression because it can be induced in naive transgenic mice by passive transfer of T but not B cells from normal mice immunized with HBsAg-expressing DNA. The T-cell effect is mediated by a noncytolytic mechanism because there is no elevation of liver enzymes in the blood, nor is there any histological evidence of liver necrosis at the time that circulating HBsAg is rapidly decreasing. Rather, it is probably caused by a cytokine-mediated effect. In a similar transgenic model it has been shown that passive transfer of HBsAg-specific CD8+ CTL into the mice causes a transient down-regulation of the HBV transgene expression which is mediated in a predominantly noncytolytic fashion by IFN-γ and tumor necrosis factor-α (TNF-α) (Guidotti *et al.*, 1994).

It is difficult to explain how DNA-based immunization can break tolerance or anergy to HBsAg in these transgenic mice in view of the fact that the DNA vaccine encodes a gene product identical to the transgene and that the amount of antigen expressed in the muscle subsequent to injection of DNA would be a very small fraction of that synthesized in the liver from the transgene. Injection of pure recombinant HBsAg protein has no effect on these mice unless it contains a heterologous epitope (*e.g.*, HIV V3 loop) as a fusion protein, is from a heterologous strain, or is given in Freund's adjuvant (Mancini *et al.*, 1993). This suggests that, to break tolerance, epitopes must appear different from those seen during pre- and early postnatal development or they must be associated with unrelated helper epitopes. For example, mice immunized with hepatitis C virus (HCV) nucleocapsid-expressing plasmids exhibit no anti-HCV responses unless the capsid protein is expressed as a fusion protein with HBsAg (Major *et al.*, 1995). It is possible that expression of HBsAg in muscle results in the appearance of different or modified epitopes or results in a different mode of antigen presentation, possibly because different APC are involved.

Regardless of the mechanism involved, the results with DNA-based immunization of transgenic mice may have important clinical significance for immunotherapeutic treatment of HBV chronic carriers. In such individuals, the absence of an immune response that resolves the viral infection may result from a lack of helper function from HBV-specific CD4+ T-cells, which are found in all patients who clear the virus but not in those who do not (Ferrari *et al.*, 1990). On the other hand, B cells from HBV chronic carriers produce antibodies when stimulated *in vitro* with a low dose of antigen. Thus, in individuals who have chronic hepatitis may be deficient in the T-cell repertoire which results in nonresponsiveness to the HBV envelope protein. Nevertheless, DNA-mediated immunization overcomes B- and T-cell nonresponsiveness in mice. Similar results in humans could provide an effective therapy for the estimated 350 million HBV chronic carriers in the world. Likewise, DNA vaccines may prove useful for treating individuals chronically infected with other viruses (*e.g.*, HIV, HCV).

3.2. Immunotherapy for Cancer

The ability to break tolerance to an antigen and induce CTL in transgenic mice opens up the possibility of DNA-based immunotherapy against cancer cells. Mice immunized with HBsAg-expressing DNA reject HBsAg-expressing P815 tumor cells transplanted following immunization (J. Reimann, University of Ulm, Germany, personal communication). In addition, mice immunized against a carcinoembryonic antigen (CEA) are fully protected against challenge with syngeneic CEA-expressing colon carcinoma cells six weeks after administering DNA (Conry *et al.*, 1995b,c). Further studies are required to determine whether effective immune responses are induced against tumor proteins once the tumor is already established.

In related studies, Stevenson *et al.* (1995) attempted DNA immunization against B-cell lymphoma in mice by using idiotypic antigen-coding sequences. Idiotype antigens are tumor-associated antigens. Despite the fact that they are produced by the individual and are therefore "self" proteins, an immune response after DNA immunization was induced and anti-idiotypic antibodies were detected. Human clinical trials are underway using this DNA-based immunization/anticancer approach. Similarly, a number of centers have human trials underway wherein the transferred DNA encodes HLA-B7, a self-antigen which is linked to graft rejection in transplant patients. By injecting tumors with the DNA encoding HLA-B7 and producing this self-antigen at an ectopic site, researchers have detected CMI responses, and preliminary reports of tumor shrinkage have been announced.

4. MECHANISM OF INDUCTION OF IMMUNE RESPONSES

4.1. Antigen Presentation and T-Cell Responses

The mechanism by which CMI is induced following DNA-based immunization is not clear. This is especially true of IM injection with DNA, because transfected muscle fibers would not be expected to express accessory molecules (*e.g.*, B-7), which, it is thought, are required to activate CD8+ cells.

By transplanting myoblasts or bone marrow cells from a DNA-immunized mouse of one H-2 haplotype into a naive F1 mouse chimeric for that and another H-2 haplotype, it has been shown that transfected muscle cells by themselves cannot prime an immune response but that bone-marrow derived cells can (M. Liu, Merck, personal communication). This suggests that the immune response following injection of DNA into muscle results from (1) simultaneous direct transfection of some nonmuscle cells (presumably APC such as dendritic cells) and/or (2) transfer of antigen from the transfected muscle cell to APC.

Nevertheless, DNA immunization of mice by the IM route induces longer lasting immune responses than those obtained with ID injection. This suggests that the relatively large amount of antigen synthesized by transfected muscle fibers may play a role in maintaining memory, even if it does not directly prime an immune response. It is possible that antigen secreted or released (*e.g.*, by cytolytic attack) from transfected muscle fibers may be stored in the germinal centers (for example, on follicular dendritic cells) and thus help to maintain a strong memory response (Gray *et al.*, 1991).

4.2. B-Cell Responses with Secreted and Nonsecreted Antigens

B cells may be primed to produce antibodies upon meeting circulating antigen secreted by transfected cells. Indeed, many of the vectors used for DNA-based immunization include a signal sequence to ensure secretion of the antigenic protein. However, humoral responses are possible even if the antigen is not secreted. For example, it has been found that in mice immunized with HBsAg-expressing DNA, a humoral response is seen, although the appearance of antibodies is delayed for a few weeks if the HBsAg is not secreted (Michel *et al.*, 1995). In addition, protective levels of circulating antibodies are induced in rabbits following IM immunization with cottontail rabbit papilloma virus major capsid protein (L1)-encoding DNA, despite the fact that L1 contains a nuclear localization signal and is thought to be targeted to the cell nucleus (Donnelly *et al.*, 1996). In these cases, B cells are presumably not activated until the expressed antigen is released from transfected (muscle) cells upon lysis by antigen-specific CTL.

5. SAFETY CONSIDERATIONS

5.1. Possibility of Tolerance to Foreign Antigen

One of the attractive features of DNA-based immunization is that the antigenic protein is continuously expressed over a period of time. This "self-boosting" effect is probably responsible, at least in part, for the extremely efficient and long-lasting immune responses induced by the DNA approach. On the other hand, there has been concern that prolonged expression of low levels of antigen might actually induce immunological tolerance. Fortunately, this does not occur. In mice DNA-immunized against HBsAg, high titers of antibody are induced which persist for at least 17 months. Nevertheless, it was still possible to boost the humoral response after nine months by a second injection of HBsAg-encoding DNA or by administering recombinant HBsAg protein (Davis *et al.*, 1996a). In fact, there is evidence now that antigen expression is sustained for only about two weeks following injection of DNA. HBsAg-expressing muscle fibers in DNA-immunized mice were completely destroyed between 10 and 20 days after injection of the DNA. This results from an immune response, most likely CTL, because it does not occur in mice which have severe combined immune deficiency (SCID) (Davis, Brazolot Millan and Watkins, unpublished results).

5.2. Possibility of an Integrative Event

When considering vaccination of human populations, the most important safety concern is the possibility that the DNA taken up by cells may integrate into the host's chromosomal DNA and cause an insertional mutagenic event by activating a proto-oncogene or by inactivating a tumor-suppressive gene. Even though the amounts of plasmid injected in a typical experiment contain 10^{10} to 10^{12} molecules of DNA, the likelihood of an insertional mutagenic event is low. First, most injected DNA is rapidly degraded after injection and only an extremely small fraction actually enters the host's cells. Second, for the limited number of cells that do take up plasmid DNA, the probability of integration is very low because the plasmid DNA vectors are designed to remain episomal and most nonintegrated DNA would soon be lost during subsequent cell division. In muscle fibers, which are permanently postmitotic, integration is a particularly remote possibility. Then, even if integration into the host genome did occur, it would occur randomly and because of a cell's complement of greater than 10^9 bases of DNA, the possibility that such events would involve an oncogene or tumor-suppressive gene is very remote. Finally, because most tumor formation requires at least two independent genetic events, the risk of having two deleterious insertions in the same cell is again considerably smaller.

It has been calculated that the probable risk of tumor formation secondary to integration, based on the rate of tumor formation resulting from insertion of a viral oncogene by a retroviral vector, is 10^{-16} per μg of DNA (R. Kurth, Paul-Ehrlich-Institut, Germany, personal communication). Because retroviruses are specifically designed to integrate into the host's genome and plasmids are specifically designed to remain episomal, the risk of an insertional mutagenic event with a DNA vaccine would be much less than this. Indeed, it is estimated to be less than the risk of spontaneous mutagenesis.

5.3. Possibility of Immune Response to DNA and Autoimmunity

Another safety concern is the possibility that the DNA introduced may induce the production of anti-DNA antibodies, which in turn could contribute to undesired autoimmune reactions against the host's DNA. Although bacterial genomic DNA sequences can be immunogenic and humans normally have some antibodies against bacterial DNA, there is no evidence that injecting vaccines composed of plasmid DNA induces the appearance of anti-DNA antibodies. This may result in part because the plasmid DNA vectors are double-stranded and antibodies are induced almost exclusively against single-stranded DNA (Pisetsky, 1995).

5.4. Other Possible Responses to Injected DNA

DNA *per se* can act as a nonspecific immune stimulant (Pisetsky, 1995). This is not necessarily undesirable, and indeed such an adjuvant type effect may be partly responsible for the highly efficient immune responses obtained from DNA vaccines. Nevertheless, this should be taken into consideration when evaluating safety for human use.

Safety concerns may also relate to contaminants in the purified DNA. Traditionally, plasmid DNA has been purified from bacterial lysates by cesium chloride density gradient centrifugation. This method involves using various organic solvents. Localizing the DNA-containing band is usually accomplished by using ethidium bromide, which is highly carcinogenic. The use of dangerous reagents and chemicals is completely avoided if the DNA is purified by using anion exchange chromatographic resins. On the other hand, anion exchange-purified DNA may have higher levels of contaminating endotoxin, but now it is possible to remove it by one simple additional step (Schorr *et al.*, 1994). It has been shown that DNA prepared on anion exchange columns is equivalent in efficiency to cesium chloride doubly purified DNA used for immunization (Davis *et al.*, 1996d).

6. SUMMARY AND FUTURE DIRECTIONS

DNA-based immunization has been demonstrated in numerous different animal models. These are based on direct gene transfer using plasmid DNA into one or more tissues. The DNA is usually introduced IM or ID as a saline solution (*i.e.*, "naked") or into the epidermis by "gene-gun" delivery of DNA coated onto gold particles. It is clear that this new method of immunization is highly efficient in inducing rapid, potent, and long-lasting humoral and cell-mediated immune responses and confers protection against live pathogenic challenge. In cases where such a comparison is possible, the immune response from a DNA vaccine is superior to that obtained from traditional antigen-based vaccines, especially in cellular immunity. For other diseases, for which it was not previously possible to develop an antigen vaccine, it has been possible to induce protective immunity with a DNA vaccine.

Although progress has been impressive over the short time since DNA vaccines were first described, it is important to realize that much of the work described to date has been the initial development and demonstration of specific disease models. Only recently have efforts been made to optimize and refine the technology, and doubtlessly much progress will yet be realized. Such work must continue to develop easy and efficient ways to induce appropriate immune responses in humans with low doses of DNA. This will include developing and testing new techniques and formulations to improve DNA transfer, increase the efficiency and longevity of gene expression, and improve or alter the immune response induced by the expressed protein. For example, better expression could be obtained by improved vector design, including modification of promoter and enhancer elements or the inclusion of introns and other untranslated sequences to increase transcription levels or enhance mRNA stability. Other issues which remain to be examined before widespread application to humans are those of safety.

The DNA-mediated induction of an immune response to a protein produced *in situ* has initiated a new era of vaccine research. DNA-based immunization offers an extremely powerful tool to molecular immunologists for studying the immune system and for developing new vaccines and other immunotherapeutic approaches. One can easily and rapidly clone and modify genes in plasmid DNA expression vectors, allowing many new constructs to be produced and tested in a short period of time. Indeed, entire expression libraries can be cloned and injected in a "shotgun" fashion to identify immunoprotective epitopes. Using this novel approach, protection against mycoplasma has been demonstrated in mice (Barry *et al.*, 1995; Lai *et al.*, 1995). In contrast to the rapidity of the DNA cloning approach, the preparation of viral vectors or the production and purification of recombinant proteins from bacteria, yeast, or stably transfected mammalian cell lines can take many months to develop.

7. IMPLICATIONS FOR GENE THERAPY

Finally, the phenomenal success of DNA-based immunization has important and possibly ominous implications for gene therapy. With DNA-based immunization, the primary goal is to induce an immune response against the expressed protein, chosen specifically for its antigenic properties. On the other hand, if a gene is to be expressed for long-term production of a desired protein, then it is essential that the immune system not attack and destroy the transfected cells. Immune responses against the expressed protein are distinctly undesirable when direct or indirect gene transfer is carried out for gene augmentation or gene replacement, for example, in treating an inborn error of metabolism or other inherited disorder.

An immune response against a therapeutic gene product is particularly likely when a protein has never been previously seen by the host's immune system and thus for which there will not be immune tolerance. This may occur, for example, when introducing a nonhuman gene (*i.e.*, drug delivery by gene therapy) or when the genetic defect is such that all or a large portion of the endogenous protein is not expressed. If antibodies are produced, the gene product could be neutralized in the circulation, and this could result in loss of biological function even with continued expression (*e.g.*, with gene therapy for factor IX). Induction of CTL could result in a direct attack on the transfected cells and loss of expression. Transfected cells could also be destroyed by complement-mediated lysis if the expressed protein is localized at the surface. If these immune responses were similar to those seen with DNA-based immunization, transfected cells would not survive for more than a few weeks. In such cases, the failure of therapy would not be expected to cause additional harm to the patient.

More worrying, however, is the possibility of inducing an immune response against a protein already expressed by the cells of the host. If a truncated version of the protein results from the genetic defect, it is possible that expression of the complete protein could result in an immune response against those epitopes of the protein encoded by the truncated genomic DNA. If this were the case, then the outcome with a completely new protein, could be the same as that discussed previously, namely, destruction of the transfected cells. However, because clonal deletion in the induction of self-tolerance usually occurs only with dominant epitopes, it is possible that immunity may be induced to previously cryptic epitopes and this in turn could induce an autoimmune disorder with potentially harmful effect on the patient. For example, an immune response to dystrophin could induce severe myopathy in a patient who has Becker muscular dystrophy, where a truncated version of dystrophin is normally present.

Although one would not expect any immunological problems by augmenting abnormally low production of a complete gene product (*e.g.*, growth hormone), the breaking of tolerance to HBsAg in transgenic mice, as discussed previously, suggests that prudence should still be exercised if the transferred gene is being expressed from an ectopic site (*i.e.*, a tissue other than that which normally produces it).

In view of these various concerns, it is prudent to design experiments for evaluating potential immune responses before conducting human clinical trials of gene therapy.

8. REFERENCES

Anderson, R., Gao, X.-M., Papakonsantinopoulou, A., Fairwether, N., Roberts, M., and Dougan, G. 1997, Immunization of mice with DNA encoding fragment C of tetanus toxin. *Vaccine* **15:**827–829.

Babinet, C., Farza, H., Morello, D., Hadchouel, M., and Pourcel, C., 1985, Specific expression of hepatitis B surface antigen (HBsAg) in transgenic mice, *Science* **230:**1160–1163.

Barnett, S. W., Rajasekar, S., Legg, H., Doe, B., Fuller, D., Haynes, J., Walker, C. M., and Steimer, K. S., 1997, Vaccination with HIV-1 gp 120 DNA induces immune responses that are boosted by a recombinant gp 120 protein subunit, *Vaccine* **15:**869–873.

Barry, M. A., and Johnston, S. A., 1996, Biological features of genetic immunization, *Vaccine,* in press.

Barry, M. A., Lai, W. C., and Johnston, S. A., 1995, Protection against mycoplasma infection using expression-library immunization, *Nature* **377:**632–635.

Bourne, N., Stanberry, L. R., Bernstein, D. I., and Lew, D., 1995, DNA immunization against experimental genital herpes simplex virus infection, *J. Infect. Dis.* **173:**800–807.

Brunham, R. C., McClarty, G., Shen, C., Zhong, D. J., Berry, J., and Yang, X., 1996, A DNA vaccine for trachoma, *Proceedings of the EC/FDA/NIAID/WHO Meeting on Nucleic Acid Vaccines for the Prevention of Infectious Diseases*, Washington, DC.

Conry, R. M., LoBuglio, A. F., Wright, M., Sumerel, L., Pike, M. J., Johanning, F., Benjamin, R., Lu, D., and Curiel, D. T., 1995a, Characterization of a messenger RNA polynucleotide vaccine vector, *Cancer Res.* **55:**1397–1400.

Conry, R. M., LoBulio, A. F., Loechel, F., Moore, S. E., Sumerel, L. A., Barlow, D. L., and Curiel D. T., 1995b, A carcinoembryonic antigen polynucleotide vaccine has *in vivo* antitumor activity, *Gene Ther.* **2:**59–65.

Conry, R. M., LoBulio, A. F., Loechel, F., Moore, S. E., Sumerel, L. A., Barlow, D. L., Pike, J., and Curiel D. T., 1995c, A carcinoembryonic antigen polynucleotide vaccine for human clinical use, *Cancer Gene Ther.* **2:**33–38.

Cox, G. J., Zamb, T. J., and Babiuk, L. A., 1993, Bovine herpes virus 1: Immune responses in mice and cattle injected with plasmid DNA, *J. Virol.* **67:**1164–1168.

Dale, J. H., Lew, A. M., Strugnell, R. A., and Panaccio, M., 1996, Use of nucleic acid vaccines to control porcine proliferative enteritis, *Proceedings of the EC/FDA/NIAID/WHO Meeting on Nucleic Acid Vaccines for the Prevention of Infectious Diseases*, Washington, DC.

Davis, H. L., and Whalen, R. G., 1995, DNA-based immunization, in *Molecular and Cell Biology of Human Gene Therapeutics* (G. Dickson, ed.), Chapman and Hall, London, pp. 368–387.

Davis, H. L., Demeneix, B. A., Quantin, B., Coulombe, J., and Whalen, R. G., 1993a, Plasmid DNA is superior to viral vectors for direct gene transfer in adult mouse skeletal muscle, *Human Gene Ther.* **4:**733–740.

Davis, H. L., Michel, M.-L., and Whalen, R. G., 1993b, DNA-based immunization for hepatitis B induces continuous secretion of antigen and high levels of circulating antibody, *Hum. Mol. Genet.* **2:**1847–1851.

Davis, H. L., Whalen, R. G., and Demeneix, B. A., 1993c, Direct gene transfer into skeletal muscle *in vivo*: Factors affecting efficiency of transfer and stability of expression, *Hum. Gene Ther.* **4:**151–159.

Davis, H. L., Michel, M.-L., Mancini, M., Schleef, M., and Whalen, R. G., 1994, Direct gene transfer in muscle with plasmid DNA for the purpose of nucleic acid immunization, *Vaccine* **12:**1503–1509.

Davis, H. L., Schirmbeck, R., Reimann, J., and Whalen, R. G., 1995, DNA-mediated immunization in mice induces a potent MHC class-I restricted cytotoxic T lymphocyte response to the hepatitis B envelope protein, *Hum. Gene Ther.* **6:**1447–1456.

Davis, H. L., Mancini, M., Michel, M.-L., and Whalen, R. G., 1996a, DNA-mediated immunization to hepatitis B surface antigen: Longevity of primary response and effect of boost, *Vaccine* **14:**910–915.

Davis, H. L., McCluskie, M. J., Gerin, J. L., and Purcell, R. H., 1996b, DNA vaccine for hepatitis B: Evidence for immunogenicity in chimpanzees and comparison with other vaccines, *Proc. Natl. Acad. Sci. USA* **93:**7213–7218.

Davis, H. L., Michel, M.-L., and Whalen, R. G., 1995b, Use of plasmid DNA for direct gene transfer and immunization, *Ann. N.Y. Acad. Sci.* **772:**21–29.

Davis, H. L., Schleef, M., Moritz, P., Mancini, M., Schorr, J., and Whalen, R. G., 1996c, Comparison of plasmid DNA preparation methods for direct gene transfer and genetic immunization, *BioTechniques* **21:**92–99.

Donnelly, J. J., Friedman, A., Martinez, D., Montgomery, D. L., Shiver, J. W., Motzel, S. L., Ulmer, J. B., and Liu, M. A., 1995, Preclinical efficacy of a prototype DNA vaccine: Enhanced protection against antigenic drift in influenza virus, *Nat. Med.* **1:**583–587.

Donnelly, J. J., Martinez, D., Jansen, K. U., Ellis, R. W., Montgomery, D. L., and Liu, M. A., 1996, Protection against papillomavirus with a polynucleotide vaccine, *J. Infect. Dis.* **173:**314–320.

Ferrari, C., Penna, A., Bertoletti, A., Valli, A., Antoni, A. D., Giuberti, T., Cavalli, A., Petit, M.-A., and Fiaccodori, F., 1990, Cellular immune response to hepatitis B virus-encoded antigens in acute and chronic hepatitis B virus infection, *J. Immunol.* **145:**3442–3449.

Fynan, E. F., Robinson, H. L., and Webster, R. G., 1993a, Use of DNA encoding influenza hemagglutinin as an avian influenza vaccine, *DNA Cell. Biol.* **12:**785–789.

Fynan, E. F., Webster, R. G., Fuller, D. H., Haynes, J. R., Santoro, J. C., and Robinson, H. L., 1993b, DNA vaccines: Protective immunizations by parental, mucosal, and gene-gun inoculations, *Proc. Natl. Acad. Sci. USA* **90:**11478–11482.

Fynan, E. F., Webster, R. G., Fuller, D. H., Haynes, J. R., Santoro, J. C., and Robinson H. L., 1995, DNA vaccines: A novel approach to immunization, *Int. J. Immunopharmacol.* **17:**79–83.

Ghiasi, H., Cai, S., Slanina, S., Nesburn, A. B., and Wechsler, S. L, 1995, Vaccination of mice with herpes simplex virus type 1 glycoprotein D DNA produces low levels of protection against lethal HSV-1 challenge, *Antiviral Res.* **28:**147–157.

Gramzinski, R. A., Maris, D. C., Doolan, D., Charoenvit, Y., Obaldia, N., Rossan, R., Hobart, P., Margalith, M., and Hoffman, S., 1997, Malaria DNA vaccine in Aotus monkeys, *Vaccine* **15:**913–915.

Gramzinski, R. A., Brazolot Millan, C. L., Obaldia, N., Hoffman, S. L., and Davis, H. L., 1998, Immune response to a hepatitis B DNA vaccine in *Aotus* monkeys: a comparison of vaccine formulation, route, and method of administration. *Molec. Med.* **4:**109–118.

Gray, D., Kosco, M., and Stockinger, B., 1991, Novel pathways of antigen presentation for the maintenance of memory, *Int. Immunol.* **3:**141–148.

Guidotti, L. G., Ando, K., Hobbs, M. V., Ishikawa, T., Runkel, L., Schreiber, R. D., and Chisari, F. V., 1994, Cytotoxic T lymphocytes inhibit hepatitis B virus gene expression by a non-cytolytic mechanism in transgenic mice, *Proc. Natl. Acad. Sci. USA* **91:**3764–3768.

Harrison, R. A., and Bianco, A. E., 1996, Immunization of rodents with DNA encoding protective antigens of *Onchocerca volvulus, Proceedings of the EC/FDA/NIAID/WHO Meeting on Nucleic Acid Vaccines for the Prevention of Infectious Diseases*, Washington, DC.

Haynes, J. R. delete from reference list and replace text references with Fynan *et al.* 1993b.

Chen, S. C., Fynan, E. F., Robinson, H. L., Lu, S., Greenberg, H. B., Santoro, J. C., and Herrmann, J. E., 1997, Protective immunity induced by rotavirus DNA vaccines, *Vaccine* **15:**899–902.

Hoffman, S. L., and Miller, L. H., 1996, Perspectives on Malaria Vaccine Development, *Hoffman SL*, ed. Malaria Vaccine Development: A Multi-Immune Response Approach: *Amer. Soc. Microbiol.* **••:**1–13.

Inchauspé, G., Major, M. E., Nakano, I., Vitvitski, L., and Trépo, C., 1997, DNA vaccination for the induction of immune responses against hepatitis C virus protein, *Vaccine* **15:**853–856.

Phillpotts, R. J., Venugopal, K., and Brooks, T., 1996, Immunization with DNA polynucleotides protects mice against lethal challenge with St. Louis encephalitis virus, *Arch. Virol.* 141, 743.

Justewicz, D. M., Morin, M. J., Robinson, H. L., and Webster, R. G., 1995, Antibody-forming cell response to virus challenge in mice immunized with DNA encoding the influenza virus hemagglutinin, *J. Virol.* **69:**7712–7717.

Kuby, J., 1994., *Immunology*, 2nd ed., Freeman, New York.

Lagging, L. M., Meyer, K., Hoft, D., Houghton, M., Belshe, R. B., and Ray, R., 1995, Immune responses to plasmid DNA encoding the hepatitis C virus core protein, *J. Virol.* **69:**5859–5863.

Lai, W. C., Bennett, M., Johnston, S. A., Barry, M. A., and Pakes, S. P., 1995, Protection against *Mycoplasma pulmonis* infection by genetic vaccination, *DNA Cell Biol.* **14:**643–651.

Lanzavecchia, A., 1993, Identifying strategies for immune intervention, *Science* **260:**937–944.

Iwasaki, A., Stiernholm, B. J. N., Chan, A. K., Berinstein, N. L., and Barber, B. H., 1997, Enhanced CTL responses mediated by plasmid DNA immunogens encoding costimulaotry molecules and cytokines, *J. Immunol.* **158:**4591–4601.

Ray, N. B., Ewalt, L. C., and Lodmell, D. L., 1997, Nanogram quantities of plasmid DNA encoding the rabies virus glycoprotein protect mice against lethal rabies virus infection, *Vaccine* **15:**892–895.

Lowrie, D. B., Tascon, R. E., Colston, M. J., and Silva, C. L., 1994, Towards a DNA vaccine against tuberculosis, *Vaccine* **12:**1537–1540.

Lowrie, D. B., Silva, C. L., Colston, M., Ragno, S., and Tascon, R. E., 1997, Protection against tuberculosis by plasmid DNA vaccine, *Vaccine* **15:**834–838.

Lu, S., Santoro, J. C., Fuller, D. H., Haynes, J. R., and Robinson, H. L., 1995, Use of DNAs expressing HIV-1 env and noninfectious HIV-1 particles to raise antibody responses in mice, *Virology* **209:**147–154.

Lu, S., Manson, K., Wyand, M., and Robinson, H. L., 1997, Simian immunodeficiency virus DNA vaccine trial in macaques: post challenge necropsy in vaccine and control groups. *Vaccine* **15:**920–923.

Major, M., Vitvitski, L., Mink, M. A., Schleef, M., Whalen, R. G., Trepo, C., and Inchauspé, G., 1995, DNA-based immunization with chimeric vectors for the induction of immune responses against the hepatitis C virus nucleocapsid, *J. Virol.* **69:**5798–5805.

Mancini, M., Hadchouel, M., Tiollais, P., Pourcel, C., and Michel, M.-L., 1993, Induction of anti-hepatitis B surface antigen (HBsAg) antibodies in HBsAg producing transgenic mice: A possible way of circumventing "nonresponse" to HBsAg, *J. Med. Virol.* **39:**67–74.

Manickan, E., Rouse, R. J., Yu, Z., Wire, W. S., and Rouse, B. T., 1995, Genetic immunization against herpes simplex virus. Protection is mediated by CD4+ T lymphocytes, *J. Immunol.* **155:**259–265.

Martinon, F., Krishnan, S., Lenzen, G., Magné, R., Gomard, E., Guillet, J.-G., Lévy, J.-P., and Meulien, P., 1993, Induction of virus-specific cytotoxic T lymphocytes *in vivo* by liposome-entrapped mRNA, *Eur. J. Immunol.* **23:**1719–1722.

Martins, L. P., Lau, L. L., Assano, M. S., and Ahmed, R., 1995, DNA vaccination against persistent viral infection, *J. Virol.* **69:**2574–2582.

McClements, W. L., Armstrong, M. E., Keys, R. D., and Liu, M. A., 1997, The prophylactic effect of immunization with DNA encoding herpes simplex virus glycoproteins on HSV-induced disease in guinea pigs, *Vaccine* **15:**857–860.

Michel, M.-L., Davis, H. L., Schleef, M., Mancini, M., Tiollais, P., and Whalen, R. G., 1995, DNA-mediated immunization to the hepatitis B surface antigen in mice: Aspects of the humoral response mimic hepatitis B viral infection in humans, *Proc. Natl. Acad. Sci. USA* **92:**5307–5311.

Michel, M.-L., Mancini, M., Davis, H. L., Hadchouel, M., Whalen, R. G., and Tiollais, P., 1997, DNA-mediated immunization to the hepatitis B surface antigen (HBsAg): A prophylactic and therapeutic approach for hepatitis B, *Viral Hepatitis and Liver Disease*, 643–647.

Milich, D. R., 1989, Synthetic T and B cell recognition sites: Implications for vaccine development, *Adv. Immunol.* **45:**195–282.

Miller, A. D., 1992, Human gene therapy comes of age, *Nature* **357:**455–460.

Montgomery, D. L., Shiver, J. W., Leander, K. R., Perry, H. C., Friedman, A., Martinez, D., Ulmer, J. B., Donnelly, J. J., and Liu, M. A., 1993, Heterologous and homologous protection against influenza A by DNA vaccination: Optimization of DNA vectors, *DNA Cell Biol.* **12:**777–83.

Mor, G., Klinman, D. M., Shapiro, S., Hagiwara, E., Sedegah, M., Norman, J. A., Hoffman, S. L., and Steinberg, A. D., 1995, Complexity of the cytokine and antibody response elicited by immunizing mice with *Plasmodium yoelii* circumsporozoite protein plasmid DNA, *J. Immunol.* **155:**2039–2046.

Okuda, K., Bukawa, H., Hamajima, K., Kawamoto, S., Sekigawa, K., Yamada, Y., Tanaka, S., Ishi, N., Aoki, I., and Nakamura, M., 1995, Induction of potent humoral and cell-mediated immune responses following direct injection of DNA encoding the HIV type 1 env and rev gene products, *AIDS Res. Hum. Retroviruses* **11:**933–943.

Pardo, O. L., Pelegrino, J. L., Guzmán, M. G., and Guillén, G., 1996, Immunization of mice with DNA encoding the pr-M protein from dengue-2 virus, *Proceedings of the EC/FDA/NIAID/WHO Meeting on Nucleic Acid Vaccines for the Prevention of Infectious Diseases*, Washington, DC.

Pertmer, T. M., Eisenbraun, M. D., McCabe, D., Prayaga, S. K., Fuller, D. H., and Haynes, J. R., 1995, Gene gun-based nucleic acid immunization: Elicitation of humoral and cytotoxic T lymphocyte responses following epidermal delivery of nanogram quantities of DNA, *Vaccine* **13:**1427–1430.

Pisetsky, D. S., 1995, Immunologic consequences of nucleic acid therapy, *Antisense Res. Dev.* **5:**219–225.

Polo, J. M., Lim, B., Govindarajan, S., and Lai, M. M., 1995, Replication of hepatitis delta virus RNA in mice after intramuscular injection of plasmid DNA, *J. Virol.* **69:**5203–5207.

Prince, A. M., Whalen, R., and Brotman, B., 1997, Successful DNA-based HBV immunization of newborn chimpanzees, against hepatitis B virus, *Vaccine* **15:**916–919.

Raz, E., Carson, D. A., Parker, S. E., Parr, T. B., Abai, A. M., Aichinger, G., Gromkowski, S. H., Singh, M., Lew, D., Yankauckas, M. A., Baird, S. M., and Rhodes, G. H., 1994, Intradermal gene immunization: The possible role of DNA uptake in the induction of cellular immunity to viruses, *Proc. Natl. Acad. Sci. USA* **91:**9519–9523.

Robinson, H. L., Hunt, L. A., and Webster, R. G., 1993, Protection against a lethal influenza virus challenge by immunization with a haemagglutinin-expressing plasmid, *Vaccine* **11:**957–960.

Romito, M., Du Plessis, D. H., Van Kleef, M., Van Wyk, A., and Viljoen, G. J., 1996, DNA-based immunization of a horse using the VP2 gene of african horsesickness virus, *Proceedings of the EC/FDA/NIAID/WHO Meeting on Nucleic Acid Vaccines for the Prevention of Infectious Diseases*, Washington, DC.

Sariol, C. A., Pardo, O., Giraldo, S., Pelegrino, J. L., Guillén, G., and Guzman, M. G., 1996, Immunization of mice with DNA encoding the envelope protein from dengue 2 virus, *Proceedings of the EC/FDA/NIAID/WHO Meeting on Nucleic Acid Vaccines for the Prevention of Infectious Diseases*, Washington, DC.

Schirmbeck, R., Bohm, W., Ando, K., Chisari, F. V., and Reimann, J., 1995, Nucleic acid vaccination primes hepatitis B virus surface antigen-specific cytotoxic T lymphocytes in nonresponder mice, *J. Virol.* **69:**5929–5934.

Schorr, J., Welzek, M., Seddon, T., and Moritz, P., 1994, Large scale purification of endotoxin-free plasmid DNA for gene therapy research, *Gene Ther.* **1:**S7.

Sedegah, M., Hedstrom, R., Hobart, P., and Hoffman, S. L., 1994, Protection against malaria by immunization with plasmid DNA encoding circumsporozoite protein, *Proc. Natl. Acad. Sci. USA* **91:**9866–9870.

Shiver, J. W., Davies, M.-E., Yasutomi, Y., Perry, H. C., Freed, D. C., Letvin, N. L., and Liu, M. A., 1996, Anti-HIV env immunities elicited by nucleic acid vaccines, *Vaccine* **15:**884–887.

Stevenson, F. K., Zhu, D., King, C. A., Ashworth, L. J., Kumar, S., and Hawkins, R. Eé., 1995, Idiotypic DNA vaccines against B-cell lymphoma, *Immunology Rev.* **145:**211–228.

Tang, D., DeVit, M., and Johnston, S. A., 1992, Genetic immunization is a simple method for eliciting an immune response, *Nature* **356:**152–154.

Ugen, K. E., Boyer, J. D., Wang, B., Bagarazzi, M., Javadian, A., Frost, P., Merva, M. M., Agadjanyan, M., Nyland, S., Williams, W. V., Coney, L., Ciccarelli, R., and Weiner, D. B., 1997, DNA vaccination using HIV-1 expression cassettes generates protective immune responses in non-human primates, *Vaccine* **15:**927–930.

Ugen, K., Agadjanyan, M., Wang, B., and Weiner, D., 1996, DNA inoculation against HTLV-1, *Proceedings of the EC/FDA/NIAID/WHO Meeting on Nucleic Acid Vaccines for the Prevention of Infectious Diseases*, Washington DC.

Ulmer, J. B., Donnelly, J. J., Parker, S. E., Rhodes, G. H., Felgner, P. L., Dwarki, V. J., Gromkowski, S. H., Deck, R. R., DeWitt, C. M., Friedman, A., Hawe, L. A., Leander, K. R., Martinez, D., Perry, H. C., Shiver, J. W., Montgomery, D. L., and Liu, M. A., 1993, Heterologous protection against influenza by injection of DNA encoding a viral protein, *Science* **259:**1745–1749.

Lozes, E., Huygen, K., Denis, O., Montgomery, D. L., Vandenbussche, J. P., Van Vooren, J.-P., Drowart,

A., Ulmer, J., Yawman, A., and Liu, M. A., 1997, Immunogenicity and efficacy of a tuberculosis DNA vaccine encoding the components of the secreted antigen 85 complex, *Vaccine* **15:**830–833.

Vogel, F. R., and Sarver, N., 1995, Nucleic acid vaccines, *Clin. Microbiol. Rev.* **8:**406–410.

Hinkula, J., Lundholm, P., and Wahren, B., 1997, Nucleic acid vaccination with HIV regulatory genes: a combination of HIV-1 genes in separate plasmids induces strong immune responses, *Vaccine* **15:**874–878.

Waine, G. J., Yang, W., Scott, J. C., McManus, D. P., and Kalinna, B. H., 1996, Progress towards a nucleic acid vaccine for schistosomiasis, *Vaccine*, in press.

Waine, G. J., Yang, W., Scott, J. C., McManus, D. P., and Kalinna, B. H., 1997, DNA based vaccination using schistosoma japonicum (Asian blood-fluke), *Vaccine* **15:**846–848.

Wang, B., Boyer, J., Srikantan, V., Coney, L., Carrano, R., Phan, C., Merva, M., Dang, K., Agadjanyan, M., Gilbert, L., Ugen, K. E., Williams, W. V., and Weiner, D. B., 1993a, DNA inoculation induces neutralizing immune responses against human immunodeficiency virus type 1 in mice and nonhuman primates, *DNA Cell Biol.* **12:**799–805.

Wang, B., Ugen, K. E., Srikantan, V., Agadjanyan, M. G., Dang, K., Refaeli, Y., Sato, A. I., Boyer, J., Williams, W. V., and Weiner, D. B., 1993b, Gene inoculation generates immune responses against human immunodeficiency virus type I, *Proc. Natl. Acad. Sci. USA* **90:**4156–4160.

Wang, B., Boyer, J., Srikantan, V., Ugen, K., Gilbert, L., Phan, C., Dang, K., Merva, M., Agadjanyan, M. G., Newman, M., Carrano, R., McCallus, D., Coney, L., Williams, W., and Weiner, D., 1995, Induction of humoral and cellular immune responses to the human immunodeficiency type 1 virus in nonhuman primates by *in vivo* DNA inoculation, *Virology* **211:**102–112.

Williams, W. V., Boyer, J. D., Merva, M., Livolsi, V., Wilson, D., Wang, B., and Weiner, D. B., 1993, Genetic infection induces protective *in vivo* immune responses, *DNA Cell Biol.* **12:**675–683.

Wolff, J. A., Malone, R. W., Williams, P., Chong, W., Acsadi, G., Jani, A., and Felgner, P. L., 1990, Direct gene transfer into mouse muscle *in vivo*, *Science* **247:**1465–1468.

World Health Organization, P. f. V. D., 1990, Potential use of live viral and bacterial vectors for vaccines, *Vaccine* **8:**425–437.

World Health Organization, International Task Force on Hepatitis BImmunization 1991, Purposes and Programmes, WHO, Beneva, Switzerland.

Xiang, Z., and Ertl, H. C. J., 1995, Manipulation of the immune response to a plasmid-encoded viral antigen by coinoculation with plasmids expressing cytokines, *Immunity* **2:**129–135.

Xiang, Z. Q., Spitalnik, S., Tran, M., Wunner, W. H., Cheng, J., and Ertl, H. C. J., 1994, Vaccination with a plasmid vector carrying the rabies virus glycoprotein gene induces protective immunity against rabies virus, *Virology* **199:**132–140.

Xiang, Z. Q., Spitalnik, S. L., Cheng, J., Erikson, J., Wojczyk, B., and Ertl, H. C., 1995, Immune responses to nucleic acid vaccines to rabies virus, *Virology* **209:**569–579.

Yang, W., Waine, G. J., and McManus, D. P., 1995, Antibodies to *Schistosoma japonicum* (Asian bloodfluke) paramyosin induced by nucleic acid vaccination, *Biochem. Biophys. Res. Commun.* **212:**1029–1039.

Yang, K., Mustafa, F., Valsamakis, A., Santoro, J. C., Griffin, D. E., and Robinson, H. L., 1997, Early studies on DNA-based immunizations for measles virus, *Vaccine* **15:**888–891.

Yankauckas, M. A., Morrow, J. E., Parker, S. E., Abai, A., Rhodes, G. H., Dwarki, V. J., and Gromkowski, S. H., 1993, Long-term anti-nucleoprotein cellular and humoral immunity is induced by intramuscular injection of plasmid DNA containing NP gene, *DNA Cell Biol.* **12:**771–776.

Yasutomi, Y., Robinson, H. L., Lu, S., Mustafa, F., Lekutis, C., Arthos, J., Mullins, J. I., Voss, G., Manson, K., Wyand, M., and Letvin, N. L., 1996, Simian immunodeficiency virus-specific cytotoxic T-lymphocyte induction through DNA vaccination of rhesus monkeys, *J. Virol.* **70:**678–681.

Yokoyama, M., Zhang, J., and Whitton, J. L., 1995, DNA immunization confers protection against lethal lymphocytic choriomeningitis virus infection, *J. Virol.* **69:**2684–2688.

Zarozinski, C. C., Fynan, E. F., Selin, L. K., Robinson, H. L., and Welsh, R. M., 1995, Protective CTL-dependent immunity and enhanced immunopathology in mice immunized by particle bombardment with DNA encoding an internal virion protein, *J. Immunol.* **154:**4010–4017.

Index